OXFORD MEDICAL PUBLICATIONS

Oxford Handbook of Obstetrics and Gynaecology

T0092304

Published and forthcoming Oxford Handbooks

OXFORD HANDBOOK OF

Obstetrics and Gynaecology

FOURTH EDITION

EDITED BY

Sally Collins

Consultant Obstetrician and Subspecialist in Maternal and Fetal Medicine, John Radcliffe Hospital, Oxford, and Professor of Obstetrics, Nuffield Department of Women's and Reproductive Health, University of Oxford, Oxford, UK

Sabaratnam Arulkumaran

Professor of Obstetrics and Gynaecology, University of Nicosia Medical School, Cyprus, Professor Emeritus, St George's, University of London, and Visiting Professor, Imperial College London, London, UK

Kevin Hayes

Consultant Obstetrician and Gynaecologist, St George's University Hospital NHS Foundation Trust, London, UK

Kirana Arambage

Consultant Gynaecologist, John Radcliffe Hospital, Oxford, and Honorary Senior Clinical Lecturer, Nuffield Department of Women's and Reproductive Health, University of Oxford, Oxford, UK

Lawrence Impey

Consultant Obstetrician and Subspecialist in Maternal and Fetal Medicine, John Radcliffe Hospital, Oxford, UK

OXFORD
UNIVERSITY PRESS

OXFORD
UNIVERSITY PRESS

Great Clarendon Street, Oxford, OX2 6DP,
United Kingdom

Oxford University Press is a department of the University of Oxford.
It furthers the University's objective of excellence in research, scholarship,
and education by publishing worldwide. Oxford is a registered trade mark of
Oxford University Press in the UK and in certain other countries

© Oxford University Press 2023

The moral rights of the authors have been asserted

First Edition published 2005
Second Edition published 2008
Third Edition published 2013
Fourth Edition published 2023

Impression: 1

Published in the United States of America by Oxford University Press
198 Madison Avenue, New York, NY 10016, United States of America

British Library Cataloguing in Publication Data
Data available

Library of Congress Control Number: 2022941170

ISBN 978–0–19–883867–8

DOI: 10.1093/med/9780198838678.001.0001

Printed and bound in China by
C&C Offset Printing Co., Ltd.

Contents

Preface

Since the previous edition of the *Oxford Handbook of Obstetrics and Gynaecology* there has been significant growth within the specialty, with new reports and guidelines that have changed the approaches involved in delivering the best-quality care for patients. In writing and developing this new edition, we have taken the latest evidence-based practice as well as our own clinical experience to help those of you who are embarking on the challenging yet rewarding field of obstetrics and gynaecology.

We are grateful to our past and present contributors, who have given both their time and expertise in writing and updating this Handbook, as well as to our readers. We hope that the information, which we have tried to present in a digestible format, will prove useful to you on the wards as well as at your desk. Where possible, we have tried to align our chapters with the Royal College of Obstetricians and Gynaecologists curriculum, but we have also included clinical tips gleaned from our practical experience. Please do let us know any suggestions or criticism related to the content of the book, and we will make every effort to improve the delivery of the content even more in the next edition.

Sally Collins
Sabaratnam Arulkumaran
Kevin Hayes
Kirana Arambage
Lawrence Impey
April 2022

Acknowledgements

We would like to thank all our second and third edition authors on whose sterling work this latest edition is built. We would also like to thank the doctors of all grades who anonymously reviewed some of the text, providing valuable feedback and further fine-tuning of the finished manuscript. To conform to the Oxford Handbook style and to avoid overlap and repetition, some contributions have been considerably edited and we thank all our authors for their understanding. We are most grateful to Prof. Basky Thilaganathan for providing many of the ultrasound images and Ms Penny Trotter for the colposcopy pictures. We cannot fail to mention the marvellous team at Oxford University Press including Elizabeth Reeve, Helen Liepman, and Caroline Smith, but especially Sylvia Warren without whose incredible patience, kindness, and expert guidance this fourth edition would not have happened. Last, but definitely not least, we would like to thank our partners and families who continue to remain so patient and supportive throughout this project, especially Berni O'Connor, 'for doing all the real work on the home front' and David, Lexi, and Bea Reynard 'for all their love and support throughout M's mad projects'.

Acknowledgements

Symbols and abbreviations

⚠	warning
▶	important
▶▶	differential diagnosis
⬤	controversial
⟿	cross-reference
ℛ	website
📹	video
1°	primary
2°	secondary
↑	increased
↓	decreased
→	leading to
±	with or without
~	approximately
+ve	positive
−ve	negative
5-FU	5-fluorouracil
ABG	arterial blood gases
ACE	angiotensin converting enzyme
ACEI	angiotensin converting enzyme inhibitor
ACTH	adrenocorticotropic hormone
ADH	antidiuretic hormone
AF	atrial fibrillation
AFI	amniotic fluid index
AFLP	acute fatty liver of pregnancy
AFP	alpha-fetoprotein
AIS	androgen insensitivity syndrome
ALP	alkaline phosphatase
ALT	alanine transaminase
AMH	anti-Müllerian hormone
ANA	antinuclear antibodies
APH	antepartum haemorrhage
APS	antiphospholipid syndrome
AREDF	absent/reversed end-diastolic flow
ARM	artificial rupture of membranes
ASD	atrial septal defect
AST	aspartate aminotransferase
AVM	arteriovenous malformation
BASHH	British Association for Sexual Health and HIV

BCG	bacillus Calmette–Guérin
bd	twice daily
BEP	bleomycin, etoposide, and cisplatin
βhCG	beta-human chorionic gonadotropin
BMD	bone mineral density
BMI	body mass index
BOT	borderline ovarian tumour
BP	blood pressure
BPD	biparietal diameter
BRCA	breast cancer gene
BSO	bilateral salpingo-oophorectomy
BV	bacterial vaginosis
CA	cancer antigen
CAH	congenital adrenal hyperplasia
CAIS	complete androgen insensitivity syndrome
CAP	chest/abdomen/pelvis
cART	combination antiretroviral therapy
CBAVD	congenital bilateral absence of the vas deferens
CD	Caesarean delivery
CEA	carcinoembryonic antigen
CF	cystic fibrosis
CGIN	cervical glandular intraepithelial neoplasia
CI	confidence interval
CIN	cervical intraepithelial neoplasia
CMV	cytomegalovirus
CNS	central nervous system
CNST	Clinical Negligence Scheme for Trusts
CO₂	carbon dioxide
COCP	combined oral contraceptive pill
COVID-19	coronavirus disease 2019
CP	cerebral palsy
CPAP	continuous positive airway pressure
CPP	chronic pelvic pain

CPR	cerebroplacental ratio *or* cardiopulmonary resuscitation
CRL	crown–rump length
CRP	C-reactive protein
CS	Caesarean section
CSF	cerebrospinal fluid
CT	computed tomography
CTG	cardiotocography
CTPA	computed tomography pulmonary angiogram
CVS	chorionic villus sampling
CXR	chest X-ray
DC	dichorionic
DCDA	dichorionic and diamniotic
DES	diethylstilbestrol
DHEAS	dehydroepiandrosterone sulphate
DIC	disseminated intravascular coagulation
DSD	disorder of sex development
DUB	dysfunctional uterine bleeding
dVIN	differentiated vulval intraepithelial neoplasia
EBL	estimated blood loss
EBRT	external beam radiotherapy
ECG	electrocardiography/ electrocardiogram
ECV	external cephalic version
EDD	expected date of delivery
EFW	estimated fetal weight
EP	ectopic pregnancy
EPAU	early pregnancy assessment unit
ESR	erythrocyte sedimentation rate
ET	endometrial thickness
ETT	endotracheal tube
EUA	examination under anaesthetic
FBC	full blood count
FBS	fetal blood sampling
FDA	Food and Drug Administration
FF	fetal fraction
FFP	fresh frozen plasma
FGM	female genital mutilation
FGR	fetal growth restriction
FH	fetal heart
FHR	fetal heart rate
FIGO	International Federation of Gynaecology and Obstetrics
FL	femur length

FM	fetal movements
FPR	false-positive rate
FSD	female sexual dysfunction
FSH	follicle-stimulating hormone
FVS	fetal varicella syndrome
GA	general anaesthesia
GABA	gamma-aminobutyric acid
GAD	generalized anxiety disorder
GAS	group A *Streptococcus*
GBS	group B *Streptococcus*
GDM	gestational diabetes mellitus
GFR	glomerular filtration rate
GMC	General Medical Council
GnRH	gonadotropin-releasing hormone
GP	general practitioner
GTD	gestational trophoblastic disease
GTN	gestational trophoblastic neoplasia
GTT	glucose tolerance test
GUM	genitourinary medicine
Hb	haemoglobin
HbA	adult haemoglobin
HbA1c	glycated haemoglobin
HBeAg	hepatitis B e antigen
HbF	fetal haemoglobin
HBsAg	hepatitis B surface antigen
HBV	hepatitis B virus
HC	head circumference
hCG	human chorionic gonadotropin
HELLP	haemolysis, elevated liver enzymes, and low platelets
HFEA	Human Fertilization and Embryology Authority
HG	high-grade serous ovarian carcinoma
HIV	human immunodeficiency virus
HLA	human leucocyte antigen
HMB	heavy menstrual bleeding
HPO	hypothalamic–pituitary–ovarian
HPV	human papillomavirus
hrHPV	high-risk human papillomavirus
HRT	hormone replacement therapy
HSG	hysterosalpingography
HSV	herpes simplex virus
HVS	high vaginal swab
HyCoSy	hysterosalpingo contrast sonography

IBD	inflammatory bowel disease
ICD-11	International Classification of Diseases, 11th Revision
ICD-MM	International Classification of Diseases for Maternal Mortality
ICG	indocyanine green
ICP	intrahepatic cholestasis of pregnancy
ICSI	intracytoplasmic sperm injection
IDS	interval debulking surgery
Ig	immunoglobulin
IHC	immunohistochemistry
IM	intramuscular
IMB	intermenstrual bleeding
IOL	induction of labour
IUCD	intrauterine contraceptive device
IUD	intrauterine death
IUI	intrauterine insemination
IUP	intrauterine pregnancy
IUS	intrauterine system
IV	intravenous
IVF	in vitro fertilization
IVU	intravenous urography
JVP	jugular venous pressure
LARC	long-acting reversible contraceptive
LDH	lactate dehydrogenase
LFT	liver function test
LGSOC	low-grade serous ovarian carcinoma
LH	luteinizing hormone
LLETZ	large loop excision of transformation zone
LMP	last menstrual period
LMWH	low-molecular-weight heparin
LN	lymph node
LNG	levonorgestrel
LVS	low vaginal swab
MBRRACE-UK	Mothers and Babies: Reducing Risk through Audits and Confidential Enquiry across the UK
MC	monochorionic
MCA	middle cerebral artery
MCDA	monochorionic and diamniotic
MCHC	mean corpuscular haemoglobin concentration
MCMA	monochorionic and monoamniotic
MCV	mean corpuscular volume
MDT	multidisciplinary team
MEA	microwave endometrial ablation
Mg	magnesium
MMR	measles, mumps, and rubella or mismatch repair
MPA	medroxyprogesterone acetate
MRI	magnetic resonance imaging
MRKH	Mayer–Rokitansky–Küster–Hauser
MSAF	meconium-stained amniotic fluid
MSU	midstream sample of urine
MTCT	mother-to-child transmission
NAAT	nucleic acid amplification test
NEC	necrotizing enterocolitis
NHSCSP	NHS Cervical Screening Programme
NHSLA	National Health Service Litigation Authority
NICE	National Institute for Health and Care Excellence
NIPT	non-invasive prenatal testing
NPV	negative predictive value
NSAID	non-steroidal anti-inflammatory drug
NT	nuchal translucency
NTD	neural tube defect
OA	occipito-anterior
OAB	overactive bladder
od	once daily
OGTT	oral glucose tolerance test
OHSS	ovarian hyperstimulation syndrome
OL	occipito-lateral
OP	occipito-posterior
PAIS	partial androgen insensitivity syndrome
PAPP-A	pregnancy-associated plasma protein-A
PAS	placenta accreta spectrum
PCB	postcoital bleeding
PCOS	polycystic ovary syndrome
PCR	protein:creatinine ratio or polymerase chain reaction
PE	pulmonary embolism

PEFR	peak expiratory flow rate
PEP	postexposure prophylaxis
PET	pre-eclampsia toxaemia
PG	prostaglandin
PGE1	prostaglandin E1
PGE2	prostaglandin E2
PID	pelvic inflammatory disease
PlGF	placental growth factor
PMB	postmenopausal bleeding
PMRT	Perinatal Mortality Review Tool
PMS	premenstrual syndrome
PO	*per os* (by mouth)
POF	premature ovarian failure
POMB/ACE	cisplatin, vincristine, methotrexate, bleomycin, dactinomycin, cyclophosphamide, and etoposide
POP	progestogen-only pill
PPH	postpartum haemorrhage
PPROM	preterm prelabour rupture of membranes
PPV	positive predictive value
PROM	prelabour rupture of membranes
PSV	peak systolic velocity
PUL	pregnancy of unknown location
PV	*per vaginam*
Q	ventilation
qds	four times daily
RCOG	Royal College of Obstetricians and Gynaecologists
RCT	randomized controlled trial
Rh	rhesus
RID	relative infant dose
RMI	risk of malignancy index
ROM	rupture of membranes
RR	rate ratio *or* relative risk
RRBSO	risk-reducing bilateral salpingo-oophorectomy
RUQ	right upper quadrant
SARC	sexual assault referral centre
SARS	severe acute respiratory syndrome
SC	subcutaneous
SFH	symphysis fundal height
sFlt-1	soluble FM-like tyrosine kinase 1
SGA	small for gestational age

SHBG	sex hormone-binding globulin
SLE	systemic lupus erythematosus
SLN	sentinel lymph node
SLNB	sentinel lymph node biopsy
SMM	surgical management of miscarriage
SNRI	serotonin and norepinephrine reuptake inhibitor
SROM	spontaneous rupture of membranes
SSRI	selective serotonin reuptake inhibitor
STI	sexually transmitted infection
STIC	serous tubal intraepithelial carcinoma
T_3	triiodothyronine
T_4	thyroxine
TAS	transabdominal scan
TB	tuberculosis
Tc	technetium
tds	three times daily
TENS	transcutaneous electrical nerve stimulation
TFT	thyroid function test
TNF	tumour necrosis factor
TOP	termination of pregnancy
TSH	thyroid-stimulating hormone
TTP	thrombotic thrombocytopenic purpura
TTTS	twin-to-twin transfusion syndrome
TV	transvaginal
TVS	transvaginal scan
TVT	tension-free vaginal tape
U&E	urea and electrolytes
UKFOCSS	UK Familial Ovarian Cancer Screening Study
UN	United Nations
UPSI	unprotected sexual intercourse
USI	urodynamic stress incontinence
USS	ultrasound scan
UTI	urinary tract infection
uVIN	usual-type vulval intraepithelial neoplasia
V/Q	ventilation/perfusion
VBAC	vaginal birth after Caesarean
VDRL	Venereal Disease Research Laboratory test
VE	vaginal examination

VEGF	vascular endothelial growth factor	VTE	venous thromboembolism
VIN	vulval intraepithelial neoplasia	vWF	von Willebrand factor
VRIII	variable rate intravenous insulin infusion	VZIG	varicella zoster immunoglobulin
VSCC	vulvar squamous cell carcinoma	WCC	white cell count
VSD	ventricular septal defect	WHO	World Health Organization
		WLE	wide local excision

Contributors

Editors

Sally Collins
Consultant Obstetrician and Subspecialist in Maternal and Fetal Medicine, John Radcliffe Hospital, Oxford, and Professor of Obstetrics, Nuffield Department of Women's and Reproductive Health, University of Oxford, Oxford, UK

Sabaratnam Arulkumaran
Professor of Obstetrics and Gynaecology, University of Nicosia Medical School, Cyprus, Professor Emeritus, St George's, University of London, and Professor, Imperial College London, London, UK

Kevin Hayes
Consultant Obstetrician and Gynaecologist, St George's University Hospital NHS Foundation Trust, London, UK

Kirana Arambage
Consultant Gynaecologist, John Radcliffe Hospital, Oxford, and Honorary Senior Clinical Lecturer, Nuffield Department of Women's and Reproductive Health, University of Oxford, Oxford, UK

Lawrence Impey
Consultant Obstetrician and Subspecialist in Maternal and Fetal Medicine, John Radcliffe Hospital, Oxford, UK

Contributors to the fourth edition

W. Catarina Ang
Consultant Gynaecologist, Royal Women's Hospital, Parkville, VIC, Australia
Chapter 21: Menopause

Ilyas Arshad
Consultant Gynaecologist, Liverpool University Hospitals NHS Trust, Liverpool, UK
Chapter 20: Contraception

Christian Becker
Associate Professor, Nuffield Department of Women's and Reproductive Health, University of Oxford, Oxford, and Honorary Consultant Gynaecologist, Subspecialist in Reproductive Medicine and Surgery, John Radcliffe Hospital, Oxford, UK
Chapter 18: Subfertility and reproductive medicine

Charlotte Bennett
Consultant Neonatologist,
Oxford University Hospitals NHS
Foundation Trust, Oxford, UK
Chapter 8: Neonatal resuscitation

Abigail Brempah
Specialty Trainee in Obstetrics
and Gynaecology, Lewisham and
Greenwich NHS Trust, London, UK
*Chapter 14: Gynaecological anatomy
and development; Chapter 15: Normal
menstruation and its disorders;
Chapter 16: Early pregnancy problems;
and Chapter 24: Miscellaneous
gynaecology*

Sarah Coleridge
Subspeciality Trainee in
Gynaecological Oncology,
Nottingham University Hospitals
Trust, Nottingham, UK
*Chapter 23: Benign and malignant
gynaecological conditions*

Ruth Curry
Consultant Obstetrician and
Subspecialist in Maternal and
Fetal Medicine, Oxford University
Hospitals NHS Foundation Trust,
Oxford, UK
*Chapter 12: Benign and malignant
tumours in pregnancy*

Charlotte Frise
Consultant Obstetric Physician,
Queen Charlotte's and Chelsea
Hospital, Imperial College
Healthcare NHS Trust, London, UK,
and Lead Consultant Obstetric
Physician for NW London
*Chapter 5: Medical disorders in
pregnancy*

Suni Halder
Consultant Obstetric Anaesthetist,
Oxford University Hospitals NHS
Foundation Trust, Oxford, UK
Chapter 7: Obstetric anaesthesia

Rumana Islam
Consultant Gynaecologist, Barts
Health NHS Trust, London, UK
*Chapter 18: Subfertility and
reproductive medicine*

Helen Jefferis
Consultant Gynaecologist/
Urogynaecologist, John Radcliffe
Hospital, Oxford, UK
Chapter 22: Urogynaecology

Shamitha Kathurusinghe
Consultant Gynaecologist, Royal
Women's Hospital, Parkville, VIC,
Australia
Chapter 21: Menopause

Bryn Kemp
Consultant Obstetrician and
Maternal Medicine Lead, Royal
Berkshire NHS Foundation Trust,
Reading, UK
*Chapter 11: Maternal and perinatal
mortality*

Kimmee Khan
Specialty Trainee in Obstetrics and
Gynaecology, Epsom and St Helier
University Hospitals NHS Trust,
London, UK
*Chapter 14: Gynaecological anatomy
and development; Chapter 15: Normal
menstruation and its disorders;
Chapter 16: Early pregnancy
problems; Chapter 19: Sexual assault;
and Chapter 24: Miscellaneous
gynaecology*

Vicky Minns
Specialty Trainee in Obstetrics and
Gynaecology, Epsom and St Helier
University Hospitals NHS Trust,
London, UK
*Chapter 14: Gynaecological anatomy
and development; Chapter 15: Normal
menstruation and its disorders;
Chapter 16: Early pregnancy problems;
and Chapter 24: Miscellaneous
gynaecology*

Jo Morrison

Consultant Gynaecological Oncologist, Musgrove Park Hospital, Somerset NHS Foundation Trust, Taunton, UK
Chapter 23: Benign and malignant gynaecological conditions

Sanyal Patel

Consultant Obstetrician and Gynaecologist, Milton Keynes University Hospital, Milton Keynes, UK
Chapter 4: Infectious diseases in pregnancy

Pathiraja Pubudu

Consultant Gynaecologist/ Gynaecological Oncologist, Addenbrooke's Hospital, Cambridge, UK
Chapter 17: Genital tract infections and pelvic pain

Jane Reavey

Senior Registrar, John Radcliffe Hospital, Oxford, UK
Chapter 17: Genital tract infections and pelvic pain

Fevzi Shakir

Consultant Gynaecologist, Royal Free Hospital, London, UK
Chapter 20: Contraception

Jasmine Tay

Consultant Obstetrician and Subspecialist in Maternal Fetal Medicine, Queen Charlotte's Hospital, Imperial College NHS Trust, London, UK
Chapter 5: Medical disorders in pregnancy

Katy Vincent

Associate Professor, Senior Fellow in Pain in Women and Honorary Consultant Gynaecologist, Nuffield Department of Women's and Reproductive Health, University of Oxford, John Radcliffe Hospital, Oxford, UK
Chapter 17: Genital tract infections and pelvic pain

Dilip Visvanathan

Consultant Gynaecologist, Barts Health NHS Trust, London, UK
Chapter 17: Genital tract infections and pelvic pain

Michael Yousif

Consultant in Liaison Psychiatry, West Middlesex University Hospital, London, UK
Chapter 13: Substance misuse and psychiatric disorders

Contributors to the second and third editions

Miss Karolina Afors
St George's Hospital, London, UK

Dr Christian Becker
John Radcliffe Hospital, Oxford, UK

Dr Amy Bennett
Department of Genitourinary Medicine, Oxford University Hospitals, NHS Trust, Oxford, UK

Mrs Rebecca Black
John Radcliffe Hospital, Oxford, UK

Dr Shabana Bora
St George's Hospital, London, UK

Dr Brian Brady
John Radcliffe Hospital, Oxford, UK

Mr Paul Bulmer
St George's Hospital, London, UK

Mr Edwin Chandraharan
St George's Hospital, London, UK

Dr Noan-Minh Chau
Specialist Registrar Rotation
in Medical Oncology, London
Deanery, UK

Dr Mellisa Damodaram
Queen Charlotte's and Chelsea
Hospital, London, UK

Miss Claudine Domoney
Chelsea and Westminster Hospital,
London, UK

Dr Stergios K. Doumouchtsis
St George's Hospital, London, UK

Dr Suzy Elniel
Chelsea and Westminster Hospital,
London, UK

Dr Cleave W. J. Gass
St George's Hospital, London, UK

Dr Ingrid Granne
John Radcliffe Hospital, Oxford, UK

Miss Catherine Greenwood
John Radcliffe Hospital, Oxford, UK

Mr Manish Gupta
John Radcliffe Hospital, Oxford, UK

Miss Pauline Hurley
John Radcliffe Hospital, Oxford, UK

Dr Nia Jones
Queens Medical Centre,
Nottingham, UK

Miss Brenda Kelly
John Radcliffe Hospital, Oxford, UK

Dr Nigel Kennea
St George's Hospital, London, UK

Dr Andy Kent
St George's Hospital, London, UK

Dr Su-Yen Khong
John Radcliffe Hospital, Oxford, UK

Dr Emma Kirk
St George's Hospital, London, UK

Dr Samatha Low
Royal Berkshire Hospital,
Reading, UK

Dr Jo Morrison
Musgrove Park Hospital,
Taunton, UK

Dr Neelanjana Mukhopadhaya
St George's Hospital, London, UK

Dr Faizah Mukri
Specialist Registrar Rotation,
London Deanery, UK

Dr Santosh Pattnayak
St George's Hospital, London, UK

Dr Natalia Price
John Radcliffe Hospital, Oxford, UK

Dr Aysha Qureshi
Royal United Hospital, Bath, UK

Dr Devanna Rajeswari
St George's Hospital, London, UK

Dr Gowri Ramanathan
St George's Hospital, London, UK

Dr Margaret Rees
John Radcliffe Hospital, Oxford, UK

Dr Jackie Sherrard
Department of Genitourinary
Medicine, Oxford University
Hospitals NHS Trust, Oxford, UK

Dr Lisa Story
John Radcliffe Hospital, Oxford, UK

Ms Louise Strawbridge
University College London,
London, UK

Mr Alex Swanton
Royal Berkshire Hospital,
Reading, UK

Dr Linda Tan
St George's Hospital, London, UK

Dr Katy Vincent
John Radcliffe Hospital, Oxford, UK

Miss Cara Williams
University College London
Hospital, UK

Dr Niraj Yanamandra
St Peter's Hospital, Chertsey, UK

Chapter 1

Normal pregnancy

Obstetric history: current pregnancy

Obstetric history taking has many features in common with most other sections of medicine, along with certain areas specific to the specialty. The basic framework can be easily learned; however, competence requires good clinical knowledge and a lot of practice. As obstetrics often requires intimate examination and discussion of sensitive information, it is important to ensure privacy, and to demonstrate respect and confidentiality. It is important to offer a health professional as a chaperone. Translation may be required and it is best to have an official translator as a family member, especially the husband/partner, translating may not divulge or may distort certain information. It is also important to ask about domestic violence when the mother is alone and offer help if appropriate.

A carefully obtained history taken in a logical sequence avoids inadvertent omission of important details, and guides the examination to follow.

Current pregnancy

Much of this information will be contained in the patient's 'hand-held' notes:
- Name.
- Age.
- Occupation.
- Relationship status.
- Gravidity (i.e. number of pregnancies, including the current one).
- Parity (i.e. number of births beyond 24wks gestation).

The expected date of delivery (EDD) can be calculated from the last menstrual period (LMP) using Naegele's rule (add 1yr and 7 days to the LMP and subtract 3mths), most often done with an obstetric calendar ('wheel'). Enquire about details that may affect the validity of the patient's EDD as calculated from her LMP including:
- Long cycles.
- Irregular periods.
- Recent use of the combined oral contraceptive pill (COCP).

▶ Dating scans between 8 and 13wks are more reliable than LMP and should be used to provide an EDD where possible.
Enquire about the current pregnancy, including:
- General health (tiredness, malaise, and other non-specific symptoms).
- If >20wks, enquire about fetal movements (FM).
- General details of pregnancy to date (previous admissions and current problems).
- Results of all antenatal (AN) blood tests—routine and specific.
- Results of anomaly and other scans (details of results can be cross-checked with the notes).
- If she is postnatal:
  - labour and delivery
  - history of the postnatal period.

An obstetric history

Should include:
- Current pregnancy details.
- Past obstetric history.
- Past gynaecological history.
- Past medical and surgical history.
- Drug history and allergies.
- Social history, including:
  - recreational drug use
  - domestic violence
  - psychiatric illness especially in the postnatal period.
- Family history especially with regard to:
  - multiple pregnancy
  - diabetes
  - hypertension
  - chromosomal or congenital malformations.

Gravidity and parity explained

The terminology used is gravida *x*, para *a+b*:
- *x* is the total number of pregnancies (including this one).
- *a* is the number of births beyond 24wks gestation.
- *b* is the number of miscarriages or termination of pregnancies before 24wks gestation.

Example

A woman who is pregnant for the 4th time with 1 normal delivery at term, 1 termination at 9wks, and 1 miscarriage at 16wks would be gravida 4, para 1+2.

Obstetric history: other relevant features

▶ History often repeats itself, so previous AN, intrapartum, or postpartum complications should influence the management of this pregnancy.

Past obstetric history includes:
- Details of all previous pregnancies (including miscarriages and terminations).
- Length of gestation.
- Date and place of delivery.
- Onset of labour (including details of induction of labour).
- Mode of delivery.
- Sex and birth weight.
- Fetal and neonatal life.
- Clear details of any complications or adverse outcomes (such as shoulder dystocia, postpartum haemorrhage, or stillbirth).

Past gynaecological/medical/surgical history
- Method of contraception before conception.
- Previous gynaecological conditions/procedures.
- Cervical smear history.
- Medical conditions, such as hypertension, epilepsy, or diabetes.
- Details of any consultations with other physicians (neurologist or endocrinologist, psychiatrists).
- Involvement of any multidisciplinary teams (MDTs).
- Details of any previous surgery.

Drug and allergy history
- Current medications.
- Medications taken at any time during the pregnancy.
- Any allergies and their severity (anaphylaxis or a rash?).

Family history
Any history of hereditary illnesses or congenital defects is important and is required to ensure adequate counselling and screening is offered.
- Familial disorders such as thrombophilias.
- Previously affected pregnancies with any chromosomal or genetic disorders, hypertensive disorders, early pregnancy loss, or preterm delivery.
- Consanguinity.

Social history
- Smoking.
- History of drug or alcohol abuse (➔ Chapter 13).
- Plans for breast-feeding.
- Social aspects, such as plans for childcare arrangements.
- Domestic violence screening.

Obstetric physical examination

At initial visit, a complete physical examination should be undertaken.

Abdominal examination: inspection

- Note the apparent size of the abdominal distension.
- Note any asymmetry.
- FM.
- Cutaneous signs of pregnancy:
  - linea nigra (dark pigmented line stretching from the xiphisternum through the umbilicus to the suprapubic area)
  - striae gravidarum (recent stretch marks are purplish in colour)
  - striae albicans (old stretch marks are silvery-white)
  - flattening/eversion of umbilicus (due to ↑ intra-abdominal pressure).
- Superficial veins (alternative paths of venous drainage due to pressure on the inferior vena cava by a gravid uterus).
- Surgical scars (a low Pfannenstiel incision may be obscured by pubic hair, and laparoscopy scars hidden within the umbilicus).

Abdominal examination: palpation

- Symphysis fundal height (SFH):
  - palpated <20wks
  - measured in centimetres >20wks.
- Estimation of number of fetuses: multiple fetal poles.
- *Fetal lie* (relationship of longitudinal axis of fetus to that of the uterus):
  - *longitudinal*—fetal head or breech palpable over pelvic inlet
  - *oblique*—the head or breech is palpable in the iliac fossa and nothing felt in the lower uterus
  - *transverse*—fetal poles felt in flanks and nothing above the brim.
- *Presentation* (part of the fetus overlying the pelvic brim):
  - cephalic (this could be vertex, face, or brow presentations determined vaginally)
  - breech
  - other (shoulder, compound).
- Amniotic fluid volume:
  - ↑ tense abdomen with fetal parts not easily palpated
  - ↓ compact abdomen with fetal parts easily palpable.

Auscultation of the fetal heart

The fetal heart (FH) is best heard at the anterior shoulder of the fetus:

- A Doppler ultrasound device (Sonicaid) from about 12wks gestation.
- A fetal stethoscope (Pinard) from about 24wks gestation.
- In a breech presentation it is often heard at, or above, the level of the maternal umbilicus.
- Rate and the rhythm of the FH should be determined over 1min.
- The recent National Institute for Health and Care Excellence (NICE) guidelines raise the need for routine fetal heart rate (FHR) auscultation in the presence of FM; but mothers enjoy listening to the FH.

General examination

- Body mass index (BMI) calculated [weight (kg)/height (m)²].
- ▶ Pregnancy complications are ↑ with a BMI <18.5 and >25.
- Blood pressure (BP) measured in the semi-recumbent position (45° tilt).
- ▶ Use an appropriate size cuff; too small a cuff gives a falsely ↑ BP.
- Auscultation of the heart and lungs:
  - flow murmurs are common and are not significant
  - cardiac murmurs may be detected for the 1st time.
- Thyroid gland (exclude a goitre).
- Breasts (exclude any lumps).
- Varicose veins and skeletal abnormalities (kyphosis or scoliosis): pregnancy associated with ↑ lumbar lordosis: ↑ lower backache.

Normal uterine size

- The uterus normally becomes palpable at 12wks gestation.
- It reaches the level of the umbilicus at 20wks gestation.
- It is at the xiphisternum at 36wks gestation.

Symphysis fundal height

▶ The SFH detects ~40–60% of small for gestational age (SGA) fetuses. Uterine size is measured from the highest point of the fundus to the upper margin of the symphysis pubis (Fig. 1.1).
Appropriate growth is usually estimated to be the number of wks gestation in centimetres (at 30wks the SFH should be 30 ± 2cm):

- ± 2cm from 20 until 36wks gestation.
- ± 3cm between 36 and 40wks.
- ± 4cm at 40wks.

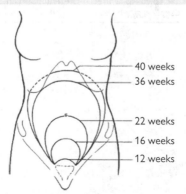

Fig. 1.1 Typical fundal heights at various stages of pregnancy. Reproduced from Wyatt JP, Illingworth RN, Graham CA, et al. (eds) (2006). *Oxford Handbook of Emergency Medicine*. Oxford: OUP. By permission of Oxford University Press.

Engagement of the fetal head

Conventionally, engagement or the passage of the maximal diameter of the presenting part beyond the pelvic inlet is estimated using the palm width of the five fingers of the hand (Fig. 1.2). If five fingers are needed to cover the head above the pelvic brim, it is five-fifths palpable, and if no head is palpable, it is zero-fifths palpable.

* Normally, the fetus engages in an attitude of flexion in the larger transverse diameter of the pelvic inlet, unless the pelvis is very roomy where it may engage in any diameter (Fig. 1.3).
* In nulliparous women, engagement usually (not in all) occurs beyond 37wks, but in multiparous women it may not occur until the onset of labour.
* Rare causes of non-engagement should always be considered and investigated with an ultrasound scan (USS) (including placenta praevia and fetal abnormality).
* In women of Afro-Caribbean origin, engagement may only occur at the onset or during the course of labour, even in nulliparous women due to the shape of the pelvic inlet.

Paulik's grip

This is a one-handed technique that uses a cupped right hand to grasp and assess the lower pole of the uterus (usually the fetal head).

▶ This can be very uncomfortable and is not necessary if the head can be palpated using two hands.

Engagement
* A head that is only two-fifths palpable is usually considered to be engaged (and therefore fixed in the pelvis; see Fig. 1.2).
* Put simply, an easily palpable head is not engaged, whereas a head more difficult to palpate is more likely to be deeply engaged.
▶ Care must be taken, as a breech presentation can sometimes be mistaken for a deeply engaged head.

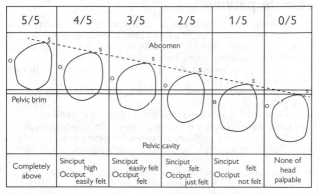

5/5	4/5	3/5	2/5	1/5	0/5
Completely above	Sinciput high Occiput easily felt	Sinciput easily felt Occiput felt	Sinciput felt Occiput just felt	Sinciput felt Occiput not felt	None of head palpable

Fig. 1.2 Clinical estimation of descent of the fetal head and engagement.

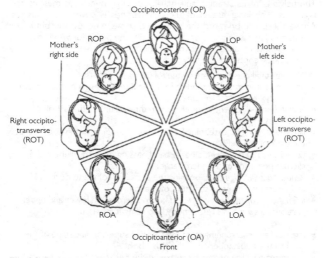

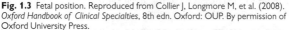

Fig. 1.3 Fetal position. Reproduced from Collier J, Longmore M, et al. (2008). *Oxford Handbook of Clinical Specialties*, 8th edn. Oxford: OUP. By permission of Oxford University Press.

Female pelvis

The bony ring of the pelvis is made up of two symmetrical innominate bones and the sacrum. Each innominate bone is made up of the ilium, ischium, and the pubis, which are joined anteriorly at the symphysis pubis and posteriorly to the sacrum at the sacroiliac joints.

The female pelvis has evolved for giving birth, and differs from the male pelvis in the following ways:

- The female pelvis is broader, and the bones more slender than those of the male.
- The male pelvic brim is heart-shaped and widest towards the back, whereas the female pelvic brim is oval-shaped transversely and widest further forwards; the sacral promontory is less prominent.
- The female pelvic cavity is more spacious and has a wider outlet than the male pelvis.
- The subpubic angle is rounded in a female pelvis (like a Roman arch) and more acute in the male pelvis (like a Gothic arch).

Pelvic muscles and ligaments

The pelvis gains its strength and stability through numerous muscles and ligaments. The inner aspect of the pelvic bones is covered by muscles. Above the pelvic brim are the iliacus and psoas muscles; the obturator internus and its fascia occupies the side walls; the posterior wall is covered by the pyriformis; and the levator ani and coccygeus, with their opposite counterparts, constitute the pelvic floor.

Pelvic ring stability is provided by the following ligaments:

- *Sacrospinous ligament:* extending from the lateral margin of the sacrum and coccyx to the ischial spine.
- *Sacrotuberous ligament:* extending from the sacrum to the ischial tuberosity.
- *Iliolumbar ligament:* extending from the lumbar spine to the iliac crest at the back of the pelvis.
- *Dorsal sacroiliac ligament:* a heavy band passing from the ilium to the sacrum posterior to the sacroiliac joint.
- *Ventral sacroiliac ligament:* bridging the sacroiliac joint anteriorly, and is an important stabilizing structure of the joint.
- *Inferior and superior pubic ligament:* a band across the lower and upper part of the symphysis respectively, providing further strength to the joint.
- *Inguinal ligament:* running from the anterior superior iliac spine of the ilium to the pubic tubercle of the pubic bone.
- The remaining ligaments that surround the pelvis are ligaments that do not provide stabilization of the pelvis.

Pelvic boundaries

The pelvis is divided by an oblique plane passing through the prominence of the sacrum, the arcuate and pectineal lines, and the upper margin of the symphysis pubis, into the greater and the lesser pelvis. The circumference of this plane is termed the pelvic brim. This pelvic brim separates the false pelvis above from the true pelvis below. The plane of the pelvis is at an angle of 55° to the horizontal.

Pelvic shapes

There are four basic shapes of the female pelvis, as illustrated in Fig. 1.4.

- *Gynaecoid:* the classical female pelvis with the inlet transversely oval and a roomier pelvic cavity.
- *Anthropoid:* a long, narrow, and oval-shaped pelvis due to the assimilation of the sacral body to the fifth lumbar vertebra.
- *Android:* the inlet is heart-shaped and the cavity is funnel-shaped with a contracted outlet.
- *Platypelloid:* a wide pelvis flattened at the brim with the sacral promontory pushed forward.

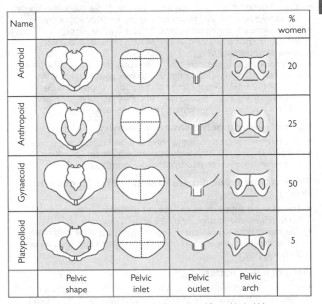

Name	Pelvic shape	Pelvic inlet	Pelvic outlet	Pelvic arch	% women
Android					20
Anthropoid					25
Gynaecoid					50
Platypolloid					5

Fig. 1.4 Basic shapes of the female pelvis. Reproduced from Abitbol M, Chervenak F, Ledger WJ. (1996). *Birth and human evolution: anatomical and obstetrical mechanics in primates.* New York: Bergin & Garvey.

Diameters of the female pelvis

The female bony pelvis is not distensible, and only very minor degrees of movement are possible at the symphysis pubis and the sacroiliac joints. Its dimensions are, hence, critical for normal childbirth.

▶ The diameters of the female pelvis vary at different parts:
• The true pelvis is bound anteriorly by the symphysis pubis (3.5cm long) and posteriorly by the sacrum (12cm long).
• The superior circumference of the true pelvis is the pelvic inlet and the inferior circumference is the outlet (Fig. 1.5).
• The true pelvis has four planes.

Plane of pelvic inlet

• This is bound anteriorly by the upper border of the pubis, laterally by the iliopectineal line, and posteriorly by the sacral promontory.
• The average transverse diameter is 13.5cm and the average anteroposterior diameter is 11cm (obstetric conjugate diameter) (transversely oblong).
• It is not possible to measure these diameters clinically, and the only diameter at the pelvic inlet amenable to clinical assessment is the distance from the inferior margin of the pubic symphysis to the midpoint of the sacral promontory (the diagonal conjugate), which is ~1.5cm greater than the obstetric conjugate diameter.

Plane of greatest pelvic dimensions/cavity

• This is the roomiest part of the pelvis and has little clinical significance.
• It is almost round in shape with an average transverse diameter of 13.5cm and an average anteroposterior diameter of 12.5cm.

Plane of least pelvic dimensions/mid-pelvis (circular in shape)

• This is bound anteriorly by the apex of the pubic arch, laterally by the ischial spines, and posteriorly by the tip of the sacrum.
• The interspinous diameter is the narrowest space in the pelvis (10cm) and represents the level at which impaction of the fetal head is most likely to occur.

Plane of pelvic outlet

• This is bound anteriorly by the pubic arch, which should have a desired angle of >90°, posterolaterally by the sacrotuberous ligaments and ischial tuberosities, leading to the coccyx posteriorly (anteroposteriorly oblong).
• The average intertuberous diameter is 11cm.

Assessment of 'pelvic adequacy'

Examination of the pelvis before labour does not accurately discriminate between those who will achieve vaginal birth and those who will not. Even computed tomography (CT) or magnetic resonance imaging (MRI) scanning, together with USS of the fetal head, is not helpful, unless there is a gross abnormality, which will be evident from the history or gait. This is because of the dynamic nature of labour, when the head 'moulds' (↓ the head circumference by a few centimetres) and the joints of the pelvis can move, ↑ the pelvic dimensions slightly.

The ideal female pelvis has the following features:
• Oval brim.
• Shallow cavity.
• Non-prominent ischial spines.
• Curved sacrum with large sciatic notches (>90°).
• Sacrospinous ligament >3.5cm long.
• Rounded subpubic arch (>90°).
• Intertuberous distance of at least 10cm.
• Diagonal conjugate diameter of at least 12cm.

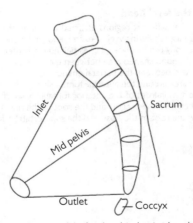

Fig. 1.5 Median sagittal section of the female pelvis showing the pelvic inlet and outlet. Reproduced from Collier J, Longmore M, et al. (2008). *Oxford Handbook of Clinical Specialties*, 8th edn. Oxford: OUP. By permission of Oxford University Press.

Fetal head

Anatomy of the fetal skull

The fetal cranium is made up of five main bones, two parietal bones, two frontal bones, and the occipital bone. These are held together by membranous areas called *sutures*, which permit movement during birth (Fig. 1.6).

- *Coronal suture:* separates the frontal bones from the parietal bones.
- *Sagittal suture:* separates the two parietal bones.
- *Lambdoid suture:* separates the occipital bone from the parietal bones.
- *Frontal suture:* separates the two frontal bones.

▶ When two or more sutures meet, there is an irregular membranous area between them called a *fontanelle* (Fig. 1.6):

- *Anterior fontanelle or bregma:* is a diamond-shaped space at the junction of the coronal and sagittal sutures; this measures about 3cm in anteroposterior and transverse diameters, and usually ossifies at ~18mths after birth.
- *Posterior fontanelle or lambda:* is a smaller triangular area that lies at the junction of the sagittal and lambdoid sutures.

▶ The positions of the sutures and fontanelles play a very important role in identifying the position of the fetal head in labour.

Regions of the fetal head

The fetal head has different regions assigned to help in the description of the presenting part felt during vaginal examination in labour.

- *Occiput:* the bony prominence that lies behind the posterior fontanelle.
- *Vertex:* the diamond-shaped area between the anterior and posterior fontanelles, and between the parietal eminences.
- *Bregma:* the area around the anterior fontanelle.
- *Sinciput:* the area in front of the anterior fontanelle, which is divided into the brow (between the bregma and the root of the nose) and the face (lying below the root of the nose and the supraorbital ridges).

Caput and moulding of the fetal head

During labour, the dilating cervix may press firmly on the fetal scalp preventing venous blood and lymphatic fluid from flowing normally. This may result in a tissue swelling beneath the skin called *caput succedaneum*. It is soft and boggy to touch and usually disappears within 24h of birth.

There is usually some alteration in the shape of the fetal head and a ↓ in the head circumference in labour by a process of overlapping of the cranial bones (a ↓ of up to 4cm is possible). This moulding is physiological and disappears a few hours after birth. The frontal bones can slip under the parietal bones and, in addition, one parietal bone can override the other and in turn slip under the occipital bone.

The degree of moulding can be assessed vaginally:
- *No moulding:* when the suture lines are separate.
- *1+ moulding:* when the suture lines meet.
- *2+ moulding:* when the bones overlap but can be ↓ with gentle digital pressure.
- *3+ moulding:* when the bones overlap and are irreducible with gentle digital pressure.

► The presence of caput and moulding can play an important part in diagnosing obstructed labour.

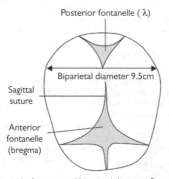

Fig. 1.6 Fontanelles, sagittal suture, and biparietal diameter. Reproduced from Collier J, Longmore M, et al. (2008). *Oxford Handbook of Clinical Specialties*, 8th edn. Oxford: OUP. By permission of Oxford University Press.

Diameters and presenting parts of the fetal head

The region that presents in labour depends on the degree of flexion or deflexion of the fetal head on presentation to the maternal pelvis. The important diameters of the fetal head as well as the presenting parts are as described below (Fig. 1.7):

- Suboccipitobregmatic diameter (9.5cm):
  - presentation of a well-flexed vertex
  - diameter extends from the middle of the bregma to the undersurface of the occipital bone where it joins the neck
  - fetal head circumference is smallest at this plane and measures 32cm.
- Suboccipitofrontal diameter (10.5cm):
  - partially flexed vertex, with diameter extending from the prominent point of the mid-frontal bone to the undersurface of occipital bone where it joins the neck.
- Occipitofrontal diameter (11.5cm):
  - presentation of a deflexed head
  - diameter extends from the prominent point of the mid-frontal bone to the most prominent point on the occipital bone
  - fetal head circumference at this plane measures 34.5cm.
- Mentovertical diameter (13cm):
  - brow presentation, with the diameter extending from the chin to the most prominent point of the mid-vertex
  - presents with the largest anteroposterior diameter.
- Submentobregmatic diameter (9.5cm):
  - face presentation, with diameter extending from just behind chin to the middle of the bregma.

▶ Other noteworthy diameters of the fetal head include:
- Biparietal diameter (BPD, 9.5cm):
  - greatest transverse diameter of the head, extending from one parietal eminence to the other.
- Bitemporal diameter (8cm):
  - greatest distance between two temporal eminences.
- Bimastoid diameter (7.5cm):
  - distance between the tips of the two mastoid processes.

⊃ Malpresentations in labour: overview, p. 351.

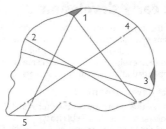

1 Suboccipitobregmatic 9.5cm
  flexed vertex presentation
2 Suboccipitofrontal 10.5cm
  partially deflexed vertex
3 Occipitofrontal 11.5cm
  deflexed vertex
4 Mentovertical 13cm brow
5 Submentobregmatic 9.5cm face

Fig. 1.7 Different presenting diameters of the fetal head. Reproduced from Collier J, Longmore M, Turmezei T, et al. (2008). *Oxford Handbook of Clinical Specialties*, 8th edn. Oxford: OUP. By permission of Oxford University Press.

Useful definitions when discussing the presenting part

- *Presentation* is the lowermost part of the fetus presenting to the pelvis. In >95% of cases the vertex is the presenting part and is called normal presentation. Any other presentation (e.g. face, brow, breech, and shoulder) is called malpresentation.
- *Denominator* is the most definable peripheral landmark of the presenting part, i.e. occiput for the vertex, mentum for the face, and sacrum for the breech presentation.
- *Position* of the presenting part is the relationship of the denominator to the fixed points of the maternal pelvis, i.e. sacrum posteriorly, pubic symphysis anteriorly, sacro-iliac joints posterolaterally, and ileo-pectineal eminences anterolaterally.
- *Station* is the relationship of the most prominent leading part of the presenting part to the ischial spines expressed as ±1,2,3cm.

▶ In the vertex presentation, >90% present in the occipito-anterior position, i.e. the occiput is in the anterior half of the pelvis and is called the normal position. If the occiput is pointing laterally or is in the posterior half of the pelvis, it is called malposition and is associated with deflexed head presenting a larger anteroposterior diameter of the vertex (11.5cm) and, hence, difficulties with progress of labour (➋ Fig. 1.3).

Placenta: early development

The placenta is the organ responsible for providing endocrine secretions and selective transfer of substances to and from the fetus. It serves as an interface between the mother and developing fetus.

Understanding the development of the placenta is important, as it is the placental trophoblasts that are critical for a successful pregnancy.

Embryological development

- After fertilization, the zygote enters the uterus in 3–5 days and continues to divide to become the blastocyst.
- Implantation of the blastocyst starts on day 7 and is finished by day 11:
  - the inner cell mass of the blastocyst forms the embryo, yolk sac, and amniotic cavity
  - the trophoblast forms the future placenta, chorion, and extraembryonic mesoderm.
- When the blastocyst embeds into the decidua, trophoblastic cells differentiate and the embryo becomes surrounded by two layers of trophoblasts:
  - the inner mononuclear cytotrophoblast
  - the outer multinucleated syncytiotrophoblast.
- The invading trophoblast penetrates endometrial blood vessels forming inter-trophoblastic maternal blood-filled sinuses (lacunar spaces).
- Trophoblastic cells advance as early or primitive villi, each consisting of cytotrophoblast surrounded by the syncytium.
- These villi mature into 2° and 3° villi, and the mesodermal core develops to form fetal blood vessels (completed by day 21).
- On days 16–17, the surface of the blastocyst is covered by branching villi which are best developed at the embryonic pole: the chorion here is known as chorionic frondosum; the future placenta develops from this area.
- Simultaneously, the lacunar spaces become confluent with one another and, by wks 3–4, form a multilocular receptacle lined by syncytium and filled with maternal blood: this becomes the future intervillous space.
- With further growth of the embryo, the decidua capsularis becomes thinner, and both villi and the lacunar spaces in the decidua are obliterated, converting the chorion into chorionic levae.
- The villi in the chorionic frondosum show exuberant division and subdivision, and with the accompanying proliferation of the decidua basalis, the future placenta is formed.
- This process starts at 6wks and the definitive numbers of stem villi are established by 12wks.

Placenta: later development

- Placental growth continues to term.
- Until wk 16, the placenta grows both in thickness and circumference due to growth of the chorionic villi with accompanying expansion of the intervillous space.
- After 16wks, growth occurs mainly circumferentially.

Placental villi

- Functional units of the placenta.
- There are ~60 stem villi in human placenta with each cotyledon containing 3–4 major stem villi.
- Despite their close proximity (0.025mm), there is no mixing of maternal and fetal blood.
- Placental barrier is made of outer syncytiotrophoblast, which is in direct contact with maternal blood, the cytotrophoblast layer, basement membrane, stroma containing mesenchymal cells, and the endothelium and basement membrane of fetal blood vessels.

The placenta at term

- Circular, diameter 15–20cm, thickness ~2.5cm at the centre.
- Weight ~500g (ratio of fetal:placental weight at term is about 6:1).
- Occupies ~30% of the uterine wall at term and has two surfaces.

Fetal surface

- Covered by a smooth, glistening amnion with the umbilical cord usually attached at or near its centre.
- Branches of the umbilical blood vessels are visible beneath amnion as they radiate from the insertion of the cord.
- Amnion can be peeled off from underlying chorion, except at insertion of cord.

Maternal surface

- Rough and spongy appearance, divided into several velvety bumps called cotyledons (15–20) by septa arising from the maternal tissues.
- Each cotyledon may be supplied by its own spiral artery.
- Numerous small greyish spots may be visible on the maternal surface representing calcium deposition in degenerated areas.

Umbilical cord

- Vascular cable that connects the fetus to the placenta.
- Varies from 30 to 90cm long, covered by amniotic epithelium.
- Contains two umbilical arteries and one umbilical vein embedded into the Wharton's jelly.
- Arteries carry deoxygenated blood from fetus to placenta and the oxygenated blood returns to fetus via the umbilical vein.
- In a full-term fetus, blood flow in the cord is ~350mL/min.

Placenta: circulation

The placental circulation consists of two distinctly different systems—the uteroplacental circulation and the fetoplacental circulation.

Uteroplacental circulation

- Uteroplacental circulation is the maternal blood circulating through the intervillous space (Table 1.1).
- Intervillous blood flow at term is estimated to be 500–600mL/min, and blood in the intervillous space is replaced 3–4 times/min.
- Pressure and concentration gradients between fetal capillaries and intervillous space favours placental transfer of oxygen and other nutrients to the fetus.

Arterial system

- Spiral arteries respond to the ↑ demand of blood supply to the placental bed by becoming low-pressure, high-flow vessels.
- They become tortuous, dilated, and less elastic by trophoblastic invasion, which starts early in pregnancy and occurs in two stages:
  - in 1st trimester, the decidual segments of the spiral arterioles are structurally modified
  - in 2nd trimester, 2nd wave of trophoblastic invasion occurs, resulting in invasion of myometrial segments of spiral arteries.

▶ Failure of this physiological change, particularly 2nd wave of trophoblastic invasion, is implicated in development of pre-eclampsia and fetal growth restriction.

Venous system

- Blood entering the intervillous space from the spiral artery becomes dispersed to reach the chorionic plate and gradually the basal plate, being facilitated by mild movements of villi and uterine contractions.
- From basal plate, uterine veins drain the deoxygenated blood.
- Venous drainage only occurs during uterine relaxation.
- Spiral arteries are perpendicular and veins are parallel to uterine wall, making large volumes of blood available for exchange at the intervillous space even though the rate of flow is ↓ during contraction, i.e. the veins are blocked for a longer time to allow pooling of blood in the retroplacental area.

Fetoplacental circulation

(See Table 1.2.)

- Two umbilical arteries carry deoxygenated blood from the fetus and enter the chorionic plate underneath the amnion.
- Arteries divide into small branches and enter the stem of the chorionic villi, where further division to arterioles and capillaries occurs.
- The blood then flows to the corresponding venous channel and subsequently to the umbilical vein.
- Maternal and fetal bloodstreams flow side by side, in opposite directions, facilitating exchange between mother and fetus.

Table 1.1 Haemodynamics of uteroplacental circulation

Volume of blood in the intervillous space	150mL
Blood flow in the intervillous space	500–600mL/min
Pressure changes in the intervillous space	
Height of uterine contraction	30–50mmHg
Uterine relaxation	10–15mmHg
Pressure in the spiral artery	70–80mmHg
Pressure in the uterine veins	8–10mmHg

Table 1.2 Haemodynamics of fetoplacental circulation

Fetal blood flow through placenta	400mL/min
Pressure	
In the umbilical artery	60–70mmHg
In the umbilical vein	10mmHg
Oxygen saturation and partial pressure of oxygen	
In the umbilical artery	60%; 20–25mmHg
In the umbilical vein	70–80%; 30–40mmHg

Placenta: essential functions

The placenta is directly responsible for mediating and/or modulating the maternal environment necessary for normal fetal development.

The placenta as an endocrine organ

As an active endocrine organ, the placenta produces a number of hormones, growth factors, and cytokines. The production of human chorionic gonadotropin (hCG), oestrogens, and progesterone by the placenta is vital for the maintenance of pregnancy.

Human chorionic gonadotropin
* 1° produced by syncytiotrophoblasts.
* Detected from 6 days after fertilization:
  * forms basis of modern pregnancy testing.
* Concentrations reach a peak at 10–12wks gestation, then plateau for remainder of the pregnancy.

The placenta as a barrier

The placenta acts as a barrier for the fetus against pathogens and the maternal immune system.

Infection
The placenta forms an effective barrier against most maternal blood-borne bacterial infections. However, some important organisms, such as syphilis, parvovirus, hepatitis B and C, rubella, Zika, human immunodeficiency virus (HIV), and cytomegalovirus (CMV), can cross it and infect the fetus during pregnancy. Although rare, there are cases of coronavirus transmission via the placenta as shown by placental inflammation and neonatal viraemia.

Drugs
Many drugs administered to the mother will pass across the placenta into the fetus; exceptions include low-molecular-weight heparin (LMWH).

Some drugs may have little effect on the fetus and be considered 'safe' (e.g. paracetamol), but others (e.g. warfarin) may significantly affect development, structure, and function of the fetus—a process known as *teratogenesis*.

Recently, a hormonal pregnancy testing drug, Primodos, used decades ago, has been incriminated in the causation of terminal limb reduction malformation. This is similar to thalidomide which was prescribed for vomiting in early pregnancy and caused phocomelia. Neither drug is used in pregnancy today.

Before prescribing any drug to a pregnant woman, it is the prescriber's obligation to ensure its benefit outweighs any risks to the pregnancy.

(➔ Common drugs: safety and usage, inside front and back covers.)

Principal functions of the placenta
- To anchor the fetus and establish the fetoplacental unit.
- To act as an organ for gaseous exchange.
- Endocrine organ to bring the needed changes in pregnancy.
- Transfer of substances to and from the fetus.
- Barrier against infection.

Placental transfer

Although the placenta acts as a barrier to most substances, it allows exchange of gases, transfer of fetal nutrition, and removal of waste products in a highly effective manner. Speed of exchange and concentration of substance exchanged depend upon:
- Concentration of the substance on each side of the placenta.
- Molecular size.
- Lipid solubility.
- Ionization.
- Placental surface area.
- Maternofetal blood flow.

A low-molecular-weight lipid-soluble substance with a high concentration gradient across the placenta, for example, will be transferred quickly to the fetus. Actual transfer occurs by simple diffusion, facilitated diffusion, active transport, and/or endocytosis (Table 1.3).

Table 1.3 Transfer mechanisms across the placenta for common anabolites and catabolites

Substance	Transfer mechanism(s)	Direction of transfer
Oxygen	Simple diffusion	To fetus
Carbon dioxide	Simple diffusion	From fetus
Glucose	Simple and facilitated diffusion	To fetus
Amino acids	Facilitated diffusion	To fetus
Iron	Endocytosis	To fetus
Fatty acids	Facilitated diffusion	To fetus
Water	Simple diffusion	To and from fetus
Electrolytes	Counter-transport mechanism	To and from fetus
Urea and creatinine	Simple diffusion	From fetus

Physiology of pregnancy: endocrine

Physiological and anatomical changes occur during the course of pregnancy to provide a suitable environment for the growth and development of the fetus. Early changes are due, in part, to metabolic demands brought on by the fetus, placenta, and uterus, and, in part, to ↑ levels of pregnancy hormones, particularly those of progesterone and oestrogen. Later changes are more anatomical in nature and are caused by mechanical pressure from the expanding uterus.

Endocrine changes

Progesterone ↑ throughout pregnancy

- Synthesized by the corpus luteum until 35 days and by the placenta thereafter.
- Progesterone promotes smooth muscle relaxation (gut, ureters, uterus) and raises body temperature.
- It is the principal hormone that prevents preterm labour and is now ↑ administered to prevent preterm labour.

Oestrogens—mainly oestradiol (90%)

- ↑ Breast and nipple growth, and pigmentation of the areola.
- Promote uterine blood flow, myometrial growth, cervical softening.
- ↑ Sensitivity and expression of myometrial oxytocin receptors.
- ↑ Water retention and protein synthesis.

Human placental lactogen (hPL)

- Has a structure and function similar to growth hormone.
- Modifies maternal metabolism to ↑ the energy supply to the fetus.
- ↑ Insulin secretion, but ↓ insulin's peripheral effect (liberating maternal fatty acids and sparing glucose enabling it to be diverted to the fetus).

The pituitary gland in pregnancy

- Enlarges mainly due to changes in the anterior lobe.
- Prolactin levels ↑ substantially, probably due to oestrogen stimulation of the lactotrophs.
- Gonadotropin secretion is inhibited, while plasma adrenocorticotropic hormone (ACTH) levels ↑.
- Maternal plasma cortisone output ↑, but the unbound levels remain constant.
- The posterior pituitary releases oxytocin principally during the 1st stage of labour and during suckling.

Effect of pregnancy on the thyroid

- The maternal thyroid gland enlarges due to ↑ demand in pregnancy.
- ↑ Renal clearance of iodine results in a relative iodide deficiency.
- The thyroid responds by tripling its iodide uptake from the blood, which results in follicular enlargement.
- Thyroid-binding globulin (TBG) is doubled by the end of the 1st trimester due to high oestrogen levels.
- As a result, total T_3 (triiodothyronine) and T_4 (thyroxine) levels rise early in pregnancy, then ↓ to remain within normal non-pregnant range.
- Thyroid-stimulating hormone (TSH) may ↓ slightly in early pregnancy, but tends to remain within the normal range.
- T_3 and T_4 cross the placental barrier in very small amounts.

▶ Iodine, antithyroid drugs, and long-acting thyroid stimulator (LATS) or antibodies associated with Graves' disease can cross the placenta and affect the fetal thyroid function, which starts as early as 12wks.

Physiology of pregnancy: haemodynamics

Plasma volume

- ↑ By 10–15% at 6–12wks of gestation.
- Expands rapidly until 30–34wks.
- Total gain at term ~1100–1600mL (total plasma volume of 4700–5200mL, a 30–50% ↑ from the non-pregnant state).
- Acute excessive weight gain is commonly due to oedema.

Red cell volume (or red cell mass)

- ↑ From 1400 to 1640mL at term (↑ 18%).
- With iron and folate supplements, an ↑ of 30% has been reported.

▶ The discrepancy between the rate of ↑ of plasma volume and that of red cell mass results in a relative haemodilution or 'physiological anaemia' with the haemoglobin (Hb) concentration, haematocrit, and red cell counts all ↓ (particularly in the 2nd trimester).
▶ Mean corpuscular Hb concentration remains constant.

Total white cell count

- ↑ Mainly due to the ↑ in neutrophil polymorphonuclear leucocytes, which peaks at 32wks.
- A further massive neutrophilia occurs during labour.
- Eosinophils, basophils, and monocytes remain relatively constant, but there is a profound ↓ in eosinophils during labour, being virtually absent at delivery.
- Although lymphocyte count and the number of B and T cells remain constant, lymphocyte function and cell-mediated immunity are profoundly depressed, giving rise to lowered resistance to viral infections.

Platelets

- ↓ Slightly during pregnancy.
- Platelet function is unchanged.

Clotting factors

- Pregnancy is a hypercoagulable state.
- Most clotting factors ↑, especially fibrinogen.

▶ Erythrocyte sedimentation rate (ESR) levels can also be elevated up to 4-fold in pregnancy.

Physiology of pregnancy: cardiorespiratory

Cardiovascular changes

Major changes occur in the cardiovascular system in pregnancy; the most significant of these changes occur within the 1st 12wks.

- Cardiac output ↑ from 5 to 6.5L/min by ↑ stroke volume (10%) and pulse rate (~15 beats/min).
- During labour, contractions may ↑ cardiac output by 2L/min, probably due to injection of blood from the intervillous space.
- With progressive enlargement of the uterus, the heart and diaphragm are displaced upwards.
- The heart enlarges and ↑ in volume by 70–80mL due to ↑ diastolic filling and muscle hypertrophy.

▶ Pregnancy may proceed normally even when the mother has an artificial cardiac pacemaker, with compensation occurring mainly from ↑ stroke volume.

Blood pressure in pregnancy

- Peripheral resistance ↓ by nearly 50% (probably due to the ↑ production of vasodilator prostaglandins).
- BP (most noticeably diastolic) ↓ mid-pregnancy by 10–20mmHg and ↑ to non-pregnant levels by term.
- Profound ↓ can occur late in pregnancy when lying supine, due to compression of the inferior vena cava leading to ↓ venous return and ↓ cardiac output (supine hypotension syndrome).
- Aortic compression may also occur causing a difference between brachial and femoral pressures giving a pressure difference of 10–15% from the supine to the lateral position.
- The balance of vasoconstrictor and vasodilator factors regulating peripheral resistance may be the basis of BP regulation in pregnancy and implicated in pregnancy-induced hypertension.
- Vasodilatation and hypotension also stimulate renin–angiotensin release, which plays a part in BP regulation.

Respiratory system changes

- The level of the diaphragm rises in pregnancy and the intercostal angle ↑ from 68° in early pregnancy to 103° in late pregnancy: breathing becomes more diaphragmatic than costal.
- Tidal volume ↑ ~40% (500–700mL) due to effect of progesterone.
- Inspiratory capacity (tidal volume plus inspiratory reserve volume) ↑ progressively in late pregnancy.
- Respiratory rate changes slightly, hence the resting pregnant woman ↑ ventilation by breathing more deeply and not more frequently.
- Breathlessness is common in pregnancy as maternal partial pressure of carbon dioxide (pCO_2) is set lower to allow the fetus to offload CO_2.

Physiology of pregnancy: genital tract and breast

Uterus

- Undergoes a 10-fold ↑ in weight to 1000g at term.
- Muscle hypertrophy occurs up to 20wks, after which stretching of the muscle fibres occurs.
- Uterine blood flow has been shown to ↑ from ~50mL/min at 10wks to 500–700mL/min at term.
- The uterine and ovarian arteries and branches of the superior vesical arteries undergo massive hypertrophy.

- The uterus is divided functionally and morphologically into three sections:
  - Cervix.
  - Isthmus (which later develops into the lower segment).
  - Body of the uterus (corpus uteri).

Cervix

- ↓ In cervical collagen towards term enables its dilatation.
- Hypertrophy of cervical glands leads to the production of profuse cervical mucus, and the formation of a thick mucus plug or operculum that acts as a barrier to infection.
- Vaginal discharge ↑ due to cervical ectopy (proliferation of columnar epithelium into vaginal portion of the cervix) and cell desquamation.

Uterine body

- ↑ In size, shape, position, and consistency.
- Uterine cavity expands from 4 to 4000mL.

Vagina

- A rich venous vascular network in connective tissue surrounds vaginal walls with blood and gives rise to slightly bluish appearance.
- High oestrogen levels stimulate glycogen synthesis and deposition:
  - action of lactobacilli on glycogen in vaginal cells produces lactic acid
  - lactic acid lowers the vaginal pH to keep the vagina relatively free from any bacterial pathogens.

Breast changes in pregnancy

- The lactiferous ducts and alveoli develop and grow under the stimulus of oestrogen, progesterone, and prolactin.
- From 3–4mths of pregnancy, colostrum (thick, glossy, protein-rich fluid) can be expressed from the breast.
- Prolactin stimulates the cells of the alveoli to secrete milk:
  - effect is blocked during pregnancy by the peripheral action of oestrogen and progesterone
  - shortly after delivery the sudden ↓ in these hormones enables prolactin to act uninhibited on the breast, and lactation begins.
- Suckling further stimulates prolactin and oxytocin release:
  - oxytocin stimulates contraction of the myoepithelial cells to cause ejection of milk.

Physiology of pregnancy: other changes

Urinary tract

Various anatomical and physiological changes occur in pregnancy:
- Kidney size ↑ by about 1cm in length.
- Marked dilatation of the calyces, renal pelvis, and ureter from 1st trimester.
- Vesicoureteric reflux occurs sporadically: a combination of reflux and ureteric dilatation leads to urinary stasis and ↑ incidence of infection.
- Although bladder muscle relaxes in pregnancy, residual urine is not normally present after micturition.
- Uric acid clearance ↑ from 12 to 20mmol/mL, causing ↓ in plasma uric acid levels: as pregnancy progresses, the filtered load of uric acid ↑, while the excretion remains constant, resulting in plasma levels returning to non-pregnant values.
- Renal blood flow ↑ by 30–50% in the 1st trimester, in line with the ↑ in cardiac output that occurs, and remains elevated:
  - results in ↑ glomerular filtration rate (GFR) and effective renal plasma flow, causing a ↓ in plasma levels of urea and creatinine
  - plays an important role in the variable glycosuria (due to exceeding the tubular maximum of absorption caused by more volume filtered) and urinary frequency that occurs in pregnancy.

⚠ Creatinine within the normal range for non-pregnant women may indicate renal impairment in pregnancy.

Alimentary system

- ↓ Tone of oesophageal sphincter and displacement through the diaphragm due to ↑ abdominal pressure causes reflux oesophagitis (heartburn).
- Gastric mobility is low and gastric secretion is ↓, resulting in delayed gastric emptying.
- Gut motility is generally ↓, and with possible ↑ sodium and water absorption in the large bowel, there is a tendency to constipation.

Skin

- Pigmentation in linear nigra, nipple, and areola or chloasma (brown patches of pigmentation seen especially on the face).
- Palmar erythema and spider naevi are also common.
- Incidence of striae varies in different populations:
  - represents the effect of disruption of collagen fibres in the subcuticular zone
  - probably related to the effect of ↑ production of adrenocortical hormones, as well as to the actual stress in the skin associated with relatively rapid expansion of the abdomen.

Preparing for pregnancy

A woman's body undergoes significant changes in pregnancy, with the developing fetus making ↑ demands. Preparation for pregnancy should begin before conception, as fetal development begins from the 3rd wk after the LMP. Damaging effects (e.g. exposure to drugs) may occur before the woman is even aware she is pregnant. Being as fit and healthy as possible before conception maximizes chances of a healthy pregnancy, but not all poor obstetric outcomes can be avoided. Pre-pregnancy counselling by a specialist team is recommended where specific risks and diseases are identified.

Specific risks for older mothers

- Advanced maternal age is a risk factor for adverse outcome.
- A woman >35yrs old has a ↓ chance of conceiving:
  - this rate of decline drops very quickly by 40yrs.
- Age also carries an ↑ risk of chromosomal abnormalities in the baby (most common abnormality being trisomy 21).
- Older mothers are more likely to develop complications in pregnancy, e.g. pre-eclampsia and diabetes mellitus.

Exercise and stress

- Moderate exercise should be encouraged, as it improves a woman's cardiovascular and muscular fitness.
- Women should be reassured that beginning or continuing a moderate course of exercise during pregnancy is not associated with adverse outcome.
- Best exercises are low-impact aerobics, swimming, brisk walking, and jogging.
- Contact and high-impact and vigorous racquet sports that may involve the risk of abdominal trauma should be avoided.
- Exercise is also associated with higher self-esteem and confidence.
- Relaxation and avoiding stress should be encouraged when planning for pregnancy.

⚠ Scuba diving may result in fetal birth defects and fetal decompression disease and, therefore, is not recommended.

Stopping contraception

- There is no delay in return to fertility after stopping the pill or having the coil removed.
- Women using contraceptive injection may experience a delay of several months.
- It is often recommended that women wait 3mths after stopping the pill before trying to conceive.

Supplements and lifestyle advice

Supplements

Folic acid

Only vitamin supplement that is recommended for use before pregnancy and up to 12wks gestation for women who are otherwise eating a healthy balanced diet.

Iron

- Routine supplementation is not necessary and should be only prescribed when medically indicated:
  - may be considered routine in areas where incidence of iron-deficiency anaemia is high.
- The amount of elemental iron in an adult female is 5g:
  - she will need 1mg/day before menstrual age
  - 2mg/day during reproductive age
  - 3mg/day during pregnancy.

Calcium

Supplementation may be necessary if intake of calcium is low; however, the ideal is ↑ calcium by dietary intake.

Iodine

Deficiency is endemic in some parts of the world, and can cause cretinism and neonatal hypothyroidism. Supplementation with iodized salt or oil should be considered.

Zinc

Low serum levels have been associated with an ↑ risk of preterm labour and growth restriction, but ↑ intake from dietary sources, such as milk and dairy products, should be sufficient.

Vitamin A

⚠ Vitamin A supplementation (intake >700 micrograms/day) might be teratogenic and should be avoided, as should consumption of products high in vitamin A, such as liver and pâté.

Alcohol, smoking, and recreational drugs

Excessive alcohol intake has been conclusively shown to cause fetal malformations. The exact threshold of alcohol that will cause malformation in the fetus has not been established.

⚠ Avoid alcohol or limit consumption to <1U/day.

Smoking during pregnancy has an adverse effect on the developing fetus (e.g. preterm labour, low birth weight). Women should be encouraged to stop and supported through smoking cessation. If they cannot stop, ↓ should be promoted.

▶ Stopping smoking at any stage has a beneficial effect.

⚠ Recreational and illegal drugs cause significant problems including miscarriage, preterm birth, poor fetal development, and intrauterine death. Help and support for dealing with any addiction should be sought from the appropriate agencies.

Recommended doses of folic acid

- 400 micrograms/day folic acid has been shown to ↓ the occurrence of neural tube defects.
- For women at higher risk (e.g. previous affected child, women with epilepsy, diabetes, and obesity), a dose of 5mg/day is recommended.

Weight and diet

- Fertility may be ↓ in women who are significantly overweight (BMI >30) or underweight (BMI <18.5).
- Obesity is the most common nutritional disorder in the industrialized world, with ↑ risks including gestational diabetes and hypertension; also, monitoring and assessment may be difficult during pregnancy and labour (➜ Obesity in pregnancy: maternal risks, p. 294).
- Malnutrition, on the other hand, is a major life hazard in the developing world and is a cause of other problems such as anaemia that has its own inherent risk for both mother and fetus.
- Poor nutrition in pregnant women is associated with the delivery of low birth weight (<2500g) babies, and improving the nutritional status and maternal weight can have a positive effect on the birth outcome.
- Weight gain should be around 11–16kg during pregnancy, and women should consume an additional 350kcal (1500kJ) a day.
- A nutritious, well-balanced diet includes foods rich in protein, dairy foods (which supply calcium), starchy foods, and plenty of fruit and vegetables that supply vitamins and fibre.
- It is best to avoid a lot of sugary, salty, or fatty foods.
- Food delicacies such as undercooked meats and eggs, pâtés, soft cheeses, shellfish and raw fish, and under-pasteurized milk should be avoided as they are potential sources of *Listeria* and *Salmonella* that could lead to adverse perinatal outcome.

⚠ Listeriosis in pregnancy is a known but rare cause of poor obstetric outcome and fetal death.

General health check

Planning a pregnancy provides a good opportunity for a general health check by the general practitioner (GP) and may identify any potential obstetric risk factors well in advance.

> ## Pre-pregnancy general health check
> May include:
> * A general examination including BP, heart, and lungs.
> * Family history of inherited disorders or congenital abnormalities.
> * Urine dipstick.
> * Blood tests such as thalassaemia and sickle cell disease may be offered if at risk.
> * Rubella (and hepatitis) status should be ascertained and vaccination given if not immune (women should be advised to avoid pregnancy for 3mths after immunization).
> * HIV screening if at risk.
> * Dental examination.

Pre-existing medical disorders

Pregnancy can have an adverse effect on pre-existing medical disorders (➔ Medical disorders in pregnancy, p. 215).
* The effect may be transient, returning to normal after delivery (e.g. diabetes mellitus), or it may be permanent and progressive, leading to maternal mortality (e.g. severe renal impairment or severe cardiac disease).
* For a woman with a pre-existing disorder contemplating pregnancy, the advice of a specialist should be sought early:
  * if the risk is very high, pregnancy may be discouraged altogether (e.g. Eisenmenger's complex—ventricular septal defects (VSDs) with pulmonary hypertension).
* Optimal control of certain diseases before conception may be very important to avoid the risk of fetal malformation or adverse outcome (e.g. diabetes mellitus).
* Some medications may be changed before conception to ↓ the risk of teratogenesis (e.g. antiepileptics).
* Pregnancy undertaken when the illness is in remission, stable, or cured will ensure a better outcome.

Medication

In general, both prescription drugs and over-the-counter medication should be used as little as possible. Most drugs carry warnings about use in pregnancy. However, the benefit may outweigh the risks, even in pregnancy, so a doctor should be consulted before stopping or starting any medication in pregnancy or before conception.

Working during pregnancy

- Women should be reassured that it is safe to continue working before and during pregnancy.
- Some workplaces are more likely to present hazards (e.g. chemical factories, operating theatres, X-ray departments); hence, precautions may be necessary—specific advice should be sought from the employer's occupational health department.
- Women should be reassured that use of computers and video display units has not been proven to be linked with any adverse outcome.
- ➲ Vaccination in pregnancy, p. 214.

Diagnosis of pregnancy

The most obvious symptom of pregnancy is cessation of periods, i.e. a period of amenorrhoea in a woman having regular menstruation.

Other common symptoms of early pregnancy

Nausea and vomiting (morning sickness)
- Common in the 1st trimester.
- May occur at any time of the day.
- May sometimes persist throughout pregnancy.

Frequency of micturition
- ↑ In plasma volume leads to ↑ urine production.
- Pressure effect of the uterus on the bladder.
- Make sure the frequency is not associated with dysuria, which may denote possible infection.

Excessive lassitude or fatigue
- Common in early pregnancy.
- Tends to disappear after 12wks gestation.

Breast tenderness or 'heaviness'
Often seen early in pregnancy, particularly in the month after the 1st period is missed.

Fetal movements or quickening
- ~20wks gestation in the nullipara.
- 18wks in the multipara.
- Many women may experience FM earlier than this and some may not perceive movements until term.
▶ Occasionally, a pregnant woman may experience an abnormal desire to eat something abnormal (such as dirt)—this is known as pica.

Clinical examination

- The vagina and cervix have a bluish tinge due to blood congestion.
- The size of the uterus may be estimated by bimanual examination (reasonably accurate in early pregnancy).
- After 12wks the uterus is palpable abdominally and the FH may be heard using a hand-held Doppler.

The pregnancy test
- The hormone hCG is secreted by trophoblastic tissue:
  - ↑ Exponentially from 8 days after ovulation (2× every 2nd day)
  - peaks at 8–12wks gestation.
- hCG levels can be measured in blood or urine.
- Test kits are available commercially (home pregnancy tests):
  - can show a positive result with urinary hCG levels >50IU/L
  - some 'early' pregnancy test kits will detect levels of >25IU/L
  - can confirm pregnancy within 1wk of a missed period.

Dating of pregnancy

Menstrual history

- The 1st day of the LMP may be used to calculate the gestational age and the EDD (➔ Obstetric history: current pregnancy, p. 2), but this may be inaccurate as:
  - many women may not be certain of their LMP
  - ovulation does not always occur on day 14 and the proliferative phase may vary in shorter or longer menstrual cycles.
- The EDD can be calculated using Naegele's formula (➔ Obstetric history: current pregnancy, p. 2).
- About 40% of women will deliver within 5 days of the EDD and about 2/3 within 10 days.

⚠ 11–42% of gestational age estimates from LMP may be inaccurate.

▶ Pregnancies resulting from *in vitro* fertilization (IVF) can be dated using the day of embryo transfer.

Dating ultrasound scan

- Between 8 and 13wks USS provides the most accurate measure of gestational age and, where possible, should be used to calculate EDD.
- Before 8wks it is unreliable due to the small size of the gestation sac and fetal pole.
- After 13wks other factors may affect fetal growth; therefore, although an estimate can be made using BPD and femur length (FL), it may be unreliable.

Crown–rump length

Crown–rump length (CRL; Fig. 1.8) is used to calculate gestation between 8 and 13wks. It is measured from one fetal pole to the other along its longitudinal axis in a straight line.

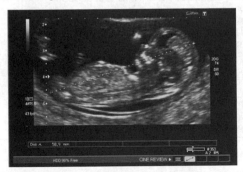

Fig. 1.8 Ultrasound image of a 12wk fetus measuring the CRL.

Ultrasound assessment of fetal growth

Any clinical suspicion that the fetus may be small or large for gestational age should be followed by a formal ultrasound assessment of fetal growth and amount of amniotic fluid (liquor volume).

The measurements used are given in Fig. 1.9:

Biparietal diameter and head circumference

- The anatomical landmarks used to ensure the accuracy and reproducibility of the measurement are a midline falx, the thalami symmetrically positioned on either side of the falx, the visualization of the cavum septum pellucidum at 1/3 the fronto-occipital distance, and the lateral ventricles with their anterior and posterior horns identifiable.
- The calipers are placed between the leading edge of the proximal and distal skull bones (BPD) and circumferentially around the head (HC).

Abdominal circumference

- The abdominal circumference (AC) is the single most important measurement in assessing fetal size and growth.
- It is measured where the image of the stomach and the portal vein is visualized in a tangential section.

Femur length

By convention, measurement of the FL is considered accurate only when the image shows two blunted ends.

⚠ FL can be underestimated if the correct plane is not obtained.

→ Fetal growth restriction: definitions, p. 144.

Uterus measurement anomalies

The uterus may measure small for dates because of:
- Wrong dates.
- Oligohydramnios.
- Fetal growth restriction.
- Presenting part deep in the pelvis.
- Abnormal lie of the fetus.

The uterus may measure large for dates because of:
- Wrong dates.
- Macrosomia.
- Polyhydramnios.
- Multiple pregnancy.
- Presence of fibroids.

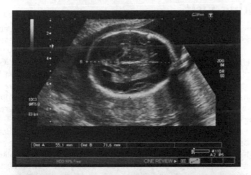

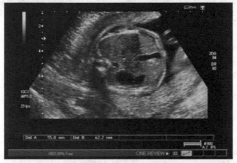

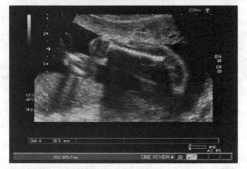

Fig. 1.9 Ultrasound measurement of biparietal diameter (top), abdominal circumference (middle), and femur length (bottom).

Booking visit

The needs of each pregnant woman should be assessed at the 1st appointment and a plan of care made for her pregnancy. This should be reassessed at each appointment as new problems can arise at any time. Many women in the UK have 'shared obstetric care' whereby the woman's GP and community midwife undertake most of the obstetric care, with a limited number of visits to the hospital.

Routine involvement of an obstetrician in the care of an uncomplicated pregnancy does not appear to improve perinatal outcomes compared with involving obstetricians when complications arise.

There should be continuity of care throughout the AN period and this should be provided by a small group of carers with whom the woman feels comfortable. The environment in which AN appointments take place should enable women to discuss sensitive issues, such as domestic violence, sexual abuse, psychiatric illness, and illicit drug use. Women should be given the information needed to choose between giving birth at home, in a midwifery-led unit, or in hospital.

Booking should ideally be early in pregnancy (before 12wks) in order to take full advantage of AN care. However, many women are seen for the 1st time in the 2nd trimester.

⚠ Children born to very late bookers or unbooked women have a higher risk of perinatal mortality (4–5×) and morbidity, with an attendant ↑ in maternal morbidity and mortality.

Booking visit: history

A comprehensive history should be elicited (➔ Obstetric history: current pregnancy, p. 2) and a full physical examination undertaken (➔ Obstetric physical examination, p. 6).
- Risk factors from past history should be highlighted.
- It is essential to obtain past obstetric notes if this information may change the management.
- History of inheritable diseases in close relatives should be sought, and history of migration and travel may identify risk for diseases such as haemoglobinopathies, some forms of hepatitis, and HIV.
- Histories of alcohol abuse, smoking, and addictive drug use are useful behavioural markers of potential risks (e.g. fetal abnormalities, impaired fetal growth, preterm labour, and neonatal drug withdrawal problems).
- It is important to identify women at risk of postnatal depression:
  - women should be asked about previous and family history of psychiatric disorders, and social problems including domestic violence and previous self-harm
  - women at risk should have psychiatric care and social support.
- Advice and support should be given on healthy lifestyles (including diet and exercise), pregnancy care services available, maternity benefits, and sufficient information to enable informed decision making following screening tests.

1st contact with healthcare professionals

Ensure the woman is given information on:
- Folic acid supplementation.
- Low-dose aspirin if meets criteria.
- Lifestyle advice.
- AN screening.
- Booking appointment.

Booking appointment (usually with a midwife in the UK)
- Identify high-risk women who need additional care.
- Calculate BMI.
- Measure BP.
- Dipstick test urine (protein, glucose, blood, etc.).
- Check an ultrasound appointment has been made for confirmation of viability, gestational age, and aneuploidy screening (if desired).
- Take blood tests for:
  - haemoglobinopathies
  - rubella
  - Venereal Disease Research Laboratory (VDRL) test
  - HIV
  - hepatitis B virus
  - red cell allo-antibodies
  - Hb for anaemia.
- Give information on:
  - AN classes
  - pregnancy care pathway
  - nutrition, diet, and vitamin supplementation
  - maternity benefits
  - how baby develops.

Antenatal care: planning

The basic aims of AN care are:

- To provide evidence-based information and support to women and their partners, to enable them to make informed decisions regarding their care.
- To advise on minor problems and symptoms of pregnancy.
- To assess maternal and fetal risk factors at the onset of pregnancy.
- To facilitate provision of prenatal screening and subsequent management of any abnormalities detected.
- To monitor fetal and maternal well-being throughout pregnancy and screen for commonly occurring complications (most notably BP and urine check at every visit to detect signs of developing pre-eclampsia and diabetes).
- To determine timing and mode of delivery when complications arise or if pregnancy continues after the EDD.

▶ The needs of each pregnant woman should be assessed at each appointment as new problems can arise at any stage in pregnancy.

⚠ Urine should be dipstick tested and BP measured at every AN visit.

Screening for chromosomal and structural abnormalities

- Ideally, screening should be offered to all women at the time of booking.
- Detailed, unbiased, written information should be provided about the conditions being screened for, types of test available, and the implications of the results.

⚠ It is important for a woman to understand that a negative result in any screening test does not guarantee that her baby does not have that or another abnormality.

For full details on current UK screening ➔ Prenatal diagnosis: overview, p. 104.

Antenatal appointment schedule

A schedule of AN appointments and what needs to be done at each visit has been described in the recent NICE antenatal care guidelines and is summarized below.

16wks
- Discuss screening results.
- Investigate if Hb level <11g.
- Offer information and arrange anomaly scan (18–20wks).

25wks (nulliparous women only)
- BP, urine dip, plot SFH.

28wks
- Screening for anaemia and atypical red cell allo-antibodies.
- Anti-D prophylaxis to rhesus (Rh) –ve women.
- BP, urine dip, plot SFH.

31wks (nulliparous women only)
- BP, urine dip, and plot SFH.

34wks
- Discuss labour and birth (including pain relief and birth plan).
- Give anti-D if Rh –ve and cell-free fetal DNA testing demonstrates a +ve fetus.
- BP, proteinuria, plot SFH.

36wks
Discuss:
- Breast-feeding.
- Vitamin K prophylaxis.
- Postnatal self-care.
- Awareness of baby blues and postnatal depression.
- BP, urine dip, plot SFH.

38wks
- BP, urine dip, plot SFH.

40wks
- BP, urine dip, plot SFH.
- Give information about prolonged pregnancy.

41wks
- Membrane sweep.
- Book induction of labour to occur by 42wks.

Further reading
NICE (2021). Antenatal care. ℘ https://www.nice.org.uk/guidance/ng201

Antenatal care: routine blood tests

AN care starts once the pregnancy is confirmed, and a referral is made by the GP to the community midwife for booking.

Routine blood tests

Full blood count (FBC)

- Physiological anaemia means the lower limit for a 'normal' Hb is 10.5g/dL in pregnancy.
- Commonest cause of anaemia is iron deficiency—investigate by assessment of haematinic indices, such as ferritin and total iron-binding capacity (TIBC) in microcytic hypochromic anaemia, serum and red cell folate, and serum vitamin B_{12} levels in macrocytic anaemia.

Blood grouping and antibody screen

Determining the blood group makes it possible to identify Rh –ve women who are at risk of Rh isoimmunization and to detect abnormal antibodies such as Kell and Duff (➋ Rhesus isoimmunization (immune hydrops), p. 130).

Rubella screen

Around 2% of nulliparous and 1% of multiparous women are not immune to rubella. It is recommended that these women receive postpartum rubella vaccination.

Syphilis screen

- Although the incidence of syphilis in the UK is low, outbreaks do occur.
- Early treatment can prevent congenital syphilis in the neonate and screening and treatment is cost-effective.

Hepatitis B screen

- Screening for hepatitis B is performed on all women in pregnancy at booking so that effective postnatal intervention can be offered.
- In adults, the virus is cleared within 6mths in 90% of those infected.
- In neonates, 90% become chronic carriers with risk of post-infective hepatic cirrhosis and hepatocellular carcinoma—hence the need to screen and prevent.
- Active immunization with hepatitis vaccine may be adequate for those neonates where the mother was surface (s) antigen +ve, but passive and active immunization is recommended for those who are core (e) antigen +ve.

HIV screen

- The recommendation for all maternity units in the UK is for universal screening for HIV at the booking visit ('opt out' policy):
  - vertical transmission from mother to fetus can be significantly ↓ (by 2/3) by treatment of mother with antiretrovirals in pregnancy and labour, and infant for 6wks postnatally
  - risk of transmission is ↓ by CD in cases of high viral load and avoidance of breast-feeding (➋ HIV and pregnancy, p. 206).

Antenatal care: specific blood tests

Haemoglobin electrophoresis

This should be routinely performed in women of minority ethnic or racial origins with high incidence of haemoglobinopathies.

Some ethnic origins at high risk of thalassaemia

- Cyprus.
- Eastern Mediterranean.
- Middle Eastern.
- Indian subcontinent.
- South-east Asia.

▶ Women of African or Afro-Caribbean origin are at risk of sickle cell disease or trait.

▶ If a woman is affected, testing her partner's status would enable appropriate counselling and further prenatal testing.

⚠ Persistent anaemia, of undiagnosed cause, may be an indication for Hb electrophoresis in any woman, regardless of racial origin.

Miscellaneous tests

A variety of other blood tests may be indicated on an individual basis. For example, thyroid function tests (TFTs, history of thyroid disease), glycated Hb (HbA1c; to assess long-term control of diabetes), or baseline urea and creatinine (in chronic hypertensives with renal complications).

Screening for gestational diabetes

💣 There is little consensus as to who, when, how, or even whether to screen for gestational diabetes mellitus (GDM). At present, there is insufficient evidence to support routine screening for GDM. The timing of any screening is equally controversial as the later the test is performed, the higher the detection rate since glucose tolerance progressively deteriorates. On the other hand, the earlier in pregnancy GDM is diagnosed and hyperglycaemia treated, the greater the likelihood of positively influencing the outcome. Most units currently use targeted screening based on known risk factors as recommended by NICE.

Risk factors for gestational diabetes

- Previous GDM.
- Family history of diabetes (1st-degree relative with diabetes).
- Previous macrosomic baby.
- Previous unexplained stillbirth.
- Obesity (BMI >30).
- Glycosuria on more than one occasion.
- Polyhydramnios.
- Large for gestational age fetus in current pregnancy.

Antenatal care: preparing for delivery

- In the early 3rd trimester, women are seen monthly and, at each visit, BP, urinalysis, and fundal height measurement, as well as enquiry about maternal well-being and fetal activity, are recorded.
- FBC and antibody screen is repeated at 28 and 34wks gestation, and Rh –ve women are offered anti-D prophylaxis at these times.
- From 36wks onwards, fetal presentation as well as growth are assessed, and an ultrasound assessment performed if indicated.
- Preparation for labour and delivery should be discussed.
- The final routine visit between 40 and 41wks includes discussions on induction of labour after 41wks gestation.
- In women who wish to avoid induction, the risks of prolonging pregnancy should be discussed and a plan for ↑ fetal surveillance with cardiotocography (CTG) and ultrasound assessment of fetal growth and liquor volume can be made.

Chapter 2

Pregnancy complications

Minor symptoms of pregnancy: gastrointestinal

Minor symptoms of pregnancy are mostly related to hormonal, physiological, and ↑ weight-bearing aspects of pregnancy.

Although usually mild and self-limiting, some women may experience severe symptoms, which can affect their ability to cope with activities of daily living (➲ Further reading).

Nausea and vomiting (morning sickness)

- Most common complaint, especially in the 1st trimester:
  - Nausea: 80–85%
  - Vomiting: 52%.
- Believed to be caused by hormones of pregnancy especially hCG.
- ↑ In multiple and molar pregnancies.
- May be severe enough to warrant hospital admission—hyperemesis gravidarum (➲ Hyperemesis gravidarum, p. 622).
- Not usually associated with poor pregnancy outcome.
- Tends to resolve spontaneously by 16–20wks.

Management
- Lifestyle modification (e.g. eat small meals, ↑ fluid intake) acupressure (P6).
- Antiemetics (prochlorperazine, promethazine, metoclopramide, ondansetron).

Gastro-oesophageal reflux (heartburn)

- Very common complaint at all stages of pregnancy:
  - 1st trimester—22%; 2nd trimester—39%; 3rd trimester—72%.
- Progesterone relaxes oesophageal sphincter allowing gastric reflux, which gradually worsens with ↑ intra-abdominal pressure from the growing fetus.

Management
- Lifestyle modification (e.g. sleep propped up, avoid spicy food).
- Alginate preparations and simple antacids.
- If severe, proton pump inhibitors (omeprazole).

Constipation

- Common complaint that appears to ↓ with gestation:
  - progesterone ↓ smooth muscle tone, affecting bowel activity
  - often made worse by iron supplementation.

Management
- Lifestyle modification (e.g. ↑ fruit, fibre, and water intake).
- Fibre supplements.
- Osmotic laxatives (lactulose).

Further reading

NICE (2021). Antenatal care. NICE guideline [NG201].
⌖ www.nice.org.uk/guidance/ng201

Minor symptoms of pregnancy: musculoskeletal and vascular

Symphysis pubis dysfunction or pelvic girdle pain

- Describes a collection of signs and symptoms producing pelvic pain.
- Usually mild, but can present with severe and debilitating pain.
- Incidence up to 10%.

Management

- Physiotherapy advice and support.
- Simple analgesia.
- Limit abduction of legs at delivery.
- Caesarean delivery (CD) not indicated.

(See ⅋ www.pelvicpartnership.org.uk.)

Backache and sciatica

- Common complaint, attributed to hormonal softening of ligaments exacerbated by altered posture due to the weight of the uterus.
- Prevalence estimated between 35% and 61%.
- Neurological symptoms (sciatica) may occur.

Management

- Lifestyle modification (e.g. sleeping positions).
- Alternative therapies including relaxation and massage.
- Physiotherapy (e.g. back care classes) and simple analgesia.

Carpal tunnel syndrome

- Occurs due to oedema compressing the median nerve in the wrist.
- Usually resolves spontaneously after delivery.

Management

- Sleeping with hands over the side of the bed may help.
- Wrist splints may be of benefit.
- If evidence of neurological deficit, surgical referral indicated.

Haemorrhoids

- Tend to occur in the 3rd trimester.
- Incidence 8–30% of pregnant women.

Management

- Avoid constipation from early pregnancy.
- Ice packs and digital reduction of prolapsed haemorrhoids.
- Suppositories and topical agents for symptomatic relief.
- If thrombosed, may require surgical referral.

Varicose veins

- Common complaint, which ↑ with gestation.

Management

- Regular exercise and compression hosiery.
- Consider thromboprophylaxis if other risk factors are present.

Minor symptoms of pregnancy: genitourinary and others

Urinary symptoms

- Frequency in the 1st trimester results from ↑ GFR and the uterus pressing against the bladder.
- Stress incontinence may occur in the 3rd trimester as a result of pressure on the pelvic floor.

▶ Urinary tract infections (UTIs) are common in pregnancy.

Management

- Screen for UTI (urine dipstick testing: nitrite analysis is best).
- Avoid caffeine and fluid late at night.

Vaginal discharge

- ↑ Due to ↑ blood flow to the vagina and cervix.
- Should be white/clear and mucoid:
  - offensive, coloured, or itchy may indicate an infection
  - profuse and watery may indicate ruptured membranes.

Management

- Exclude ruptured membranes.
- Exclude sexually transmitted infection (STI) and candidiasis (common in pregnancy).
- Reassurance.

Itching and rashes

- Skin changes and itching are common in pregnancy.
- Rashes are usually self-limiting and not serious.

Management

- Full history and examination to exclude infectious causes (e.g. varicella (➔ Varicella zoster, p. 172) and intrahepatic cholestasis (➔ Intrahepatic cholestasis of pregnancy, p. 252).
- Emollients and simple over-the-counter 'anti-itch creams'.
- Reassurance—most will resolve after delivery.
- Referral to dermatologist if severe.

Other common minor symptoms of pregnancy

- *Breast enlargement and pain:* helped with supportive underwear.
- *Mild breathlessness on exertion*: important to exclude pulmonary embolus and anaemia.
- *Headaches:* important to exclude pre-eclampsia or (rare) neurological cause.
- Tiredness.
- Insomnia.
- Stretch marks.
- Labile mood.
- Calf cramps.
- Braxton Hicks contractions.

Antepartum haemorrhage: overview

Antepartum haemorrhage (APH) is bleeding from the genital tract in pregnancy at ≥24wks gestation before onset of labour.

Women with placenta praevia or placental abruption may present with typical symptoms and signs and with recognized risk factors.
⚠ However, there may be minimal or no *per vaginam* (PV) loss in a large abruption and an abruption is usually, but not always, painful

Causes of antepartum haemorrhage
- Unexplained (80%): usually marginal placental bleeds (i.e. minor placental abruptions).
- Placenta praevia.
- Placental abruption.
- Others, including:
  - maternal:
    - incidental (cervical erosion/ectropion)
    - local infection of cervix/vagina
    - a 'show', usually light and pink or brown
    - genital tract tumours, particularly cervical carcinoma
    - varicosities
    - trauma.
  - fetal: vasa praevia.

⚠ There may be rapid and severe haemorrhage from a placenta praevia.

⚠ Most bleeding from an abruption is concealed.

Vasa praevia
- This occurs when the fetal vessels run in membranes below the presenting fetal part, unsupported by placental tissue or umbilical cord.
- Incidence of ruptured vasa praevia is 1:2500–2700.
- May present with PV bleeding after rupture of fetal membranes followed by rapid fetal distress (from exsanguination).
- Reported fetal mortality of rupture 33–100%.
- Risk factors include:
  - low-lying placenta
  - multiple pregnancy
  - IVF pregnancy
  - bilobed and especially succenturiate lobed placentas.

Antepartum haemorrhage: assessment

Initial assessment

Rapid assessment of maternal and fetal condition is a vital 1st step as it may prove to be an obstetric emergency.

History

A basic clinical history should establish:
- Gestational age.
- Amount of bleeding (but don't forget blood may be concealed).
- Associated or initiating factors (coitus/trauma).
- Abdominal pain.
- Fetal movements.
- Date of last smear.
- Previous episodes of PV bleeding in this pregnancy.
- Leakage of fluid PV.
- Previous uterine surgery (including CD).
- Smoking and use of illegal drugs (especially cocaine).
- Blood group and Rh status (will she need anti-D?).
- Previous obstetric history (placental abruption/fetal growth restriction (FGR), placenta praevia).
- Position of placenta, if known from previous scan.

Maternal assessment

This should include:
- BP.
- Pulse.
- Other signs of haemodynamic compromise (e.g. peripheral vasoconstriction or central cyanosis).
- Uterine palpation for size, hardness/contractions, tenderness, fetal lie, presenting part.

⚠ Remember, never perform a vaginal examination (VE) in presence of PV bleeding without 1st excluding a placenta praevia ('No PV until no PP').

Once a placenta praevia is excluded, a speculum examination should be undertaken to assess degree of bleeding and possible local causes of bleeding (trauma, polyps, ectropion), and to determine if membranes are ruptured. A digital examination ascertains cervical changes indicative of labour.

Fetal assessment
- Establish whether a FH can be heard.
- Ensure that it is fetal and not maternal (remember, the mother may be very tachycardic).
- If the FH is heard and gestation is estimated to be 26wks or more, FHR monitoring should be commenced.

Placenta praevia and low-lying placenta
(See Fig. 2.1.)

Definitions
- *Placenta praevia* (formerly major or grade III–IV): the placenta is over the internal cervical os.
- *Low lying placenta* (formerly minor or grade I–II): the placenta is within 20mm of the internal os.

Incidence
About 0.5% of pregnancies at term.

Diagnosis
Transvaginal USS is safe and is more accurate than transabdominal USS in locating the placenta, particularly if posterior.

⚠ Establish that there has been no previous CD (➔ Placenta accreta spectrum: overview, p. 138).

Management
- Consider admission in women with major placenta praevia who have bled.
- Offer steroids if <35wks.
- Women with asymptomatic major placenta praevia may remain at home if they
  - are close to the hospital
  - are fully aware of the risks to themselves and their baby
  - have a constant companion.
- Delivery is likely to be by CS if the placental edge is <2cm from the internal os.
- If recurrent PV bleeding: deliver immediately if massive, otherwise electively at 34–36wks.
- If asymptomatic, consider delivery by 37wks.
- Cross-match blood and ensure senior surgeon.

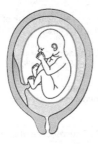
Normal placenta

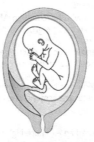
Low-lying placenta

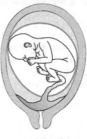
Placenta previa

Fig. 2.1 Placenta praevia.

Antepartum haemorrhage: management

> **Antepartum haemorrhage categories**
> Following full assessment, women will fall into one of two categories:
>
> *Bleeding heavy and continuing*
> - Mother or fetus is/soon will be compromised.
> - This is an emergency—manage as per massive obstetric haemorrhage.
> - ➔ Massive obstetric haemorrhage: management, p. 416.
>
> *Bleeding minor, or settling, and neither mother nor fetus compromised*
> - This is a limited APH (see following section).

Limited antepartum haemorrhage

Maternal management
- FBC.
- Kleihauer testing, if woman known to be RhD –ve and fetal blood group unknown or RhD +ve, to determine extent of fetomaternal haemorrhage and if more anti-D is required.
- Group and save (G&S).
- Coagulation screen and renal function if suspected abruption.

> ▶ All RhD –ve women whose baby is RhD +ve or whose baby's RhD status is unknown require 500IU of anti-D immunoglobulin.
> (➔ Rhesus isoimmunization, p. 130).

Fetal management
- USS to establish fetal well-being (growth/volume of amniotic fluid) and to confirm placental location.
- Fetal Doppler measurement (the function of the placenta may be compromised even by small abruptions).

Ongoing antenatal management
- Most units admit women who have had an APH for 24h, as the risk of further bleeding is estimated to be greatest during that time.
- Offer steroids if <35wks
- If the bleeding settles and mother is discharged, a clear plan for the remaining pregnancy should be made including extra fetal surveillance of growth and well-being.
- Management must be individualized according to suspected cause of bleeding, gestation, fetal assessment, and continuing maternal risk factors.

> ⚠ All women who have had an APH are high risk: ↑ surveillance of both mother and fetus.
>
> ⚠ History of APH ↑ risk of bleeding at delivery: 'APH = postpartum haemorrhage (PPH)'.

Placental abruption

Definition
Placenta separates partly or completely from uterus before delivery of fetus. Blood accumulates behind placenta in uterine cavity or is lost through cervix.

Incidence
0.5–1.0% of pregnancies.

Types
- *Concealed:* no external bleeding evident (<20%).
- *Revealed:* vaginal bleeding.

Presentation
- Usually present with abdominal pain.
- Typically, sudden onset, constant, and severe, may have backache.
- The uterus is tender on palpation.
- Uterine activity is common, may later be hard ('woody').
- Many will be in labour (up to 50% on presentation).
- Bleeding is very variable, often dark.
- Maternal signs of shock.
- Fetal distress is common and precedes fetal death.

⚠ *Remember, extent of the maternal haemorrhage may be much greater than apparent vaginal loss.*

Diagnosis
- Made clinically.
- USS is of use only to exclude placenta praevia.

Management
- Intravenous (IV) access and bloods (➔ Massive obstetric haemorrhage: management, p. 416).
- Establish immediate fetal well-being with CTG.
- Admit all with vaginal bleeding or unexplained abdominal pain.
- Arrange USS.
- Give steroids if <35wks.
- If fetal distress or maternal compromise, resuscitate, give magnesium sulfate ($MgSO_4$) if <30–32wks, and deliver.
- If no fetal distress, and bleeding and pain cease, consider delivery by term.

If placenta low lying at 20wk/anomaly scan
- Warn about PV bleeding, but advise that most placentas will move by term.
- Ensure no previous CD (➔ Placenta accreta spectrum: diagnosis and managment p. 142).
- Repeat scan at 32wks; if still low, repeat at 36wks.

Further reading
RCOG (2018). Placenta praevia and placenta accreta. Green-top guideline no. 27a.
🕮 www.rcog.org.uk/en/guidelines-research-services/guidelines/gtg27a/

Blood pressure in pregnancy: physiology

Basic physiology

BP is directly related to systemic vascular resistance and cardiac output, and follows a distinct course during pregnancy:
- ↓ In early pregnancy until 24wks due to ↓ in vascular resistance.
- ↑ After 24wks until delivery via ↑ in stroke volume.
- ↓ After delivery, but may peak again 3–4 days postpartum.

⚠ Most women book in 1st trimester. Be aware of the pregnant woman with a high booking BP, who may have previously undetected chronic hypertension—especially important in older pregnant women.

Blood pressure measurement

BP must be measured correctly to avoid falsely high or low readings that may influence clinical management:
- BP should be measured sitting with the upper arm at the level of the heart.
- Use the correct cuff size:
  - a normal adult cuff is usually for an upper arm of ≤34cm
  - a cuff too small may lead to a falsely high reading.
- The diastolic BP should be taken as Korotkoff V (the absence of sound), rather than Korotkoff IV (muffling of sound), which was previously used, unless the sound is heard all the way down to 0.

Classification of hypertension

- Hypertension (previously mild–moderate) BP ≥140/90.
- Severe hypertension BP ≥160/110.

Blood pressure in pregnancy: hypertension

Pre-eclampsia

→ Pre-eclampsia: overview, p. 60.

Pregnancy-induced hypertension

Defined as hypertension (≥140/90) in the 2nd half of pregnancy in the absence of proteinuria or other markers of pre-eclampsia.

- Affects 6–7% of pregnancies.
- At ↑ risk of going on to develop pre-eclampsia (15–26%).
- Risk ↑ with earlier onset of hypertension.
- Delivery should be after 37wks.
- BP usually returns to pre-pregnancy limits within 6wks of delivery.

Chronic hypertension

- Complicates 3–5% of pregnancies.
- Pregnant women who have a high BP (≥140/90) prior to 20wks or are on treatment for hypertension.
- ↑ risk of developing pre-eclampsia.
- Delivery should be after 37wks.

▶ Now more common because of an older pregnant population.

⚠ If BP very high, important to exclude a 2° cause, rather than attributing it to essential hypertension.

Postnatal hypertension

- New hypertension may arise in the postpartum period.
- It is important to determine whether this is physiological, pre-existing chronic hypertension, or new-onset pre-eclampsia.

▶ Remember, BP peaks on the 3rd to 5th day postpartum.

⚠ Symptoms such as epigastric pain or visual disturbance and new-onset proteinuria are suggestive of postpartum pre-eclampsia.

Postnatal management of hypertension

See Table 2.1.
- Daily BP monitoring up to 5 days is wise
- Captopril can be used (up to 50mg (by mouth (PO)) tds), or enalapril.
- Nifedipine (10mg PO bd up to 30mg PO qds) may also be used.

▶ Women should be told that breastfeeding is safe with these drugs.
- GP can follow up the BP in the community and titrate the medication to the BP.
- Women on medication should be offered a postnatal follow-up appointment 6wks postnatally.
- ↑ BP usually resolves by 6wks.
- If still ↑ after this, it is important to look for 2° causes of hypertension.

Table 2.1 Antihypertensive medications

Medication	Dose	Side effects	Breast-feeding
Labetalol	100mg bd up to 600mg qds	Avoid in asthma	Yes
	IV infusion for severe refractory hypertension		Yes
Methyldopa	250mg bd up to 1g tds	Depression change postnatally. No longer 1st line antenatal	Yes
Nifedipine	10mg bd up to 30mg tds	Tachycardia, flushing, headache	Yes
Hydralazine	25mg tds up to 75mg qds	Tachycardia, pounding heartbeat, headache, diarrhoea	Yes
Atenolol	50–100mg od	Avoid in asthma	Yes
Angiotensin-converting enzyme inhibitors (ACEIs)	Postpartum only, as fetotoxic		Captopril or enalapril safe

---

Hypertension in pregnancy treatment principles

⚠ Treatment of BP is urgently required for maternal safety at levels of 160/110 and non-urgently if BP ≥140/90.

• Escalation may be required (Table 2.1).
• Treatment should aim for BP levels of 135/85.

▶ Treatment of BP protects women from the adverse effects of ↑ BP but does not alter the course of pre-eclampsia.

2° causes of hypertension

• Renal disease.
• Cardiac disease, e.g. coarctation of the aorta.
• Endocrine causes, e.g. Cushing's syndrome, Conn's syndrome, or rarely a phaeochromocytoma.

▶ Women with chronic hypertension are at risk of:

• Exacerbation of hypertension.
• Superimposed pre-eclampsia.
• Fetal growth restriction.
• Placental abruption.

Pre-eclampsia: overview

Pre-eclampsia is a multisystem disorder characterized by hypertension and, usually, proteinuria. It arises from the placenta. However, it can present in a wide variety of ways and not always in the classical fashion. It has a wide spectrum of severity ranging from mild to severe (e.g. haemolysis, elevated liver enzymes, and low platelets (HELLP) syndrome or eclampsia). It remains a cause of maternal morbidity and mortality in the UK. It is a common cause of prematurity and hospital admission and has huge economic implications.

Incidence

• Pre-eclampsia affects 3–5% of pregnancies (usually in mild form).
• Severe pre-eclampsia affects up to 1% of pregnancies.

Prediction of pre-eclampsia

History

• An ↑ (7×) chance of pre-eclampsia in subsequent pregnancies in women who have had pre-eclampsia before.
• Risk ↑ with earlier onset (Box 2.1), ↑ severity, and after HELLP syndrome (➋ Eclampsia and haemolysis, elevated liver enzymes, and low platelets (HELLP) syndrome, p. 66).
• Presence of other risk factors, e.g. medical disease, family history.
• Blood tests:
  • low pregnancy-associated plasma protein-A (PAPP-A) (➋ Common screening tests, p. 108) associated with ↑ risk.
  • raised uric acid and creatinine, low platelets, and high Hb may help differentiate pre-eclampsia from pregnancy-induced hypertension.
  • between 20 and 35wks, soluble FM-like tyrosine kinase 1 (sFlt-1)/ placental growth factor (PlGF) ratio <38 virtually excludes pre-eclampsia within next 2wks.
• USS: uterine artery Dopplers at 11–13wks or 20wks are predictive of early-onset or severe pre-eclampsia.

Integrated testing

The combination of independent risk factors such as history, mean arterial BP, PAPP-A, and uterine artery Dopplers at 12wks ± other biomarkers can also be used.

🔾 This combination of markers to define at risk women is more effective at ↓ the incidence of pre-eclampsia than using history alone, but is not yet in common usage.

Prevention of pre-eclampsia

Low-dose aspirin (150mg PO od) from 12wks (should be <16wks) is advised in women at ↑ risk (Box 2.1).

Definition of pre-eclampsia

Owing to its heterogeneous nature, it can be difficult to define. The new international consensus criteria define it as:
- New hypertension BP ≥140/90.
  And
- Either urinary protein:creatinine ratio (PCR) ≥30 (~2+ on dipstick testing.
  Or
- Evidence of end-organ dysfunction including abnormal renal or liver function, or placental dysfunction.

▶ This wider definition acknowledges that proteinuria may be absent at presentation but is vague regarding specific criteria for end-organ dysfunction.

Box 2.1 Risk factors for and prevention of pre-eclampsia

Advise low-dose aspirin (150mg) from 12wks if:

1 major risk factor
- Hypertensive disease during a previous pregnancy.
- Chronic kidney disease (CKD).
- Autoimmune disease, e.g. systemic lupus erythematosus (SLE) or antiphospholipid syndrome.
- Type 1 or type 2 diabetes.
- Chronic hypertension.
  Or

>1 minor risk factors
- 1st pregnancy.
- Age ≥40yrs.
- Pregnancy interval of >10yrs.
- BMI of ≥35kg/m² at 1st visit.
- Family history of pre-eclampsia.
- Multi-fetal pregnancy.

▶ Note additional later risk factors for pre-eclampsia:
- Fetal hydrops.
- Hydatidiform mole.

Further reading
NICE (2019). Hypertension in pregnancy: diagnosis and management. NICE guideline [NG133].
℅ www.nice.org.uk/guidance/ng133

Pre-eclampsia: clinical features and investigations

Pre-eclampsia can present with a wide variety of signs and symptoms. It presents to the clinician a diagnostic dilemma and never ceases to surprise. However, most women with pre-eclampsia are asymptomatic.

Symptoms
- Headache (common in pregnancy).
- Visual disturbance (esp. flashing lights) (common in pregnancy).
- Epigastric or right upper quadrant (of abdomen) (RUQ) pain.
- Nausea and vomiting.
- Rapid oedema (esp. face).

⚠ Symptoms usually occur only with severe disease.

Signs
- Hypertension (>140/90; severe if ≥160/110).
- Proteinuria (PCR ≥30).
- Facial oedema.
- Epigastric/RUQ tenderness suggests liver involvement and capsule distension.
- Confusion or cortical blindness.
- Uterine tenderness or vaginal bleeding from a placental abruption.
- Fetal growth restriction on USS, particularly if <36wks.

Laboratory investigations
FBC
- Relative high Hb due to haemoconcentration.
- Thrombocytopaenia.
- Anaemia if haemolysis (➔ Eclampsia and haemolysis, elevated liver enzymes, and low platelets (HELLP) syndrome, p. 66).

Biochemistry
- ↑ Urate, ↑ urea, and ↑ creatinine.
- Abnormal liver function tests (LFTs; ↑ transaminases) and ↑ lactate dehydrogenase (LDH; a marker for haemolysis).
- ↑ Proteinuria (PCR ≥30).
- sFlt-1/PlGF ratio (between 20 and 35wks) <38 virtually excludes pre-eclampsia in next 2wks; ratio >85 mean pre-eclampsia very likely.

Coagulation profile
- Usually normal unless very severe.

Pre-eclampsia: management

Pre-eclampsia has several severe complications (Box 2.2). Cure is delivery of placenta. Management depends on several issues, including maternal and fetal well-being and gestational age.

Box 2.2 Severe complications of pre-eclampsia

- Eclampsia.
- HELLP.
- Cerebral haemorrhage.
- FGR and fetal compromise.
- Renal failure.
- Placental abruption.

Management and admission with pre-eclampsia

Hypertension 140/90–159/109 and no maternal or fetal compromise
- Treat BP if ≥140/90, aim for BP of 135/80.
- Outpatient monitoring:
  - warn about development of symptoms
  - 3/wk review of BP
  - 1–2/wk review of FBC and biochemistry
  - regular USS assessment (fortnightly if remains normal).
- Deliver by 37wks unless criteria for immediate delivery.

Hypertension 160/110+ or maternal or fetal compromise
- Treat BP, aim for BP of 135/85.
- Admission is often advised but is not always indicated. If admitted:
  - 4-hourly review of BP.
  - 3/wk review of FBC and biochemistry.
  - daily CTG
  - regular USS assessment (fortnightly growth and twice-weekly Doppler/liquor volume depending on severity of pre-eclampsia).
- Deliver by 37wks unless criteria for immediate delivery.

▶ Medication does not cure the condition, but aims to prevent hypertensive complications of pre-eclampsia.

Severe pre-eclampsia: management

⚠ Defined as the occurrence of BP ≥160 systolic or ≥110 diastolic in the presence of significant proteinuria (PCR ≥30), *or* if maternal complications occur.

▶ Senior obstetric, anaesthetic, and midwifery staff should be informed and involved in the management of a woman with severe pre-eclampsia.

Treatment

* The only treatment is delivery, but this can sometimes be delayed with intensive monitoring if <34wks.
* Pre-eclampsia often worsens for 24h after delivery.

Indications for immediate delivery

* Worsening liver or renal function or thrombocytopaenia.
* Severe maternal symptoms, especially epigastric pain with abnormal LFTs, e.g. HELLP syndrome.
* Pulmonary oedema, e.g. oxygen saturation <90%.
* Eclampsia or abnormal neurological findings.
* Evidence of placental abruption.
* Fetal reasons such as abnormal CTG; role of USS parameters dependent on gestation

Management

Blood pressure

* BP needs to be stabilized with antihypertensive medication (aim for 135/85, every 30min until <160/110).
* Initially use PO nifedipine 10mg: can be given twice 30min apart.
* If BP remains high after 2–3 nifedipine doses:
  * start IV labetalol infusion
  * ↑ infusion rate until BP is adequately controlled.
* Start maintenance therapy, usually labetalol; methyldopa if asthmatic.

Other management

* Take bloods for FBC, urea and electrolytes (U&E), LFTs, and clotting profile.
* Strict fluid balance chart.
* CTG monitoring of fetus until condition stable.
* USS of fetus:
  * evidence of FGR, estimate weight if severely preterm
  * assess condition using fetal and umbilical artery Doppler.

⚠ If <34wks, steroids should be given and the pregnancy may be managed expectantly unless the maternal or fetal condition worsens.

Eclampsia and haemolysis, elevated liver enzymes, and low platelets (HELLP) syndrome

Eclampsia

Eclampsia is defined as the occurrence of a tonic–clonic seizure in association with a diagnosis of pre-eclampsia.

- Complicates ~1–2% of pre-eclamptic pregnancies.
- May be the initial presentation of pre-eclampsia, and may occur before hypertension or proteinuria.
- Fits may occur antenatally (38%), intrapartum (18%), or postnatally usually within the 1st 48h (44%).

⚠ Every hospital in the UK should have an eclampsia protocol and eclampsia box with all the drugs for treatment.

⚠ When new to a hospital, familiarize yourself with protocol and whereabouts of the drug box.

⚠ Eclampsia is a sign of severe disease: most women who die with pre-eclampsia or eclampsia do so from other complications, such as blood loss, intracranial haemorrhage, or HELLP.

HELLP syndrome

This is a serious complication regarded by most as a variant of severe pre-eclampsia which manifests with haemolysis (H), elevated liver enzymes (EL), and low platelets (LP).

- Incidence is estimated at 5–20% of pre-eclamptic pregnancies; milder versions without haemolysis most common.
- Maternal mortality is estimated at 1%; perinatal mortality is 10–60%.
- Liver enzymes ↑ and platelets ↓ before haemolysis occurs.
- Usually self-limiting, but permanent liver or renal failure may occur.
- Symptoms include:
  - epigastric or RUQ pain (65%)
  - nausea and vomiting (35%)
  - urine is 'tea-coloured' due to haemolysis.
- Signs include:
  - tenderness in RUQ
  - ↑ BP and other features of pre-eclampsia.
- Eclampsia may coexist.
- Delivery is indicated.
- Treatment is supportive and as for eclampsia ($MgSO_4$) is indicated).
- Although platelet levels may be very low, platelet infusions are only required if bleeding, or for surgery and <40.

⚠ Beware of epigastric pain in any pregnant and immediately postnatal women: always check the BP, urine, and liver enzymes.

Management of eclampsia

⚠ Call for help—obstetric senior and junior specialist registrars (SpRs) and consultant; anaesthetic SpR and consultant; delivery suite coordinator.
- Basic principles of airway, breathing, and circulation plus IV access.
- Most eclamptic fits are short-lasting and terminate spontaneously.
- $MgSO_4$ is the drug of choice for both control of fits and preventing (further) seizures.
- A loading dose of 4g should be given over 5–10min followed by an infusion of 1g/h for 24h.
- If further fits occur, a further 2g can be given as a bolus (the therapeutic range for magnesium (Mg) is 2–4mmol/L).
- In repeated seizures use diazepam (if still fitting, the patient may need intubation and ventilation and imaging of the head to rule out a cerebral haemorrhage).
- Strict monitoring of the patient is mandatory: pulse, BP, respiration rate, and oxygen saturations every 15min; urometer and hourly urine.
- Assessment of reflexes every hour for Mg toxicity (usually knee reflexes, but use biceps if epidural *in situ*).
- Half/stop infusion if oliguric (<20mL/h) or raised creatinine and seek senior/renal advice.
- Mg toxicity is characterized by confusion, loss of reflexes, respiratory depression, and hypotension.
- If toxic give 1g calcium gluconate over 10min.
- If hypertensive give BP-lowering drugs:
  - oral nifedipine
  - IV labetalol (avoid in asthmatics).
- Fluid restrict the patient to 80mL/h or 1mL/kg/h due to the risk of pulmonary oedema (even if oliguric the risk of renal failure is small); monitor the renal function with the creatinine.
- A central venous pressure line may be needed if there has been associated maternal haemorrhage and fluid balance is difficult or if the creatinine rises.
- The fetus should be continuously monitored with CTG.
- Deliver fetus once the mother is stable.
- Vaginal delivery is not contraindicated if cervix is favourable.
- If HELLP syndrome coexists, consider involvement of renal and liver physicians.
- Third stage should be managed with 5–10U oxytocin, rather than Syntometrine® or ergometrine because of ↑ in BP.

Further reading

NICE (2019). Hypertension in pregnancy: diagnosis and management. NICE guideline [NG133].
🖱 www.nice.org.uk/guidance/ng133

Multiple pregnancy: overview

Incidence

- About 1 in 34 babies born in the UK is a twin or triplet.
- Incidence of multiple pregnancy was ↑, but now appears to be stable at:
  - twins—15:1000
  - triplets—1:5000
  - quadruplets—1:360 000.
- Higher multiples than this are extremely rare, but do occur: a surviving set of quintuplets was born in the UK in 2007.

Aetiology

Multiple predisposing factors including:
- Previous multiple pregnancy.
- Family history.
- ↑ parity.
- ↑ maternal age:
  - <20yrs: 6:1000
  - >35yrs: 22:1000
  - >45yrs: 57:1000.
- Ethnicity:
  - Nigeria: 40:1000
  - Japan: 7:1000.
- Assisted reproduction—incidence of multiple pregnancy:
  - clomifene: 10%
  - intrauterine insemination (IUI): 10–20%
  - IVF with two-embryo transfer: 20–30%.

▶ In an attempt to ↓ this complication, the Human Fertilization and Embryology Authority (HFEA) recommend that no more than two embryos should be transferred per IVF cycle.

Further reading

Human Fertilization and Embryology Authority.
🖰 www.hfea.gov.uk
The Multiple Births Foundation.
🖰 www.multiplebirths.org.uk

Multiple pregnancy: types

Dizygotic twins

Dizygotic twins result from two separate ova being fertilized by different sperm, simultaneously implanting and developing.

Consequently, these fetuses will have separate amniotic membranes and placentas (dichorionic and diamniotic—DCDA). Twins may be different sexes. This mechanism of twinning accounts for 2/3 of multiple pregnancies; this type is most affected by predisposing factors, such as age and ethnicity.

Monozygotic twins

Monozygotic twins result from division into two of a single, already developing, embryo and will be genetically identical and, therefore, always the same sex. Whether they share the same amniotic membrane and/or chorion depends on the stage of development when the embryo divides. About 2/3 are monochorionic diamniotic.

See Fig. 2.2 for an explanation of the mechanism of twinning.

> **Timing of division in monozygotic twins**
> - <3 days → DCDA 30%.
> - 4–7 days → monochorionic, diamniotic (MCDA) 70%.
> - 8–12 days → monochorionic, monoamniotic (MCMA) <1%.
> - >12 days → conjoined twins (very rare).

The worldwide monozygotic twinning rate appears to be constant at about 3.5 per 1000. However, the rate is slightly greater than expected with IVF treatment.

Diagnosis

There are several signs and symptoms associated with multiple pregnancy including:
- Hyperemesis gravidarum.
- Uterus is larger than expected for dates.
- Three or more fetal poles may be palpable at >24wks.
- Two FHs may be heard on auscultation.

However, most are diagnosed on USS in the 1st trimester (at a dating or nuchal translucency scan). As most women in the UK now have USS at some stage in their pregnancy, diagnosis is rarely missed.

Chorionicity

Determining chorionicity allows risk stratification for multiple pregnancy and is best done by USS in the 1st trimester or early in the 2nd. The key indicators are:
- Obviously widely separated sacs or placentae—DC.
- Membrane insertion showing the lambda (λ) sign—DC.
- Absence of λ sign <14wks diagnostic of MC.
- Fetuses of different sex—DC (dizygotic).

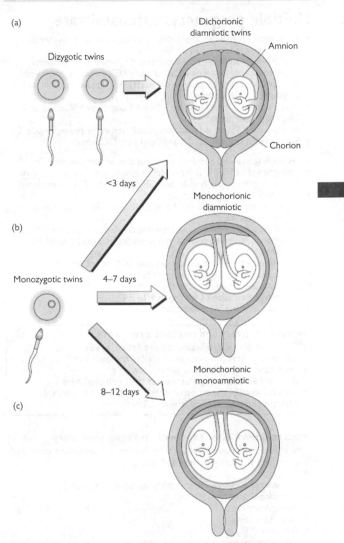

Fig. 2.2 Mechanism of twinning. Dizygotic twins (a) are always DCDA, but with monozygotic twins (a, b, and c), the type will depend on the time of the division of the conceptus.

Multiple pregnancy: antenatal care

- All multiple pregnancies are by definition 'high risk' and the care should be consultant led.
- Establish chorionicity—most accurately diagnosed in 1st trimester (absence of λ sign diagnostic), so an early USS should be considered with any indications of multiple pregnancy (e.g. fundus palpable <12wks or exaggerated symptoms of early pregnancy).
- Iron and folate supplements are advised if additional FBC check at 20–24wks shows anaemia.
- Advise aspirin 150mg od if additional risk factors for pre-eclampsia.
- Serial growth scans at 28, 32, and 36wks for DC twins.

- ♦ A 24wk scan is also recommended but is of limited benefit.
- Management of FGR is as for singleton pregnancies but risk of iatrogenic preterm birth of a non-FGR co-twin should be considered.
- Size discordance is calculated as:
  - (estimated fetal weight (EFW) larger fetus − EFW smaller fetus) ÷ EFW largest fetus.
- Surveillance needs to be more intensive (2-weekly scans) for MC twins, or higher multiples, so referral to a specialist fetal medicine team is advisable.
- More frequent antenatal checks because of ↑ risk of pre-eclampsia.
- Advise of risks and signs of preterm birth.
- Discuss mode, timing, and place of delivery.
- Establish presentation of leading twin by 34wks.
- Offer delivery at 37wks: induction or CD.

Preterm delivery and multiple pregnancy

(➔ Preterm labour: prevention and prediction, p. 96).
- Incidence ↑: principal cause of morbidity and mortality.
- Predictable with transvaginal cervical scanning.
- Beneficial effect of progesterone less than with singletons.
- Cervical cerclage controversial: only if additional risk factors for preterm birth, e.g. cervical length <15mm

---

Maternal risks associated with multiple pregnancy

The risks of pregnancy appear to be heightened with twins compared with singletons, leaving mothers at ↑ risk of:
- Anaemia.
- Pre-eclampsia (5× greater risk with twins than singletons).
- Gestational diabetes.
- Polyhydramnios.
- Placenta praevia.
- APH and PPH.
- Operative delivery.

Fetal risks associated with multiple pregnancy

⚠ All fetal risks ↑ with MC twins.

↑ *Risk of miscarriage*
- Especially with MC twins.

↑ *Risk of congenital abnormalities*
- Only in MC twins.

FGR
- Up to 25% of twins.

Preterm labour
- Main cause of perinatal morbidity and mortality:
  - 40% of twins deliver before 37wks
  - 10% of twins deliver before 32wks.

↑ *Perinatal mortality*
- Singletons 5:1000.
- DC twins 18:1000; MC twins higher.
- Triplets 53:1000.

↑ *Risk of intrauterine death (stillbirth)*
- Singletons 8:1000.
- DC twins 31:1000; MC twins higher.
- Triplets 84:1000.

↑ *Risk of disability*
- Mainly, but not entirely, due to prematurity and low birth weight).

↑ *Incidence of cerebral palsy (CP)*
- Singletons 2:1000.
- DC twins 7:1000; MC twins higher.
- Triplets 27:1000.

Vanishing twin syndrome
- One twin apparently being reabsorbed at an early gestation (1st trimester).

Monochorionic, diamniotic twins

The shared circulation of MC twins can lead to several problems.

Twin-to-twin transfusion syndrome (TTTS)

This affects about 5–25% of MC twin pregnancies and left untreated has an 80% mortality rate. It may occur acutely at any stage or more commonly take a chronic course, which, at its worst, leads to severe fetal compromise at a gestation too early to consider delivery. It is caused by vascular anastomoses within the placenta, which redistribute the fetal blood, leading to fluid overload in the 'recipient' and hypovolaemia in the 'donor' twin.

▶ MC twins require intensive monitoring, usually in the form of serial USSs every 2wks from 16wks until delivery. The treatment options potentially available include:

- Laser ablation to completely separate the circulations. This method is associated with lowest risk of neonatal handicap.
- Selective feticide by cord occlusion is reserved for refractory disease.

▶ TTTS managed by laser treatment leads to survival of at least one in 80% and both twins in 50%.

Twin anaemia polycythaemia sequence (TAPS)

- Marked difference in Hb values between MC twins with TTTS.
- Usually complicates inadequate separation of circulations at laser treatment for TTTS.
- Management is controversial; early delivery should be considered.

Selective fetal growth restriction

- Growth discordance (even without TTTS), is more common.
- Defined as >20% size difference or where one twin is <10th centile.
- Very variable pattern of umbilical artery Doppler signals (intermittent absent/reversed end-diastolic flow: ↑ AREDF) indicates a high risk of sudden demise.
- Treatment: if >32wks delivery is safest; if <28wks, selective termination or laser ablation should be considered.
- Selective termination requires closure of the shared circulation so is normally performed using diathermy cord occlusion.

Twin reversed arterial perfusion (TRAP)

In this rare condition, one of an MC twin pair is structurally very abnormal with no or a rudimentary heart, and receives blood from the other (umbilical artery flow direction is reversed), which is called the 'pump twin'.

This normal twin may die of cardiac failure, and unless the abnormal twin is very small or flow to it ceases, selective termination using radiofrequency ablation is indicated.

Termination of pregnancy issues

- Although MC twins may be discordant for structural abnormalities, genetically they are identical.
- Selective termination of pregnancy requires closure of the shared circulation so is normally performed using diathermy cord occlusion.

Effects of twin-to-twin transfusion on the fetus

Donor twin
- Hypovolaemic and anaemic.
- Oligohydramnios: appear 'stuck' to the placenta or uterine wall.
- Growth restriction.

Recipient twin
- Hypervolaemic and polycythaemic.
- Large bladder and polyhydramnios.
- Cardiac overload and failure.
- Evidence of fetal hydrops (ascites, pleural, and pericardial effusions).
- This twin is often more at risk than the donor.

Intrauterine death of a twin
- DC:
  - the death of one twin in the 1st trimester or early part of the 2nd does not appear to adversely affect the remaining fetus
  - preterm birth follows in >50%.
- MC:
  - because of the shared circulation, subsequent death or neurological damage from hypovolaemia follows in up to 25%, where one of the pair dies
  - delivery does not ↓ the risk of brain injury
  - preterm birth follows in >50% when occurs in the 3rd trimester.

Further reading
NICE (2019). Twin and triplet pregnancy. NICE guideline [NG137]
℘ www.nice.org.uk/guidance/ng137

Multiple pregnancy: labour

- For all multiple pregnancies mode of delivery is debated.
- The 2nd twin is at ↑ risk of perinatal mortality, but it is not currently the case that all twins are delivered by CS.
- For labour, the leading twin should be cephalic (>80%), and there should be no absolute contraindication (e.g. placenta praevia).
- Triplets and higher-order multiples are usually delivered by CS.

  For management of labour and delivery, see Box 2.3.

Intrapartum risks associated with multiple pregnancy

- Malpresentation.
- Fetal hypoxia in 2nd twin after delivery of the 1st.
- Cord prolapse.
- Operative delivery.
- PPH.
- Rare:
  - cord entanglement (MCMA twins only)
  - head entrapment with each other: 'locked twins'
  - fetal exsanguination due to vasa praevia.

Box 2.3 Management of labour and delivery for twins

- Twins are usually offered delivery at 37wks gestation, but 40% will have delivered spontaneously before then.
- CD is offered if the leading twin is not cephalic.
- The woman should have IV access and a G&S.
- Fetal distress is more common in twins; continuous fetal monitoring with CTG is important throughout labour, particularly after the 1st twin has delivered to avoid hypoxia in the 2nd.
- It may be helpful to monitor the leading twin with a fetal scalp electrode and the other abdominally.
- An epidural may be helpful, especially if there are difficulties delivering the 2nd twin, but is not essential.
- Many units choose to deliver twins in theatre as there is more space available and it provides immediate recourse to surgical intervention if required.
- Importance of support for mother cannot be overestimated.
- Leading twin should be delivered as for a singleton, but with care to ensure adequate monitoring of the 2nd throughout.
- After delivery of 1st baby, the lie of the 2nd twin should be checked and gently 'stabilized' by abdominal palpation while a VE is performed to assess the station of the presenting part.
- It is helpful to have an ultrasound scanner available in case of concerns about malpresentation of the 2nd twin.
- Once the presenting part enters the pelvis, the membranes can be broken; the 2nd twin is usually delivered within 20min of the 1st.
- Judicious use of oxytocin may help if the contractions diminish after delivery of the 1st twin.
- If fetal distress occurs in the 2nd twin, or there is excessive delay, delivery may be expedited with either forceps or ventouse.
- If this is inappropriate, the choice is between CD and breech extraction (often after internal podalic version).
- Breech extraction involves gentle and continuous traction on one or both feet, and must only be performed by an experienced obstetrician.
- As there is an ↑ risk of uterine atony, Syntometrine® and prophylactic oxytocin infusion is recommended.

Breech presentation: overview

Breech presentation occurs when the baby's buttocks lie over the maternal pelvis. The lie is longitudinal, and the head is found in the fundus. This becomes ↓ common with gestation, such that breech presentation at term occurs with only 3–4% of fetuses, but is much more common preterm.

Types of breech
- Extended breeches (70%):
  - both legs extended with feet by head; presenting part is the buttocks.
- Flexed breeches (15%):
  - legs flexed at the knees so that both buttocks and feet are presenting.
- Footling breeches (15%):
  - one leg flexed and one extended.

Causes and associations of breech presentation
- Idiopathic (most common).
- Preterm delivery.
- Previous breech presentation.
- Uterine abnormalities, e.g. fibroids/Müllerian duct abnormalities.
- Placenta praevia and obstructions to the pelvis.
- Fetal abnormalities.
- Multiple pregnancy.

Consequences of breech presentation
Fetal
- There is an ↑ risk of hypoxia and trauma in labour.
- Irrespective of the mode of delivery, neonatal and longer-term risks are ↑—reasons are incompletely understood but may be due to:
  - association with congenital abnormalities
  - many preterm babies are breech at the time of delivery.

Maternal
Most breeches are delivered by CS.

Diagnosis of breech presentation
- Before 36wks it is not important unless the woman is in labour.
- Breech presentation is commonly undiagnosed before labour (30%).
- On examination:
  - lie is longitudinal
  - the head can be palpated at the fundus
  - the presenting part is not hard
  - the FH is best heard high up on the uterus.
- USS confirms the diagnosis and should also assess growth and anatomy because of the association with fetal abnormalities.

External cephalic version

External cephalic version (ECV) is a method for manually turning a breech or transverse presentation into a cephalic one. It is performed from 36wks in nulliparous women and 37wks in multiparous ones. The intention is to ↓ the need for delivery by CS.

- *Method:* after USS, a forward roll technique is used. The breech is elevated from the pelvis, and pushed to the side where the back is; the head is then pushed forward and the roll completed. Excessive force must not be used. After the attempt, CTG is performed and anti-D given if the mother is Rh −ve. See Fig. 2.3.
- *Efficacy:* the success rate is about 50%. Spontaneous reversion to breech presentation occurs in 3%. Attempting ECV halves the chance of non-cephalic presentation at delivery and greatly ↓ the risk of CS. Nulliparity, difficulty palpating the head, high uterine tone, an engaged breech, less amniotic fluid, and white ethnicity are associated with more difficulty.
- *Facilitation:* success rates are ↑ by the use of tocolysis, such as salbutamol, given either electively or if a 1st attempt fails. Epidural or spinal analgesia occasionally used.
- *Safety:* ~0.5% will require immediate delivery by CS due to FHR abnormalities or vaginal bleeding.
  - Theoretical or minor risks include pain, precipitation of labour, placental abruption, fetomaternal haemorrhage, and cord accidents.
  - The chances of CD during labour are slightly higher than with a fetus that has always been cephalic.
- *Other methods:* so-called natural methods of version (postural methods, acupuncture, moxibustion) remain unproven.

Contraindications to external cephalic version

Absolute
- CD already indicated.
- APH.
- Fetal compromise.
- Oligohydramnios.
- Rhesus isoimmunization.
- Pre-eclampsia.

Relative
- One previous CD.
- Fetal abnormality.
- Maternal hypertension.

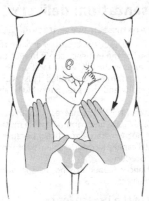

1. Gently disimpact the breech from the pelvis, guiding it towards the iliac fossa.

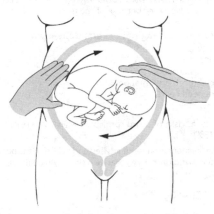

2. Continue to guide the breech upwards until the baby is transverse, then gentle pressure on the occiput helps to complete the forward roll.

Fig. 2.3 External cephalic version.

Breech presentation: delivery

Mode of delivery of breech presentation

- If ECV is declined or fails, or the breech is undiagnosed, the parents should be appraised of the evidence about breech birth.
- Most breech deliveries in the UK, USA, and Europe are by CS, because a meta-analysis of randomized controlled trials (RCTs) has shown this to ↓ neonatal mortality and short-term morbidity, although not longer-term morbidity.
- The risk of mortality (↑ ~3×) compared with elective CD is still relatively low at 2–3/1000 and parental choice must be respected.
- Elective CD does not ↑ maternal morbidity because attempting a vaginal delivery still carries a considerable risk of emergency CD, which is a more risky procedure.
- The breech in advanced labour, or who is a 2nd twin, or preterm is not necessarily best delivered by CS.

Vaginal delivery of the breech fetus

💣 Knowledge and experience of this remains important because breech delivery requires skill and will occasionally be inevitable because of diagnosis in advanced labour or because of the mother's wishes.

> ### Ideal selection for vaginal breech delivery
> - Fetus is not compromised.
> - EFW is <3.8kg.
> - Spontaneous onset of labour.
> - Extended breech presentation.
> - Non-extended neck.

⚠ There is a risk of cord prolapse which is greatest in footling breeches (15%).

⚠ Oxytocin augmentation is not advised and failure of the buttocks to descend after full dilatation is a sign that delivery may be difficult.

Vaginal breech delivery technique

- Maternal effort should be delayed until the buttocks are visible.
- After delivery of the buttocks the baby is encouraged to remain back upwards but should not otherwise be touched until the scapula is visible.
- The arms are then hooked down by the index finger at the fetal elbow, bringing them down the baby's chest.
- The body is then allowed to hang.
- If the arms are stretched above the chest and cannot be reached, *Løvset's* manoeuvre is required.
  - this involves placing the hands around the body with the thumbs on the sacrum and rotating the baby 180° clockwise and then counterclockwise with gentle downward traction.
  - this allows the anterior shoulder and then the posterior shoulder to enter the pelvis and for the arm to be delivered from below the pubic arch.
- When the nape of the neck is visible, delivery is achieved by placing two fingers of the right hand over the maxilla and two fingers of the left at the back of the head to flex it (*Mauriceau–Smellie–Veit* manoeuvre) and maternal pushing is encouraged.
- If this fails to deliver the head, forceps should be applied before the next contraction.
- The all-fours position for delivery is ↑ advocated by experienced attendants as birth may require less help.

Further reading

RCOG (2017). Management of breech presentation. Green-top guideline no. 20b.
⌕ www.rcog.org.uk/en/guidelines-research-services/guidelines/gtg20b/

Transverse, oblique, and unstable lie

Definition

- A transverse or oblique lie occurs when the axis of the fetus is across the axis of the uterus:
  - common preterm
  - occurs in only 1% of fetuses after 37wks.
- Unstable lie occurs when the lie is still changing:
  - usually several times a day
  - may be transverse or longitudinal lie, and cephalic or breech presentation—see Fig. 2.4.

Assessment

- Ascertain stability from the history:
  - has the presentation been changing?
- Ascertain fetal lie by palpation.
- Neither the head nor buttocks will be presenting.
- Also assess the laxity of the uterine wall.
- Does the presenting part move easily?
- USS should be performed to help ascertain the cause.

Management of abnormal lie

- Admission to hospital from 39wks is often recommended with unstable lie, so that CD can be carried out if labour starts or the membranes rupture and the lie is not longitudinal.
- With ↑ gestation the lie will usually revert to longitudinal and in these circumstances the woman can be discharged.
- If the lie does not stabilize, a CD is usually performed at 41wks.
- If the lie is stable but not longitudinal, CD should be considered at 39wks.

💣 Some advocate a stabilizing induction whereby the fetus is turned to cephalic and an amniotomy immediately performed. This requires expertise.

Risks of abnormal lie

- Labour with a non-longitudinal lie will result in obstructed labour and potential uterine rupture.
- Membrane rupture risks cord prolapse because with longitudinal lie, the presenting part usually prevents descent of the cord through the cervix.

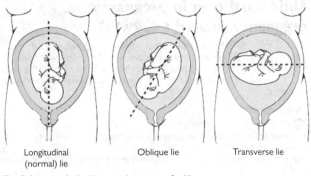

Longitudinal   Oblique lie   Transverse lie
(normal) lie

Fig. 2.4 Longitudinal, oblique, and transverse fetal lie.

Causes and associations of abnormal fetal lie
- Multiparity (particularly >para 2) with lax uterus (common).
- Polyhydramnios.
- Uterine abnormalities, e.g. fibroids and Müllerian duct abnormalities.
- Placenta praevia and obstructions to the pelvis.
- Fetal abnormalities.
- Multiple pregnancy.

Abdominal pain in pregnancy: pregnancy related (<24wks)

It is often difficult to differentiate between gynaecological, non-gynaecological, and pregnancy-related causes of abdominal pain. Some of the routine surgical investigations and procedures carry a risk to the fetus but this needs to be balanced against the risk of delayed diagnosis and treatment.

Miscarriage

(→ Miscarriage: management, p. 606.)

- Lower abdominal dull ache to severe continuous or colicky pain.
- Vaginal bleeding is present in most cases.
- Positive urine pregnancy test, pelvic examination, and USS are helpful in diagnosis.

Ectopic pregnancy

(→ Ectopic pregnancy: diagnosis, p. 610.)

- Usually unilateral lower abdominal pain at <12wks gestation.
- Associated with brownish vaginal bleeding.
- Shoulder tip pain may be haemoperitoneum (bleeding ectopic).
- Serum hCG, USS, and laparoscopy are diagnostic.

Constipation

Physiological changes result in the slowing of gut peristalsis.

Signs and symptoms

- Varied but colicky lower abdominal pain (L > R) is common.

Management

- High-fibre diet.
- Osmotic laxatives.
- Glycerol suppositories.

Round ligament pain

This pain is attributed to stretching of the round ligaments.

Incidence

- 20–30% of pregnancies.

Signs and symptoms

- Commonly presents in 1st and 2nd trimester.
- Pain is often bilateral and located on the outer aspect of the uterus.
- Radiating to the groin.
- Aggravated by movement (especially getting up from a chair or turning over in bed).

Management

- Reassurance.
- Simple analgesia.
- Support belts may help.

Urinary tract infection
UTIs are more common in pregnancy and are an important association of preterm labour.

Signs and symptoms
- Suprapubic/lower abdominal pain.
- Dysuria, nocturia, and frequency.

Investigations
- Urine dipstick:
  - nitrites strongly suggest a UTI
  - blood, leucocytes, and protein raise index of suspicion.
- Midstream sample urine (MSU).

Management
- Antibiotics.
- Analgesia.
- ↑ Fluid intake.

Fibroid red degeneration
Uterine fibroids occur in 20% of women of reproductive age. They may ↑ in size during pregnancy, compromising blood supply to central areas and causing pain. This is known as red degeneration.

Incidence
- 15% of pregnant women who have fibroids.

Signs and symptoms
- Usually occurs between the 12th and 22nd wk of pregnancy.
- Constant pain localized to one area of the uterus coinciding with the site of the fibroid (may be severe pain).
- May have a low-grade pyrexia.

Investigations
- USS (identifies fibroids but cannot confirm red degeneration).
- FBC (may show leucocytosis).

Treatment
- Analgesia (pain should resolve in 4–7 days; however, it may be severe and prolonged, so advice from pain specialists should be sought).

▶ Placental abruption differs in that the fibroid uterus is soft, and only the site of the fibroid is tender.

⚠ Myomectomy must not be performed in pregnancy as it will bleed ++ (the only exception being for a torted pedunculated fibroid).

Abdominal pain in pregnancy: pregnancy related (>24wks)

Labour

Signs and symptoms
- Usually presents with regular painful contractions.
- Preterm labour may present with a history of vague abdominal pain which the woman may not associate with uterine activity.

⚠ Consider a VE in pregnant women with abdominal pain.

Symphysis pubis dysfunction/pelvic girdle pain

Signs and symptoms
Pubic pain relating to upper thighs and perineum:
- Aggravated by movement.
- Difficulty walking resulting in a waddling gait.

Treatment
- Analgesia and physiotherapy.

Reflux oesophagitis

Relaxation of the oesophageal sphincter occurs in pregnancy and the pressure of the gravid uterus on the distal end of the oesophagus results in an ↑ incidence of reflux oesophagitis. Gastric ulceration is less common due to ↓ gastric acid secretion.

Incidence
- 60–70% of pregnant women.

Risk factors
- Polyhydramnios.
- Multiple pregnancy.

Signs and symptoms
- Epigastric/retrosternal burning pain exacerbated by lying flat.

Management
- Exclude pre-eclampsia.
- Antacids, proton pump inhibitors.
- Dietary and lifestyle advice (avoidance of supine position).

Uterine rupture

This usually occurs during labour but has been reported antenatally.

Risk factors
- Previous CD or other uterine surgery.
- Congenital abnormalities of the uterus.
- Induction or use of oxytocin in labour.
- Failure to recognize obstructed labour.

Signs and symptoms
- Tenderness over sites of previous uterine scars.
- Fetal parts may be easily palpable.
- Fetus not palpable on VE.
- Vaginal bleeding may be evident.
- Signs of maternal shock may be present.

⚠ CTG may show fetal distress and change in apparent uterine activity (contractions may seem to disappear on the tocograph).

Investigations
- FBC.
- Cross-match blood.

Management
- Maternal resuscitation.
- Urgent laparotomy to deliver fetus and repair uterus.

Other causes of abdominal pain in pregnancy
- Placental abruption.
- Pre-eclampsia/HELLP.

Braxton Hicks contractions

These are spontaneous benign contractions of the uterus, commonly occurring in the 3rd trimester.

Signs and symptoms
- Painless and infrequent tightenings of the uterus.
- VE reveals uneffaced and closed cervix.

Investigations
- Exclusion of precipitants of preterm labour (dipstick/MSU for UTI).
- Fibronectin assay if uncertain whether preterm labour
  (➔ Preterm labour: overview, p. 94).

Treatment
- Reassurance.

Abdominal pain in pregnancy: bowel related

Appendicitis

This is the most common surgical emergency in pregnant patients. Its incidence is 1:1500–2000 pregnancies with equal frequency in each trimester. Pregnant women have the same risk of appendicitis as non-pregnant women.

Signs and symptoms
- Classically periumbilical pain shifting to right lower quadrant.

⚠ Pain moves towards the RUQ during the 2nd and 3rd trimesters due to displacement of the appendix by a gravid uterus.
- Nausea and vomiting.
- Anorexia.
- Guarding and rebound tenderness present in 70% of patients.

⚠ Rovsing's sign and fever are often absent in the pregnant patient.

Investigations
- White cell count (WCC) and C-reactive protein (CRP) are often ↑.
- USS: to exclude other causes of pain.
- CT/MRI should be considered.

Management
Diagnostic laparoscopy/laparotomy and appendicectomy.

⚠ Fetal loss is 3–5% with an unruptured appendix, ↑ to 20% if ruptured.

Intestinal obstruction

It is the 3rd most common non-obstetric reason for laparotomy during pregnancy. It complicates 1:1500–3000 pregnancies. Incidence ↑ as the pregnancy progresses. Adhesions are the most common cause.

Signs and symptoms
- Acute abdominal pain.
- Vomiting.
- Constipation.
- Pyrexia.

Diagnosis
- Erect abdominal X-ray showing gas-filled bowel with little gas in large intestine.
- USS (abdominal and pelvic).

Treatment
- Conservative treatment ('drip and suck').
- Surgery for any acute obstructive cause or when not responding to conservative management.

Causes of intestinal obstruction
- Adhesions from surgery, e.g. myomectomy.
- Volvulus.
- Intussusception.
- Hernia.
- Neoplasm.

Abdominal pain in pregnancy: other causes

Acute cholecystitis

This is the 2nd most common surgical condition in pregnancy (progesterone ↓ smooth muscle tone and predisposes to cholestasis leading to gallstone formation). The incidence of gallstones is 7% in nulliparous and 19% in multiparous women. The incidence of acute cholecystitis is 1–8:10,000 pregnancies.

Signs and symptoms
- Colicky epigastric/RUQ pain.
- Nausea and vomiting.
- Murphy's sign may be positive in acute cholecystitis.
- Jaundice (indicating obstruction of the common bile duct).
- Signs of systemic infection (fever and tachycardia).

Investigations
- FBC, LFTs, CRP (WCC and alkaline phosphatase are ↑ anyway).
- ↑ Bilirubin (identifies concomitant biliary tree obstruction).
- USS biliary tract (may demonstrate calculi or a dilated biliary tree).

Management
- Conservative approach is the most common management.
- Analgesics and antiemetics.
- Hydration.
- Antibiotics.
- Cholecystectomy preferably by laparoscopic approach may be indicated in women with recurrent biliary colic, acute cholecystitis, and obstructive cholelithiasis (usually after delivery).

Adnexal torsion

This occurs when an enlarged ovary twists on its pedicle.

⚠ *Torsion of the ovary and other adnexal structures is more common in pregnant than non-pregnant women.*

Signs and symptoms
- Sudden-onset unilateral colicky lower abdominal pain.
- Nausea and vomiting.
- There may be systemic symptoms such as fever.

Investigations
- WCC and CRP: may be elevated.
- USS of pelvis may show an adnexal mass and Doppler studies may show impaired blood flow.

Management
- If suspected, urgent laparotomy should be performed to either remove or untwist the adnexa.
- This may either preserve the ovary or present a non-viable ovary from becoming gangrenous.

Pancreatitis

Occurs most frequently in 3rd trimester and immediate postpartum period. It can occur in early pregnancy associated with gallstones.

⚠ Although rare, it is more common in pregnancy than in non-pregnant women of a similar age.

Incidence
1:5000 pregnancies.

Risk factors
• Gallstone disease.
• High alcohol intake.
• Hyperlipidaemia.

Signs and symptoms
• Epigastric pain commonly radiating to the back.
• Pain exacerbated by lying flat and relieved by leaning forwards.
• Nausea and vomiting.

Investigations
• Serum amylase and lipase levels. FBC, glucose.
• USS to establish presence of gallstones.

Management
Conservative treatment is the mainstay:
• IV fluids. Electrolyte replacement.
• Consider IV antibiotics.
• Parenteral analgesics, e.g. morphine (pethidine is contraindicated).
• Bowel rest with or without nasogastric suction.

⚠ Early surgical intervention is recommended for gallstone pancreatitis in all trimesters as >70% will relapse before delivery.
• Laparoscopic/open cholecystectomy.
• Endoscopic retrograde cholangiopancreatography (ERCP) has a limited role in pregnancy because of radiation exposure to the fetus.

⚠ If pancreatitis is severe, liaise with high dependency/intensive care unit.

Non-abdominal causes of abdominal pain

Other conditions unrelated to abdominal structures may also present with abdominal pain:
• Lower lobe pneumonia.
• Diabetic ketoacidosis.
• Sickle cell crisis.

▶ Women with social problems and domestic abuse may repeatedly attend with undiagnosable pain and it is important to ask them about this directly but sympathetically.

Preterm labour: overview

Preterm birth is defined as delivery between 24 and 37wks.

- Delivery <34wks is a more useful definition as severe adverse outcomes are rare after then.
- 1/3 medically indicated (e.g. PET), and 2/3 spontaneous.
- Accounts for 5–10% of births but >50% of perinatal deaths.
- It also causes long-term handicap—blindness, deafness, and CP:
  - risk is higher the earlier the gestation.
- Incidence is ↑ worldwide.
- >50% of women with painful preterm contractions will not deliver preterm: fetal fibronectin/transvaginal USS may help in diagnosis.

Acute preterm labour

- Preterm labour associated with cervical weakness (avoid the term 'incompetence') classically presents with ↑ vaginal discharge, mild lower abdominal pain, and bulging membranes on examination.
- Preterm labour associated with factors such as infection, inflammation, or abruption presents with lower abdominal pain, painful uterine contractions, and vaginal loss.
- Spontaneous rupture of membranes (SROM) is a common presentation of/antecedent for preterm labour.

▶ In practice, it is often less clear-cut than this, and infection and cervical weakness are related and often coexist.

History
- Ask about pain/contractions—onset, frequency, duration, severity.
- Vaginal loss: SROM or PV bleeding.
- Obstetric history (check hand-held notes).

Examination
- Maternal pulse, temperature, respiratory rate.
- Uterine tenderness (suggests infection/abruption).
- Fetal presentation.
- *Speculum*: look for blood, discharge, liquor—take swabs.
- Gentle VE.

Investigations
- FBC, CRP (raised WCC and CRP suggest infection).
- Swabs, MSU.
- USS for fetal presentation (malpresentation common) and EFW.
- Fetal fibronectin/transvaginal USS if available (➲ Management of preterm labour, p. 95).

Risk factors for preterm delivery

- Previous preterm birth or late miscarriage.
- Multiple pregnancy.
- Cervical surgery.
- Uterine anomalies.
- Medical conditions, e.g. renal disease.
- Pre-eclampsia and FGR (spontaneous and iatrogenic).

Management of preterm labour

- Establish whether threatened or 'real' preterm labour:
  - transvaginal cervical length scan (>15mm unlikely to labour)
  - fibronectin assay: if −ve, unlikely to labour.
- Admit if risk high.
- Inform neonatal unit.
- Arrange *in utero* transfer to tertiary level unit if <27wks, or <EFW <800g, or multiple <28wks.
- Check fetal presentation with USS.
- Steroids (12mg betamethasone intramuscularly (IM)—two doses 24h apart).
- Consider tocolysis (drug treatment to prevent labour and delivery) not >24h and not in presence of sepsis:
  - allow time for steroid administration and/or *in utero* transfer
  - currently used tocolytics include nifedipine, and atosiban IV.

◐※ Aim should be not just prolongation of gestation (a surrogate measure) but improvement in perinatal morbidity and mortality. Trials of tocolysis have not shown improvement in these substantive outcome measures, so some prefer to avoid them.

- Liaison with senior obstetricians and neonatologists is essential, especially at the margins of viability (22–26wks).
- A clear plan needs to be made about:
  - mode of delivery
  - monitoring in labour
  - presence of paediatrician/appropriate intervention at delivery.
- Give IV antibiotics but only if labour confirmed.
- Administer magnesium 4g diluted in 20mL normal saline over 10min if <30–32wks—↓ the risk of CP.

Further reading

NICE (2015, updated 2022). Preterm labour and birth. NICE guideline [NG25].
℘ www.nice.org.uk/guidance/ng25

Preterm labour: prevention and prediction

Prevention

Treatment of bacterial vaginosis (BV)

Some evidence suggests this ↓ the incidence of preterm prelabour rupture of membranes (PPROM) and low birth weight in women with previous preterm birth if given at <16wks.

Progesterone

- In high-risk women (e.g. previous history of late miscarriage/preterm birth) ↓ recurrence.
- In low-risk women with a short cervix, ↓ preterm birth (this may mean screening for preterm birth with cervical scanning may become universal).
- Less effective in twin pregnancies.
- Cream or pessaries used.

Cervical sutures (cerclage)

- ◆ May be of benefit in selected cases.
- Elective (women with previous loss from cervical weakness).
- USS indicated (in response to short cervix on transvaginal scan (TVS)).
- Rescue (in response to cervical dilatation).

Cervical pessary (e.g. Arabin®)

◆ The evidence concerning these is controversial.

Reduction of pregnancy number

Selective reduction of triplet or higher-order multiple pregnancies (to two) ↓ the risk of preterm labour while slightly ↑ the risk of early miscarriage.

Types of cervical cerclage

Vaginal

- As elective in pregnancy <13wks or if cervix found to be short.
- 'Shirodkar' (bladder dissection required) or 'MacDonald' usual types:
  - Prolene® or Mersilene® tape used.
- Rescue cerclage if non-infected when the cervix is open with bulging membranes may prevent extreme preterm birth in 50%.

Abdominal (laparoscopic or open)

- As elective procedure prior to pregnancy or <13wks.
- Effective but invasive.
- Usually reserved for refractory cases, or where no cervix is present in vagina.
- Delivery by CS is indicated.

Preterm prelabour rupture of membranes: overview

- Complicates 1/3 of preterm deliveries.
- About 1/3 is associated with overt infection (more common at earlier gestations) often at time of presentation.

History

- Ask about vaginal loss:
  - gush
  - constant trickle or dampness.

⚠ Chorioamnionitis may cause few symptoms but is associated with significant neonatal morbidity and mortality.

⚠ Chorioamnionitis is associated with significant risks to the mother and is a cause of maternal mortality.

Features suggestive of chorioamnionitis

History

- Fever/malaise.
- Abdominal pain, including contractions.
- Purulent/offensive vaginal discharge.

Examination

- Maternal pyrexia and tachycardia.
- Uterine tenderness.
- Fetal tachycardia.
- Speculum: offensive vaginal discharge—yellow/brown.

▶ Avoid VE as this ↑ the risk of introducing infection.

Investigations

- FBC, CRP:
  - ↑ WCC and CRP indicate infection but are not 100% sensitive.
- Swabs:
  - high vaginal swab (HVS)
  - low vaginal swab (LVS).
- MSU.
- USS for fetal presentation, EFW, and liquor volume.
- Maternal lactate estimation if sepsis suspected.

Preterm prelabour rupture of membranes: management

- If evidence of chorioamnionitis:
  - sepsis bundle including lactate estimation
  - broad-spectrum antibiotic cover
  - steroids (betamethasone 12mg IM)
  - deliver whatever the gestation.
- If no evidence of chorioamnionitis, manage conservatively:
  - admit
  - steroids (12mg betamethasone IM—two doses 24h apart)
  - antibiotics (erythromycin).

▶ Use of antibiotics ↓ major markers of neonatal morbidity but without long-term benefits. The ORACLE trial showed erythromycin to be beneficial.

⚠ Co-amoxiclav is associated with an ↑ risk of necrotizing enterocolitis (NEC) and should be avoided.

Prognosis

Depends on:
- Gestation at delivery.
- Gestation at PPROM:
  - PPROM at <20wks—few survivors
  - PPROM at >22wks—survival up to 50%.
- Reason for PPROM:
  - prognosis better if PPROM 2° to invasive procedure (e.g. amniocentesis), rather than spontaneous.

Risks to fetus from PPROM
- Prematurity.
- Infection.
- Pulmonary hypoplasia.
- Limb contractures.

Further reading

NICE (2015, updated 2022). Preterm labour and birth. NICE guideline [NG25].
℗ www.nice.org.uk/guidance/ng25

Prolonged pregnancy: overview

Prolonged pregnancy is a cause of anxiety for both women and obstetricians. It is a common occurrence and is a recognized cause of ↑ fetal morbidity and mortality.

Definition of prolonged pregnancy

According to the International Federation of Gynaecology and Obstetrics (FIGO), prolonged pregnancy is defined as any pregnancy that exceeds 42wks (294 days) from the 1st day of the LMP in a woman with regular 28-day cycles. Different terminologies are used generally in day-to-day practice, such as postdates, post-term, and post-maturity.

Incidence

- The incidence of pregnancy lasting ≥42wks is 3–10%.
- With one previous prolonged pregnancy there is a 30% chance of another one.
- With a history of two this rises to 40%.

Maternal risks

- Maternal anxiety and psychological morbidity.
- ↑ intervention:
  - induction of labour
  - operative delivery with ↑ risk of genital tract trauma.

Fetal risks of prolonged pregnancy

Perinatal mortality ↑ after 42wks of gestation

- Antepartum and intrapartum deaths are 4× more common.
- Early neonatal deaths are 3× more common.
- Risks are ↑ even in normally grown fetuses as deterioration in placental function may be rapid and unpredictable.

Other risks

- Meconium aspiration and assisted ventilation.
- Oligohydramnios.
- Macrosomia, shoulder dystocia, and fetal injury.
- Cephalhaematoma.
- Fetal distress in labour.
- Neonatal:
  - hypothermia
  - hypoglycaemia
  - polycythaemia
  - growth restriction.

Fetal post-maturity syndrome
- This is used to describe post-term infants who show signs of intrauterine malnutrition.
- The neonate has a scaphoid abdomen, little subcutaneous fat on the body or limbs, peeling skin over the palm and feet, overgrown nails, and an anxious, alert look.
- The baby's skin is also stained with meconium.
- This condition constitutes only a small proportion of babies born after 42wks.

⚠ These features can be seen at an earlier gestation in babies with FGR. Hence, the term prolonged pregnancy is preferred to post-maturity for pregnancy beyond 42wks.

Prolonged pregnancy: management

- Attempt to confirm the EDD as accurately as possible:
  - EDD based on CRL from 10–13+6wk USS is best unless the pregnancy is the result of IVF.
- Assess any other risk factors which may be an indication to induce:
  - pre-eclampsia
  - diabetes
  - ↑ maternal age
  - APH
  - FGR associated with placental insufficiency.
- Offer 'stretch and sweep' by 41wks.
- Offer induction of labour from 41wks:
  - this slightly ↓ perinatal mortality
  - it also ↓ the risk of CD
  - but it 'medicalizes' many labours
  - if declined, ensure adequate fetal surveillance.

Fetal monitoring

USS has minimal prognostic value and daily CTG should be offered from 42wks. They should also be advised to report any ↓ in fetal movements.

(⊖ Monitoring the high-risk fetus: cardiotocography, p. 157.)

Counselling

Most units in the UK advise induction of labour by 42wks because of the ↑ perinatal mortality and morbidity beyond this time.

▶ This does not lead to an ↑ in the risk of CD.

⚠ Those mothers who prefer to await spontaneous onset of labour should have appropriate counselling regarding ↑ fetal mortality and morbidity.

Further reading

NICE (2021). Antenatal care. NICE guideline [NG201].
℗ www.nice.org.uk/guidance/ng201

Chapter 3

Fetal medicine

Prenatal diagnosis: overview

Benefits

Congenital abnormalities affect ~2% of newborn babies in the UK, and account for ~21% of perinatal and infant deaths, as well as causing significant disability and morbidity later in life.

Although some pregnancies are known to be at high risk, e.g. for mothers with type 1 diabetes or parents with a previously affected child, the vast majority of congenital defects occur unexpectedly in otherwise uncomplicated pregnancies. Prenatal identification in such situations can help in a multitude of ways:

- Enabling decision on timing, mode, and place of delivery (e.g. in a unit that provides paediatric surgery).
- Preparing parents to cope with an affected child.
- Introducing parents to specialist neonatal services.
- Ensuring fetal surveillance, such as later USSs to monitor the condition and ensure the best possible outcome.
- Potentially allowing *in utero* treatment (rarely available at present).
- Giving parents the option of terminating the pregnancy in severe cases.

Counselling

The news that there is a problem with their unborn child is often devastating for parents. How they respond to the situation will vary with such factors as age, social background, and religious belief. Not all parents will wish to terminate the pregnancy: many will choose to go on, even in the face of abnormalities incompatible with life. Some parents report that the opportunity to hold their child enabled them to grieve. Counselling must be supportive, informative, and non- directional. Care must also be taken to counsel adequately before any screening tests. If parents have no intention of having the riskier diagnostic tests performed then there is little benefit in screening and anxiety may be generated. Detailed written information should always be provided beforehand.

Trisomy 21 (Down syndrome)

Most common identifiable cause of learning disability. Usually occurs as a result of non-disjunction of chromosome 21 at meiosis (95%). May also be due to balanced translocation in parents (4%). 1% is estimated to be due to mosaicism. Around 50% will have one or more serious congenital abnormality. Around 10% will die before age of 5yrs, and current life expectancy is 50–55yrs.

Risk of trisomy 21 ↑ with maternal age
- <25yrs: 1:1500.
- 30yrs: 1:910.
- 35yrs: 1:380.
- 40yrs: 1:110.
- 45yrs: 1:30.

- Natural prevalence 1:600 live births, but incidence is now 6:10,000 due to *in utero* diagnosis and termination of pregnancy (TOP).
- *Typical appearance:*
  - flat nasal bridge
  - epicanthic folds
  - single palmar crease.
- *Intellectual impairment:*
  - 80% profound or severe
  - mean mental age at 21yrs is 5yrs
  - ↑ risk of early-onset dementia.
- *Congenital malformations:*
  - cardiac abnormalities (46%, e.g. VSD, atrial septal defect (ASD), and tetralogy of Fallot)
  - gastrointestinal atresias are common (e.g. duodenal atresia).
- ↑ risk of other medical conditions, including:
  - leukaemia
  - thyroid disorders
  - epilepsy.

Genetic counselling after diagnosis of trisomy 21
- If the karyotype indicates straightforward trisomy 21 from non-disjunction, the risk of recurrence is ~1% above the risk from maternal age alone.
- If there is a chromosomal translocation, the recurrence risk is 1:10 if the mother carries it and 1:50 if it is the father.

Support group
Down Syndrome Medical Interest Group: ℬ www.dsmig.org.uk

Other types of aneuploidy

Trisomy 18 (Edwards' syndrome)

Second-most common autosomal trisomy. Most due to non-disjunction at meiosis. Most will die soon after birth; survival to 1yr is anecdotal.

- Incidence 1:6000 live births (prevalence estimated at 1:3000).
- Risk ↑ with ↑ maternal age.
- *Features:*
  - craniofacial abnormalities including small facial features, small chin, and low-set ears
  - rocker bottom feet
  - clenched fists.
- *Congenital malformations:*
  - cardiac abnormalities in almost all fetuses (usually VSD)
  - gastrointestinal abnormalities
  - urogenital abnormalities.

Trisomy 13 (Patau's syndrome)

Least common autosomal trisomy; ~75% due to non-disjunction. Babies die soon after birth.

- Incidence 1:10,000 live births.
- Risk ↑ with ↑ maternal age.
- *Features:* craniofacial, including cyclopia with proboscis located on forehead; microcephaly.
- *Congenital malformations (midline):*
  - holoprosencephaly (failure of cleavage of embryonic forebrain)
  - gastrointestinal abnormalities, especially exomphalos
  - cleft lip and palate (midline).

See ℜ www.rarechromo.org

Turner's syndrome (45 XO)

This affects only females and is due to the loss of an X chromosome. It is one of the few chromosomal abnormalities that does not result in mental impairment. Almost all women with Turner's syndrome will have short stature and loss of ovarian function, but the extent of the other features varies enormously.

- Incidence 1:2500 live female births.
- *Features:*
  - short stature, webbed neck, and wide carrying angle
  - non-functioning 'streak' ovaries
  - coarctation of the aorta.

See ℜ www.tss.org.uk

Klinefelter's syndrome (47 XXY)

Affects only males and is caused by non-disjunction of the X chromosomes. The individual is almost always sterile and may have hypogonadism. They are phenotypically tall with occasionally ↓ IQ.

- Incidence 1:700 live male births.

Screening for chromosomal abnormalities

Ideally, screening should be offered to all women at the time of booking. In the UK, almost all units use the 'combined test' to screen for Down syndrome, the most common chromosomal abnormality. This has a detection rate of 75% with a false +ve rate (FPR) of no more than 3%. This means that a risk of 1 in 150 or less is considered 'high risk'.

Counselling

Detailed, unbiased, written information should be provided about the condition itself, types of test available, and the implications of the results. It is important for a woman to understand that a −ve result does not guarantee that her baby does not have an abnormality.

Screening relies on the integration of different independent risk factors, such as maternal age, blood hormone levels, and scan findings. These findings are slightly dependent on other factors including maternal weight, ethnicity, IVF pregnancies, smoking, multiple pregnancy, and diabetes, and calculations are modified according to these.

Powerful arguments have been made by many that prenatal screening, and ultimately often termination, of fetuses with conditions such as Down syndrome is often done by parents with inadequate information, impairs diversity, and can prevent the life of individuals who may be happy and enrich their family and society as a whole.

Screening versus diagnostic tests

Care must always be taken to explain the difference between the types of test available including their advantages, disadvantages, and limitations.

Screening tests
- Should be cheap and widely available.
- Non-invasive, safe, and acceptable.
- Have good sensitivity (high detection rate) and specificity (low FPR).
- Provide a measure of the risk of being affected by a certain disorder (e.g. 1 in 100 risk of Down syndrome).
- Must have a suitable diagnostic test for those identified as 'high risk'.

Diagnostic tests
- Need to definitely confirm or reject the suspected diagnosis (e.g. the fetus does, or does not, have Down syndrome).
- Must be as safe as possible.
- Must have high sensitivity and specificity.
- The implications of the disorder tested for must be serious enough to warrant an invasive test.

Common screening tests

Combined test

When

Scan and blood test at 11–13+6wks.

How

- USS (nuchal) measurement of the subcutaneous tissue between the skin and the soft tissue overlying the cervical spine with the fetus in the neutral position (Fig. 3.1).
- A blood test measuring:
  - PAPP-A
  - β-hCG.

Summary

- Now the recommended and most commonly used screening test.
- Performance enhanced by use of additional risk factors:
  - nasal bone
  - tricuspid regurgitation.
- Careful USS at the same time can identify many structural abnormalities.

Risk of trisomy 21

Calculated by multiplying the background maternal age and gestation-related risk by a likelihood ratio derived from the nuchal translucency (NT) measurement and the two blood tests.

Triple and quadruple tests

When

Blood tests at 15–20wks.

How

- Dating scan (but not nuchal scan).
- Blood tests measuring:
  - oestriol
  - hCG
  - α-fetoprotein (AFP)
  - inhibin A (not if triple).

Summary

- Recommended if NT scan not possible or gestation too advanced.
- Less operator dependent (scan) than the combined test.

Combined test

Advantages
- Performance ~90% detection for 5% FPR (75% for 3%).
- May detect other abnormalities such as anencephaly.
- An ↑ NT is also a marker for structural defects, e.g. cardiac malformations.
- Result usually available in 1st trimester, allowing surgical TOP.
- Acceptable detection rate for all trisomies.

Disadvantages
- Expensive and difficult to perform nuchal scan.

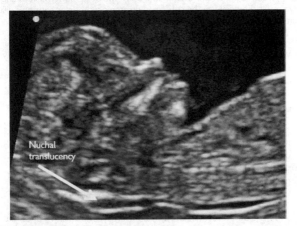

Fig. 3.1 Nuchal translucency at 11–13+6wk USS.

Other 11–13+6wk markers
- Fetuses with Down syndrome are more likely to have an absent or hypoplastic nasal bone, a reversed a-wave in the ductus venosus, and have significant tricuspid regurgitation at 11–13+6wks.
- Other structural abnormalities such as exomphalos may be seen.
- Only in conjunction with a nuchal scan can the presence or absence of these be used to modify the risk of a combined test.
- They may considerably ↑ the accuracy of the combined test.
- These are not commonly used because they require skill and time to detect accurately.

Cell-free DNA testing (non-invasive prenatal testing)

Fetal DNA (placental in origin) is detectable in the maternal circulation and can now be tested for chromosomal, and even some single gene, abnormalities. Maternal blood is taken from 10wks; the test itself is therefore virtually risk free, barring false-positive results. However, it remains expensive.

- Sensitivity approaches 100% for trisomies, with FPRs of <0.5% (0.1% for Down syndrome).
- Both the false +ve and false −ve rates are much higher for other abnormalities including sex chromosome abnormalities and microdeletions such as di George.

⚠ Therefore, the tests are of limited usage for other abnormalities and a +ve result should always be confirmed on amniocentesis or chorionic villus sampling (CVS).

- Whether to test is commonly dependent on the prior risk from a cheaper widely available screening test such as the combined test (e.g. where the result is not entirely reassuring, such as a risk of aneuploidy calculated as 1 in 100–300).

When

Blood test at 10–21wks.

How

- Counselling regarding test performance is essential.
- Cell-free fetal DNA is measured from a maternal blood test.
- Non-invasive prenatal testing (NIPT) should always be combined with ultrasound.

When not to do NIPT

- Before 10wks.
- Where the NT is >3.5mm or a structural abnormality is visible.
- Where the risk of aneuploidy is very high, as even with a risk of 1 in ≤100, 3% of fetuses will have a chromosomal abnormality it does not detect.

Summary

Best screening test for aneuploidies but limited by cost and by false +ves and −ves for other chromosomal abnormalities.

NIPT: fetal fraction (FF)
- The amount of fetoplacental DNA in the maternal circulation is variable.
- FF is the percentage of total maternal plasma cell-free DNA that is of fetoplacental origin.
- FF is highest between 10 and 21wks.
- Most normal pregnancies will have a FF of 10–15%.
- FF in the sample must be >2–4% to obtain an accurate result
- Low FF results in a test failure or 'no call' result:
  - occurs in 2–6% of tests
  - 50–60% will have an appropriate FF on a 2nd blood draw
  - high BMI is a risk factor
  - if genuinely low is associated with a 2+-fold ↑ risk of aneuploidy
  - failure rates are higher in twins and IVF pregnancies.

Diagnosis of structural abnormalities

This should be offered to all women in the UK at the time of booking and usually takes the form of the 'anomaly scan', a detailed USS undertaken at around 18–21wks gestation. The aim is to identify specific structural malformations.

The detection of malformations may vary and is dependent on:
- The anatomical system affected.
- Gestational age at the time of the scan.
- Skill of the operator.
- Quality of the equipment.
- BMI of the mother.

Management of structural fetal abnormalities: principles

Most are isolated abnormalities although chromosomal abnormalities and other conditions are more commonly present. Referral to a tertiary centre is required in many cases.
- Establish if isolated (e.g. other abnormalities, consider amniocentesis) and consider genetics review.
- Establish severity (features specific to abnormality).
- Counsel, with neonatologist, with paediatric surgeon/relevant postnatal specialist if appropriate regarding prognosis.
- Discuss TOP if considered legal.
- Consider risk of preterm birth (e.g. polyhydramnios).
- Offer referral to consider *in utero* surgery if appropriate (e.g. spina bifida, diaphragmatic hernia).
- Fetal medicine follow-up in addition to usual pregnancy care.
- Neonatal liaison, alert, and MDT.
- Establish time, place, and mode of birth.

UK (2018) fetal conditions to be screened at anomaly scan, with minimum detection rates

- Anencephaly: 98%.
- Open spina bifida: 90%.
- Cleft lip: 75%.
- Congenital diaphragmatic hernia: 60%.
- Lethal skeletal abnormality: 60%.
- Gastroschisis: 98%
- Exomphalos: 80%
- Bilateral renal agenesis: 84%
- Cardiac abnormalities (➔ Cardiac defects (congential heart disease), p. 116): 50%.

See NHS Screening Programme:
🔗 https://phescreening.blog.gov.uk/2018/09/17/national-fetal-anomaly-screening-guidance-updated/

Essential parts of the anomaly scan

Fetal normality
- Skull shape and internal structures: cavum pellucidum, cerebellum, ventricular size at atrium <10mm.
- Nuchal fold.
- Spine—longitudinal and transverse views.
- Abdominal shape and contents at the level of stomach.
- Kidneys.
- Umbilicus/abdominal wall.
- Bladder.
- Arms (three bones and hand).
- Legs (three bones and foot).
- Heart:
  - four-chamber view
  - outflow tracts—pulmonary artery and aorta
  - three-vessel and trachea view.
- Face and lips.

Liquor volume
- Depth of deepest cord-free vertical pool.

Placental site
- Location relative to the cranio-caudal axis of the uterus:
  - anterior
  - posterior
  - left/right lateral.
- Position relative to the internal cervical os:
  - over the internal os: 'placenta praevia'
  - edge <20mm from the internal os: 'low-lying placenta'.

Other findings
- Uterine normality:
  - an abnormally shaped uterus should be recorded, but most will not be detected at this scan due to the late gestation.
- Location of the cord insertion is not routinely recorded but should be looked for if the placenta is in the lower segment of the uterus, especially if there is a succenturiate lobe, in order to detect those at risk of vasa praevia.
- Uterine artery Doppler can be used as a screen for pre-eclampsia and FGR—practice varies throughout the UK.

Neural tube defects

Craniospinal defects occur early in development when the neural tube fails to close properly. Type and severity depend on degree and site of defect. There is growing evidence that prevalence is declining, possibly due to ↑ use of folate supplementation.

- Spina bifida and anencephaly make up >95% of neural tube defects (NTDs).
- Incidence 2:1000 in England (3:1000 in Scotland).

Anencephaly

Absence of skull vault and cerebral cortex. It is incompatible with life, with babies rarely living more than a few hours if they are not stillborn.

Spina bifida: meningocele/myelomeningocoele

Incomplete fusion of vertebrae potentially allowing herniation of part of spinal cord.

- If exposed, neural tissue is damaged *in utero*.
- Cerebellum usually herniated, often causing CSF obstruction and hydrocephalus.
- Prognosis varies from near-normal neurological function to severe disability.
- Coexisting abnormalities relatively uncommon.
- Physical symptoms dependent mostly on height (e.g. T1), and size of the lesion, and include bladder, bowel, and sexual dysfunction as well as mobility issues.
- Mental impairment more common if cerebral ventriculomegaly present.
- Requires referral tertiary referral for evaluation and birth and postnatal care.
- Consider *in utero* surgery.

⚠ *Dietary supplementation with folic acid ↓ the incidence of NTDs.*
Recommended doses:
- 400 micrograms/day for 3mths before conception, continued to 12wks.
- 5mg/day for women with previously affected child, with a high BMI or those taking anticonvulsants.

Specific USS findings with some neural tube defects

* *Anencephaly:*
  * absence of cranium and bulging eyes ('frog-like' appearance)
  * 99% will be detected by 20wks (Fig. 3.2).
* *Spina bifida:* findings vary according to the severity of the lesion:
  * defect seen in the vertebral bodies or tissue overlying the spine
  * frontal bone scalloping ('lemon sign')
  * abnormally shaped cerebellum due to herniation ('banana sign')
  * up to 95% detection rate for major defects.

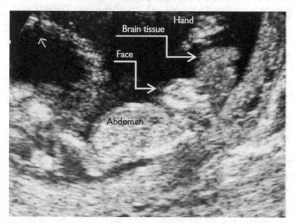

Fig. 3.2 Ultrasound of anencephaly at 12wks.

Open *in utero* surgery for spina bifida

* Open surgery for open spina bifida can be undertaken between 19 and 26wks in a small number of specialist centres.
* Hysterotomy is used; a 'keyhole' approach is not recommended.
* Both the fetus and the pregnancy must meet specific criteria, e.g. singleton with T1–S1 lesion, isolated abnormality, low prior risk of preterm birth.
* Surgery appears to improve short- to intermediate-term outcomes, despite ↑ the risk of preterm birth.
* A principal concern is rupture, in the index or subsequent pregnancies, of the vertical uterine scar that is required.

Cardiac defects (congenital heart disease)

- Most common major malformation in children, with an estimated incidence of 6–8:1000.
- The most commonly seen abnormalities are VSDs (Fig. 3.3).
- May be associated with a chromosomal abnormality, commonly trisomy 21 or 18, and with many other congenital abnormalities.
- Where isolated, many can be surgically corrected at birth, leading to a good quality of life, although those where a univentricular circulation results are associated with neurodevelopmental delay.
- Some require urgent treatment at birth, so detection is important.
- Place of birth is an important consideration:
  - some babies will require a prostaglandin E1 (PGE1) infusion to keep the ductus arteriosus open
  - others will require birth in a centre with paediatric cardiac surgery facilities.

Common cardiac abnormalities for which detection rates are calculated in the UK are:
- Transposition of the great arteries (TGA).
- Atrioventricular septal defect (AVSD).
- Tetralogy of Fallot (TOF).
- Hypoplastic left heart syndrome (HLHS).

Risk factors for cardiac abnormalities

- Family history of congenital heart disease in 1st-degree relative (recurrence risk 3%).
- Previous affected child (risk depends on type).
- Drug exposure, particularly anticonvulsants and lithium.
- Maternal diabetes mellitus.
- Other congenital abnormalities.
- ↑ NT (>3.5mm).

Timing of cardiac scans

- In skilled hands, many cardiac abnormalities can be seen at 12–13wks.
- Many cardiac abnormalities are missed at routine anomaly scans.
- The detection rate improves with training and specifically if 'three-vessel', 'outflow tract', and 'trachea' views are found in addition to the four-chamber view (Fig. 3.4).
- Evolution of defects change and later scanning, e.g. at 32wks, may be beneficial.

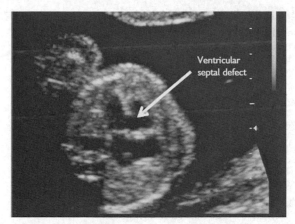

Fig. 3.3 USS of ventricular septal defect.

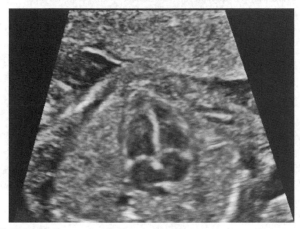

Fig. 3.4 USS of a normal cardiac four-chamber view.

Urinary tract defects

Renal agenesis

- Bilateral renal agenesis is lethal because anhydramnios causes lung hypoplasia.
- It may not be evident until >16wks because amniotic fluid is not all urinary before this time.

Lower urinary tract obstruction

- This is most common in male fetuses where folds of mucosa block the bladder neck causing outflow obstruction (posterior urethral valve syndrome).
- The severity is variable; back pressure may cause irreversible renal damage and oligohydramnios.
- The use of *in utero* suprapubic catheterization (shunt) remains controversial.

Hydronephrosis

- Accounts for 75% of fetal renal abnormalities.
- At least 40% resolve spontaneously in the neonatal period.
- It is usually due to pelviureteric obstruction, vesicoureteric reflux, ureterocoele, or bladder obstruction (Fig. 3.5).
- Most cases can be treated postnatally so the prognosis is excellent unless there is bladder obstruction or severe bilateral abnormalities.

Specific USS findings with some urinary tract defects
- *Lower urinary tract obstruction due to valves:*
  - thick-walled dilated bladder with 'keyhole' sign of upper urethral dilatation
  - hydronephrosis
  - variable degrees of oligohydramnios according to severity.
- *Ureterocele:*
  - cystic area of prolapsed ureter in bladder.

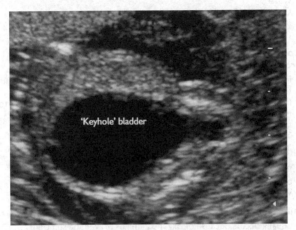

'Keyhole' bladder

Fig. 3.5 USS of posterior urethral valve syndrome (keyhole bladder).

Lung defects

Diaphragmatic hernia

- A defect in the diaphragm results in the abdominal contents herniating into the chest. 90% are left sided.
- There is a 30% incidence of aneuploidy and a strong association with other malformations.
- The prognosis is related to the amount of visible contralateral lung measured using the ratio of lung area to head circumference (LHR), and to whether the liver is also in the chest. Right-sided lesions also do worse.
- Overall, ~40% will die postnatally; all will require postnatal surgery.
- *In utero* treatment for severe cases, using tracheal obstruction (fetoscopic tracheal occlusion) should be considered.

Congenital pulmonary airway malformation (CPAM)/ bronchopulmonary sequestration

- In congenital pulmonary airway malformation, part of the lung alveolar tissue is replaced by a proliferation of cysts resembling bronchioles.
- In bronchopulmonary sequestration, a segment of lung unconnected to the bronchial tree is supplied by an aberrant artery.
- In practice, many are mixed lesions.
- The prognosis is good, and most are born asymptomatic.
- In <10%, *in utero* hydrops develops with subsequent death, or there is insufficient lung for postnatal survival.
- Routine late postnatal surgery is widely but not uniformly advised to prevent infection and possible neoplastic change.
- Where there are neonatal symptoms, early surgery is usual.

Lung hypoplasia

- Usually occurs because of oligohydramnios preventing sufficient circulation of amniotic fluid through the lungs around 20wks.
- Most commonly therefore it is due to preterm previable rupture of membranes or to renal anomalies.
- Fetuses are asymptomatic *in utero* but are unable to maintain gaseous exchange after birth.

Specific ultrasound findings with some lung defects

Diaphragmatic hernia
- Stomach or liver is seen within chest cavity
- With a left-sided hernia, the heart may be deviated to the right.
- Abdominal circumference is often smaller than expected.
- Usually detectable at 20wks.

CPAM
- Cystic lesions or solid mass present within the lung parenchyma.
- Usually detectable at 20wks (Fig. 3.6).

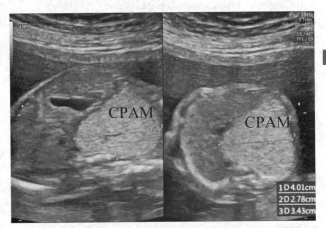

Fig. 3.6 USS of (solid) CPAM, in sagittal and transverse—it appears as a bright, space-occupying lesion in the chest and can be solid, cystic, or a combination of both.

Gastrointestinal defects

Exomphalos (omphalocele)

- Failure of the gut to return into the abdominal cavity after the normal embryological extrusion and rotation; the bowel and often liver are contained within a sac and the umbilical cord arises from the apex of this sac (Table 3.1).
- ~1/3 occur with chromosomal abnormalities and up to 50% of the remainder have other malformations (e.g. cardiac).
- Prognosis depends on the presence of other abnormalities, and the size of the lesion.
- Requires referral to a fetal medicine centre, and postnatal surgery.
- The large exomphalos requires Caesarean delivery (CD).

Gastroschisis

- This involves protrusion of the gut through an anterior abdominal wall defect, usually to the right of the umbilical cord; the bowel is not covered by a sac and floats freely (Table 3.1).
- Usually occurs in very young women—rare after 25yrs.
- There is no ↑ risk of chromosomal abnormalities.
- The gastrointestinal tract may become obstructed or atretic.
- ~1 in 10–20 will die, prognosis is good in remainder.
- Requires referral to a fetal medicine centre and postnatal surgery.
- Vaginal delivery is not necessarily contraindicated.

Gastrointestinal obstruction

- Usually causes polyhydramnios, worse with upper gastrointestinal obstructions.
- *Duodenal atresia:* 30% have trisomy 21.
- *Oesophageal atresia:* 15% have aneuploidy.
- *Bowel obstruction:* may cause polyhydramnios. Prognosis poorer if multiple obstructions.
- *Cystic fibrosis (CF):* common with bowel obstruction (Fig. 3.7).

Table 3.1 Comparison of the features of exomphalos and gastroschisis

	Exomphalos	Gastroschisis
Viscera within a sac	Yes, unless ruptured	No
Insertion of umbilical cord	At apex of sac	Next to the defect
Evisceration of:	Liver ± intestinal loops, spleen	Usually, intestinal loops only
Chromosomal abnormalities	30%	<1%
Other malformations	50%	<5%
Mortality	30%	5%

Specific USS findings with some gastrointestinal defects

Anterior abdominal wall defects
- Bowel is seen outside the abdominal wall.

Duodenal atresia
- Distension of stomach and proximal duodenum ('double bubble') (Fig. 3.8).
- May not be apparent by 20wks, but usually seen by 25wks.
- Polyhydramnios.

Oesophageal atresia
- Absence of stomach bubble and polyhydramnios.
- Tracheo-oesophageal fistula common.
- Commonly coexists with other abnormalities

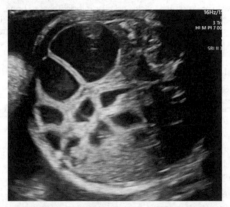

Fig. 3.7 Fetal bowel obstruction.

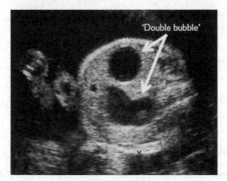

Fig. 3.8 USS of duodenal atresia ('double bubble').

Normal variants and 'soft markers'

Some features at 20wks may themselves be of limited significance, but are nevertheless slightly more common in chromosomally abnormal fetuses. They can therefore be used to modify the risk of aneuploidy. However, these features may cause considerable parental anxiety as they are often, mistakenly, seen as abnormalities. Furthermore, they may ↑ the FPR of screening. In the UK the term 'soft markers' is not recommended.

Mild renal pelvic dilatation

- Dilatation of >7mm at 20wks.
- Slightly ↑ (~1.5-fold) risk of chromosomal abnormalities.
- Repeat scan in 3rd trimester (to ensure not enlarged) and neonatal follow-up is recommended.

Echogenic bowel

- Bowel with areas of echogenicity similar in brightness to bone.
- Moderate association (~5-fold ↑) with chromosomal abnormalities.
- Although usually benign, occasionally associated with ↑ perinatal risk, CF, and bowel obstruction.
- Consider referral for expert opinion.

↑ Nuchal fold

- 20wk equivalent of NT (>6mm in transverse section).
- ↑ risk of chromosomal abnormalities (~10-fold).
- Amniocentesis for chromosomal abnormalities is usually offered.
- Early sign of hydrops.

Mild ventriculomegaly

- Dilatation of posterior horn of lateral cerebral ventricle >10mm.
- Slightly ↑ risk of chromosomal abnormalities.
- Refer for expert opinion for including neurosonography.

Small measurements

- Measurements <5th centile are considered significant.
- Most have no detectable abnormality and form part of the normal range.
- Consider referral for expert review.

Variants that do not require reporting

Choroid plexus cysts, fetal intracardiac foci, two-vessel cord, and dilated cisterna magna are no longer considered significant.

Further reading

Public Health England (2021). Fetal anomaly screening programme: standards.
℘ https://www.gov.uk/government/publications/fetal-anomaly-screening-programme-standards

Diagnostic tests

These tests require fetal samples. Non-invasive prenatal testing has meant they are less commonly performed (➜ Cell-free DNA testing (non-invasive prenatal testing), p. 110).

Methodologies for analysis fetal/trophoblast cells

Polymerase chain reaction (PCR)

Using PCR, millions of copies of a DNA sample are made to allow more detailed study. Usually used where there is a high risk of aneuploidies, the results are available in <24h.

Microarray

This chromosomal analysis compares the DNA of the sample with that of a normal control. It detects deletions of duplications and detects down to 0.2Mb. Results may take 2wks.

Exome sequencing

A panel of genes is tested. This can be targeted according to the phenotype.

Chorionic villus sampling

This is usually performed between 11 and 13wks and involves aspiration of some trophoblastic cells from the placenta. The amount of tissue obtained is small, but PCR allows rapid analysis (Fig. 3.9). It requires ultrasound guidance and is usually performed transabdominally and occasionally transcervically.

Indications

- For PCR if 1st trimester screening is high risk for aneuploidy.
- For microarray also if the NT is >3.5mm or a structural abnormality is seen.
- For DNA analysis if parents are carriers of an identifiable gene mutation such as CF or thalassaemia.

Benefits

- Allows 1st-trimester TOP if an abnormality is detected which can be performed surgically.

Amniocentesis

This is only undertaken from 15wks onwards. It involves aspiration of amniotic fluid which contains fetal cells shed from the skin and gut. It is performed transabdominally with ultrasound guidance (Fig. 3.10).

Indications

- For PCR if screening tests suggest aneuploidy.
- For DNA analysis if parents are carriers of an identifiable gene mutation, such as CF or thalassaemia.
- For microarray if the NT is >3.5mm or a structural abnormality is seen.
- For diagnosis of fetal infections such as CMV and toxoplasmosis.

Benefits

- Lower procedure-attributed miscarriage rate than CVS (0.5%).
- Less risk of maternal contamination or placental mosaicism.

Risks of CVS and amniocentesis

- Miscarriage in <1%:
  - lower in expert hands
  - slightly lower with amniocentesis than CVS.
- ↑ Risk of vertical transmission of blood-borne viruses such as HIV and hepatitis B.
- False −ve results (rare) from contamination with maternal cells—especially with DNA analysis requiring PCR.
- Failure to culture cells ~0.5%.
- Placental mosaicism (CVS only) produces misleading results (estimated at <1%).

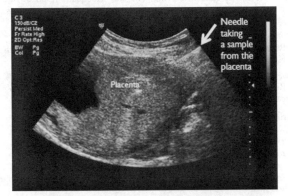

Fig. 3.9 Chorionic villus sampling.

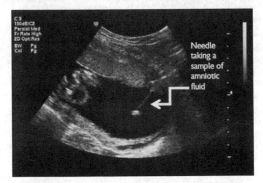

Fig. 3.10 Amniocentesis.

Fetal hydrops: overview

Definition

- The abnormal accumulation of serous fluid in two or more fetal compartments. This may be pleural or pericardial effusions, ascites, skin oedema, or placental oedema, usually with polyhydramnios.
- Divided into non-immune and immune causes.

Incidence

- Occurs in ~1:2000 births.

Pathophysiology

The mechanism for the development of hydrops appears to be due to an imbalance of interstitial fluid production and inadequate lymphatic return. This can result from congestive heart failure, obstructed lymphatic flow, or ↓ plasma osmotic pressure.

Immune hydrops

- Results from blood group incompatibility between the mother and the fetus causing fetal anaemia.

Non-immune hydrops

- Results from other causes, including fetal anaemia that is due to other causes such as fetal infection.

Non-immune fetal hydrops

Ultrasound

- The diagnosis is made by USS.
- Associated structural abnormalities may be seen.
- Fetal echocardiography is required to diagnose cardiac lesions.
- Peak systolic velocity (PSV) in middle cerebral artery (MCA) shows fetal anaemia.

Fetal blood or amniotic fluid sampling

- Fetal blood sampling if anaemia is suspected (with blood ready for *in utero* transfusion).
- Amniotic fluid or fetal blood for chromosome analysis ± virology.

Maternal blood testing

- Kleihauer test for fetomaternal haemorrhage.
- Antibody screen must be performed to exclude immune hydrops.
- Virology (parvovirus, CMV, toxoplasmosis).
- Consider haemoglobin electrophoresis for α-thalassaemia trait.

Treatment

- Prognosis depends on the underlying cause.
- Where treatment is not possible, the option of TOP should be discussed.
- In the 3rd trimester, delivery may be a better alternative than *in utero* treatment.

Non-immune fetal hydrops: principal causes

Severe anaemia
- Congenital parvovirus B19 infection.
- α-Thalassaemia major (common in areas such as South-east Asia).
- Massive fetomaternal haemorrhage.
- Glucose-6-phosphate dehydrogenase deficiency.

Cardiac abnormalities
- Structural abnormalities.
- Fetal tachyarrhythmia (SVT or atrial flutter).
- Congenital heart block.

Chromosomal abnormalities
- Trisomies 13, 18, and 21.
- Turner's syndrome (45 XO).

Other genetic syndromes
Multiple other syndromes, e.g. achondrogenesis, Noonan's syndrome, Fryns' syndrome, myotonic dystrophy.

Other infections
- Toxoplasmosis (➔ Toxoplasmosis, p. 204).
- Rubella (➔ Rubella, p. 160).
- CMV (➔ Cytomegalovirus, p. 166).
- Varicella (➔ Varicella zoster, p. 172).

Other structural abnormalities
- CPAM.
- Diaphragmatic hernia.
- Pleural effusions.
- Fetal tumour, e.g. sacrococcygeal teratoma.

Twin-to-twin transfusion syndrome
- Recipient from volume overload and donor from anaemia (➔ Twin-to-twin transfusion syndrome (TTTS), p. 74).

Placental
- Chorioangioma.

Non-immune fetal hydrops: treatable causes

Fetal anaemia
- *In utero* blood transfusion may be performed.

Pleural effusions or large cystic CPAM
- *In utero* percutaneous drainage and subsequent insertion of shunt to drain into amniotic fluid may be possible.

Twin-to-twin transfusion syndrome
- Laser photocoagulation of placental anastomoses.

Cardiac
- Tachyarrhythmias may be treated with drugs, e.g. flecainide.

Rhesus isoimmunization (immune hydrops)

Definition/pathology

- Occurs when a maternal antibody response is mounted against fetal red cells.
- These immunoglobulin antibodies (IgG) cross the placenta and cause fetal red blood cell destruction.
- The ensuing anaemia, if severe, precipitates fetal hydrops, which is often referred to as immune hydrops.

Rhesus blood groups

- Consists of three linked gene pairs; one allele of each pair is dominant: *C/c*, *D/d*, and *E/e*. There are only five antigens (d is not an antigen; it merely implies absence of D).
- Inheritance is Mendelian.
- *D* gene is the most significant cause of isoimmunization, because ~16% of white mothers are RhD –ve (*d/d*).
- Incidence lower in Afro-Caribbean and Asian populations.
- Other significant antigens include c, E, and atypical Kell antibody. because of success of anti-D prophylaxis, these now account for up to 1/2 of cases.

Pathophysiology of rhesus disease

- Fetal cells cross into the maternal circulation in normal pregnancy; the amount is ↑ during particular 'sensitizing events'.
- The fetus may carry the gene for an antigen which the mother does not have—with RhD, the fetus may be *D/d* (RhD +ve), but the mother *d/d* (RhD –ve).
- Individuals exposed to a 'foreign' antigen mount an immune response (sensitization); initially, this is immunoglobulin (IgM), which cannot cross the placenta so the index pregnancy is not at risk.
- Re-exposure in a subsequent pregnancy causes the primed memory B cells to produce IgG, which actively crosses into fetal circulation.
- IgG binds to fetal red cells, which are destroyed in the reticuloendothelial system.
- Causes a haemolytic anaemia (if erythropoiesis is inadequate to compensate, severe anaemia causes high-output cardiac failure, 'fetal hydrops,' and, ultimately, death).
- In milder cases, haemolysis leads to neonatal anaemia or jaundice from ↑ bilirubin levels.

Prevention of rhesus (D) disease

Theory

If sufficient anti-D immunoglobulin is given to the mother it will bind to any fetal red cells in her circulation carrying the D antigen. This prevents her own immune system from recognizing them and therefore becoming sensitized.

Prophylaxis

- Anti-D (1500IU) is given to all women who are Rh −ve (d/d) in whom NIPT has shown the fetus to be Rh +ve (D/d or D/D) or in whom the Rh status is unknown:
  - routinely at 28wks
  - within 72h of any potentially sensitizing event
  - after delivery.

Sensitizing events

- A Kleihauer test should be performed if there is any suspicion of a fetomaternal haemorrhage as the standard dose of anti-D may not be sufficient to prevent sensitization.
- This should be routinely undertaken at delivery if the neonate is RhD +ve.

▶ The use of anti-D, together with smaller family sizes, mean that Rh disease is now rare.

Rhesus disease: management

- All women should be checked for antibodies (Rh and atypical) at booking, 28, and 34wks.
- If antibodies are detected, identifying the partner's status will help determine the potential fetal blood group and risk to the fetus.
- PCR of fetal cells in maternal blood (NIPT) may also determine the fetus's blood group: this is now routine in all Rh −ve women.
- Positive, but low levels of antibodies should prompt repeat testing at least every 4wks.
- If levels are >4–10IU/mL, assessment for fetal anaemia is required.

⚠ Amniocentesis or fetal blood sampling based on antibody levels or history alone is now obsolete.

- PSV of the MCA should be measured, once/wk.
- The MCA PSV will become abnormal before the baby becomes hydropic.
- If it is ↑ (>1.5 multiples of median) fetal blood sampling is indicated, with blood available for transfusion.
- Gestation-corrected nomograms for the MCA are widely available, one such online calculator can be found at:
  - ℅ www.perinatology.com/calculators/MCA.htm

Treatment

- If fetal haematocrit is <30, irradiated, Rh −ve, CMV −ve packed red cells are transfused into the umbilical vein at the cord insertion, or into the hepatic vein.
- Can be performed from 18wks onwards (>35wks delivery is preferable).
- Haemolysis will continue and the transfusion is repeated either every 2wks or when the MCA becomes abnormal again.

⚠ Risk of fetal loss, or need for urgent delivery if >26wks, is 1–3% per transfusion in skilled hands.

Postnatal management

- Anaemia may persist and is corrected by blood transfusion.
- Hyperbilirubinaemia and jaundice occur because *in utero* the mother cleared this red blood cell breakdown product, but the immature neonatal liver is unable to cope (this usually needs phototherapy, but may require exchange transfusion).

⚠ Antibodies may persist for wks, causing continued haemolysis in the neonate; this requires careful monitoring.

Oligohydramnios

- After 20wks amniotic fluid largely consists of fetal urine.
- The volume depends on:
  - urine production
  - fetal swallowing
  - absorption.
- Normal volume varies with gestation (nomograms are available), and is highest between 24 and 36wks.

Definition of oligohydramnios

- ↓ in amniotic fluid volume.
- Amniotic fluid volume is measured by ultrasound, by:
  - measuring the deepest vertical pool
  - by adding up the deepest pools in the four quadrants of the uterus to give the amniotic fluid index (AFI).
- As a general rule the diagnosis is made if there is a:
  - deepest pool of <2cm
  - AFI of <8cm.

Causes of oligohydramnios

Leakage of amniotic fluid

- SROM.
  ⚠ Infection can both cause, and result from, ruptured membranes.

↓ *Fetal urine production*

- Utero placental insufficiency.
- Fetal renal failure or abnormalities.
- Post-dates pregnancy.
- Twin–twin transfusion syndrome (donor twin).

Obstruction to fetal urine output

- Fetal abnormalities such as posterior urethral valves.

Investigations

- USS of fetus, including Doppler.
- Speculum examination to look for ruptured membranes.
- If suspected SROM: CRP, FBC, and vaginal swabs should be taken.
- Point-of-care tests have good sensitivity for SROM, e.g. AmniSure®.

Complications of oligohydramnios

Related to cause

- Preterm rupture of the membranes is commonly followed by:
  - intrauterine infection
  - delivery (spontaneous or iatrogenic if infection detected).
- Uteroplacental insufficiency may result in FGR.

Related to ↓ volume

- Lung hypoplasia if it occurs <22wks.
- Limb abnormalities, e.g. talipes, if prolonged.
- ⚠ Oligohydramnios before 22wks has a very poor prognosis.

Management of oligohydramnios

If SROM at >34wks

- Induce labour unless CD is indicated for another reason.

If SROM <34wks

- Exclude infection (chorioamnionitis); treat and deliver if present.
- Give prophylactic oral erythromycin if no infection.
- Monitor for signs of infection (4-hrly temperature and pulse).
- Consider induction at 34–36wks.

If FGR

- Manage according to umbilical artery Doppler and CTG.

If apparently isolated oligohydramnios

- Reconsider cause.
- Intervention is not usual if fetal/umbilical artery Dopplers are normal.

If fetal renal tract abnormality

- Refer to fetal medicine centre.

Polyhydramnios

Definition

- ↑ in amniotic fluid volume.
- Amniotic fluid volume is measured by ultrasound, by:
  - measuring the deepest vertical pool
  - by adding up the deepest pools in the four quadrants of the uterus to give the AFI.
- As a general rule the diagnosis is made if there is a:
  - deepest pool of >8cm
  - AFI of >22cm.

Complications

- Preterm delivery, presumably because of uterine stretch.
- Of the cause, e.g. duodenal atresia is associated with trisomy 21.
- Malpresentation at delivery because of ↑ room for fetus to move.
- Maternal discomfort because of abdominal distension.

Investigations

- Exclude maternal diabetes, e.g. glucose tolerance test (GTT).
- Ultrasound examination of fetus.
- Offer amniocentesis.

Causes of polyhydramnios

↑ Fetal urine production

- Maternal diabetes.
- TTTS (recipient twin).
- Fetal hydrops.

Fetal inability to swallow or absorb amniotic fluid

- Fetal gastrointestinal tract obstruction (e.g. duodenal atresia, tracheo-oesophageal fistula).
- Fetal neurological or muscular abnormalities (e.g. myotonic dystrophy, anencephaly).
- Other rare abnormalities or syndromes (e.g. facial obstruction).
- Idiopathic (usually mild).

Management of polyhydramnios
- Severe polyhydramnios is usually associated with fetal abnormality:
  - refer to fetal medicine centre
  - amnioreduction (drainage of excess fluid with a needle)—rarely indicated
  - non-steroidal anti-inflammatory drugs (NSAIDs)—rarely considered as can constrict the ductus arteriosus: close supervision is therefore indicated.
- TTTS is best managed in a fetal medicine centre, usually with laser ablation of placental anastomoses.
- If preterm, assess risk of delivery with cervical scan and/or fibronectin assay, and consider steroids.
- If unstable or transverse lie at term, admit to hospital: CD if labour ensues with an abnormal lie.

Placenta accreta spectrum: overview

Placenta accreta spectrum (PAS) disorder describes a situation where the placenta does not detach spontaneously after delivery and cannot be forcibly removed without causing potentially life-threatening bleeding. It is one of the most dangerous obstetric conditions being significantly associated with maternal morbidity and mortality.

The actual incidence of PAS is disputed, with estimates ranging from 1:533 to 1.7:10,000, and is ↑ worldwide. This is most likely due to the ↑ rates of CD, which is the single greatest risk factor for PAS in future pregnancies.

Although it is a spectrum ranging from a 'sticky' placenta to a highly vascular, surgically complex condition, it is often divided into three categories: accreta (abnormally adherent), increta, and percreta (abnormally invasive). See Fig. 3.11.

This has been described clinically by FIGO (Table 3.2).

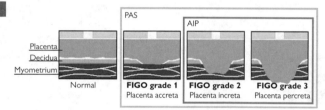

Fig. 3.11 Nomenclature used for PAS. Reproduced with permission from Morlando M and Collins S (2020) 'Placenta Accreta Spectrum Disorders: Challenges, Risks, and Management Strategies' *Int. J. Womens Health* 12: 1033–1045.

Risk factors for PAS

History of
- Previous abnormally invasive placenta.
- CD.
- ≥2 episodes of endometrial curettage (including ERPC and surgical TOP).
- Uterine surgery involving the endometrium (e.g. myomectomy which breached the cavity or resection of uterine septum).
- Endometrial ablation.
- Asherman's syndrome.

Further reading

RCOG (2018). Placenta praevia and placenta accreta: diagnosis and management. Green-top guideline no. 27a.
⚘ www.rcog.org.uk/en/guidelines-research-services/guidelines/gtg27a/

Table 3.2 FIGO classification of PAS

Grade	Definition	
	Clinical criteria	*Histologic criteria*
1 Abnormally adherent placenta (accreta)	At vaginal delivery—no separation with synthetic oxytocin and gentle controlled cord traction; attempts at manual removal of the placenta results in heavy bleeding from the placenta implantation site requiring mechanical or surgical procedures	Microscopic examination of the placental bed samples from hysterectomy specimen shows extended areas of absent decidua between villous tissue and myometrium with placental villi attached directly to the superficial myometrium. The diagnosis cannot be made on just delivered placental tissue nor on random biopsies of the placental bed.
	If laparotomy is required (including for caesarean delivery): same as above—macroscopically, the uterus shows no obvious distension over the placental bed (placental 'bulge'), no placental tissue is seen invading through the surface of the uterus and there is no or minimal neovascularity	
2 Abnormally invasive placenta (increta)	At laparotomy: abnormal macroscopic findings over the placental bed—bluish/purple colouring, distension (placental 'bulge'); significant amounts of hypervascularity (dense tangled bed of vessels or multiple vessels running parallel craniocaudally in the uterine serosa); gentle cord traction results in the uterus being pulled inwards without separation of the placenta (the so-called dimple sign)	Hysterectomy specimen or partial myometrial resection of the increta area shows placental villi within the muscular fibres and sometimes in the lumen of the deep uterine vasculature (radial or arcuate arteries)

Table 3.2 *Continued*

Grade		Definition	
3 Abnormally invasive placenta (percreta)	3a Limited to the uterine serosa	At laparotomy: abnormal macroscopic findings on uterine serosal surface (as above) and placental tissue seen to be invading through the surface of the uterus; no invasion into any other organ, including the posterior wall of the bladder (a clear surgical plane can be identified between the bladder and uterus)	Hysterectomy specimen showing villous tissue within or breaching the uterine serosa
	3b With urinary bladder invasion	At laparotomy: placental villi are seen to be invading into the bladder but no other organs; clear surgical plane cannot be identified between the bladder and uterus	Hysterectomy specimen showing villous tissue breaking the uterine serosa and invading the bladder wall tissue or urothelium
	3c With invasion of other pelvic tissue or organs	At laparotomy: placental villi are seen to be invading into the broad ligament, vaginal wall, pelvic sidewall, or any other pelvic organ (with or without invasion of the bladder)	Hysterectomy specimen showing villous tissue breaching the uterine serosa and invading pelvic tissue/ organs (with or without invasion of the bladder)

Reproduced with permission from Jauniaux E, et al. FIGO classification for the clinical diagnosis of placenta accreta spectrum disorders. *Int J Gynaecol Obstet.* 2019;146(1):20–24. Copyright 2019 John Wiley and Sons.

Placenta accreta spectrum: diagnosis and management

⚠ Maternal and neonatal outcomes are generally improved when diagnosis is made before delivery, and the woman is managed by an MDT with expertise in the condition.

Placenta previa with PAS: a toxic combination

PAS of all grades can occur anywhere within the uterus where there is scar tissue. However, the combination of previa with PAS remains the most dangerous because of:
- ↑ Risk of PV bleeding and emergency delivery.
- Poor contractility of the lower segment.
- Difficult access to the fetus without transecting the placental bed.
- Close proximity to other structures including the bladder and ureters.
- Blood supply from below the uterine artery making vascular control harder.

Screening for PAS

As the single greatest risk factor is CD with a dose-related effect clearly seen, the RCOG and FIGO recommend the following strategy for screening:
- Always look at placental location at the 18–20wk 'anomaly' USS.
- If it is anterior and low lying/previa ask one single question:
  - 'Have you had a Caesarean delivery?'
- If the answer is yes, refer to someone with experience in diagnosing PAS, usually at a fetal medicine centre.

Diagnosis of PAS

- USS is highly accurate when performed by a skilled operator with experience in diagnosing PAS.
- Refer women with any ultrasound features suggestive of PAS to a specialist unit with imaging expertise.
- The diagnostic value of MRI and USS imaging is similar when performed by *experts*.
- MRI may be used to complement USS to assess the depth of invasion and lateral extension of myometrial invasion, especially with posterior placentation and/or in women with USS signs suggesting parametrial invasion.

⚠ No imaging modality can rule out a degree of 'sticky' (abnormally adherent) placenta.

Management of PAS

- Women diagnosed with PAS should be cared for by an MDT in a specialist centre with expertise in managing invasive placentation.
- In the absence of risk factors for preterm delivery, planned delivery at 35+0 to 36+6wks provides the best balance between fetal maturity and the risk of unscheduled delivery.

PAS management strategies
- Hysterectomy with the placenta *in situ*.
- Local resection of the affected area.
- Conservative management (intentional placental retention).

⚠ The mainstay of management is to not disturb the placental bed the choice of strategy depends on:
- severity of PAS
- experience of operator
- maternal social situation (access to healthcare) and preference (including desire for future fertility).

The undiagnosed PAS at 2am

Uterus not yet open

⚠ Call for help/2nd opinion and consider the options:
- Is it really safe to continue?
- Can you ↑ the safety for the patient? If so, how quickly?
- Deferring delivery is an option if it means you can:
  - reopen with all precautions in place
  - transfer to a specialist unit.

Baby delivered and no separation
- Don't panic.
- Don't dig! The unseparated PAS does not bleed.
- Get senior help URGENTLY, both obstetric and gynaecologist/gynae oncologist.
- Tell the anaesthetist, theatre staff, and haematologist to instigate local massive obstetric haemorrhage protocol.

Holding patterns until help arrives

At CD
- If open and unseparated don't dig it out, apply as much pressure as possible to the placental bed with large swabs and wait.
- If bleeding:
  - don't remove any placenta left inside, just pack the cavity very tightly as a tamponade and apply external pressure
  - consider applying a Foley catheter around the lower segment of the uterus (as low as possible) and pull it tight to form a tourniquet
  - worst-case scenario: apply internal pressure to the aorta.

At manual removal of placenta
- If possible don't remove the placenta.
- Don't try to remove the significantly adherent pieces.
- Tamponade with an intrauterine balloon + bimanual compression.
- Worst-case scenario: apply external pressure to the aorta.

Fetal growth restriction: definitions

The fetus has an inherent growth potential which under ideal conditions should produce a healthy baby of the appropriate size. Where growth is suboptimal, fetal well-being may be compromised. This problem is analogous to 'failure to thrive' in children and is termed fetal growth restriction (FGR). If the suboptimal growth is due to poor placentation this is often referred to as uteroplacental insufficiency.

Definitions

Fetal growth restriction

This is a baby that is *pathologically* smaller than it should be, often <10th centile. However, FGR might not result in the baby being small if it was genetically predestined to be large. FGR can sometimes be detected by the observation that the growth velocity has slowed, 'dropping centiles'. Again, this may not always be seen if the uteroplacental insufficiency has been short-lived or is rapidly evolving; as is seen in post-dates babies. Defining and identifying FGR is therefore difficult: combinations of growth, including slowing of growth velocity, and Doppler abnormalities have been suggested as a solution to this difficulty.

Small for gestational age

Most epidemiological studies use SGA as a surrogate marker for FGR. The most common definition of SGA is where the estimated weight of the fetus is <10th percentile for its gestational age. This method is imperfect as it includes small, but healthy babies, and excludes average-sized FGR babies that should have been born bigger or have 'uteroplacental insufficiency' that is less long-standing.

Early FGR

- ~50% of stillbirths occur before 37wks.
- Pre-eclampsia commonly coexists, particularly <34wks.
- More likely to be SGA, and have abnormal umbilical artery Doppler indices; therefore, easier to identify.
- Management involves balancing the risk of *in utero* decompensation and death versus the risk of preterm birth.

Late-onset FGR

- Less likely to be small; SGA babies are still over-represented.
- Less likely to be associated with maternal pre-eclampsia.
- Umbilical artery Doppler alone is less predictive.
- Delivery poses less risk because the gestation is greater.

△ Even early term birth (i.e. 37wks) carries greater infant risk than birth at 39wks.

Importance of FGR

For FGR fetuses compared with normally grown population

- Perinatal mortality is 6–10× ↑.
- Incidence of CP is 4× ↑.
- 20% of all stillborn infants are SGA; ~50% are FGR.

FGR fetuses are also more likely to have

- Intrapartum fetal distress and asphyxia.
- Meconium aspiration.
- Emergency CD.
- Necrotizing enterocolitis.
- Hypoglycaemia and hypocalcaemia.

Further reading

Gordijn SJ et al. (2016). Consensus definition of fetal growth restriction: a Delphi procedure. *Ultrasound Obstet Gynecol*. 48:333–339.
🔗 https://obgyn.onlinelibrary.wiley.com/doi/full/10.1002/uog.15884

Identifying growth potential

Customized growth charts

By adjusting for physiological (rather than pathological) factors that could affect fetal size, it may be possible to identify babies who are pathologically small. This 'customization' of individual fetal size can adjust for:

- Maternal height and, to a lesser extent, paternal height.
- Maternal weight in early pregnancy.
- Parity.
- Ethnic origin.
- Sex of the fetus.

Some of these factors have been used to generate customized growth charts which aim to identify the optimal growth curve for an individual fetus. These are freely available at ⅊ www.gestation.net.

💣 Some data suggest that this method improvements the detection of babies that are actually FGR.

Universal growth standards

An alternative school of thought suggests that all healthy babies should grow in a similar fashion and that physiological influences such as ethnicity are more complex. This has led to the production of 'standards' of fetal growth.

💣 Do not use size alone as a predictor of adverse outcome, especially after 34wks.

Further reading

Perinatal Institute (2011). Fetal growth assessment & implementation of customised charts. ⅊ www.perinatal.org.uk

Fetal growth restriction: risk factors

Maternal
- Chronic maternal disease:
  - hypertension
  - cardiac disease
  - chronic renal failure.
- Substance abuse:
  - alcohol
  - recreational drug use.
- Smoking.
- Autoimmune diseases, including antiphospholipid antibody syndrome.
- Genetic disorders, including phenylketonuria.
- Poor nutrition.
- Low socioeconomic status.

Placental (placental insufficiency)
- Abnormally shallow trophoblast invasion (also causes pre-eclampsia).
- Infarction.
- Abruption.
- Tumours: chorioangiomas (placental haemangiomas).
- Abnormal umbilical cord or cord insertion: two-vessel cord.

Fetal
- Genetic abnormalities, including:
  - trisomy 13, 18, or 21
  - Turner's syndrome
  - partial hydatidiform mole
  - triploidy.
- Congenital abnormalities, including:
  - cardiac, e.g. tetralogy of Fallot, transposition of the great vessels
  - gastroschisis.
- Congenital infection, including:
  - CMV
  - rubella
  - toxoplasmosis.
- Multiple pregnancy.

▶ In practice, placental insufficiency is commonly the result of maternal factors, so placental and maternal should be considered as one, uteroplacental insufficiency.

Fetal growth restriction: risk assessment

The principle is to identify the pregnancy at high risk and monitor fetal growth with serial USSs. See Fig. 3.12. This is done at booking on the basis of history and investigations, and reassessed later in pregnancy if new risk factors (e.g. pre-eclampsia) develop. Those pregnancies considered low risk undergo only clinical examination, with recourse to ultrasound if the baby is clinically thought to be small.

Booking risk factors
- Past obstetric history.
- Maternal medical conditions.
- BMI.
- Smoking status.
- Blood pressure.
- PAPP-A.

▶ Uterine artery Doppler can be used but is not always performed.

Risk factors at 20wks
- Uterine artery Doppler.
- Ultrasound markers such as echogenic bowel or small size.

Risk factors seen later in pregnancy
- Complications developing such as:
  - pre-eclampsia
  - vaginal bleeding
  - gestational diabetes
  - maternal illness.

◆ In the future, screening for placental function using serum markers, history, and ultrasound will become routine.

Considerations for management of FGR

The only management strategy for FGR is delivery of the baby to prevent stillbirth. Yet preterm birth is a major risk factor for neonatal and infant death, CP, and low IQ. Therefore, a balance of risk *in utero* versus postnatal risk must be achieved. However, the risk of infant mortality, CP, and low IQ is lowest at 39–40wks, so even delivering at 37wks could ↑ these risks.

Further, there may be more subtle long-term consequences, including up to 1/3 of children not reaching their predicted adult height, and having childhood attention and performance deficits. The effects appear to last into adulthood, with a stimulus or insult at a critical, sensitive period of early life having permanent effects on structure, physiology, and metabolism. People who were small or disproportionate (thin or short) at birth have been found to have higher rates of heart disease, high blood pressure, high cholesterol, and abnormal glucose-insulin metabolism (Barker hypothesis).

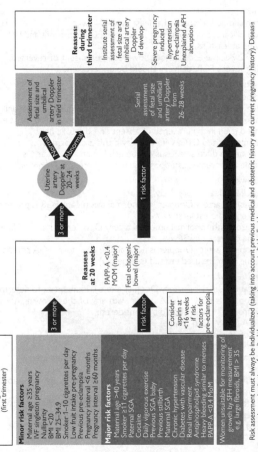

Booking assessment (first trimester)

Minor risk factors
Maternal age ≥35 years
IVF singleton pregnancy
Nulliparity
BMI <20
BMI 25–34.9
Smoker 1–10 cigarettes per day
Low fruit intake pre-pregnancy
Previous pre-eclampsia
Pregnancy interval <6 months
Pregnancy interval ≥60 months

Major risk factors
Maternal age >40 years
Smoker ≥11 cigarettes per day
Paternal SGA
Cocaine
Daily vigorous exercise
Previous SGA baby
Previous stillbirth
Maternal SGA
Chronic hypertension
Diabetes with vascular disease
Renal impairment
Antiphospholipid syndrome
Heavy bleeding similar to menses
PAPP-A <0.4 MoM

Women unsuitable for monitoring of growth by SFH measurement e.g. large fibroids, BMI > 35

3 or more

1 risk factor

Consider aspirin at <16 weeks if risk factors for pre-eclampsia

Reassess at 20 weeks
PAPP-A <0.4 MOM (major)
Fetal echogenic bowel (major)

3 or more

1 risk factor

Uterine artery Doppler at 20–24 weeks

Normal / Abnormal

Assessment of fetal size and umbilical artery Doppler in third trimester

Serial assessment of fetal size and umbilical artery Doppler from 26–28 weeks

Reassess during third trimester
Institute serial assessment of fetal size and umbilical artery Doppler if develop
Severe pregnancy induced hypertension
Pre-eclampsia
Unexplained APH
abruption

Risk assessment must always be individualized (taking into account previous medical and obstetric history and current pregnancy history). Disease progression or institution of medical therapies may increase an individual's risk.

Fig. 3.12 Example of FGR risk assessment tool. Reproduced from Green-top Guideline No. 31: The Investigation and Management of the Small-for-Gestational-Age Fetus.

Fetal growth restriction: management

Monitoring and criteria for delivery

In common practice, FGR without SGA is frequently undetected; therefore, most algorithms are for the management of SGA and SGA with features of FGR.

See Fig. 3.13.

SGA <34wks

- The scan should be repeated at least every 2–3wks.
- If the umbilical artery Doppler is abnormal, FGR is present and USS should be at least 2×/wk.
- If, from 32wks, the end-diastolic flow becomes absent or reversed, denoting severe FGR, delivery should be undertaken.

FGR <32wks (SGA with AREDF)

- Should be managed in a fetal medicine centre, and if <27wks or weighing <800g, be delivered in a level 3 neonatal intensive care unit.
- At this more severely preterm gestation, the FGR pregnancy may be prolonged even in the presence of absent end-diastolic flow.
- Daily computerized CTG, with delivery if this is abnormal.
- Doppler of the ductus venosus can be used as an adjunct and is preferable at extreme gestations (<26wks) where CTG is not validated.

SGA 32–36wks

- Repeat USS at least every 2–3wks.
- If the umbilical artery Doppler is abnormal this means FGR is present and USS should be at least 2×/wk.
- SGA fetuses with abnormal umbilical artery Doppler (but not AREDF) should be delivered by 36wks.
- If the umbilical artery Doppler is normal, the near-term SGA criteria for expediting birth are used instead (see below).

SGA from 36–37wks

At this gestation, umbilical artery Doppler alone is inadequate to determine which SGA baby is FGR. In SGA babies with any of the following risk factors, birth from 37+0wks should be considered:

- Very SGA (EFW <3rd centile).
- Slowing of growth rate of the abdominal circumference (AC).
- Low cerebroplacental ratio (CPR; <5th centile).
- Abnormal (>90th centile) 20wk or 3rd-trimester uterine artery Doppler.
- Other risk factors, e.g. high maternal age, low PAPP-A, hypertension, or gestational diabetes.
- Fetuses that are SGA but without these risk factors should not usually be delivered before 39+0wks and induction of labour may not be indicated at all.

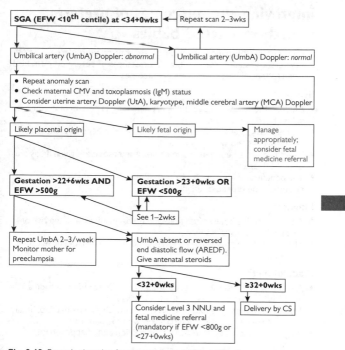

Fig. 3.13 Example algorithm for management of SGA at <34wks.

Improving the outcomes of preterm growth-restricted babies

Beyond getting the difficult balance of severity of uteroplacental insufficiency versus gestation correct, the circumstances of severe preterm birth can lead to tangible improvements in outcomes.

Steroids

- Antenatal steroids improve the short- and long-term outcomes for babies born at <35wks.
- Beyond this gestation the evidence is poorer, the benefits are less, and potential risks less well understood.
- Steroids such as betamethasone or dexamethasone are given IM as two doses, 24h apart.
- The benefits are greatest >24h and <7 days later, and as these should not usually be repeated, timing is crucial.

Magnesium

- An antenatal Mg bolus, often followed up by an infusion, ↓ the risk of CP in babies born at <32wks.
- The benefits are greatest within 12h of administration; the dose can be repeated.

Place of birth

- A severely FGR (<800g) or preterm fetus (<27wks) born outside a level 3 NICU has an ↑ risk of death and disability.
- The decision regarding extreme preterm birth should be made by fetal medicine specialists after full discussion with the parents.
- Pregnancies should be transferred for opinion and, if appropriate, delivery.

Mode of birth

- Where birth is expedited for an FGR fetus <34wks, it is usual to perform a CD.
- The cord is left intact for >1min and the newborn kept warm.

Clinical identification of the high-risk fetus

Symphysis fundal height (SFH)

Use

In low-risk pregnancy to identify SGA only.

Indications

All pregnancies, at each visit >24wks:
- Measurement of the SFH (in cm).
- Sequential measurements can reveal changes in fetal growth.
- Detection rate of SGA is improved by using serial measurements plotted on a graph.
- If size or growth is suspected to be abnormal, USS is indicated.

Routine monitoring of fetal movement

Use

To try to prevent stillbirth.

Indications

Commonly advocated for all pregnancies:
- Mothers should be advised to contact their midwife or the hospital for further assessment if there is a ↓ in FM.
- 'Recurrent episodes' often thought to imply risk but little evidence this is the case.

🌑 The fetus only stops moving as pre-terminal event so reliance on FM monitoring for general fetal well-being is thought illogical by some.

Auscultation of the fetal heart

Use

To confirm the fetus is alive.

🌑 It provides no predictive information done (with hand-held Doppler or a Pinard stethoscope) as part of a standard antenatal examination.

Monitoring the high-risk fetus: ultrasound

B-mode (greyscale) ultrasound

Use
- To estimate the fetal weight (using an algorithm based on fetal biometry measurements).
- Serial USS allows assessment of growth velocity.
- Assessment of presentation, amniotic fluid volume, placental location, and gross fetal anomalies.

Indications
- Screening the high-risk fetus for changing growth velocity (↑ or ↓).
- Where SFH is ↑ or ↓ than expected for gestation.
- Changes in maternal health e.g. development of gestational diabetes.

✒ Universal' serial growth scans is ↑ practised but the benefits are as yet unproven.

Uterine artery Doppler

Use
- As a screening test for early-onset pre-eclampsia and FGR (can be done at any gestation but most often used at 20wks).
- To help to determine if SGA is fetal or placental in origin (useful in severe early-onset growth restriction).
- To help differentiate between SGA and FGR fetuses after 34wks.

Indications
- Screening for an ↑ risk of early-onset pre-eclampsia or FGR.
- Early-onset severe growth restriction.
- In the late 3rd trimester to help identify FGR in the SGA fetus.

Umbilical artery Doppler

↑ Resistance in the umbilical artery is an indicator of placental failure. Using this in high-risk pregnancies ↓ risk of fetal death and the need for interventions around birth, such as CD.

Use
- To diagnose and monitor uteroplacental insufficiency.
- To help to determine whether the cause of observed SGA is placental or not.

Indications
- Assess the severity of uteroplacental insufficiency in an SGA fetus.
- In very preterm babies Doppler can be used to decide intensity of monitoring and timing of expedited birth.

Understanding umbilical artery Dopplers

- When the placenta is functioning normally, flow through the umbilical artery is not impeded by end organ resistance; therefore, blood continues to flow forwards (away from the heart) during cardiac diastole, seen on Doppler waveform as 'end-diastolic flow' (Fig. 3.14).
- As the uteroplacental unit begins to fail, the vascular resistance ↑ and the forward flow in diastole begins to be ↓ (this can be numerically quantified and used for monitoring).
- When the resistance is very high, blood no longer flows forwards in diastole: this is called 'absent end-diastolic flow' (AEDF) (Fig. 3.15).
- As this situation worsens, the resistance is so great that blood may flow back towards the heart during diastole: this is called 'reversed end-diastolic flow' (REDF) (Fig. 3.16).

Middle cerebral artery Doppler

This vessel will demonstrate a ↓ resistance in the compromised baby as a result of 'head sparing'. The PSV ↑ in an anaemic fetus.

Uses
- As an adjunct to other Doppler measurements to determine placental/ fetal health, particularly after 34wks (CPR).
- To detect fetal anaemia in at-risk pregnancies (e.g. Rh disease).

Indications
- To diagnose or monitor suspected placental failure or anaemia.

Cerebroplacental ratio

- CPR = MCA pulsatility index/umbilical artery pulsatility index.
- A low value is a better predictor of poor neonatal outcome than either vessel alone at >34wks.
- ⚠ It is not usually used alone in deciding timing of delivery.

Ductus venosus Doppler

The waveform in this vein is a surrogate for cardiac function.

Use

To monitor cardiac function in high-risk fetuses.

Indications
- Monitoring for TTTS.
- To time delivery in severely compromised, very preterm babies as an adjunct to CTGs and umbilical artery.
- In fetuses <26wks, where CTG is not validated, it may be used alone to determine delivery.

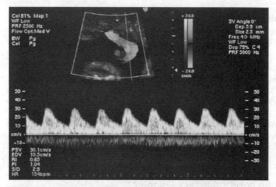

Fig. 3.14 Example of normal umbilical artery Doppler waveform.

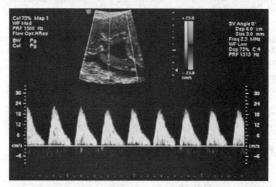

Fig. 3.15 Example of umbilical artery Doppler waveform with absent end-diastolic flow (AEDF).

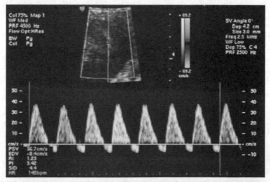

Fig. 3.16 Example of umbilical artery Doppler waveform with reversed end-diastolic flow (REDF).

Monitoring the high-risk fetus: cardiotocography

- CTG is the output of electronic monitoring of the FHR, correlated with any uterine contractions.
- Analysis by inspecting the CTG is difficult, but it is more reproducible when done by computerized algorithms, e.g. the Dawes–Redman criteria.

Normal antenatal cardiotocography

- The baseline FHR is between 110 and 160 beats/min and varies from that baseline by 5–25 beats/min.
- The heart rate should speed up by at least 15 beats/min for at least 15s (accelerations).
- Two accelerations should be seen in 20min (reactive).
- There should be no slowing of the FHR from the baseline (decelerations).

▶ The most useful features in assessing the fetus's health are the variability and presence or absence of accelerations.

Abnormal antenatal cardiotocography

Caused by a failure of autonomic regulation of the heart rate, this is an end-stage event, so the lead-time between uteroplacental insufficiency causing an abnormal CTG and fetal death or long-term damage is short, and this limits its usefulness in antenatal screening.

◆ Routine antenatal CTG has not been found to be useful in low-risk populations.
   CTG is used to exclude current compromise:
- In acute conditions known to cause fetal compromise, e.g. abruption and in women reporting ↓ FMs or abdominal pain.
- Daily in the surveillance of chronic conditions that are associated with uteroplacental insufficiency such as pre-eclampsia, and in FGR when there is AEDF.

⚠ Because the CTG only becomes abnormal at a very late stage in FGR, less frequent than daily CTGs should not be relied upon as a method of monitoring.

Further reading

NICE (2021). Antenatal care. NICE guideline [NG201].
🔊 www.nice.org.uk/guidance/ng201

Infectious diseases in pregnancy

Rubella

Background

- RNA togavirus.
- Respiratory droplet spread—person to person (highly infectious).
- Incubation 14–21 days.
- Infectious for 7 days before and after appearance of rash.
- Reinfection can occur mostly with vaccine-induced immunity.

Clinical features

Symptoms are only present in 50–75% of infected individuals:
- Mild febrile illness.
- Maculopapular rash.
- Arthralgia.
- Lymphadenopathy.

Diagnosis

Paired serology (acute phase and then repeated 10–14 days later) consistent with infection if:
- Appearance of IgM antibodies.
- ≥4× ↑ in IgG antibody titres or ↑ IgG avidity.

Congenital defects associated with rubella

- Major malformations are most likely during organogenesis, with severity ↓ with advancing gestation (Table 4.1).
- Defects include:
  - sensorineural deafness
  - cardiac abnormalities (e.g. VSD and patent ductus arteriosus)
  - eye lesions (cataracts, microphthalmia, and glaucoma)
  - microcephaly and intellectual disability.
- Late-developing sequelae include:
  - diabetes mellitus
  - thyroid disorders
  - progressive panencephalitis.

Prevention

- 'Herd immunity' is maintained by widespread vaccination.
- Uptake has ↓ following concern over safety of the measles, mumps, and rubella (MMR) vaccine.
- Ideally women should be tested before pregnancy, but screening at booking identifies those at risk and in need of postnatal vaccination.

⚠ Vaccine is a live-attenuated virus and contraindicated in pregnancy.

▶ Pregnancy should be avoided for 10–12wks after vaccination.

Management of pregnant women with rubella

- Supportive treatment; hospital admission is rarely required.
- Fetal medicine assessment should be arranged urgently (Table 4.1).

Pregnant women in contact with rubella

▶ Rapidly confirm rubella in the contact.

No action required if the woman has had
- Two documented doses of rubella vaccine.
- One documented dose of vaccine followed by at least one test that has detected rubella antibody ≥10IU/mL.
- At least two previous rubella screening tests that have detected antibody, at least one where rubella antibody >10IU/mL.

⚠ However, she must be advised to return if she develops a rash.

▶ If these criteria are not met → test for IgM and IgG.

Rubella IgG is detected and IgM is NOT detected
- Reassure.
- Advise to return if she develops a rash.

Rubella IgM is detected (irrespective of IgG result)
- Consistent with acute infection.
- Inform the local health protection team as rubella is a notifiable disease in the UK.
- Obtain further serum for IgG and IgM plus avidity.
- Reference testing is recommended.

Neither rubella IgG nor IgM is detected
- Send further sample 1mth after contact or if illness develops and interpret results as above.
- Advise MMR vaccine after delivery.

Table 4.1 Risk of congenital defects in 1° rubella infection

Gestation	Risk of transmission	Risk of congenital abnormality	Treatment
<13wks	80%	Almost all infected fetuses	Termination of pregnancy may be offered without invasive prenatal diagnosis
13–16wks	50%	About 35% of those infected (mainly deafness)	Fetal blood sampling may be later offered to confirm infection
>16wks	25%	Rarely causes defects	Reassurance

Further reading

Public Health England (2011, updated 2019). Viral rash in pregnancy.
🔗 https://www.gov.uk/government/publications/viral-rash-in-pregnancy

Measles

Background
- RNA paramyxovirus.
- Respiratory droplet spread—person to person (highly infectious).
- Incubation 9–12 days.
- Infectious for 2–5 days before and after appearance of rash.
- Rare in the UK following the introduction of the MMR vaccine, however is now ↑ following a ↓ in MMR uptake.

Clinical features
- Significant fever.
- Generalized maculopapular erythematous rash (appears 2–4 days after onset of symptoms).
- Pathognomonic Koplik's spots inside the mouth.
- Symptoms such as cough, coryza, and conjunctivitis can also occur.

Diagnosis
- Viral RNA detection in saliva is one way of confirming diagnosis.
- Alternatively, paired serology (acute phase and then repeated 10–14 days later) consistent with infection if:
  - IgM in serum taken >4 days but <1mth after the onset of rash.

Maternal risks
- Pneumonia.
- Acute encephalitis.
- Corneal ulceration → scarring.
- A rare complication called subacute sclerosing panencephalitis can develop later in life.

⚠ *Measles in pregnancy can cause maternal death.*

The effect of maternal measles infection on the fetus

This is associated with:
- Fetal loss.
- Preterm delivery.
- ▶ But is *not* associated with congenital malformations.

If rash appears between 6 days pre and 6 days post delivery:
- Administration of human normal immunoglobulin to the neonate is recommended immediately after birth or exposure (as neonatal measles has been associated with subacute sclerosing panencephalitis).

Management of a pregnant woman with measles

Treatment is generally supportive, with hospital admission rarely being required.

Pregnant woman in contact with measles

▶ Try to rapidly confirm measles in the person the pregnant woman was in contact with.

- Factors ↑ likelihood of the contact having measles include:
  - contact took place when abroad
  - person with suspected measles had travelled abroad
  - person had not been vaccinated against measles
  - person has recently been hospitalized.
- Reassure measles risk is remote if she has had:
  - two documented doses of measles vaccine, or
  - previous test demonstrating immunity.

⚠ She must be advised to return if she develops a rash.

▶ If these criteria are not met then send serum for IgG.

Measles IgG detected
- Reassure and no further tests required.

Measles IgG not detected
- Inform the local health protection team as this is a notifiable disease in the UK.
- Human normal immunoglobulin as soon as possible.
- Advise immunization with MMR vaccine after delivery.
- Fetal medicine assessment should be arranged urgently.

Further reading

Public Health England (2011, updated 2019). Viral rash in pregnancy.
𝒮 https://www.gov.uk/government/publications/viral-rash-in-pregnancy

Parvovirus B19

Background

- DNA virus.
- Respiratory droplet spread—person to person.
- Incubation 4–20 days.
- Seroprevalence: ~50% of UK women immune.
- Incidence of 1° infection in pregnancy <1:100.

Clinical features

- Often asymptomatic.
- Typical 'slapped cheek' rash (erythema infectiosum).
- Maculopapular rash.
- Fever.
- Arthralgia.

Diagnosis

- Paired serology (acute phase and then repeated 10–14 days later) consistent with recent infection if:
  - appearance of IgM antibodies
  - ↑ IgG antibodies.

Maternal risks

- Fit and healthy: minimal.
- Immunocompromised: risk of sudden haemolysis potentially severe enough to require blood transfusion.

The effect of maternal parvovirus B19 infection on the fetus

- Fetal infection rate is thought to be ~30%.
- The virus causes suppression of erythropoiesis sometimes with thrombocytopenia and direct cardiac toxicity, eventually resulting in cardiac failure and hydrops fetalis.
- No congenital defects associated with parvovirus infection.

⚠ ~10% of fetuses infected at <20wks will die.

Management of parvovirus B19 in pregnancy
• Care in specialist fetal medicine unit to monitor for development of fetal anaemia (by serial measurement of the PSV of the fetal MCA on USS) as this may develop many wks after the initial infection.
• Consideration of *in utero* red blood cell transfusion in severely anaemic, hydropic fetuses to prevent fetal demise.
• Consideration of platelet transfusion if significantly thrombocytopenic to ↓ the risk of fetal bleeding at the time of the *in utero* transfusion.

Pregnant women in contact with parvovirus B19
• Send serum for parvovirus B19 IgM and IgG:

Parvovirus B19 IgG is detected and IgM is not detected
• Reassure.
• Advise to return if mother develops a rash.

Parvovirus B19 IgM is detected (irrespective of IgG result)
• Consistent with acute infection.
• Send the sample for confirmatory testing.
• Obtain further serum (reference testing is recommended).
• Refer for management at fetal medicine unit.

Neither parvovirus B19 IgG nor IgM is detected
• Send further sample 1mth after contact or if illness develops and act on results as above.
• Refer for specialist advice.

Further reading
Public Health England (2011, updated 2019). Viral rash in pregnancy.
🔗 https://www.gov.uk/government/publications/viral-rash-in-pregnancy

Cytomegalovirus

Background
- Herpes virus.
- Transmitted in bodily fluids—low infectivity.
- Can remain dormant within host for life; reactivation common.
- Seroprevalence: ~50% of UK women.
- Incidence of infection in pregnancy ~1:100.

Clinical features
- Asymptomatic in 95% of cases but may present with:
  - fever
  - malaise
  - lymphadenopathy
  - bloods may show atypical lymphocytosis, and mononucleosis.

Diagnosis
Maternal infection
- Paired serology (acute phase and then repeated 10–14 days later) consistent with infection if:
  - significant ↑ in IgM antibodies (may persist for up to 8mths)
  - ↑ IgG antibody titres.
- Culture/PCR of maternal urine can also be diagnostic but is not widely available.

Fetal infection
- Culture/PCR of amniotic fluid (after 20wks).

CMV-associated congenital defects
- FGR.
- Microcephaly.
- Hepatosplenomegaly and thrombocytopenia.
- Jaundice.
- Chorioretinitis.
- Later sequelae include:
  - psychomotor retardation—reported to account for as much as 10% of intellectual disability in children <6yrs old.
- Sensorineural hearing loss.

Risk of fetal infection with 1° maternal infection
- 40% of fetuses will be infected (irrespective of gestation).
- 90% of these are normal at birth, of whom 20% will develop late, usually minor sequelae.
- 10% of these are symptomatic, of whom:
  - 33% will die
  - 67% will have long-term problems.

Management of CMV in pregnancy

- As most fetuses will be unaffected, counselling about management (including termination of pregnancy) is difficult even in the face of confirmed fetal infection.
- Close monitoring of fetal growth and well-being is indicated, with appropriate paediatric follow-up.

Further reading

Public Health England (2011, updated 2019). Viral rash in pregnancy.
🔗 https://www.gov.uk/government/publications/viral-rash-in-pregnancy

Herpes simplex

Background

- Herpes simplex virus (HSV)-1 is a DNA virus that most commonly causes mucosal lesions such as cold sores, but is ↑ being associated with genital herpes.
- HSV2 is a DNA virus that most commonly causes genital infection.
- Spread by person-to-person contact.
- After the initial infection the virus remains latent and can be reactivated, often in response to a stress or immunocompromise.
- Incubation ~2–7 days.
- Individual may be infectious even when apparently asymptomatic.

Clinical features

1° infection

- Most are asymptomatic.
- Typical vesicular lesions can be very painful and last for 10–14 days.
- Distribution of lesions is usually isolated to one area of the body.
- Systemic symptoms can occur at the time of initial infection and include fever and lethargy/malaise.
- 1° genital infection can cause vulvitis that can be severe enough to cause urinary retention.

Recurrent infection

- Systemic symptoms are less common.
- Local lymphadenopathy can occur.
- Appearance of typical lesions is usually heralded by prodromal symptoms such as tingling or pain.
- Episodes are of shorter duration than 1° infection.

Other manifestations (more commonly seen with HSV1 than HSV2)

- Vesicles may be absent.
- Encephalitis (➲ Box 4.1, p. 170).
- Fulminant hepatitis.
- Sacral radiculopathy.
- Transverse myelitis.
- 1° ocular infection.

⚠ Immunocompromised individuals are more at risk of disseminated infection and ↑ frequency of reactivation.

Diagnosis

- Usually made on the history appearance of the typical rash.
- Vesicle swabs can be diagnostic.
- Viral PCR assays can also be used.
- Acute and convalescent antibody levels can be performed but may be difficult to interpret.

Management of 1° genital herpes in pregnancy

- Refer to genitourinary medicine (GUM) to confirm diagnosis with PCR.
- 5 days of aciclovir (400mg tds) may ↓ severity and duration of the 1° attack (IV if immunocompromised or severe infection).
- Paracetamol and 2% lidocaine gel for symptomatic relief.
- Assess for other sexually transmitted infections (STIs).

1st or 2nd trimester infection

- Refer for obstetric care.
- If undelivered for 6wks, manage expectantly and anticipate vaginal delivery if genital lesions are no longer present.
- Offer further aciclovir from 36wks (↓ herpetic lesions at term and hence the need for delivery by CD).
- No evidence for management of women with rupture of membranes at term, but expediting delivery to minimize the duration of potential exposure to HSV is often advised.

3rd trimester infection

- Aciclovir 400mg tds PO should be continued until delivery.
- CD should be recommended for those developing 1° genital herpes in the 3rd trimester, particularly those developing symptoms <6wks of expected delivery, as the risk of neonatal transmission is very high at 41%.
- Aciclovir should be given intrapartum (IV 5 mg/kg tds) and to the neonate (IV 20 mg/kg tds) if vaginal delivery.

⚠ 15% presenting with 1° infection will actually have recurrent herpes so type-specific HSV antibody testing is advisable.

▶ Presence of antibodies of the same type as the HSV isolated from genital swabs would confirm the episode to be a recurrence.

Management of recurrent genital herpes in pregnancy

- Risk of neonatal HSV is low, even if lesions present at the time of delivery (0–3% for vaginal delivery).
- Vaginal delivery should be anticipated in the absence of other obstetric indications for CD.
- Consider daily suppressive aciclovir (400mg tds) from 36wks (32wks if HIV +ve).
- Fetal blood sampling or fetal scalp electrode may ↑ the risk of neonatal HSV infection; however, given the small background risk (0–3%) of transmission, the ↑ risk associated with invasive procedures is unlikely to be clinically significant so they may be used if required.
- In the case of PPROM <34wks, expectant management is appropriate, including oral aciclovir 400 mg tds.

Further reading

BASH, RCOG (2014). Management of genital herpes in pregnancy.
⅋ www.rcog.org.uk/globalassets/documents/guidelines/management-genital-herpes.pdf

Herpes simplex: complications

Maternal

- Often presents with encephalitis, hepatitis, disseminated skin lesions, or a combination of these.
- More common in pregnant and/or immunocompromised women.
- Maternal mortality is high.
- Co-infection with HIV results in an ↑ replication of both viruses.

Box 4.1 HSV encephalitis (more commonly HSV1)

- Associated with significant morbidity and mortality if untreated.
- Tends to occur in later pregnancy.
- Symptoms include:
  - confusion and/or ↓ conscious level
  - fever
  - seizures
  - severe headache or altered behaviour.
- Empirical treatment is required (high-dose IV aciclovir) and empirical antibiotics will usually be given alongside this.
- Urgent lumbar puncture should be performed with cerebrospinal fluid (CSF) sent for viral PCR.

Fetus

- Infection has not been shown to cause congenital defects but has been associated with miscarriage and preterm delivery.

Neonate

- 1° genital herpes infection in the 3rd trimester is associated with transmission to the neonate in ~41% of women.
- With recurrent genital herpes should be informed that the risk of neonatal herpes is low, even if lesions are present at the time of delivery (0–3% for vaginal delivery).

Neonatal herpes infection

- Occurs in 1st 2wks of life.
- 25% limited to eyes and mouth only.
- 75% widely disseminated, of whom:
  - ~70% will die
  - many of the survivors will have long-term problems including neurodevelopmental difficulties.

Varicella zoster

Background
- DNA virus.
- 1° infection known as varicella or 'chicken pox'.
- Spread by respiratory droplets and contact with vesicle fluid.
- Incubation 10–21 days.
- Infectious from 2 days before rash until all vesicles are crusted.
- Seroprevalence: ~90% of UK women immune.
- Incidence of 1° infection in pregnancy ~3:1000.
- Reactivation after initial infection known as zoster or 'shingles'.

Clinical features
- Fever.
- Malaise.
- Maculopapular rash which becomes vesicular then crusts over.

Diagnosis
- This is a clinical diagnosis based on a history of contact with chicken pox/shingles and the development of a typical rash.

Maternal risks

⚠ *Varicella in pregnancy is often more severe and may be life-threatening as a consequence of*:
- Varicella pneumonia.
- Hepatitis.
- Encephalitis.

Fetal risks
- Fetal infection rate is thought to be ~25% in all trimesters.
- If <20wks there is a 2% risk of FVS with congenital defects (Table 4.2) including:
  - skin scarring
  - limb hypoplasia
  - eye lesions (congenital cataracts, microphthalmia, chorioretinitis)
  - neurological abnormalities (intellectual disability, microcephaly, cortical atrophy, and dysfunction of bladder and bowel sphincters).

Neonatal risks
▶ Neonatal varicella is seen in babies whose mothers contracted the infection in the last 4wks of pregnancy.

⚠ If maternal rash appears 5 days before delivery or up to 2 days afterwards, the neonate requires varicella zoster immunoglobulin (VZIG) as soon as possible (this is when severe infection is most likely in the neonate, which can be fatal).

Management of varicella in pregnancy

1° infection, with no evidence of complications
- Oral aciclovir (800mg five times per day for 7 days) starting within 24h of symptom onset is likely to be beneficial.

1° infection, evidence of complications such as pneumonitis
- Admit to hospital.
- Consider IV antiviral therapy.

All cases
- Arrange follow-up for fetal monitoring (Table 4.2).

⚠ Contact with non-immune pregnant women should be avoided.

Table 4.2 Fetal risks from 1° maternal varicella infection

Gestation	Risk to fetus	Management
<20wks	2% develop FVS	• Detailed USS at 16–20wks, may consider TOP if evidence of FVS seen • Neonatal ophthalmic examination
>20 to <28wks	Very small risk of FVS	• Detailed USS 5wks after infection • Neonatal ophthalmic examination
>28wks	Not associated with congenital abnormality	• Fetal and neonatal surveillance
Within 4wks of delivery	~20% will develop neonatal varicella infection	• VZIG as soon as possible • 14 days monitoring for signs of infection, with aciclovir if varicella develops

Further reading

RCOG (2015). Chickenpox in pregnancy. RCOG green-top guideline no. 13.
🔗 www.rcog.org.uk/en/guidelines-research-services/guidelines/gtg13/

Varicella contact and shingles

⚠ Significant contact with varicella is defined as being in the same room for ≥15min, face-to-face contact, or contact in the setting of a large open ward.

Exposure to varicella *and* **no history of previous infection**
- Send for varicella zoster virus serology testing.

If IgG detected within 10 days of exposure
- Assume immunity.

If IgG not detected within 10 days of exposure
- Mother requires VZIG as soon as possible.
- Oral aciclovir should be prescribed if >20wks and the rash appeared within preceding 24h.
- Oral aciclovir should be considered if <20wks and the rash appeared within preceding 24h.

Shingles in pregnancy
- Reactivation of varicella zoster virus is known as shingles.
- Painful vesicular rash in a dermatomal distribution.
- Low risk of transmission as affected areas are often not exposed; however, viral shedding may be greater if areas exposed (e.g. ophthalmic) or if the woman is immunocompromised.
- Treatment with oral aciclovir (800mg five times per day for 7–10 days) should be prescribed.

⚠ Contact with non-immune pregnant women should be avoided.

Varicella zoster virus vaccination
- Live attenuated vaccine, so should not be used during pregnancy.
- Administration after delivery should be recommended to women who are identified to be non-immune.

Hepatitis B

Background
- DNA virus.
- Spread by infected blood, blood products, or sexual contact.
- Incubation 2–6mths.
- Incidence of carrier status in UK women is ~1:100.

Clinical features
- Acute infection has a prodrome of non-specific systemic and gastrointestinal symptoms followed by an episode of jaundice.
- Those with chronic infection are usually asymptomatic.

Diagnosis
Based on clinical picture and serology (Tables 4.3 and 4.4).

Maternal risks
- Pregnancy does not alter the course of acute infection, and so prognosis is similar to that of non-pregnant individuals:
  - 65% subclinical disease with full recovery
  - 25% develop acute hepatitis
  - 10% become chronic carriers
  - <0.5% fulminant hepatitis (associated with significant mortality).

Fetal risks
Severe acute infection may → miscarriage or preterm labour, but no related congenital defects have been identified.

> **Management of chronic hepatitis B in pregnancy**
> ▶ In the UK all women should be screened at booking as detection of infection has important consequences for ↓ of mother-to-child transmission (MTCT).
> - Nucleoside analogues (i.e. entecavir/tenofovir) are advised in highly viraemic women (viral load (VL) >1,000,000IU/mL) to ↓ MTCT (usually started in the 2nd/3rd trimester).
> - No evidence that CD prevents vertical transmission.
> - Breast-feeding is not contraindicated.

Neonatal risks of hepatitis B

- Transmission usually occurs at delivery, but <5% may be due to transplacental bleeding *in utero*.
- Neonatal infection may be fatal, and usually results in chronic carrier status with significant lifelong risks of cirrhosis and hepatocellular carcinoma.
- The carrier status of the mother at delivery determines the risk of vertical transmission:
  - HBsAg and HBeAg +ve: ~95% risk
  - HBsAg +ve *and* HBeAg −ve *and* VL <100,000: <15% risk.

⚠ Babies whose mothers have acute or chronic HBV should receive HBV vaccination ± HBV IgG if high VL within 24h of delivery (this is up to 95% effective at preventing neonatal HBV infection).

Table 4.3 Diagnostic tests for hepatitis B infection

HBsAg	Hepatitis B surface antigen
HBeAg	Hepatitis B e antigen
HBV DNA	Hepatitis B virus DNA
Anti-HBs	Antibody to Hep B surface antigen
Anti-Hbe	Antibody to Hep B e protein
Anti-HBc	Antibody to Hep B core antigen

Table 4.4 Interpreting test results for hepatitis B infection

Diagnosis	Positive	May be +ve or −ve
Vaccination	• Anti-HBs	
Incubation period		• HBsAg • HBeAg • HBV DNA
Acute infection	• HBsAg • HBeAg • HBV DNA • Anti-HBc IgM	
Past infection	• Anti-HBs • Anti-HBc	• HBV DNA • Anti-HBe
Chronic infection	• HBsAg • HBV DNA	• HBeAg • Anti-HBe

Hepatitis C

Background

- RNA virus.
- Main method of transmission is IV drug abuse.
- In the last decade, there have been advances in treatment and a ↓ risk of complications such as cirrhosis and hepatocellular carcinoma.
- Older treatments were of limited benefit and associated with adverse effects (peginterferon alfa and ribavirin).
- Oral direct antiviral agents were introduced after 2011 and have transformed the treatment of hepatitis C with shorter treatment duration (8–16wks) and they are much better tolerated with a 95% cure rate.
- Drug regimens are available that work across all genotypes.

Clinical features

- Acute infection is normally asymptomatic.
- Chronic infection is identified either through screening or when cirrhosis is diagnosed.
- Up to 30% clear the virus spontaneously after the acute episode.
- Cirrhosis and liver failure can occur.
- Many extra-hepatic manifestations have been described including membranoproliferative glomerulonephritis, cryoglobulinaemia, and thyroid disease.

Diagnosis

- Serological testing for anti-hepatitis C antibody (remains +ve after successful treatment).
- Positive viral RNA confirms infection.
- ▶ If RNA +ve, then genotyping should be performed.
- LFTs are of limited value as can be normal even in the presence of significant cirrhosis.
- Liver USS may identify abnormal liver appearance, and/or the presence of complications such as splenomegaly.
- Liver biopsy can be performed to assess fibrosis, but non-invasive tests are preferred (Fibroscan®, or transient elastography).

New identification of hepatitis C antibody positivity in pregnancy

- Thorough history for potential source.
- Send blood for viral RNA level.
- If −ve:
  - likely to have spontaneously cleared infection or been treated.
- If +ve:
  - ensure also tested for HIV and hepatitis B.
  - arrange liver ultrasound (for cirrhosis, portal hypertension).
- Refer to hepatology for review with respect to treatment.

Management of hepatitis C in pregnancy

- Anti-hepatitis C antibodies are not routinely screened for but should be measured in women assessed to be at risk (see below).
- Hepatitis C virus (HCV) infection is not a contraindication to vaginal delivery or breast feeding, although women with high VLs have greater vertical transmission rates.
- Invasive fetal monitoring and prolonged labour should be avoided.
- Infected women should be referred for treatment after delivery.
- Newer treatments are not currently recommended in pregnancy due to a lack of safety and efficacy data.

Women who warrant screening for hepatitis C

- History of IV drug use.
- Recipient of blood products before 1992.
- Haemophilia carriers who received factor concentrates before 1987.
- History of haemodialysis.
- Unexplained elevated alanine transaminase (ALT).
- HIV +ve.

Other viruses that cause hepatitis in pregnancy

Hepatitis A

- Pregnancy does not alter the course or outcome.

Hepatitis E

- Acute self-limiting illness in the non-pregnant population.
- Can cause severe infection with fulminant liver failure in pregnancy.
- Treatment is supportive and there is no evidence for efficacy of specific antiviral therapy.

Other viruses

- Abnormal liver function can be seen with:
  - acute HSV
  - CMV
  - EBV.

Influenza

Background

- In pregnancy is associated with ↑ mortality compared to non-pregnant women.
- Varies with the strain of virus and uptake of vaccination.
- Underlying medical conditions including asthma ↑ risk of severe infection.

Clinical features

- Appear 2–3 days after exposure:
  - sore throat
  - fatigue
  - loss of appetite
  - cough
  - headache
  - weakness
  - muscle ache
  - insomnia
  - shortness of breath.

Influenza vaccination

- Advised for all:
  - pregnant women at any gestation to provide both maternal protection and passive immunity to neonate
  - healthcare professionals involved in care of pregnancy.
- Inactivated vaccines are preferred.

Management of suspected influenza in pregnancy

Assess severity

- Examination including:
  - hypoxia
  - tachypnoea
  - abnormalities on chest auscultation.
- Chest X-ray (CXR):
  - bilateral infiltrates
  - evidence of consolidation suggestive of $2°$ bacterial infection.

Mild infection

- Diagnosis is clinical.
- Supportive with hydration.
- Paracetamol to relieve symptoms.
- Rest, stay off work.

Potentially severe infection

⚠ Consider hospital admission if woman is breathless, has an abnormal CXR, signs of severe infection, or has an underlying medical condition predisposing her to severe infection.

- Swabs of throat, nose, or nasopharynx for viral PCR; point-of-care rapid antigen tests are available in some hospitals.
- Blood cultures.
- Empirical antibiotics.
- Antivirals (oseltamivir or zanamivir) are ideally started within 48h of symptom onset but can be considered if symptoms started between 3 and 5 days prior to presentation.

COVID-19

Novel coronavirus (severe acute respiratory syndrome coronavirus 2 (SARS-CoV-2)) is a new strain of coronavirus causing coronavirus disease 2019 (COVID-19), first identified in China at the end of 2019.

Like other human coronavirus such as Middle East respiratory syndrome coronavirus (MERS-CoV) and SARS coronavirus (SARS-CoV), it can cause mild to moderate upper-respiratory tract illnesses.

See Fig. 4.1.

Transmission

- Can be readily isolated from respiratory droplets or secretions, faeces, an d fomites (objects).
- Transmission known to occur most often through close contact with an infected person (within 2 metres) or from contaminated surfaces.
- Pregnant women are not more likely to contract the infection than the general population.
- There is growing evidence that pregnant women are at ↑ risk of severe illness especially in the 3rd trimester.

● There is no clear evidence regarding vertical transmission for virus from mother to baby or of ↑ congenital abnormalities.

Signs and symptoms

- Majority of cases will be asymptomatic.
- Those who are symptomatic are mostly mild or moderate and suitable for non-hospital symptom management.
- ~10% will be classed as severe/critical and require inpatient multidisciplinary care.
- Main symptoms are recognized as:
  - cough
  - pyrexia
  - loss of smell/taste
  - shortness of breath
  - other flu-like symptoms may occur as well as gastrointestinal symptoms.

Risk factors for hospital admission

- Black, Asian, or minority ethnicity.
- Overweight or obesity.
- Pre-existing comorbidity.
- Maternal age >35yrs.
- Living in ↑ socioeconomic deprivation.
- Working in healthcare or other public-facing occupations.

Fetal risks

- Maternal infection is associated with:
  - a 2× ↑ risk of stillbirth
  - FGR
  - Preterm birth (mostly iatrogenic).

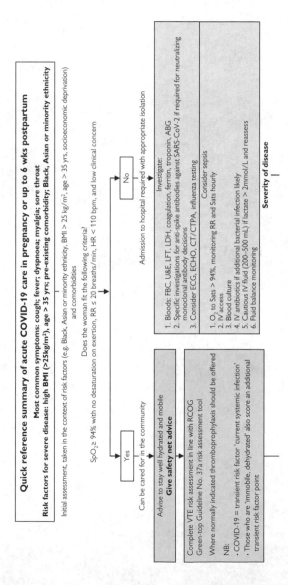

Quick reference summary of acute COVID-19 care in pregnancy or up to 6 wks postpartum

Most common symptoms: cough; fever; dyspnoea; myalgia; sore throat

Risk factors for severe disease: high BMI (>25kg/m²), age > 35 yrs; pre-existing comorbidity; Black, Asian or minority ethnicity

Initial assessment, taken in the context of risk factors (e.g. Black, Asian or minority ethnicity, BMI > 25 kg/m², age > 35 yrs, socioeconomic deprivation) and comorbidities

Does the woman fit the following criteria?

$SpO_2 \geq$ 94% with no desaturation on exertion, RR ≤ 20 breaths/min, HR < 110 bpm, and low clinical concern

Yes

Can be cared for in the community

Advise to stay well hydrated and mobile
Give safety net advice

Complete VTE risk assessment in line with RCOG Green-top Guideline No. 37a risk assessment tool

Where normally indicated thromboprophylaxis should be offered

NB:
• COVID-19 = transient risk factor 'current systemic infection'
• Those who are 'immobile, dehydrated' also score an additional transient risk factor point

No

Admission to hospital required with appropriate isolation

Investigate:
1. Bloods: FBC, U&E, LFT, LDH, coagulation, ferritin, troponin, ABG
2. Specific investigations for anti-spike antibodies against SARS-CoV-2 if required for neutralizing monoclonal antibody decisions
3. Consider ECG, ECHO, CT/CTPA, influenza testing

Consider sepsis
1. O_2 to Sats > 94%, monitoring RR and Sats hourly
2. IV access
3. Blood culture
4. IV antibiotics if additional bacterial infection likely
5. Cautious IV fluid (200–500 mL) if lactate > 2mmol/L and reassess
6. Fluid balance monitoring

Severity of disease

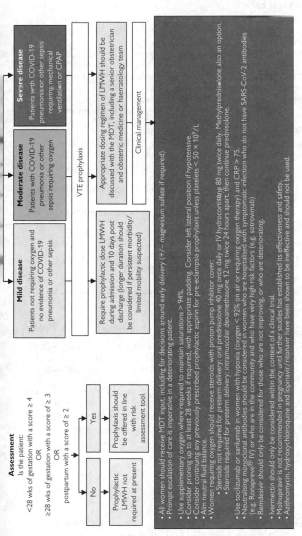

Assessment

Is the patient:

<28 wks of gestation with a score ≥ 4
OR
≥28 wks of gestation with a score of ≥ 3
OR
postpartum with a score of ≥ 2

- No → Prophylactic LMWH not required at present
- Yes → Prophylaxis should be offered in line with risk assessment tool

Mild disease	Moderate disease	Severe disease
Patients not requiring oxygen and no evidence of COVID-19 pneumonia or other sepsis	Patients with COVID-19 pneumonia or other sepsis requiring oxygen	Patients with COVID-19 pneumonia or other sepsis requiring mechanical ventilation or CPAP

VTE prophylaxis

Require prophylactic dose LMWH during admission and 10 days post discharge (longer duration should be considered if persistent morbidity/limited mobility suspected)

Appropriate dosing regimen of LMWH should be discussed with the MDT, including a senior obstetrician and obstetric medicine or haematology team

Clinical management

- All women should receive MDT input, including for decisions around early delivery (+/− magnesium sulfate if required).
- Prompt escalation of care is imperative in a deteriorating patient.
- Use supplementary oxygen where required to maintain saturations > 94%
- Consider proning up to at least 28 weeks if required, with appropriate padding. Consider left lateral position if hypotensive.
- Consider continuing any previously prescribed prophylactic aspirin for pre-eclampsia prophylaxis unless platelets < 50×10^9/L
- Aim neutral fluid balance.
- Women requiring oxygen should receive steroids with proton pump inhibitor cover:
  - Steroids not required for preterm delivery: oral prednisolone 40 mg once daily or IV hydrocortisone 80 mg twice daily. Methylprednisolone also an option.
  - Steroids required for preterm delivery: intramuscular dexamethasone 12 mg twice 24 hours apart, then continue prednisolone.
- Use tocilizumab or sarilumab in women with hypoxia (oxygen < 92% on air or requiring oxygen therapy) and CRP > 75.
- Neutralising monoclonal antibodies should be considered in women who are hospitalised with symptomatic infection who do not have SARS-CoV-2 antibodies (e.g. Ronapreve® IV) or who are in the community and who have very high risk factors (e.g. sotrovimab)
- Remdesivir should only be considered for those who are not improving, or who are deteriorating.
- Ivermectin should only be considered within the context of a clinical trial.
- Molnupiravir is not recommended in pregnancy until further studies has established its effectiveness and safety
- Azithromycin, hydroxychloroquine and lopinavir/ritonavir have been shown to be ineffective and should not be used.

Fig. 4.1 Management of COVID-19 in the pregnant patient. Reproduced from RCOG and RCM: Coronavirus (COVID-19) Infection in Pregnancy. https://www.rcog.org.uk/media/xsubnsma/2022-03-07-coronavirus-covid-19-infection-in-pregnancy-v15.pdf

COVID-19: management

Antenatal care

- Service adjustment is required to ensure women can practise social distancing measures.
- Women should receive routine antenatal care.
- Attention should be paid to social situation as domestic abuse and mental health issues have been shown to ↑ during the pandemic.
- All admitted with COVID-19 should be offered LMWH while they are an inpatient and for 10 days after discharge.
- Low-dose aspirin should be discontinued for the duration of COVID-19 infection due to the risk of COVID-19-associated thrombocytopenia.

Labour

- Asymptomatic COVID-19 +ve women should be cared for in the same manner as the general obstetric population.
- Non-critical symptomatic women are recommended to deliver in an obstetric unit with:
  - assessment of the severity of COVID-19 symptoms by the most senior available clinician
  - maternal observations including temperature, respiratory rate, and oxygen saturation
  - confirmation of the onset of labour, as per standard care.
  - Continuous electronic fetal monitoring using CTG.
  - involvement of the MDT—consultant obstetrician, anaesthetist, midwife-in-charge, and neonatal consultant
  - effort should be made to minimize staff entering the room and the appropriate personal protective equipment should be worn
  - care should be according to standard obstetric practice
  - water-birth is contraindicated.

Postnatal care

- Women who have suspected, probable, or confirmed COVID-19:
  - should be supported to breast-feed if they choose
  - should be supported and enabled to remain together with their babies and to practise skin-to-skin/kangaroo care.
- For a woman who has suspected or confirmed COVID-19 and whose baby needs to be cared for on the neonatal unit, a precautionary approach should be adopted to minimize any risk of women-to-infant transmission.

Further reading

RCOG, RCM (2022). Coronavirus (COVID-19) infection in pregnancy.
🔗 https://www.rcog.org.uk/guidance/coronavirus-covid-19-pregnancy-and-women-s-health/coronavirus-covid-19-infection-in-pregnancy/

COVID-19 vaccination

- Vaccination is strongly recommended and can be given at any time during pregnancy.
- It should be offered to pregnant women at the same time as the rest of the population, based on age and clinical risk.
- Pregnant women should be offered the Pfizer–BioNTech or Moderna vaccines unless they have already had one dose of the Oxford–AstraZeneca vaccine, in which case they should complete the course with Oxford–AstraZeneca.
- Antibodies have been found in cord blood suggesting that vaccination confers some passive immunity to the neonate.
- Breast-feeding can continue.
- There is no evidence that it affects fertility.

Care for pregnant patients who are critically deteriorating with COVD-19

⚠ The priority is to stabilize the woman's condition and appropriate chest imaging must not be delayed.

⚠ Care must be escalated urgently for any signs of decompensation, these include:
- ↑ O_2 requirements or FiO_2 >35%
- ↑ respiratory rate >25 breaths/min
- rapidly ↑ respiratory rate despite O_2 therapy
- ↓ urine output or evidence of acute kidney injury
- drowsiness.
- An MDT meeting should be urgently arranged.
- O_2 should be titrated to saturations of 94–98% using escalation through nasal cannula → face mask → venturi mask → non-rebreather mask → non-invasive positive airway pressure, e.g. continuous positive airway pressure (CPAP) → intubation and intermittent positive-pressure ventilation (IPPV) → extracorporeal membrane oxygenation (ECMO).
- Careful neural fluid balance with boluses of 250–500mL if needed.
- Corticosteroid therapy should be given for 10 days, or up to discharge, for women requiring O_2.
- Steroids for fetal lung maturation should be given.
- Tocilizumab should be used if required.
- Remdesivir should only be considered in pregnant women who are not improving or who are deteriorating.
- Hydroxychloroquine, lopinavir/ritonavir, and azithromycin should not be used as they are ineffective in treating COVID-19.

✱ Molnupiravir is not recommended in pregnancy until further studies have established its effectiveness and safety

Zika

Background

- Flavivirus, 1st discovered in Uganda in 1947.
- Spread by day-biting mosquitoes.
- Small number of cases found to be spread by sexual transmission, risk is very low.
- Usually a mild and short-lived illness (2–7 days); severe disease is uncommon.

Clinical features

Symptoms include:
- Fever.
- Headache.
- Red sore eyes and conjunctivitis.
- Joint pain and/or swelling.
- Muscle pain.
- Rash.
- Itching.

Prevention

- 50% DEET-based mosquito repellents are the most effective and are safe in pregnancy and breast-feeding.
- Avoid unnecessary travel to areas affected by Zika if pregnant or planning pregnancy (see UK Government advice: ℘ www.gov.uk/guidance/zika-virus-country-specific-risk)

Fetal abnormalities

See Table 4.5.

Table 4.5 Fetal abnormalities in congenital Zika infection

Cranial abnormalities	Extracranial abnormalities
Microcephaly	Fetal growth restriction
Cerebral and/or ocular calcification	Oligohydramnios
Ventriculomegaly	Talipes
Periventricular cysts	
Callosal abnormalities	
Microphthalmia	
Cerebellar atrophy	
Vermian agenesis	
Blake's cyst	
Mega cisterna magna	
Choroid plexus cyst	
Brain atrophy → microcephaly	
Cortical and white matter abnormalities	

Management of pregnant woman with possible infection

See Fig. 4.2.

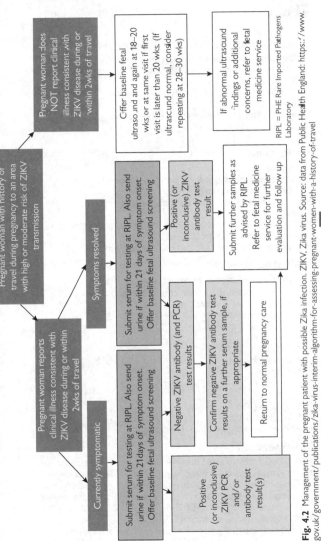

Fig. 4.2 Management of the pregnant patient with possible Zika infection. ZIKV, Zika virus. Source: data from Public Health England: https://www.gov.uk/government/publications/zika-virus-interim-algorithm-for-assessing-pregnant-women-with-a-history-of-travel

Ebola

If the diagnosis of Ebola is being considered
- Liaise with public health providers (and local ID/micro services) before the patient arrives in hospital, or as soon as possible after risk identified.
- Maximize the safety of all staff who are working within the high-risk area.
- Follow strict infection control procedures using full personal protective equipment.

Background
- Filovirus 1st recognized in 1976.
- Interaction with pregnancy is poorly understood.
- Incubation period is up to 21 days.
- Efficient human-to-human transmission through mucosal contact with infected body fluids.
- Risk of transmission continues after death so corpses must be handled with full infection control procedures.
- Can cross the placenta so likely to transmit it to the fetus.

Clinical features
Consistent with infection in an area of suspected infection
- Fever + contact with a known case of Ebola.
- Fever + three of the following:
  - Headache
  - Myalgia or arthralgia
  - Dysphagia
  - Hiccups
  - Loss of appetite
  - Dyspnoea
  - Diarrhoea
  - Lethargy
  - Vomiting
  - Dyspepsia.
- Any person with unexplained bleeding.

Treatment
- IV access early (to avoid sharps injury if patient distressed).
- Supportive care with focus on electrolyte and fluid replacement.
- If possible, treat complications such as refractory shock, hypoxia, haemorrhage, septic shock, multiorgan failure, and disseminated intravascular coagulation (DIC).
- Manage distressing symptoms.
- Consider empirical antibacterial and antimalarial treatment.
- No curative treatment available, some experimental therapies and vaccinations are being developed.
- Manage pregnancy after patient has tested −ve for Ebola (after 4 days of being symptomatic).

Postnatally

- No evidence that women who survive and subsequently become pregnant pose a risk for virus transmission.
- Semen in men who survive continues to contain virus for at least 3mths following recovery.

Obstetric management in women with Ebola infection

⚠ Likelihood of baby surviving in an infected mother is very low therefore fetal monitoring is not advised and emergency CD is not indicated for fetal reasons.

It is recommended to

- Deliver in high-risk area.
- Anticipate vaginal delivery, healthcare practitioner to be to one side to avoid direct splash of bodily fluids.
- Minimize vaginal examinations and avoid artificial rupture of membranes.
- Do not perform an episiotomy.
- Active 3rd stage.
- Not to suture if there is a vaginal tear, use pressure instead.

In utero death

- Do not induce labour until serology −ve and woman is well.
- If planned emptying of the uterus (at any stage of pregnancy) it is recommended to use mifepristone and/or misoprostol.
- Placenta and stillborn child must be disposed of in accordance with high-risk material protocol.

Live birth

- Unlikely.
- Assume baby is Ebola +ve and highly contagious.

Lactation

- Breast milk is likely to be infected, consider lactation suppressant, e.g. cabergoline.
- If not feasible, provide breast pump with clear instructions for safe disposal of the infected milk, and a weaning technique with the aim of ceasing lactation.
- Mother can nurse and breast-feed baby.
- Appropriate counselling on high chance of neonatal death.
- On discharge give supplies to assist with re-entry into community:
  - medicines including iron supplements
  - nutritional supplements
  - clothing
  - hygiene pads
  - contraception.

Further reading

WHO. Ebola: case management, infection prevention, and control.
🔗 www.who.int/teams/health-care-readiness/ebola

Other viral infections

Epstein–Barr virus (EBV)

- Infectious mononucleosis is a common presentation of 1° EBV.
- A generalized maculopapular rash may occur (particularly if ampicillin or a similar antibiotic has been taken).
- 1° infection in pregnancy carries no specific risk to the fetus.

Enteroviruses

- Coxsackie virus groups A and B, echovirus, and enterovirus 68–71.
- Wide range of manifestations including:
  - meningitis
  - rash
  - febrile illness
  - myocarditis.
- No clear causal relationship evident for adverse fetal or neonatal outcome.

▶ Hand, foot, and mouth is caused by an enteroviral infection.
- 1° infection or contact with it in pregnancy is not known to have any adverse consequences for the fetus.

Group A *Streptococcus*

Background
- *Streptococcus pyogenes*—an aerobic Gram +ve coccus.
- Most common bacterial cause of acute pharyngitis ('strep throat').
- Up to 30% of population are asymptomatic carriers (skin or throat).
- Easily spread—person to person or droplet.

⚠ Can cause severe illness in pregnancy that can be insidious in onset, can cause a rapid deterioration, and can be fatal, therefore a high index of suspicion is required.

Diseases caused by group A *Streptococcus* (GAS)
- Pharyngitis.
- Impetigo.
- Cellulitis and other infections of soft tissue and muscle.
- Scarlet fever.
- Rheumatic fever.
- Toxic shock syndrome.
- Postpartum endometritis.

Clinical features
- Often a personal or family history of sore throat or respiratory illness.
- Symptoms can be non-specific but include vomiting, diarrhoea, and fever.
- Complications including septic shock, DIC, and multiorgan failure can occur.

Advice about prevention of GAS in pregnancy
- There may be transfer from the throat or nose to the perineum via the hands when using the toilet or changing sanitary towels.
- Antenatal education should raise awareness of this and the importance of good personal hygiene including washing hands *before*, as well as after, using the toilet or changing sanitary towels.

Fetal risks
⚠ If maternal peripartum infection with invasive GAS, inform neonatologist and start prophylactic antibiotics for the neonate.

Management of GAS in pregnancy
- A high clinical suspicion is required and empirical antibiotics started early if GAS infection is suspected.
- Early involvement of intensive care services.
- A decision about delivery timing and mode has to be individualized, and depends on:
  - gestation
  - assessment of fetal well-being
  - degree of maternal resuscitation required

Further reading

RCOG (2012). Bacterial sepsis in pregnancy. Green-top guideline no. 64a.
℘ https://www.rcog.org.uk/media/ea1p1r4h/gtg_64a.pdf
RCOG (2012). Bacterial sepsis following pregnancy. Green-top guideline no. 64b.
℘ https://www.rcog.org.uk/media/bfnkzznd/gtg_64b.pdf

Group B *Streptococcus*

Background
- Common bowel commensal.
- Vaginal carriage occurs in up to 20% of women.
- Most frequent cause of early-onset, severe neonatal infection (incidence 1:2000 live births).
- Up to 70% of babies from affected mothers will be colonized at delivery but only 1% of these develop symptoms of sepsis.

Clinical features
No signs or symptoms.

Diagnosis
- Carriage is confirmed by culture from an LVS or perianal swab.
- Active infection is confirmed by culture of the organism on culture of blood, urine, or CSF.

Fetal risks
Associated with PPROM and preterm delivery.

Neonatal risks

⚠ Early-onset Group B *Streptococcus* (GBS) infection (<4 days from delivery) has ~20% mortality rate and may present with:
- Pneumonia.
- Septicaemia.
- Meningitis.

⚠ Late-onset infection (>7 days) is not associated with maternal GBS carriage.
- Carries a mortality rate of ~20%
- Of those surviving, 50% will have serious neurological sequelae, such as cortical blindness and deafness.

Management of GBS in pregnancy

⚠ Routine antenatal screening: not currently recommended by the RCOG.

Intrapartum prophylaxis advised if
- History of previous neonatal GBS infection.
- Incidental finding of GBS in urine or on vaginal swab.

Intrapartum prophylaxis (in absence of +ve swabs) should be considered if
- Prematurity (<37wks).
- Prolonged rupture of membranes (>18h).
- Pyrexia in labour.

Intrapartum antibiotics
- IV benzylpenicillin as soon as possible after onset of labour and at least 2h before delivery.
- IV clindamycin if penicillin allergic.

Further reading

RCOG (2012). Bacterial sepsis in pregnancy. Green-top guideline no. 64a.
⅏ https://www.rcog.org.uk/media/ea1p1r4h/gtg_64a.pdf
RCOG (2012). Bacterial sepsis following pregnancy. Green-top guideline no. 64b.
⅏ https://www.rcog.org.uk/media/bfnkzznd/gtg_64b.pdf

Listeria

Background
- Caused by *Listeria monocytogenes*, a Gram +ve, rod-shaped bacterium.
- Rare, affecting ~1:10,000 pregnancies in the UK.
- Found in soft cheese, pâté, undercooked meat, and shellfish.
- ↑ incidence of infection in pregnant women.

Clinical features
- Non-specific so a high clinical suspicion is required.
- Produces gastroenteritis often accompanied by flu-like symptoms.
- Can cause meningitis.

Diagnosis
- Confirmed by culture of the organism from bodily fluid samples.
- Stool culture not routinely required for suspected systemic infection, and should only be sent if gastroenteritis is present (special culture medium required so essential to mention possible diagnosis).
- Listeria meningitis can be confirmed by CSF culture.
- MRI advised where listeria meningitis is suspected.

Fetal risks
- Crosses the placenta causing chorioamnionitis, and miscarriage or preterm labour.

Neonatal risks
- Neonatal infection may be:
  - generalized septicaemia
  - pneumonia
  - meningitis.

Management of listeria in pregnancy
- High index of suspicion.
- Treatment is with high-dose amoxicillin.
- In penicillin allergy, alternatives such as trimethoprim–sulfamethoxazole can be used.
- Fetal monitoring depending on gestation.

Syphilis

Background
- Caused by *Treponema pallidum*, a spirochaete bacterium.
- STI.
- Currently relatively rare in the UK, but incidence ↑.
- At-risk groups include women who have another sexually transmitted disease, sex workers, or those living in an area with high prevalence.

Clinical features
- Infected individuals can be asymptomatic (particularly with 1° infection as they may not notice a cervical or vaginal chancre).

1° infection
- Painless ulcer ('chancre') at site of initial infection which resolves spontaneously after 3–6wks.
- Often associated with regional lymphadenopathy.

2° infection
- Systemic infection, occurring wks to mths after the 1° infection.
- Features include lymphadenopathy, systemic symptoms (fever, malaise, myalgia), rash, liver abnormalities, transient proteinuria.
- Spontaneous resolution is common.

Late infection (tertiary syphilis)
- Can occur up to 30yrs after initial infection, and in the absence of a clinically apparent 1° or 2° infection.
- Cardiovascular (aortitis), neurological (tabes dorsalis), and granulomatous lesions ('gumma') can occur.

Diagnosis
- All pregnant women: routine screening at the 1st antenatal visit.
- High risk: repeat later in pregnancy (e.g. 28 and 32wks).

Fetal risks
- The spirochaete can cross the placenta and is associated with preterm delivery and stillbirth.
- Congenital syphilis defects include:
  - 8th nerve deafness
  - Hutchinson's teeth
  - saddle nose
  - sabre shins.

Management of syphilis in pregnancy
- Treatment with penicillin:
  - <16wks—prevents virtually all congenital infection
  - >16wks—still effective in most cases.
- Contact tracing with testing ± treatment should be offered.
- Assess for other STIs ± refer to GUM clinic.

Testing for syphilis
Non-treponemal specific tests
- VDRL test.
- Rapid plasma reagin.

Treponemal-specific tests
- *T. pallidum* haemagglutination assay.
- Fluorescent treponemal antibody absorption.
- *T. pallidum* enzyme immunoassay.

⚠ False +ve results are common and can occur in SLE, tuberculosis (TB), leprosy, malaria, or IV drug users.

▶ A reactive result requires further confirmatory testing, ideally a treponemal-specific test looking at a different antigen.

Malaria

Background
- Protozoan infection (75% *Plasmodium falciparum*, others include *P. vivax*, *P. ovale*, *P. malariae*).
- Not endemic in the UK but commonly imported.
- Spread by the sporozoite-bearing female *Anopheles* mosquito.

Clinical features
There are often no specific symptoms or signs, with the infection presenting with a 'flu-like' illness, but may include:
- Fever (cyclical 'spiking').
- Rigors/chills/sweats.
- Muscle pain and general malaise.
- Confusion, drowsiness, lethargy.

Box 4.2 Features of severe malaria

Clinical features
- Impaired consciousness/prostration.
- Respiratory distress and/or pulmonary oedema.
- Seizures.
- Circulatory collapse.
- Abnormal bleeding, DIC.
- Jaundice.
- Haemoglobinuria (in absence of glucose-6-phosphate dehydrogenase deficiency).

Laboratory tests
- Severe anaemia (Hb <80g/L).
- Thrombocytopenia.
- Hypoglycaemia (<2.2mmol/L).
- Acidosis (pH <7.3).
- Hyperlactataemia.
- Hyperparasitaemia (>2% parasitized red blood cells).

Diagnosis
- Rapid antigen testing is now in widespread use.
- Thick and thin blood films can also be diagnostic:
  - >3 −ve smears, 12–24h apart to exclude the diagnosis.

Maternal risks
- Pregnancy ↑ the risk of developing severe disease.

⚠ Infection in pregnancy can be *fatal*.

Fetal risks
- Stillbirth, miscarriage, or preterm delivery.
- Congenital malaria.
- Low birth weight (2° to prematurity or FGR).

Management of malaria in pregnancy

⚠ Malaria in pregnancy should be treated as an emergency.
- Should be admitted to hospital.
- Assessment of severity (Box 4.2).
- Lumbar puncture if suspicion of cerebral malaria.
- Quinine and clindamycin is the treatment of choice for non-severe *P. falciparum* infection in the 1st trimester.
- IV artesunate should be used for non-severe *P. falciparum* infection in the 2nd and 3rd trimesters, and all severe cases.
- Antipyretics as needed.
- Close monitoring for severe malaria.
- Delivery plans entirely depend on the severity of the maternal illness, assessment of fetal well-being, and gestation, but usually malaria is not an indication for delivery.

⚠ Placental sequestration of parasites can occur, so the placenta should be sent for histological examination after delivery.

⚠ Risk of neonatal infection so paediatrics team should be informed at delivery.

⚠ Notifiable condition in the UK and needs reporting to the local health protection team.

Malaria prophylaxis in pregnancy
- Appropriate antimalarials should be taken (proguanil and chloroquine are most commonly used).
- Avoidance of exposure to mosquito bites:
  - mosquito nets
  - long sleeves and trousers (tucked into socks)
  - insect repellents—50% DEET-based mosquito repellents are the most effective and are safe in pregnancy and breast-feeding.

Further reading
RCOG (2010). The diagnosis and treatment of malaria in pregnancy. Green-top guideline no. 54b.
🕮 www.rcog.org.uk/media/rfrerkjz/gtg_54b.pdf

Toxoplasmosis

Background

- Caused by protozoan parasite *Toxoplasma gondii*.
- Spread by contact with cat faeces and by eating undercooked meat.
- Incubation <2 days.
- ~20% of UK women are immune.
- Incidence of 1° infection in pregnancy ~1:500.

Clinical features

Asymptomatic in ~80% of cases but may present with:
- Fever.
- Lymphadenopathy.

Diagnosis

Maternal infection

- Paired serology (acute phase and then repeated 10–14 days later) consistent with recent infection if:
  - isolated very high titres of IgM antibodies (may persist up to 1yr)
  - concurrent high IgM and IgG antibodies
  - 4-fold ↑ in IgG antibodies.

Fetal infection

- Diagnosed by the presence of IgM antibodies in amniotic fluid or fetal blood.
- Amniocentesis is accurate only after 20wks.
- Although ultrasound signs such as cerebral ventriculomegaly can occur, most affected fetuses have a normal scan.

Fetal risks

- Spontaneous miscarriage is common with infection in the 1st trimester (Table 4.6).
- Defects associated with 1° infection include:
  - chorioretinitis
  - microcephaly and hydrocephalus
  - intracranial calcification
  - intellectual disability.

Table 4.6 Risk of congenital defects by gestation

Gestation	Risk of transmission	Risk of congenital abnormality in Infected fetuses
<12wks	~17%	75%
12–28wks	~25%	25%
>28wks	65%	<10%

Management of toxoplasmosis in pregnancy

- Fit and healthy women have minimal risk.
- Immunocompromised women have a risk of severe disseminated illness with chorioretinitis and encephalitis.
- Spiramycin for maternal infection may ↓ the risk of fetal infection.
- If vertical transmission occurs, combination anti-toxoplasmosis therapy is used.
- Neonatal follow-up should include an ophthalmic review and cranial radiological studies.
- It is usually recommended that future pregnancies are delayed until maternal IgM antibodies have been cleared.

HIV and pregnancy

Background

- In the UK, >10% of the estimated total of individuals living with HIV are unaware of their infection.
- Those diagnosed late have an ↑ risk of death in the 1st yr after diagnosis compared to those diagnosed early.
- The risk of MTCT in the UK is <0.1% and improved after the introduction of routine antenatal screening in 1999.
- High VLs ↑ rate of MTCT.
- Pregnancy does not alter the course of the infection.
- Antiretroviral Pregnancy Registry provides the best data on teratogenicity and 1st-trimester antiretroviral therapy exposure.

⚠ Many partners of HIV +ve women are unaware of the diagnosis, so care needs to be taken when communicating in pregnancy with judicious documentation in hand-held notes, and a local system to flag the information should the mother be admitted as an emergency.

Classes of antiretroviral drugs are covered in Table 4.7.

Further reading

Antiretroviral Pregnancy Registry.
🖱 www.apregistry.com
British HIV Association (BHIVA). Current guidelines.
🖱 www.bhiva.org/guidelines.aspx

Table 4.7 Classes of antiretroviral drugs

Class of drug	Examples	Potential problems
Nucleoside analogue reverse transcriptase inhibitors	• Zidovudine (ZDV, previously AZT) • Lamivudine (3TC) • Didanosine (ddI) • Stavudine (d4T) • Abacavir (ABC) • Tenofovir • Emtricitabine	• All generally well tolerated, but reported case of: • anaemia • nausea, and vomiting • ↑ transaminases • hyperglycaemia • Lactic acidosis is a possibility when d4T and ddI are combined
Non-nucleoside analogue reverse transcriptase	• Nevirapine (NVP) • Delavirdine • Efavirenz inhibitors	• Greatest experience is with NVP, but although well tolerated there is an association with deranged liver function in women with good CD4 counts. • Rash is also reported
Protease inhibitors	• Ritonavir • Indinavir • Nelfinavir • Saquinavir	• Hyperglycaemia is a risk with new-onset diabetes or exacerbation of existing diabetes • Diarrhoea, with nausea, vomiting, and altered taste • Altered liver function reported
HIV-1 integrase strand transfer inhibitor		• Depression • Hyperglycaemia • Changes in body fat distribution

HIV: pre-pregnancy counselling

This depends on both the status of their partner and their individual VL (Table 4.8).

Table 4.8 Pre-pregnancy counselling for couples with HIV

	Positive woman, negative man	Positive man, negative woman	Positive woman, positive man
Antiretroviral therapy	Recommended but not essential if using AI	Recommended	Recommended for both
Timed ovulatory condomless sex	Recommended only if VL <50 copies/mL	Recommended only if VL <50 copies/mL	Recommended unless one or both partner detectable HIV RNA + discordant resistance
Pre-exposure prophylaxis for conception	Consider if HIV +ve partner's HIV RNA not suppressed	Consider if HIV +ve partner's HIV RNA is not suppressed	Note recommended
Artificial insemination using non-spermicidal condoms	Recommended	N/A	NA
Sperm washing	Not recommended	Not recommended unless detectable HIV RNA (suppressive ART 1st choice)	Not recommended
Sperm donor	Consider if ♂ subfertility	Consider if ♂ subfertility	Consider if ♂ subfertility
Egg donor	Consider if ♀ subfertility	Consider if ♀ subfertility	Consider if ♀ subfertility

Source: data from BHIVA/BASHH/FSRH guidelines for the sexual & reproductive health of people living with HIV. www.bhiva.org/file/zryuNVwnXcxMC/SRH-guidelines-for-consultation-2017.pdf

HIV: antenatal management

Combination antiretroviral therapy (cART)

- All HIV +ve women should start cART during pregnancy and continue lifelong (regardless of CD4 count).
- cART should be commenced:
  - within the 1st trimester if VL >100,000 copies/mL (c/mL) and/or CD4 cell count <200 cells/mm^3
  - as soon as they are able to do so in the 2nd trimester, by 24wks at the latest.
- Treatment is started as recommended in the BHIVA guidelines.
- An integrase inhibitor-based regimen is suggested as the 3rd agent of choice with high baseline VL (>100,000c/mL), where cART is being started late in pregnancy or where it is failing to suppress the virus.
- No dose alterations are routinely advised in pregnancy.
- Zidovudine monotherapy can be used in women declining cART who have a baseline VL of <10,000c/mL and a CD4 >350 cells/mm^3 and who consent to a CD.

Hepatitis B or C co-infection

- Requires management alongside a clinician experienced in co-infection, with hepatology input if significant cirrhosis.
- Vaginal delivery can be supported if the woman has fully suppressed HIV VL on cART, irrespective of HBV/HCV VL.

Special circumstances

- Invasive prenatal diagnostic testing should not be performed until after maternal HIV status is known, and ideally deferred until VL<50c/mL.
- If not on cART and the invasive diagnostic test procedure cannot be delayed until VL<50c/mL, can start cART to include raltegravir and be given a single dose of nevirapine 2–4h prior to the procedure.
- ECV can be performed in HIV +ve women.

Late presentation

- Women presenting in labour/with rupture of membranes/requiring delivery without a documented HIV result must be recommended to have an HIV diagnostic point-of-care test.
- A reactive point-of-care test result must prompt interventions to prevent MTCT without waiting for formal serological confirmation.
- If presenting after 28wks start cART without delay as per BHIVA guidelines.

⚠ An untreated women presenting in labour at term should be given a combination of treatments (see BHIVA guidelines in 'Further reading').

Antenatal management of HIV

▶ All cases of HIV in pregnancy (diagnosed before or during pregnancy) in the UK should be reported to the national study of HIV in pregnancy and childhood (even if the pregnancy is not continued to term).
▶ Cases can be reported online at:
🖰 www.ucl.ac.uk/nshpc/pregnancies-hiv-positive-women-0

* Newly-diagnosed women do not require other baseline tests in addition to routine antenatal screening.
* HIV resistance testing prior to treatment initiation (except in women presenting late).
* Sexual health screening with treatment of infection according to British Association for Sexual Health and HIV (BASHH) guidelines.
* Encouraged to continue cART post delivery.
* Women who conceive on cART should have a minimum of one CD4 count at baseline and one at delivery.
* When cART is started in pregnancy:
  * CD4 cell count should be performed at initiation
  * VL should be performed 2–4wks later, at least once every trimester, at 36wks, and at delivery
  * LFTs should be performed at initiation of cART and at each antenatal visit.
* If VL not suppressed (to <50c/mL) at 36wks with cART:
  * review adherence and concomitant medication
  * perform resistance testing if appropriate
  * consider therapeutic drug monitoring
  * optimize to best regimen
  * consider intensification.
* Fetal USS should be carried out as per national guidance.
* The combined screening test for trisomy 21 is recommended as this has the best sensitivity and specificity and will minimize the number of women who may need invasive testing.
* Non-invasive prenatal testing should be considered for women with a high-risk result as this may ↓ the need for invasive procedures.

Further reading
BHIVA. Current guidelines.
🖰 www.bhiva.org/guidelines.aspx
BASHH. BASHH guidelines.
🖰 www.bashh.org/guidelines

HIV: intrapartum

Mode of delivery

- This should depend on:
  - VL at 36wks
  - presence/absence of obstetric complications
  - chronology of an individual's treatment and response to treatment.

⚠ Vaginal delivery does not require any modifications to standard intrapartum care.

VL <50c/mL

- No obstetric complications → support vaginal delivery (including vaginal birth after Caesarean (VBAC)).
- CD for obstetric indication only.

VL 50–399c/mL

- Consider elective CD (depending on factors including VL and trajectory, treatment duration, adherence, obstetric issues).

VL ≥400c/mL

- Elective CD advised at 38–39wks.

Rupture of membranes (ROM)

⚠ In all cases of *term* prelabour ROM, delivery should be expedited.

VL <50c/mL

- Immediate induction of labour is recommended.
- Low threshold for treatment of intrapartum pyrexia.

VL 50–999c/mL

- Consider CD (depending on factors including actual VL and trajectory, treatment duration, adherence, obstetric issues).

VL >1000c/mL

- Immediate CD recommended.

⚠ If ROM between 34 and 37wks, GBS prophylaxis advised.

PPROM at <34wks

- IM steroids administered as per national guidelines.
- Optimize virological control.
- Delivery timing and mode based on MDT discussion.

Intrapartum IV zidovudine if

- VL >1000c/mL + labour/ROM/admission for elective CD.
- VL unknown + not on treatment + labour/ROM.

▶ *Not* required if VL<1000c/mL + on cART.

HIV: postnatal concerns

Neonatal management

- Post-exposure prophylaxis (PEP) should be started within 4h of birth.
- Neonate should be risk stratified by the paediatric team so as to decide length and type of PEP treatment.
- Co-trimoxazole prophylaxis for *Pneumocystis jirovecii* pneumonia is recommended from 1mth of age if HIV PCR is +ve at any stage or if the infant is confirmed to be diagnosed with HIV,

⚠ This should only be stopped if HIV infection is subsequently excluded.

Postnatal management and follow-up

- All women are recommended to continue cART postpartum.
- Should be followed up at 4–6wks.

Breast-feeding

- Use of formula milk eliminates the risk of HIV exposure after birth.
- If not breast-feeding, the use of cabergoline to suppress lactation should be considered.
- Women on cART with VL<50mL and good adherence, who choose to breast-feed can be supported in this, but there is a low risk of MTCT.

Further reading

BHIVA. Current guidelines.
💾 www.bhiva.org/guidelines.aspx

BASHH. BASHH guidelines.
💾 www.bashh.org/guideline

Vaccination in pregnancy

Vaccination

- Live-attenuated vaccines (e.g. rubella, polio, MMR, varicella zoster virus) are contraindicated in pregnancy.
- Passive immunization with specific human immunoglobulin is safe and may provide important protection (e.g. VZIG).
- Women who are HBsAg −ve but considered at high risk should be offered vaccination in pregnancy.
- Vaccinations for travel should be considered on an individual basis, and the small risk from the vaccine compared with the risk from contracting the disease.
- See Table 4.9 for an overview.

Table 4.9 Vaccinations in pregnancy

Infection	Issues
COVID-19	Recommended at any stage of pregnancy
Pneumococcus	Inactivated virus, so can be used in pregnancy
Cholera	Limited efficacy therefore not recommended
Hepatitis A	Low risk, but consider human normal immunoglobulin for short periods
Meningococcus	Safety unknown, consider if high risk
Rabies	Consider immunoglobulin for PEP
Tetanus	Safe in pregnancy
Yellow fever	Safety unknown, consider if high risk

Medical disorders in pregnancy

Epilepsy: overview

- 0.6% of pregnant women have epilepsy.
- Most women have been diagnosed before conception.
- If a seizure occurs for the 1st time in pregnancy there is a wide differential diagnosis (Box 5.1).
- Seizure frequency can ↑ (37%), ↓ (13%), or remain unchanged (50%).
- Women with poorly controlled epilepsy and those who stop medication are at the highest risk of ↑ seizure frequency.

⚠ The fetus usually tolerates seizures without long-term sequelae, but there is ↑ risk of fetal death with status epilepticus.

Fetal risks

There is an ↑ risk of major congenital anomalies (2–5%) in women with epilepsy. Most of this risk is due to anticonvulsant medication; however, women not on antiepileptic drugs still have a higher risk than the general population. The use of multiple drugs carries a higher risk to the fetus than monotherapy. Higher doses lead to ↑ risk. Dividing doses and ↓ peak blood levels may be beneficial. Ideally, any change in anticonvulsant therapy should be undertaken before pregnancy.

▶ Folic acid (5mg daily) should be advised for all women as this ↓ the risk of some anomalies.

Fetal risks of anticonvulsant therapy

- Teratogenicity: congenital anomalies or fetal anticonvulsant syndrome.
- Neonatal withdrawal.
- Vitamin K deficiency (enzyme inducers) and haemorrhagic disease of newborn.
- Developmental delay and behavioural problems.

Drugs used in treatment of epilepsy

These have varying risks of congenital anomalies and can be divided according to their ability to induce liver enzymes.

Enzyme-inducing anticonvulsants

- Carbamazepine.
- Topiramate.
- Phenobarbital.
- Phenytoin.
- Primidone.

Non-enzyme-inducing anticonvulsants

- Lamotrigine.
- Levetiracetam.
- Valproate (Box 5.1)
- Gabapentin.
- Ethosuximide.

Box 5.1 Differential diagnosis of 1st seizure in pregnancy
- Eclampsia.
- Epilepsy.
- Infection:
  - encephalitis
  - abscess.
- Metabolic:
  - drug or alcohol withdrawal
  - drug toxicity
  - hypoglycaemia
  - electrolyte imbalance (e.g. ↓ Na, ↓ Ca).
- Space-occupying lesion.
- Vascular:
  - cerebral venous sinus thrombosis
  - thrombotic thrombocytopenic purpura (TTP)
  - cerebral infarction or haemorrhage.

💣 All patients who present with their 1st seizure in pregnancy should have imaging of the brain with CT or, preferably, MRI and be reviewed by a neurologist.

Use of valproate in women of childbearing age

Doctors in the European Union are advised not to prescribe valproate for epilepsy or bipolar disorder in pregnant women, in women who can become pregnant, or in girls, unless other treatments are ineffective or not tolerated.

Those for whom valproate is the only option for epilepsy or bipolar disorder should be advised on the use of effective contraception, and treatment should be started and supervised by a doctor experienced in treating these conditions.

Epilepsy: management

Pre-pregnancy counselling

- Involve a neurologist if clarity about diagnosis is required.
- Optimize treatment, achieve seizure control, and educate patient.
- Use the least number of drugs at the lowest dose to control seizures to minimize risk of congenital anomalies.
- In conjunction with epilepsy team, consider stopping drugs if seizure free for >2yrs (warn of risk of seizures and implications for driving).
- All women should take folic acid 5mg daily for at least 12wks before conception and continue until delivery (↓ risk of neural tube defects).
- Risk of epilepsy in the child (4% if one parent affected, 15% if both parents affected).

Antenatal care

- Do not change medication in pregnancy if well controlled, and emphasize the importance of compliance with medication.
- Detailed anomaly scan (neural tube defects, facial clefts, and cardiac abnormalities).
- Consider fetal echocardiography at 22–24wks in patients requiring multiple antiepileptic medications.
- Insufficient evidence for routine 3rd trimester maternal vitamin K.
- General advice (showers rather than baths, avoid sleep deprivation).
- The levels of some antiepileptics, particularly lamotrigine, may ↓ precipitously and often require a 30–50% ↑ in dose by 12–20wks.

💧 There is no role for *routine* monitoring of drug levels (it may be useful in women with ↑ seizure frequency, suspected non-compliance, concern over toxic side effects, or polypharmacy).

Intrapartum care

- Aim for vaginal delivery (CD should be for obstetric indications; seizures are not an indication unless in status epilepticus).
- Labour is associated with ↑ risk of seizures due to:
  - sleep deprivation
  - ↓ absorption of drugs
  - hyperventilation.

▶ Additional medication at delivery is not routinely required in women with epilepsy.

- Control seizures with benzodiazepines.
- Ensure usual anticonvulsants are taken at the correct time.

Postnatal care

- Neonatal vitamin K to ↓ risk of haemorrhagic disease of the newborn.
- Breast-feeding is encouraged.
- If the anticonvulsant dose was ↑ in pregnancy, it should be ↓ back to pre-pregnancy levels slowly postpartum.
- Contraception with enzyme-inducing drugs:
  - COCP containing 50 micrograms oestrogen with a shorter pill-free interval
  - progestogen-only pill (POP) is less effective
  - intrauterine contraceptive device (IUCD) is ideal.
- General advice (bathing and feeding) to minimize risk of harm to baby from seizures.
- ↑ awareness regarding risk from sudden unexplained death in epilepsy (SUDEP).

Further reading

Epilepsy Foundation.
℘ www.epilepsy.com.

Epilepsy Society.
℘ www.epilepsysociety.org.uk/

Women With Epilepsy.
℘ www.womenwithepilepsy.co.uk

Stroke

- Ischaemic and haemorrhagic stroke are rare in women of reproductive age, but there is an ↑ risk in the postpartum period.
- 9-fold ↑ risk for ischaemic and 28-fold ↑ for haemorrhagic stroke in the 1st 6wks postpartum compared with non-pregnant women.
- Symptoms include:
  - abrupt onset of weakness
  - sensory loss
  - dysphasia.

Common risk factors for ischaemic stroke at all ages include:
- Smoking.
- Diabetes.
- Hypertension.
- Hypercholesterolaemia.

See Box 5.2.

Cryptogenic stroke

- Defined as an infarction not clearly attributable despite extensive investigation to a definite:
  - cardioembolism
  - large artery atherosclerosis
  - or small artery disease.
- More common in young people.

Management in pregnancy

Individuals who have previously had a stroke are unlikely to have a further event in pregnancy, unless stroke was caused by dissection (usually vertebral artery).

Ischaemic
- Antiplatelet agent throughout pregnancy.
- If atrial fibrillation (AF) present, anticoagulation may be appropriate.
- Look for underlying causes.

Haemorrhagic
- Look for underlying structural cause and treat if possible.
- Venous thromboembolism (VTE) risk assessment (LMWH likely to be contraindicated in acute setting).

Box 5.2 Causes of stroke in pregnancy

Ischaemic
- Pre-eclampsia/eclampsia
- Central nervous system (CNS) vasculitis.
- Carotid artery dissection.
- Emboli:
  - mitral stenosis
  - peripartum cardiomyopathy
  - ondocarditis
  - paradoxical emboli.
- Coagulopathies:
  - thrombophilia
  - antiphospholipid syndrome.
- TTP.
- Cerebral vein thrombosis.

Haemorrhagic
- Pre-eclampsia/eclampsia.
- DIC.
- Arteriovenous malformation (AVM).
- Ruptured aneurysm.
- CNS vasculitis.

Investigations

A neurologist should be involved in the investigation and management:
- MRI or CT scan of head.
- Cerebral angiography ± venography.
- Echocardiogram and consideration of bubble study.
- Carotid Dopplers.
- Thrombophilia screen and antiphospholipid antibodies.
- Homocysteine level/methylenetetrahydrofolate reductase (MTHFR) screen.

Subarachnoid haemorrhage

Outside pregnancy the most common cause is a ruptured berry aneurysm, but AVMs may dilate in pregnancy due to the effect of oestrogen, resulting in a similar incidence.

Presentation

- Headache.
- Vomiting.
- Loss of or impaired consciousness.
- Neck stiffness.
- Focal neurological signs.

Management

- Early treatment is recommended to ↓ the chance of subsequent bleeding (the risk is high for AVM).
- Surgery is usually recommended, excision of the AVM, coiling, or clipping.
- Tight BP control recommended.

Delivery

- Labour is a high-risk time for bleeding, so elective CD should be recommended if the lesion is inoperable.
- If the lesion has been successfully treated, vaginal delivery is recommended (a longer passive 2nd stage with early use of assisted delivery may ↓ the risk of rebleeding).
- Epidural anaesthesia is contraindicated with a recent subarachnoid haemorrhage due to ↑ intracranial pressure.

Cardiac disease: management

The pattern of heart disease in pregnancy has changed over the past few decades. Congenital heart disease is now more common than rheumatic and ischaemic heart disease has become a common cardiac cause of death in pregnancy.

⚠ Normal pregnancy is associated with significant haemodynamic changes which may not be tolerated in women with heart disease.

Antenatal management

- MDT management with an obstetrician, cardiologist, anaesthetist, and cardiothoracic surgeon if required.
- Preconception counselling should be offered to:
  - optimize maternal cardiovascular status (may involve surgery)
  - modify medication
  - discuss maternal and fetal risks of pregnancy.
- The ability of a woman to tolerate pregnancy depends on:
  - exercise tolerance (New York Heart Association (NYHA) class)
  - presence of pulmonary hypertension or left heart obstruction
  - presence of cyanosis.
- Consider whether discussion about TOP is appropriate (e.g. for women with pulmonary hypertension).
- Correct factors that may lead to decompensation (anaemia, infection, hypertension, and arrhythmias).
- Monitor for signs of heart failure and consider serial maternal echo.
- Monitor fetal growth by serial USS as risk of FGR and death *in utero*, especially with maternal cyanosis.

Intrapartum and postpartum management

- A clear intrapartum care plan should be agreed before labour.
- Aim for a vaginal delivery usually with a short active 2nd stage.

⚠ CD is indicated with an aortic root >4.5cm, left ventricular ejection fraction <30%, aortic dissection, or aneurysm.

- In labour, maternal cardiac ± invasive monitoring may be required (the fetus should be continuously monitored).
- Avoid aortocaval compression.
- Blood loss should be minimized by active management of 3rd stage followed by an infusion of oxytocin, but ergometrine and prostaglandin F2α (PGF2α, dinoprost) should be avoided.
- Epidural analgesia may ↓ changes in heart rate and BP associated with pain (low-dose epidural is usually well tolerated, but may cause serious complications with restricted cardiac output).
- Strict fluid balance is mandatory as there is a much higher risk of pulmonary oedema the 1st few days postpartum.
- Discuss contraception before discharge.

⚠ Risk of congenital heart disease in fetus is 3–5% if either parent is affected. Some conditions carry higher risk. It is higher if mother rather than father is affected. Arrange for fetal echocardiography at 22wks.

Haemodynamic changes in normal pregnancy

• Peripheral vasodilatation leads to a ↓ in systemic vascular resistance.
• Cardiac output ↑ by:
  • 40% during pregnancy (↑ heart rate and ↑ stroke volume)
  • 15% in the 1st stage of labour
  • 50% in the 2nd stage of labour.
• Following delivery there is further ↑ cardiac output due to ↑ venous return from:
  • relief of vena caval obstruction
  • tonic uterine contraction (expels blood into systemic circulation).
• Colloid osmotic pressure ↓ leading to ↑ susceptibility to pulmonary oedema.
• Hypercoagulability.

▶ These changes start in early pregnancy around 6/40wks

Artificial heart valves

Women with artificial heart valves often have near-normal cardiac function and therefore tolerate pregnancy well. The main maternal and fetal risk is from anticoagulation, which must be continued throughout pregnancy in women with mechanical heart valves as without it there is a high morbidity (stroke) and mortality (valve thrombosis). The choice of anticoagulant should be made after discussion with the patient. Warfarin better protects against valve thrombosis, therefore is better for the mother, but heparin is preferable for the fetus.

⚠ There is a 4–12% risk of an embolic event per pregnancy.

Management

- Antenatally there are two options in women with mechanical valves:
  - continue warfarin throughout pregnancy
  - conceive on warfarin, change to LMWH from 6–12wks to minimize risk of warfarin embryopathy, then use warfarin from 12 to 36wks.
- Risk of bleeding in labour with warfarin (mother and baby) is high:
  - all patients should be changed to LMWH at 36wks (or earlier if concerns with preterm labour)
  - LMWH should be stopped in labour and restarted after delivery
  - if the woman labours within 2wks of stopping warfarin, a CD is advised
  - warfarin should be restarted 7–10 days postpartum.
- Reversal in the event of life-threatening bleeding:
  - *warfarin*—urgent administration of prothrombin concentrate and vitamin K
  - *LMWH*—protamine sulfate.
- Heparin and warfarin can safely be given to breast-feeding mothers.
- Low-dose aspirin should be given with LMWH because of its antithrombotic effects and relative safety.
- Titrate LMWH optimal dose based on anti-Xa effect, both trough (pre-dose) and 4h peak levels; check anti-Xa every 2–3wks.
- See Table 5.1.

Tissue valves

- Bioprosthetic or homograft valves do not require anticoagulation but aspirin would be advised.
- They have a shorter life expectancy than mechanical valves, so structural deterioration may occur in pregnancy.
- Anticoagulation would still be required with arrhythmias, e.g. AF.

Anticoagulant drugs and risks

Low-molecular-weight heparin
- ↓ maternal bleeding.
- No risk to fetus (does not cross the placenta).
- ↑ risk of embolic events.
- ↑ risk of valve thrombosis—may require emergency valve replacement and has a high mortality.
- Osteoporosis and heparin-induced thrombocytopenia are very uncommon side effects (compared to unfractionated heparin)

Warfarin
- ↑ risk of miscarriage.
- Risk of warfarin embryopathy (risk dose dependent: ↑ if >5mg/day).
- Maternal and fetal/neonatal bleeding (due to ↓ vitamin K level in fetus).
- Long half-life.

Table 5.1 Suggested target anti-Xa levels if on LMWH

	Peak (4–6h post dose)	Trough
Aortic valve replacement	0.8–1.2U/L	≥0.6U/L
Mitral valve or right-sided valve replacement	1.0–1.2U/L	≥0.6U/L

Further reading

European Society of Cardiology (2018). 2018 ESC Guidelines for the management of cardiovascular diseases during pregnancy.
🔗 https://academic.oup.com/eurheartj/article/39/34/3165/5078465

Acquired heart disease

Mitral stenosis

- This is the most common lesion of rheumatic heart disease (90%).
- ↑ Risk of pulmonary oedema in pregnancy, greatest in labour:
  - ↑ in heart rate in pregnancy, ↓ ventricular filling time, and ↑ pulmonary blood volume → pulmonary oedema
  - 1st-line treatment for pulmonary oedema should be diuretics. β-blockers also used to ↓ heart rate and improve left atrial emptying (add digoxin if in AF), but are less attractive in acute heart failure.
- Mitral stenosis is the most likely lesion to require treatment for pulmonary oedema, heart failure, or surgery in pregnancy.
- With severe mitral stenosis, consider surgery before pregnancy.
- Risk of thromboembolism is ~1.5% in pregnancy, higher with left atrial enlargement and AF (treat with LMWH).
- Mitral regurgitation is well tolerated in pregnancy; heart failure and endocarditis are rare.

Aortic stenosis

- Aortic valve disease is less common than mitral valve disease (it is less likely to be 2° to rheumatic disease, more likely to be due to a congenital bicuspid valve).
- Severity and risk of complications is dependent on the gradient across the valve: >100mmHg in the non-pregnant state is severe. Gradient is expected to ↑ in pregnancy due to the cardiovascular changes, the absence of this is also concerning.

⚠ Associated symptoms are chest pain, syncope, and sudden death.

Pulmonary hypertension and Eisenmenger's syndrome

- 1° pulmonary hypertension is an idiopathic abnormality of the pulmonary vasculature.
- In Eisenmenger's syndrome there is:
  - pulmonary hypertension with reversal of the initial left-to-right shunt and consequent cyanosis
  - a fixed high pulmonary vascular resistance and inability to ↑ pulmonary blood flow
  - slowly worsening hypoxaemia.

⚠ Maternal mortality is high (25%) but has improved. Death classically occurs in the 1st few days postpartum.

Management of pulmonary hypertension and Eisenmenger's syndrome in pregnancy

- Women should be advised about effective contraception, and termination discussed if pregnancy occurs.
- Pregnancy should be managed in a pulmonary hypertension centre with MDT care from cardiologists, obstetricians, and anaesthetists.
- Antenatal care includes:
  - medical treatment (dependent on underlying aetiology)
  - anticoagulation
  - oxygen
  - serial fetal growth USS.
- Avoid manoeuvres that suddenly ↑ vagal tone (causes bradycardia) and venous return, e.g. ergometrine.
- Avoid PGF2α (associated with pulmonary vasoconstriction and pulmonary hypertensive crisis).
- Delivery should be in a high dependency unit with tight control of blood pressure, fluid balance, and oxygen saturations.

💣 Mode of delivery and epidural use should be individualized.

Myocardial infarction

Myocardial infarction

Remains rare in pregnancy, but incidence has been ↑ due to ↑ age at pregnancy and lifestyle factors.

⚠ Mortality high (20% immediate, 32% overall); highest in puerperium.

- Risk factors for ischaemic heart disease include:
  - smoking
  - hypertension
  - diabetes
  - hypercholesterolaemia
  - family history
  - obesity.
- There may be atypical symptoms, such as abdominal or epigastric pain, and vomiting or dizziness.
- Diagnosis is based on history, electrocardiogram (ECG) changes, and elevated troponin.

⚠ A single normal ECG especially in a pain-free individual does not rule out ischaemia. Serial ECGs should be considered.

- Should be managed on a coronary care unit by cardiologists.
- 1° percutaneous coronary intervention is the treatment of choice for ST elevation myocardial infarction in the pregnant woman.
- Thrombolysis is associated with higher fetal loss rates, but should be considered if 1° percutaneous coronary intervention is not available.

Delivery

- Aim for a vaginal delivery with a short 2nd stage (avoid ergometrine as it can cause coronary artery spasm).

Past history of myocardial infarction

- Should have a pre-pregnancy assessment of cardiac function (echo and exercise test) with counselling on the basis of the results.
- Aspirin should be continued in pregnancy.

Peripartum cardiomyopathy

- This is a rare condition; incidence <1:2000.
- Occurs in the last few wks of pregnancy and the 1st few mths after delivery.
- ▶ A diagnosis is only made when other causes have been excluded.

Risk factors

- ↑ maternal age.
- Multiparity.
- Multiple pregnancy.
- Afro-Caribbean ethnicity.
- Poor socioeconomic class.
- Hypertension in pregnancy.

Presentation

- Breathlessness.
- Palpitations.
- Oedema.
- Poor exercise tolerance.
- Embolic phenomena.

Diagnosis

Global dilatation of all four chambers of the heart (seen on echo) with exclusion of other causes of cardiomyopathy.

Management

- Supportive:
  - should include ACEIs (after delivery)
  - anticoagulation (●⁎ immunosuppression has been tried).
- If the diagnosis is made antenatally, delivery is indicated.
- Consider heart transplantation if there is heart failure despite optimal medical therapy.

⚠ Mortality 25–50% (long-term survival likely if patient survives initial episode).

⚠ Recurrence risk high (up to 50%). Discourage further pregnancies if cardiac function does not return to normal as there is a greater chance of further morbidity and mortality in a subsequent pregnancy if this is the case.

Congenital heart disease

Marfan's syndrome

This is an autosomal dominant condition (fibrillin gene on chromosome 15) caused by a defect in fibrillin synthesis (genetic testing is available). The main risk is of aortic dissection and rupture. This risk ↑ if there is a family history of rupture and/or there is evidence of aortic root dilatation.

Management
- Monthly echo for aortic dimensions until 8wks postpartum.
- β-Blockers should be given for hypertension or aortic dilatation as they are shown to ↓ rate of dilatation and risk of dissection.
- Aim for vaginal delivery with a short 2nd stage (if aortic root dilatation is present, deliver by CD).

Risk of mortality
- <1% if aortic root <4cm.
- >25% if aortic root >4cm.
- Pregnancy is contraindicated with an aortic root >4.5cm until aortic root replacement.

Coarctation of aorta

- Usually been corrected before pregnancy.
- Main risk is of aortic dissection; this risk is highest if there is hypertension present (usually treated with β-blockers).
- Also associated with berry aneurysms, which can bleed in pregnancy causing cerebral haemorrhage.
- If uncorrected or recurrent, coarctation risks include:
  - hypertension
  - heart failure
  - angina.
- Avoid balloon angioplasty in pregnancy (↑ risk of dissection).
- CD advisable if there is associated aortic dilatation.

Fallot's tetralogy

- The majority will have had surgery and the risk will depend on not only the type of surgery but also its success.
- There are two main risks:
  - paradoxical emboli can pass through the shunt causing strokes
  - cyanosis affects the fetus → ↑ risk of miscarriage, FGR, prematurity, and death *in utero*.
- Risks are minimized by anticoagulation (prophylactic dose LMWH), bed rest, and oxygen.

Most common congenital cardiac lesions seen in pregnancy
- Patent ductus arteriosus.
- ASD.
- VSD.

Pregnancy is generally well tolerated in women with these lesions.

Further reading

European Society of Cardiology (2018). 2018 ESC Guidelines on the management of cardiovascular diseases during pregnancy.
🔗 https://academic.oup.com/eurheartj/article/39/34/3165/5078465

Anaemia

Iron-deficiency anaemia

- The most common cause of anaemia in pregnancy (90% of cases).

Diagnosis

- ↓ mean corpuscular volume (MCV), ↓ mean corpuscular haemoglobin concentration (MCHC), and ↓ ferritin.
- Often asymptomatic and detected on screening.
- Treat by oral iron supplementation:
  - vitamin C (orange juice) ↑ absorption
  - tea ↓ absorption.
- The expected improvement in Hb is ~10g/L/wk.
- In situations such as multiple pregnancy or known depletion of iron stores, consider prophylactic supplementation even if no anaemia.
- Parenteral iron should be considered in those who do not tolerate the oral preparations (corrects the anaemia more rapidly).
- If severe iron-deficiency anaemia (Hb <70g/L) is diagnosed near term, parenteral iron is advisable and blood transfusion may be required.

Folate deficiency

- Also common in pregnancy.

Risk factors

- Poor nutritional status.
- Haematological problems with a rapid turnover of blood cells, e.g. haemolytic anaemia and haemoglobinopathies.
- Drug interaction with folate metabolism, e.g. antiepileptics.

Diagnosis

- ↑ MCV, ↓ serum folate, and ↓ red cell folate.
- Folic acid given preconception and in early pregnancy to ↓ risk of neural tube defects (400 micrograms/day for general population).
- Women with high risk of neural tube defects should take 5mg folic acid daily, this includes those women:
  - on anticonvulsants
  - with a previous child affected with a neural tube defect
  - with demonstrated deficiency
  - with diabetes
  - with a BMI >35kg/m²
  - with sickle cell disease.

Vitamin B$_{12}$ deficiency

- Seen in pernicious anaemia, terminal ileum disease, and strict vegans.
- Uncommon to make a new diagnosis in pregnancy.
- The normal range for vitamin B$_{12}$ in pregnancy is ↓ than in non-pregnant individuals, so caution is required when interpreting vitamin B$_{12}$ results in pregnancy.
- Women with a previous diagnosis should continue treatment throughout pregnancy.

Physiological adaptation in pregnancy

- Plasma volume expansion (50%) greater than red cell mass ↑ (25%).
- This leads to physiological dilution with ↓ Hb and ↓ haematocrit.
- Anaemia is diagnosed if Hb <105g/L in pregnancy.
- There should be no change in MCV or MCHC in normal pregnancy.
- Normally pregnancy has:
  - 2–3-fold ↑ in iron requirements
  - 10–20-fold ↑ in folate requirements in pregnancy.

Further reading

Pavord S et al. (2012). UK guidelines on the management of iron deficiency in pregnancy. *Br J Haematol.* 156:588–600.

Sickle cell disease

Inheritance is autosomal recessive. Most commonly seen in people of Afro-Caribbean origin, but also occurs in those from the Middle East, Mediterranean, and Indian subcontinent. As diagnosis has usually been made in childhood, it is rare to make a new diagnosis in pregnancy.

Pathophysiology

Results in distortion of the shape of red cells into a rigid sickle shape. This leads to microvascular blockage, stasis, and infarction in any organ in the body. Crises can be precipitated by infection, dehydration, hypoxia, and cold.

Risks in pregnancy

- Crises are more common during pregnancy.
- ↑ Risk of pre-eclampsia.
- ↑ Risk of delivery by CS 2° to fetal distress.

Management

- MDT care with an obstetrician and haematologist.
- Pre-pregnancy counselling should involve screening of the partner (if the partner is a carrier, consider prenatal diagnosis).
- Stop iron-chelating agents before pregnancy.
- If there is a history of iron overload, arrange a maternal echo and MRI of liver.
- Folic acid 5mg/day.
- Penicillin prophylaxis for hyposplenism.
- Monitor Hb and HbS % and arrange transfusion if necessary (may have red cell antibodies from multiple transfusions).
- Screen for urine infection and proteinuria at each visit.
- Treatment of a crisis involves:
  - adequate analgesia
  - oxygen
  - rehydration
  - antibiotics if infection suspected
  - exchange transfusion may be required in severe crises.
- Regular assessment of fetal growth with USS.
- Aim for vaginal delivery ensuring adequate hydration and avoiding hypoxia (continuous fetal monitoring as ↑ risk of fetal distress).
- Consider antenatal and postnatal thromboprophylaxis.

Clinical features of sickle cell disease

- Haemolytic anaemia.
- Painful crises.
- Hyposplenism (chronic damage to the spleen results in atrophy).
- ↑ risk of infection (UTI, pyelonephritis, pneumonia, puerperal sepsis).
- Avascular necrosis of bone.
- ↑ risk of thromboembolic disease (pulmonary embolism (PE), stroke).
- Acute chest syndrome (fever, chest pain, tachypnoea, ↑ WCC, pulmonary infiltrates).
- *Iron overload:* leads to cardiomyopathy.
- Maternal mortality 2%.

Fetal risks in sickle cell disease

- Miscarriage.
- FGR.
- Prematurity.
- Stillbirth.

⚠ Perinatal mortality is ↑ 4–6× compared to the general population.

Further reading

RCOG (2011). Management of sickle cell disease in pregnancy. Green-top guideline no. 61.
⚲ https://www.rcog.org.uk/media/nyinaztx/gtg_61.pdf

Thalassaemia

Adult haemoglobin (HbA) is made up from two α- and two β-globin chains associated with a haem complex. There are four genes for α-globin and two for β-globin chain production. An adult's blood is normally made up of HbA ($\alpha_2\beta_2$, 97%), HbA$_2$ ($\alpha_2\delta_2$, 1.5–3.5%), and fetal haemoglobin (HbF) ($\alpha_2\gamma_2$, <1%). Thalassaemia is a group of genetic conditions → impaired production of the globin chains and resulting in red cells with inadequate Hb content. HbF consists of two α and two γ chains, so a fetus cannot be affected by β-thalassaemia.

α-Thalassaemia

- Caused by defects in 1–4 of the α-globin genes.
- Most common in individuals from South-east Asia.
- α-Thalassaemia trait has two ($\alpha0$) or three ($\alpha+$) normal genes: women are usually asymptomatic, but may become anaemic in pregnancy.
- In HbH disease, there is one normal gene and three abnormal:
  - unstable Hb is formed by tetramers of the β chain
  - chronic haemolysis results and iron overload is common
  - offspring will have either $\alpha0$ or $\alpha+$ thalassaemia.
- α-Thalassaemia major (Hb Barts) has no functional α genes and is incompatible with life:
  - fetuses are often hydropic and born prematurely
  - severe early-onset pre-eclampsia often complicates pregnancy.

β-Thalassaemia

- β-Thalassaemia trait has one defective gene and women are asymptomatic but may become anaemic in pregnancy.
- It is most common in individuals from Cyprus and Asia.
- Incidence of β-thalassaemia minor is 1:10,000 in the UK compared with 1:7 in Cyprus:
  - offspring have a 1:4 chance of β-thalassaemia major.
- β-Thalassaemia major has two defective genes and women are often transfusion dependent:
  - iron overload can occur
  - puberty is often delayed
  - there is subfertility and only very few pregnancies have been reported.
- Repeated transfusions cause iron overload, → endocrine, hepatic, and cardiac dysfunction:
  - heart failure is the most common cause of death
  - iron-chelating therapy can ↓ the incidence of iron overload
  - the condition can be cured by bone marrow transplant.

Management of thalassaemia in pregnancy

- Check ferritin in early pregnancy: give iron supplements only if iron deficient.
- Women need folic acid 5mg daily.
- If the woman has thalassaemia, the partner needs screening:
  - if positive, the couple need counselling on the risk of pregnancy with thalassaemia major
  - prenatal diagnosis should be offered.

Screening for thalassaemia in pregnancy

- Screen all women of Mediterranean, Middle Eastern, Indian, Asian, African, or West Indian ethnic origin by Hb electrophoresis at booking.
- In $\alpha 0$ and $\alpha +$ thalassaemia no abnormal Hb is made and there is no excess in HbA_2 or HbF:
  - Hb electrophoresis is normal
  - the diagnosis can be confirmed by globin chain synthesis studies or DNA analysis of nucleated cells.
- In α-thalassaemia there is a ↑ concentration of HbA_2 and/or HbF.
- Suspect the diagnosis of thalassaemia in the presence of:
  - low MCV
  - low MCHC
  - microcytic anaemia with normal MCHC (which differs from iron deficiency where the MCHC is also low).

Haemophilia

X-linked inherited deficiency of clotting factor VIII or IX that causes problems with bleeding. Haemophilia A (factor VIII deficiency) is 4× more common than haemophilia B (factor IX deficiency). Can vary in severity depending on the clotting factor levels: mild (>5% to <40%), moderate (1–5%), or severe (<1%). Severity tends to be similar within members of one family. The use of prophylactic recombinant factor replacement from childhood has now dramatically changed the outlook and life expectancy for affected children.

Incidence

- 15:100,000 males.
- Female carriers have one abnormal gene and do not usually have significant bleeding problems, but the clotting factor level is ~50% of normal (may be much ↓ due to lyonization).
- Female carriers have a 50% chance of having an affected son and a 50% chance of having carrier daughters.
- An affected male will produce carrier daughters and unaffected sons.
- 1/3 of newly diagnosed infants have no family history and are the result of a new mutation.

Prenatal diagnosis and antenatal care

- Manage jointly with haematologist.
- Genetic counselling and prenatal diagnosis (if the mutation is known by DNA family studies) should be offered to affected families.
- If the mutation is not known, fetal cell free DNA testing from a maternal blood sample can be used to determine fetal sex.
- Check hepatitis serology if previous exposure to blood products.
- Maternal coagulation factor activity should be checked at booking, at 28 and 34wks, and when clinically indicated (e.g. before surgery).
- ↑ risk of PPH, particularly with factor IX deficiency (factor VIII levels, but not factor IX, ↑ in pregnancy in haemophilia carriers).
- There is a rapid ↓ to pre-pregnancy levels after delivery.

Intrapartum and postpartum care

- Aim for vaginal delivery.
- Check maternal coagulation factor activity and give replacement factors if necessary.
- Send FBC, clotting screen, and group and save when in labour.
- Avoid fetal scalp electrodes, fetal blood sampling, ventouse, and rotational forceps in affected fetuses or males with unknown status.
- Epidural anaesthesia can be used if normal coagulation screen, platelet count >100 × 10⁹/L, normal bleeding time, and satisfactory clotting factor levels.
- Maintain clotting factors and give tranexamic acid for 5 days postpartum to ↓ risk of PPH.
- Avoid IM injections in neonate with possible clotting disorder.
- Send cord blood of males for clotting factor VIII or IX levels (refer to haemophilia centre if diagnosis is confirmed).

Von Willebrand disease

- Von Willebrand factor (vWF) stabilizes factor VIII and helps adherence of platelets to vessel wall.
- Autosomal dominant (types 1 and 2).
- Autosomal recessive (type 3)—more uncommon and severe.
- Diagnosis by measuring:
  - vWF antigen
  - factor VIII
  - ristocetin cofactor activity
- Levels of vWF and factor VIII ↑ in pregnancy and ↓ rapidly postpartum.
- Main risk is PPH.
- Desmopressin can be used in some type 1 cases (it stimulates the release of vWF from endothelial cells).

Further reading

Chalmers E et al. (2011). Guideline on the management of haemophilia in the fetus and neonate. *Br J Haematol*. 154:208–215.

Mumford AD et al. (2014). Guideline for the diagnosis and management of the rare coagulation disorders. *Br J Haematol*. 2014;167:304–326.

Idiopathic thrombocytopenic purpura

- Caused by antibodies to surface antigens on platelets, → platelet destruction.
- Incidence 1–3:1000 pregnancies.
- Diagnosis is by exclusion of other causes of thrombocytopenia.
- Pregnancy does not affect the disease, but due to a ↓ median platelet count in pregnancy, the platelet count with idiopathic thrombocytopenic purpura usually ↓ further in pregnancy.

Fetal risks

- IgG antiplatelet antibodies can cross the placenta and cause fetal thrombocytopenia.
- Difficult to predict whether fetus will be affected (it has no relation to maternal platelet count).
- Can lead to antenatal and intrapartum intracranial haemorrhage:
  - <2% with a history of idiopathic thrombocytopenic purpura before pregnancy
  - risk is highest if there has been a previously affected child.

Management

- FBC every 2–4wks.
- Bleeding is unlikely if platelet count is >50 × 10⁹/L (treatment is not required at this level).
- Patients with bleeding or platelet count <50 × 10⁹/L should be started on oral steroids, >75% respond within 3wks.
- Patients who fail to respond to steroids can be treated with IV immunoglobulin.
- Splenectomy is rarely performed in pregnancy.
- Platelet transfusions may be required if rapid response is needed.
- In labour, avoid:
  - fetal scalp electrodes
  - fetal blood sampling
  - ventouse delivery
  - rotational forceps delivery.
- No fetal benefit from delivery by CS, but ↑ maternal risks.
- Cord platelet count should be taken at birth:
  - the count reaches a nadir at around day 4
  - the neonate may require IV immunoglobulin.

Causes of thrombocytopenia in pregnancy

- Spurious.
- Platelet clumping.
- Gestational thrombocytopenia.
- Pre-eclampsia.
- Idiopathic thrombocytopenic purpura.
- TTP.
- DIC.
- SLE.
- Bone marrow suppression.
- Folate deficiency.

Further reading

American Society of Hematology (2018). Clinical practice guide on thrombocytopenia in pregnancy.
℞ www.hematology.org/Clinicians/Guidelines-Quality/Quick-Reference.aspx

Asthma

This is the most common respiratory disease encountered in pregnancy and affects 1–4% of women of childbearing age. It is caused by reversible bronchoconstriction of smooth muscle in the airways, with inflammation and excess mucus production. Diagnosis is based on recurrent episodes of wheeze, shortness of breath, chest tightness, or cough, and variation in peak expiratory flow rate (PEFR) of >15% after treatment with bronchodilators. Pregnancy outcomes in women with asthma are usually good.

Effect of pregnancy on asthma

1/3 of patients show no change in their asthma, 1/3 show improvement, and 1/3 deteriorate, usually in those with more poorly controlled asthma at conception. Deterioration occurs most often between 24 and 36wks. Deterioration may be due to cessation of maintenance therapy.

Effect of asthma on pregnancy

Usually there is no effect on the fetus or course of the pregnancy, but poorly controlled asthma may be associated with low birth weight and/or preterm labour.

Management

- Current therapy should continue in pregnancy, and women educated and reassured of the safety of the medication and warned not to stop their treatment.
- Women should continue to monitor their PEFR (↑ diurnal variation with ↓ PEFR in the night or early morning may be an early sign of worsening of asthma).
- Chronic and acute severe asthma should be treated as in the non-pregnant state (aim for O_2 sats >95% and administer O_2 if required).
- $MgSO_4$ is readily available in maternity services and may be used for acute severe asthma when there has not been a good initial response to inhaled bronchodilator therapy.
- Strongly encourage smoking cessation.
- CXR should be considered to look for pneumothorax or consolidation.
- ↑ Risk of gestational diabetes in women on long-term oral steroids.
- Asthma attacks are rare during labour; inhaled β-agonists can be used (there is no evidence that they interfere with uterine activity).
- Women on long-term oral steroids (prednisolone >5mg/day for >3wks) are at risk of adrenal crisis at delivery so parenteral steroids required—IV/IM hydrocortisone minimum dose of 50mg every 6h until 6h after birth (see NICE intrapartum guideline).
- PGF2α should only be used in cases of life-threatening postpartum haemorrhage because of its bronchoconstriction action.

⚠ The fetus is at greater risk from undertreated asthma than from the drugs used in its treatment.

Asthma care: British Thoracic Society recommendations
- *Step 1:* inhaled short-acting β-agonists: salbutamol or terbutaline.
- *Step 2:* inhaled steroids (up to 800 micrograms/day); beclometasone, budesonide.
- *Step 3:* long-acting beta-agonist: salmeterol or formoterol.
- *Step 4:* high-dose inhaled steroid (up to 2000 micrograms/day): oral slow-release theophylline, leukotriene antagonists.
- *Step 5:* oral steroids: review by respiratory physician if oral steroids commenced.

⚠ Leukotriene receptor antagonists are not usually commenced in pregnancy but can be continued in women who have demonstrated significant improvement in asthma control that was not achievable by other medication.

Acute severe asthma
- *Clinical findings:*
  - heart rate >110 beats/min
  - respiratory rate >25/min
  - pulsus paradoxus >20mmHg
  - PEFR <50% predicted
  - accessory muscle use
  - unable to complete sentences.
- *Medication:*
  - nebulized salbutamol and ipratropium
  - IV or PO steroids
  - IV aminophylline or IV $MgSO_4$
  - Antibiotics if evidence of infection.

⚠ Silent chest with very little wheeze is a sign of life-threatening asthma and urgent medical/critical care input is required.

Further reading

British Thoracic Society (2019). British guideline on the management of asthma.
🔗 https://www.brit-thoracic.org.uk/quality-improvement/guidelines/asthma/

Cystic fibrosis

This is one of the commonest genetic conditions, affecting 1:2000 people of European origin with a gene frequency of ~1:25. Transmission is autosomal recessive and disease is caused by defective function of the cystic fibrosis (CF) transmembrane conductance regulation (CFTR) chloride channel. The condition affects the lungs, gastrointestinal tract, pancreas, hepatobiliary system, and reproductive organs. Recurrent chest infections lead to bronchial damage and respiratory failure.

Most men are infertile owing to congenital absence of the vas deferens and women are subfertile because of unfavourable mucus, ↓ BMI, and anovulation. Advances in both treatment of CF resulting in better lung function and health, and in assisted reproductive techniques, means that more women with CF are able to successfully become pregnant.

Prenatal counselling

Offspring will receive one affected gene from the mother, so paternal status should be ascertained. There are many different gene mutations, but screening will detect ~90% of mutations. Risk of an affected child is 2–2.5% for unknown paternal carrier status. If the father's screen is negative, the risk of an affected child ↓ to 1:500. If the father is a carrier, the chance of an affected child is 1:2. Chorionic villus sampling can then be performed to check the fetus for affected genes.

Management of pregnancy with CF

- Care involves an MDT with chest physician (CF unit), obstetrician, dietitian, and physiotherapist.
- Principles of care involve control of respiratory infections, avoidance of hypoxia, maintaining nutrition, and fetal surveillance.
- Chest physiotherapy should continue as normal.
- Watch for signs of chest infection; treat aggressively with antibiotics, tailored according to sputum culture results.

⚠ Avoid tetracyclines.

- Cardiac status should be checked by echocardiography.
- In the later stages of pregnancy women can become breathless even without infections.
- High calorie intake with pancreatic enzyme supplementation is required.
- 8% of pregnant women with CF have pre-existing diabetes and 20% have diabetes by term.
- Fetal monitoring with regular growth scans (fetal risks are FGR due to maternal hypoxaemia and preterm labour).
- Aim for a vaginal delivery (limit the 2nd stage, as pneumothoraces can occur with prolonged or repeated Valsalva manoeuvres).
- Avoid general anaesthesia and inhalational analgesia if possible.
- Same thing applies with PGF2α as many women with CF have an element of obstructive airways disease.

Predictors of poor maternal or fetal outcomes in CF

- Hypoxaemia: PaO_2 <60mmHg free from infection.
- Cyanosis.
- Pulmonary hypertension.
- Poor pre-pregnancy lung function: forced expiratory volume in 1s (FEV_1) <60% predicted.
- Pancreatic insufficiency (especially diabetes) and malnutrition.
- Lung colonization with *Burkholderia cepacia*.

Respiratory infections

Pneumonia

Incidence as in the non-pregnant population: 1–2:1000 pregnancies.
* Risk factors include smoking, chronic lung disease, and immunosuppression.
* *Clinical features*: fever, cough, purulent sputum, chest pain, and breathlessness.
* *Investigations*: FBC, CRP, renal function, LFT, and CXR; arterial blood gases (ABG) if woman hypoxic.
▶ Consider urinary *Legionella* antigen if *Legionella* is a possibility.
* Fetal risks are preterm labour and possibly FGR.
* Treatment involves adequate oxygenation, hydration, and antibiotics in line with local hospital guidelines.

⚠ Varicella infection (chickenpox) causes pneumonia in 10% of cases in pregnancy. Mortality is ~10% and is highest in the latter stages of pregnancy. Women who develop varicella in pregnancy should be treated with aciclovir; they should be hospitalized if respiratory signs develop (on a non-obstetric ward with barrier nursing).

COVID-19 infection: ➔ COVID-19, p. 182.

Tuberculosis

* UK incidence of TB is ↑, especially in the immunosuppressed (HIV) and immigrant population.
* Uncommon in pregnancy, does not adversely affect the outcome if it is diagnosed and treated in the 1st 20wks.
* *Clinical features:* cough, haemoptysis, fever, weight loss, chest pain, and night sweats.
* *Investigations*—screening (active or latent infection):
  * Mantoux subcutaneous test (bacillus Calmette–Guérin (BCG) vaccination may cause false positives)
  * *in vitro* blood test based on interferon gamma release assay (QuantiFERON or T-SPOT; BCG vaccination does not cause false positives)
  * CXR (classically calcification and upper lobe abnormalities)
  * sputum microscopy with a Ziehl–Nielsen stain (culture can take 6wks)
  * bronchoscopy if no sputum
  * tissue biopsies for extrapulmonary TB.
* ↑ Risk of prematurity and FGR if treatment is inadequate or delayed.
* Transplacental spread of infection is rare.

Neonatal considerations
- MTCT after delivery (or to other caregivers) can occur if the mother remains infectious (smear +ve).
- Women usually become non-infectious (smear –ve) within 2wks of starting treatment.
- The baby should be given BCG vaccination and, if mother smear +ve, prophylaxis with isoniazid for 3mths.

Management of TB in pregnancy
- Respiratory physician and microbiologist involvement is essential.
- Treatment should be supervised to encourage and confirm compliance.
- A minimum of a 6mth course of treatment is required.
- A typical treatment regimen for pulmonary TB would involve an initial phase of therapy with isoniazid, rifampicin, ethambutol, ± pyrazinamide for 2mths, followed by a continuation phase of 4mths of isoniazid and rifampicin (and based on drug sensitivities):

Isoniazid
- Can cause demyelination and peripheral neuropathy.
- ↑ risk of hepatitis in pregnancy so monitor liver function monthly.

Rifampicin
- Can be safely used in pregnancy.
- It is a liver enzyme inducer; therefore, give vitamin K to the mother in the last 4wks of pregnancy to prevent haemorrhagic disease of the newborn.

Ethambutol
- Safe in pregnancy.

Streptomycin
- 10% risk of deafness in fetus due to damage to the 8th cranial nerve; avoid in pregnancy.

Pyrazinamide
- Considered safe after the 1st trimester, occasionally used before 14wks.

Inflammatory bowel disease

- Ulcerative colitis affects women more than men.
- Crohn's disease is equally distributed between the sexes.
- Clinical features are diarrhoea, abdominal pain, rectal bleeding, and weight loss.

Effect of inflammatory bowel disease (IBD) on pregnancy

- Infertility, miscarriage, stillbirth, and fetal anomaly rates are not ↓ in women with quiescent or well-controlled disease.
- Active disease at conception, 1st presentation in pregnancy, colonic rather than small bowel disease alone, active disease after resection, and severe disease treated by surgery are all associated with ↑ risk of miscarriage, stillbirth, prematurity, and low birth weight.

Effect of pregnancy on IBD

- If the condition is quiescent at conception, the risk of relapse is the same as in non-pregnant women.
- Conception occurring at a time of active disease is associated with persistent activity during pregnancy.

Management of IBD in pregnancy

⚠ Acute flares carry a ↑ risk of adverse outcome, treat aggressively.

▶ Most drugs used for IBD are considered low risk during pregnancy.

⚠ Methotrexate is contraindicated in pregnancy.

- Folic acid (5mg/day) should be given before conception and throughout pregnancy to women on sulfasalazine.
- Maintenance therapy may include sulfasalazine, other 5-aminosalicylic acid derivatives, and/or steroids (PO or rectally).
- Active disease should be investigated by stool culture to exclude infection (including parasites), inflammatory markers, faecal calprotectin, and sigmoidoscopy to assess disease activity in colitis.
- Azathioprine, 6-mercaptopurine, or ciclosporin may be useful in maintaining disease control.
- No adverse fetal outcomes have been associated with the use of biologic therapies such as anti-tumour necrosis factor (TNF) agents; however, women using these should be advised to avoid live vaccines for the 1st 6mths.
- Surgery is occasionally required in pregnancy when complications occur such as intestinal obstruction, haemorrhage, perforation, fistula, abscess formation, or toxic megacolon.
- CD is usually reserved for obstetric reasons but may be considered with:
  - severe perianal Crohn's disease (a scarred perineum is inelastic and tears may result in fistula formation)
  - women with ulcerative colitis and a pouch
  - women with poorly controlled disease who may need a pouch in the future.
- Breast-feeding is safe in women on steroids, sulfasalazine, other 5-aminosalicylic acid derivatives, azathioprine, and biological agents).

Drugs used to treat IBD in pregnancy (European evidence-based consensus rating)

Safe
- Oral 5-aminosalicylates.
- Mesalazine.
- Sulfasalazine.
- Corticosteroids.
- Azathioprine.
- 6-Mercaptopurine

Probably safe
- Infliximab.
- Adalimumab.
- Etanercept.
- Certolizumab.
- Ciclosporin.
- Tacrolimus.
- Budesonide.
- Metronidazole.

Contraindicated
- Methotrexate.
- Tofacitinib.

Further reading

Selinger C et al. (2020). Frontline Gastroenterology Standards for the provision of antenatal care for patients with inflammatory bowel disease: guidance endorsed by the British Society of Gastroenterology and the British Maternal and Fetal Medicine Society. *Frontline Gastroenterol*. 12:182–187.

Intrahepatic cholestasis of pregnancy

Intrahepatic cholestasis of pregnancy (ICP) affects 0.7% of pregnancies in the UK. It is more common in women of Asian ethnicity and there is geographical variation in prevalence. 1/3 of women have a family history of the condition. It most often occurs in the 3rd trimester and resolves spontaneously after delivery.

Definition

Pruritus and elevated bile acids in pregnancy in the absence of another diagnosis. Abnormal LFTs are almost always present.

Symptoms

- Pruritus of the trunk and limbs, often palms and soles, without a skin rash (often worse at night).
- Anorexia and malaise.
- Epigastric discomfort, steatorrhoea, and dark urine (less common).

Risks

Maternal risks
- Vitamin K deficiency (potentially → PPH).

Fetal risks
- Preterm labour (including iatrogenic).
- Stillbirth (actual risk yet to be determined but is likely to be small).
- ↑ Risk of meconium (delivery in a consultant-led unit is recommended).

Management of ICP

- Send LFTs and bile acids for all woman itching, without a rash.
- If normal, they should be repeated every 1–2wks if symptoms persist, as itching can predate abnormal LFTs.
- Exclude other causes of pruritus and liver dysfunction.
- Oral vitamin K should be considered in women with evidence of malabsorption such as steatorrhoea.
- Symptoms may be alleviated by topical emollients (antihistamines cause sedation but do not improve pruritus).
- Ursodeoxycholic acid (8–12mg/kg daily in two divided doses; probably safe up to 20–30mg/kg/day) ↓ pruritus between 1 and 7 days after starting, but there is no proven benefit for fetal adverse effects.
- Fetal surveillance with USS and CTG monitoring are commonly used but of no proven benefit.
- Women with bile acids >100μmol/L at any point during their pregnancy are considered to have severe ICP and are at ↑ risk of stillbirth and other obstetric complications, such as spontaneous preterm birth, gestational diabetes, and pre-eclampsia, compared to the general obstetric population.
- Postnatal resolution of symptoms and LFTs should be established.
- Recurrence risk in subsequent pregnancy is 45–70% (it can also recur with the combined contraceptive pill).

Delivery considerations with ICP

⚠ *Intrauterine death is usually sudden and cannot be predicted by biochemical results, CTG findings, or on USS.*

☝ Timing of delivery is balanced between an ↑ risk of perinatal and maternal morbidity with early intervention against protection from small risk of stillbirth; therefore, this should be discussed with the woman on an individual basis.

Women with severe ICP, particularly those with bile acids >100μmol/L despite treatment, should be counselled about the risks and benefits of early induction (sometimes as early as 35wks).

Differential diagnosis of ICP

- Gallstones.
- Acute or chronic viral hepatitis.
- 1° biliary cholangitis (antimitochondrial antibody +ve).
- Chronic active hepatitis (anti-smooth muscle antibody +ve).

Investigations for ICP

- LFTs:
  - ALT
  - aspartate amniotransferase (AST)
  - gamma-glutamyltransferase (γGT)
  - alkaline phosphatase.
- ▶ Use pregnancy-specific reference ranges.

- Clotting screen.
- Bile acids.
- Viral serology:
  - hepatitis A, B, C, E
  - CMV
  - EBV.
- Autoimmune screen:
  - antinuclear antibodies (ANA)
  - antimitochondrial and anti-smooth muscle antibodies.
- USS of the liver and biliary tree.

Further reading

Ovadia C et al. (2019).
Association of adverse perinatal outcomes of intrahepatic cholestasis of pregnancy with biochemical markers: results of aggregate and individual patient data meta-analyses. *Lancet*. 393:899–909.

Acute fatty liver of pregnancy

This is a rare condition affecting 1:10,000 pregnancies. It typically presents in the 3rd trimester and can occur at any parity. It is associated with twin pregnancy (9–25%), a male fetus ($\mathcal{O}$:$\mathcal{O}$ ratio 3:1), and mild pre-eclampsia (30–60%).

⚠ Acute fatty liver of pregnancy (AFLP) has a maternal mortality of 18%, higher if diagnosis is delayed, and fetal mortality of 23%.

- Diagnosis is based on the Swansea criteria (Box 5.3).
- Can progress rapidly to fulminant liver failure, DIC, and renal failure.
- Hypoglycaemia is common.
- Some women may have significant polyuria 2° to transient diabetes insipidus.

Investigations

FBC and film, clotting, U&E, urate, LFTs, and blood gases.

Differentiating AFLP from HELLP syndrome

Distinctive features of AFLP
- Hypertension and proteinuria may be absent or mild.
- Early coagulopathy.
- Profound and persistent hypoglycaemia.
- Marked hyperuricaemia.
- Fatty infiltration on imaging the liver (may also be normal).

Management of AFLP

- This should be in a high dependency or intensive care setting with an MDT.
- Management should involve:
  - treatment of hypoglycaemia
  - correction of coagulopathy (e.g. with IV vitamin K)
  - strict control of BP and fluid balance.
- Delivery should follow stabilization (regional anaesthesia is contraindicated in presence of thrombocytopenia (<80 × 10⁹/L) or deranged clotting).
- Bleeding complications are common.
- Fluid balance may require central line.
- Following delivery, care is supportive, and most women improve rapidly after delivery with no long-term liver damage.
- Some patients with fulminant hepatic failure may require transfer to a specialist liver unit, who should be informed as soon as the diagnosis is suspected.
- Recurrence rate is unknown but may be greater than that of HELLP.

Box 5.3 The Swansea criteria for diagnosing AFLP

Six or more are required in the absence of another cause
- Vomiting.
- Abdominal pain.
- Polydipsia/polyuria.
- Encephalopathy.
- Elevated bilirubin >14µmol/L.
- Hypoglycaemia <4mmol/L.
- Elevated urea >340µmol/L.
- Leucocytosis >11 × 10⁹/L.
- Ascites or bright liver on USS.
- Elevated transaminases aspartate aminotransferase (AAT) or ALT >42IU/L.
- Elevated ammonia >47µmol/L.
- Renal impairment; creatinine >150µmol/L.
- Coagulopathy; prothrombin time >14s or activated partial thromboplastin time >34s.
- Microvesicular steatosis on liver biopsy.

Causes of jaundice in pregnancy

Causes not specific to pregnancy
- Haemolysis.
- Gilbert's syndrome.
- Viral hepatitis (hepatitis A, B, C, E, EBV, CMV).
- Autoimmune hepatitis (1° biliary cholangitis, autoimmune hepatitis, 1° sclerosing cholangitis).
- Gallstones.
- Cirrhosis.
- Drug-induced hepatotoxicity.
- Malignancy.

Causes specific to pregnancy (10% of cases)
- Hyperemesis gravidarum.
- Pre-eclampsia/HELLP syndrome.
- AFLP.
- ICP.

Renal tract infections

More common in pregnancy because of dilatation of upper renal tract and urinary stasis. Asymptomatic bacteriuria affects 5–10% of pregnant women; untreated it can lead to symptomatic infection in 40% of cases.
- Cystitis complicates 1% of pregnancies.
- Pyelonephritis occurs in 1–2% of pregnant women and is associated with preterm labour.
- Women should be screened for asymptomatic bacteriuria with MSU sample at booking. If this is –ve, the chance of developing a urinary infection in pregnancy is <2%.

Symptoms
- *Cystitis:* urinary frequency, urgency, dysuria, haematuria, proteinuria, and suprapubic pain.
- *Pyelonephritis:* fever, rigors, vomiting, and loin and abdominal pain.

▶ Consider the diagnosis of pyelonephritis in women presenting with hyperemesis or threatened preterm labour.

Investigations
- *Urinalysis:* the most useful markers are nitrites but they may be poor predictors of positive culture in asymptomatic bacteriuria.
- *MSU:* a positive result is confirmed with a culture of >100,000 organisms/mL. Mixed growth, likely contaminant or non-significant culture—do not treat and repeat MSU.
- *Bloods:* blood cultures, FBC, U&E, and CRP.
- *Renal USS:* after a single episode of pyelonephritis or ≥2 UTI, to exclude hydronephrosis, congenital abnormality, and calculi.

⚠ 20% of pregnant women with pyelonephritis have an abnormal renal tract.

- Repeat MSU is advised after antibiotic treatment for culture-proven urinary infection to prove eradication—15% develop recurrent bacteriuria and require further treatment.

Treatment
- Oral antibiotics are recommended in asymptomatic bacteriuria and cystitis to prevent pyelonephritis and preterm labour.
- Pyelonephritis should be initially treated with IV antibiotics. IV fluids and antipyretics should also be given (manage in hospital because of risk of preterm labour).

Prevention
- ↑ fluid intake.
- Double voiding and emptying bladder after sexual intercourse.
- *Cranberry juice:* proven in non-pregnant population to ↓ bacteriuria.
- Prophylactic antibiotics: if ≥2 culture +ve urine infections + 1 risk factor.

Risk factors for urinary tract infection

Antenatal
* Previous infection (in previous pregnancy or outside pregnancy).
* Renal stones.
* Diabetes mellitus.
* Immunosuppression.
* Polycystic kidneys.
* Congenital anomalies of renal tract (e.g. duplex collecting system).
* Neuropathic bladder.

Postpartum (risk mainly associated with catheterization)
* Prolonged labour.
* Prolonged 2nd stage.
* CD.
* Pre-eclampsia.

Antibiotic options for renal tract infections

Drug of choice
Depends on antibiotic sensitivities and local antibiotics protocols.

Options include
* *Penicillins:* e.g. amoxicillin—resistance common so not recommended empirically.
* *Cephalosporin.*
* *Gentamicin:* monitor levels to minimize toxicity.
* *Trimethoprim:* avoid in 1st trimester as it is a folate antagonist.
* *Nitrofurantoin:* avoid in late 3rd trimester as risk of haemolytic anaemia in neonate with glucose-6-phosphate dehydrogenase deficiency.
* *Sulfonamides:* avoid in 3rd trimester as risk of kernicterus in neonate due to displacement of protein binding of bilirubin.

Contraindicated antibiotics
* *Tetracyclines:* cause permanent staining of teeth and problems with skeletal development.
* *Ciprofloxacin:* causes skeletal problems.

Chronic kidney disease

There are ↑ maternal and fetal risks to pregnancy with renal disease. This is dependent upon:
- Underlying cause.
- Degree of renal impairment.
- Presence and control of hypertension.
- Amount of proteinuria.
- As renal function deteriorates, so does the ability to conceive and sustain a pregnancy.

Management

- MDT care involving a renal physician.
- Baseline investigations, ideally before conception, include:
  - FBC
  - U&E
  - calcium
  - urine PCR.
- Pre-pregnancy counselling (genetic counselling if a familial disorder).
- Early and regular antenatal care is advised with the following aims:
  - *control BP*: tight control lessens chance of renal function declining
  - *monitor*: renal function and proteinuria
  - *fetal well-being*: serial growth scans
  - *early detection of complications*: anaemia, UTI, pre-eclampsia, FGR.
- Medication should be reviewed and may need altering.

⚠ ACEI should be stopped as soon as pregnancy is confirmed.
- Aspirin (75–150mg at night) should be prescribed to all women with CKD as pre-eclampsia prophylaxis.
- Erythropoietin may be required with significant renal impairment.
- Hospital admission should be considered with ↑ proteinuria or hypertension, deteriorating renal function, or symptoms of pre-eclampsia.
- Aim for vaginal delivery, but rates of CD are ↑.

⚠ Look for an underlying cause of deterioration in renal function: UTI, obstruction, dehydration, pre-eclampsia, or renal vein thrombosis.

⚠ It can be difficult to differentiate between pre-eclampsia and deterioration of renal impairment. Thrombocytopenia, FGR, and abnormal LFTs suggest the former diagnosis. PlGF-based testing may be useful in this setting but more data are needed about levels in setting of CKD.

Risks of pregnancy with chronic kidney disease

Maternal risks

- Accelerated, and possibly permanent, deterioration in renal function; this is more likely if there is also hypertension and proteinuria and significant renal impairment at conception.
- Hypertension.
- Proteinuria.
- Superimposed pre-eclampsia.
- VTE (if nephrotic level of proteinuria).
- UTI.

Fetal risks

- Miscarriage.
- FGR.
- Spontaneous and iatrogenic preterm delivery.
- Fetal death.

Commonest causes of chronic renal impairment

- Reflux nephropathy (condition may be familial).
- Diabetic kidney disease.
- Lupus nephritis.
- Chronic glomerulonephritides.
- Polycystic kidneys (adult polycystic kidney disease is inherited in an autosomal dominant manner).

Pregnancy after renal transplantation

Menstruation, ovulation, and fertility return after transplantation. Women should be informed of this and contraception discussed. Those who wish to conceive should allow 1yr of stable transplant function before trying to conceive.

The best outcomes are seen with:
- Well-controlled BP.
- No proteinuria.
- No evidence of graft rejection.
- Plasma creatinine <180µmol/L, preferably <125µmol/L.

Management of pregnancy in a transplant recipient

- MDT management with a renal physician.
- Antenatal care should be at 2–4wk intervals. Aims are:
  - serial assessment of renal function: deterioration may be caused by infection, dehydration, pre-eclampsia, drug toxicity, or rejection
  - diagnosis and treatment of graft rejection
  - BP control (avoid ACEIs)
  - prevention, early diagnosis, and treatment of anaemia
  - detection and treatment of any infection
  - serial assessment of fetus (risk of FGR)
  - regular drug level measurement if on tacrolimus.
- All women will be on immunosuppressive therapy, which must be continued; prednisolone, azathioprine, and tacrolimus are commonly used.
- Aim for vaginal delivery with continuous fetal monitoring (parenteral steroids are necessary to cover labour if on regular steroids as per NICE intrapartum guidelines, due to adrenal suppression).
- Prophylactic antibiotics are recommended for obstetric procedures.
- A transplanted kidney does not obstruct labour; CD should be for obstetric reasons—the current rate is 40% (women with pelvic osteodystrophy may need elective CD).

⚠ Mycophenolate mofetil is associated with congenital abnormalities and so this should be replaced with an alternative agent before conception.

Risks of pregnancy after renal transplantation

Maternal risks
- ↑ risk of ectopic pregnancy; as a result of pelvic adhesions 2° to surgery, peritoneal dialysis, and pelvic infection.
- 15% develop significant deterioration in renal function, which may be permanent.
- Graft rejection: ~5%—same as in non-pregnant women (pregnancy usually has no effect on graft survival or function).
- Hypertension, proteinuria, and pre-eclampsia: 30–40%.
- Infections, especially urinary tract: up to 40%.

Fetal risks
- Miscarriage and congenital anomaly rates are unchanged.
- FGR 30%, higher if the mother is on ciclosporin.
- Preterm delivery 45–60%: may be iatrogenic, spontaneous, or 2° to preterm rupture of membranes.

⚠ If maternal complications occur before 28wks the chance of a successful pregnancy outcome ↓ from 95% to 75%.

Graft rejection

Consider the diagnosis if there is deteriorating renal function with:
- Fever.
- Oliguria.
- Renal enlargement and tenderness.

▶ It can be difficult to diagnose and a renal biopsy may be required.

⚠ Blood transfusion should be avoided if possible as it ↑ likelihood of sensitization making graft rejection more of a problem.

Investigations in pregnancy following renal transplantation

At each visit
- FBC, U&E.
- MSU.
- PCR.

Every 2–4wks
- USS for fetal growth and well-being.

Every 4wks
- Drug levels of ciclosporin/tacrolimus.
- Calcium, phosphate, albumin, and LFTs.
- Urine PCR.

Acute kidney injury

Characterized by oliguria and/or ↑ urea and creatinine, and may be accompanied by hyperkalaemia, and metabolic acidosis. Rare in pregnancy, typically complicating the postpartum period. There are three phases:
* *Oliguria:* few days to several wks.
* *Polyuria:* 2 days to 2wks, dilute urine is produced, and as waste products are still not excreted, renal function still deteriorates.
* *Recovery:* urine volume returns to normal with a gradual improvement in renal function.

Management of acute kidney injury

* Seek advice from a physician or nephrologist.
* Most cases are reversible with appropriate management (permanent problems more likely with pre-existing renal disease).
* Assessment should include the following investigations:
  * FBC, coagulation, U&E, glucose, LFTs
  * blood cultures, MSU, HVS
  * urinalysis looking for the presence of blood and protein
  * ECG (looking for changes due to ↑ K⁺) and ABG
  * fetal assessment with CTG and USS
  * renal USS if obstruction suspected.
* Interventions to be considered include catheterization, central venous line, and renal biopsy if improvement is delayed; only a minority require dialysis.
* Replace fluid/blood loss but avoid fluid overload as there is a significant risk of pulmonary oedema (accurate documentation of input/output, daily weight, and may benefit from central venous pressure monitoring).
* Maintain BP at levels that allow adequate renal perfusion.
* Review medication and stop nephrotoxic drugs.
* Correct hyperkalaemia, coagulopathy, and give antibiotics if infection suspected.
* Dialysis is required for persistent hyperkalaemia, acidosis, pulmonary oedema, or uraemia.

Some causes of renal failure in pregnancy

Pre-renal (hypovolaemic)

- Haemorrhage:
  - antepartum (abruption, placenta praevia, etc.)
  - postpartum (uterine atony, genital tract trauma, etc.)
- Hyperemesis.
- Septic shock.
- AFLP.

Intrinsic

- Pre-eclampsia.
- HELLP syndrome.
- Sepsis.
- Drug reaction.
- Amniotic fluid embolus.

Post-renal

- Obstruction.
- Ureteric damage.
- Pelvic or broad ligament haematoma.

⚠ Non-pregnancy-related problems may also be the cause.

Treatment of hyperkalaemia

- Bolus of 10% calcium gluconate IV slowly, for cardioprotection.
- IV insulin and glucose infusion.
- Consider use of calcium polystyrene sulfonate.

💣 These are only temporary measures; dialysis may be required.

Systemic lupus erythematosus

More common in women than men (9:1) with a higher prevalence in the Afro-Caribbean population than in white populations (5:1). The incidence is 1:1000 and onset during the reproductive age is common. It is a connective tissue disease of relapses (flares) and remissions. Diagnosis is based on at least four features from the American Rheumatism Society Criteria present either consecutively or concurrently (Box 5.4).

Monitoring disease severity in pregnancy

- Flares can be difficult to diagnose as similar symptoms occur in normal pregnancy, e.g. fatigue, hair loss, joint aches, anaemia.
  - ESR is ↑ in normal pregnancy and CRP is not a marker of disease activity
  - C3 (↓) or anti-DNA levels (↑) are an objective index of disease activity.
- Renal disease can also be difficult to distinguish from pre-eclampsia, as hypertension, proteinuria, and thrombocytopenia are common in both conditions:
  - ↑ urate and liver transaminases are not features of SLE
  - ↓ C3 and ↑ anti-DNA levels suggest lupus nephritis
  - renal biopsy is diagnostic, but rarely performed in pregnancy
  - PlGF-based testing can be considered to differentiate between SLE flare or superimposed PET.

Maternal risks

- Long-term prognosis is not affected by pregnancy.
- There is ↑ risk of flare-up, especially in the puerperium.
- Hypertension, pre-eclampsia, and placental abruption are more common.

⚠ Do not stop hydroxychloroquine as this may precipitate a flare.

Fetal risks

- ↑ risk of miscarriage, preterm delivery, preterm rupture of membranes, FGR, and *in utero* fetal death:
  - risks are due to anticardiolipin antibodies, lupus anticoagulant, renal impairment, or hypertension
  - risk is low if all these are absent.
- Congenital heart block may occur in women with anti-Ro (or anti-La) antibodies, which cross the placenta:
  - risk of occurrence if anti-Ro +ve is 2%
  - ↑ to 18% if previously affected child.
- Transient skin lesions similar to cutaneous lupus can occur in neonates (usually in 1st 2wks of life) in 5% of babies born to anti-Ro/La mothers.

Management of SLE in pregnancy

- MDT management.
- Pre-pregnancy counselling of maternal and fetal risks based on BP, renal function, anti-Ro, and antiphospholipid antibody status.
- Treat hypertension and modify medication if necessary (➔ Blood pressure in pregnancy: hypertension, p. 58).
- Advise conception during periods of disease remission: less risk of flare.
- Obtain objective evidence of flare.
- Flare-ups should be treated by starting or ↑ dose, or steroids.
- Assess fetal growth and well-being (uterine artery Doppler at 24wks is a useful screening test).
- Refer to fetal cardiology for monitoring of fetal arrythmia.

Box 5.4 American College of Rheumatology classification criteria for SLE

4 or more of the following features are required (simultaneously or following each other)

- Malar rash ('butterfly' rash on face).
- Discoid rash.
- Serositis, e.g. pleuritis or pericarditis.
- Oral or nasopharyngeal ulceration.
- Arthritis.
- Non-erosive, migratory of two or more joints.
- Photosensitivity.
- Neurological features, e.g. seizures, psychosis.
- Haematological features:
  - Haemolytic anaemia
  - Leucopenia ($<4 \times 10^9$/L)
  - Lymphopenia ($<1.5 \times 10^9$/L)
  - Thrombocytopenia ($<100 \times 10^9$/L).
- Immunological features:
  - anti-dsDNA antibodies
  - ANA.

Source: data from Aringer M et al. (2019). 2019 European League Against Rheumatism/American College of Rheumatology classification criteria for systemic lupus erythematosus. *Arthritis Rheumatol.* 71(9):1400–1412. https://onlinelibrary.wiley.com/doi/10.1002/art.40930

Antiphospholipid antibody syndrome

This condition is diagnosed on the basis of the presence of one or more clinical features and one or more positive laboratory findings. The condition may be complicated by hypertension, pulmonary hypertension, epilepsy, thrombocytopenia, leg ulcers, and valvular problems. It is called 1° if features of connective tissue disease are absent or it can occur 2° to established connective tissue disease.

Lupus anticoagulant is an inhibitor of the coagulation pathway, and anticardiolipins are antibodies against the phospholipid components of cell walls.

Maternal risks

- These include thrombosis, thrombocytopenia, and pre-eclampsia.
- Previous poor obstetric history is an important predictor of outcome (the risk is less with just recurrent miscarriages).

Fetal risks

- Risks include early and late miscarriage, *in utero* death, FGR, placental abruption.
- Fetal outcome may be improved by:
  - MDT management
  - fetal monitoring (including serial growth scans, umbilical and uterine artery Dopplers)
  - appropriate drug therapy
  - timely delivery.
- Women with double or triple laboratory criteria positivity and/or previous thrombotic events are at highest risk of pregnancy complications.
- Possible mechanisms of fetal injury are recurrent placental infarction and direct cellular injury.

Management of antiphospholipid antibody syndrome in pregnancy

No thrombosis or pregnancy loss
- No treatment or aspirin 75–150mg.

Previous thrombosis
- Aspirin + LMWH (therapeutic).

Previous recurrent 1st-trimester miscarriages
- Aspirin + LMWH (prophylactic dose).

Previous intrauterine death (IUD) or FGR or severe pre-eclampsia
- Aspirin + LMWH (prophylactic dose).

▶ Start aspirin and LMWH when pregnancy confirmed.

▶ Liaise with anaesthetist if the woman is on LMWH (regional anaesthesia is contraindicated within 12h of a prophylactic dose of heparin and 24h of therapeutic dose).

✒ Some studies have disputed improved pregnancy outcomes with LMWH compared with aspirin alone. Consider stopping heparin if 24wk uterine artery Doppler is normal. The improved live birth rate is due to ↓ miscarriages.

⚠ Steroids are not recommended → less success and more side effects.

Antiphospholipid antibody syndrome diagnostic criteria

Clinical criteria
- *Vascular thrombosis:* arterial or venous, *or*
- Three or more consecutive miscarriages (<10wks), *or*
- One or more fetal death >10wks, *or*
- One or more preterm delivery (<34wks) due to pre-eclampsia or placental insufficiency.

And

Laboratory criteria
- Anticardiolipin antibody (IgG or IgM) in medium or high titre (in titre >99th percentile), on at least two occasions >12wks apart, *or*
- β2-glycoprotein-1 antibody (IgG or IgM) in medium or high titre (in titre >99th percentile), on at least two occasions >12wks apart, *or*
- Lupus anticoagulant present on at least two occasions >6wks apart.

Rheumatoid arthritis

This is more common in women than men, with an incidence of 1:1000–2000 pregnancies. Characterized by symmetrical chronic inflammation and destruction of synovial joints. Autoantibodies are formed to immunoglobulins, which are deposited as immune complexes in the synovial fluid and elsewhere. 80–90% have rheumatoid factor and 20–30% are ANA +ve. It is a multisystem disorder with many extra-articular features including anaemia, nodules, carpal tunnel syndrome, and eye and lung involvement.

Maternal risks

- The condition improves in pregnancy in 50% of cases, but flares are not uncommon in the puerperium.
- At this age atlantoaxial subluxation rarely causes problems during intubation.

Fetal risks

There is usually no adverse effect on pregnancy unless the woman is anti-Ro/La +ve or has antiphospholipid antibodies (5–10%).

Drugs used in the treatment of autoimmune diseases

Safe to continue in pregnancy and breast-feeding

- Paracetamol.
- Steroids.
- Hydroxychloroquine.
- Sulfasalazine (5mg folic acid daily alongside this).
- Azathioprine.
- Biological agents, such as etanercept, adalimumab, and infliximab (see national guidelines regarding use in 3rd trimester).

Discontinue/avoid in pregnancy

- *NSAIDs:* oligohydramnios, premature closure of ductus arteriosus and neonatal haemorrhage especially with 3rd-trimester use.
- *Gold:* teratogenic effect seen in animals only.
- *Penicillamine:* connective tissue abnormalities only in high doses.
- *Cyclophosphamide (alkylating agent):* can be used after 1st trimester if no suitable alternative available.
- *Methotrexate (folate antagonist):* causes miscarriage and congenital anomalies.

Myasthenia gravis

Uncommon condition; highest incidence in women of childbearing age. It is caused by autoimmune disruption of nicotinic acetylcholine receptors at the skeletal muscle motor end plate, → muscle weakness and fatigue. 90% have acetylcholine receptor antibodies. Muscles affected include eyes (ptosis, diplopia), face, neck, limbs, and trunk. Diagnosis confirmed by identification of pathological antibodies such as anti-AChR or anti-MuSK. Condition can be worsened by infection, hypokalaemia, exercise, emotion, and drugs (aminoglycosides, $MgSO_4$, local anaesthetic, β-blockers, β-agonists, narcotics, and neuromuscular blocking drugs).

Effect of pregnancy on myasthenia

- No change in 60%, improvement in 20%, deterioration in 20%.
- No consistent effect between pregnancies.
- Symptoms commonly worsen postpartum.
- Previous thymectomy associated with fewer −ve effects in pregnancy.
- Hyperemesis, delayed gastric emptying, ↑ volume of distribution of drugs, ↑ renal clearance can lead to subtherapeutic drug levels.
- ↑ doses of anticholinesterases may be required as pregnancy advances; this is best achieved by ↓ dose intervals.
- Parenteral anticholinesterases should be given in labour to avoid absorption problems.

Effect of myasthenia on pregnancy

- Preterm delivery, polyhydramnios, and FGR are all ↑.
- The 1st stage of labour is not prolonged (the smooth muscle of the myometrium is not affected by the condition).
- In the 2nd stage there can be skeletal muscle fatigue; instrumental delivery may be required to prevent maternal exhaustion.
- Neonatal myasthenia can occur following delivery in 10–20% of babies:
  - it results from transplacental passage of maternal antibodies
  - there is poor correlation between the condition and maternal disease activity or antibody levels
  - presentation is with generalized hypotonia, poor sucking/feeding, and a weak cry
  - onset is within 24h and the condition resolves by 2mths
  - treatment is with anticholinesterases.

⚠ $MgSO_4$ is contraindicated for treatment of eclampsia in myasthenia.

Management of myasthenia gravis in pregnancy

- Inform neurologist, paediatrician, and anaesthetist of pregnancy.
- ↑ Steroids can lead to respiratory deterioration, so do not amend doses without discussing with the neurologist.
- The usual treatment options have all been used in pregnancy:
  - long-acting anticholinesterases (e.g. pyridostigmine)
  - immunosuppression: steroids, azathioprine
  - immunoglobulins
  - plasmapheresis
  - thymectomy.

Further reading

Norwood F et al. (2014). Myasthenia in pregnancy: best practice guidelines from a U.K. multispecialty working group. *J Neurol Neurosurg Psychiatry*. 85:538–543.

Diabetes: established disease in pregnancy

- Established diabetes affects 1–2% of pregnancies.
- Without good glycaemic control there is ↑ fetal and neonatal morbidity and mortality.
- Management should be by an MDT including:
  - obstetrician
  - physician/diabetologist
  - diabetes specialist nurse/midwife
  - dietitian.
- Glucose metabolism is altered by pregnancy.
- Many pregnancy hormones are diabetogenic (human placental lactogen, cortisol, glucagon, oestrogen, and progesterone).
- Insulin requirements ↑ throughout and are maximal at term.

Effect of diabetes on pregnancy

- *Maternal hyperglycaemia:* leads to fetal hyperglycaemia.
- *Fetal hyperglycaemia:* leads to hyperinsulinaemia (through β-cell hyperplasia in fetal pancreatic cells) and insulin acts as a growth promoter leading to:
  - macrosomia
  - organomegaly
  - ↑ erythropoiesis
  - fetal polyuria (polyhydramnios).
- *Neonatal hypoglycaemia:* caused by the removal of maternal glucose supply at birth from a hyperinsulinaemic fetus.
- *Respiratory distress syndrome:* more common in babies born to mothers with diabetes due to surfactant deficiency occurring through ↓ production of pulmonary phospholipids.

Effect of pregnancy on diabetes

- *Ketoacidosis:* rare, but may be associated with hyperemesis, infection, tocolysis (β-sympathomimetics), or steroid therapy.
- *Retinopathy:* there is a 2× ↑ risk of development or progression of existing disease—rapid improvement in glycaemic control leads to ↑ retinal blood flow, which can cause retinopathy.

▶ All diabetic women should have assessment for retinopathy in pregnancy, and proliferative retinopathy requires treatment. Early changes usually revert after delivery.

- *Nephropathy:* affects 5–10% of women. Renal function and proteinuria may worsen during pregnancy. This is usually temporary. There is ↑ maternal risk of pre-eclampsia and fetal risk of FGR in this population and ↑ surveillance is required.
- *Ischaemic heart disease:* pregnancy ↑ cardiac workload. Women with symptoms should be assessed by a cardiologist before conception.

Complications of diabetes in pregnancy

Maternal

- UTI.
- Recurrent vulvovaginal candidiasis.
- Gestational hypertension/pre-eclampsia.
- Obstructed labour.
- Operative deliveries: CD and assisted vaginal deliveries.
- ↑ Retinopathy (15%).
- ↑ Nephropathy.
- Cardiac disease.

Fetal

- Miscarriage*
- *Congenital abnormalities:*
  - neural tube defects
  - microcephaly
  - cardiac abnormalities.
  - sacral agenesis
  - renal abnormalities.
- Preterm labour.
- Polyhydramnios (25%).
- Macrosomia (25–40%).
- FGR.
- Unexplained IUD.

Neonatal

- Polycythaemia.
- Jaundice.
- Hypoglycaemia.
- Hypocalcaemia.
- Hypomagnesaemia.
- Hypothermia.
- Cardiomegaly.
- Birth trauma: shoulder dystocia, fractures, Erb's palsy, asphyxia.
- Respiratory distress syndrome.

* In diabetics with poor control.

Diabetes: antenatal management

Pre-pregnancy counselling

Offer to all women with diabetes of reproductive age, include:
- *Achievement of optimal control:* ↑ risk of miscarriage and congenital abnormalities with poor control). Use of continuous insulin pumps, and continuous glucose monitoring devices has been very beneficial to many women with pre-existing diabetes.
- *Assessment of severity of diabetes:* check for hypertension, retinopathy (fundoscopy, ophthalmology assessment), nephropathy (U&E, urinalysis, urinary PCR), neuropathy (clinical assessment), and cardiac disease.
- *Education:* ensure understanding of effects of hyperglycaemia on fetus and need for tight control—instruct to inform doctor as soon as pregnancy confirmed; some drugs may need stopping (ACEI, statins).
- *General health:* stop smoking, optimize weight (aim for a normal BMI), minimize alcohol.
- *Folic acid:* ↑ risk of neural tube defects, so start on 5mg folic acid.
- *Rubella status:* offer vaccination if not rubella immune.
- *Contraception:* ensure effective contraception until good control achieved and pregnancy desired.

Antenatal care

Manage with an MDT including a diabetologist.
- *Control:* as for pre-pregnancy, aim for normoglycaemia. Monitor glucose at least 4×/day, usually fasting and after meals for a tighter control. Women can alter their own insulin based on their glucose. Insulin can be given as subcutaneous (SC) injections 4×/day or as a continuous infusion in an insulin pump.
- *HbA1c:* this gives an objective measurement of control over the preceding 2mths.
- *Dietitian review:* low-sugar, low-fat, high-fibre diet—low glycaemic index.
- *Dating ultrasound:* to confirm viability and gestation.
- *Anomaly scan:* 5–10× ↑ risk of congenital anomalies, risk depends on glycaemic control before conception and early pregnancy.
- *Fetal echocardiography:* consider between 20–24wks.
- *Antenatal surveillance:* individualize care. Serial USS every 2–4wks to detect polyhydramnios, macrosomia, or FGR; ↑ surveillance if problems detected. The use of umbilical artery Doppler pertinent in cases with ↓ of growth velocity.
- *Hypoglycaemia:* awareness of hypoglycaemia may be lost. Educate patient and family and supply with glucagon.

Diabetes: labour and postpartum care

Timing and mode of delivery should be individualized and based on EFW, obstetric factors (previous mode of delivery, gestation, glycaemic control, and antenatal complications), and maternal preference.

Mode of delivery

- Individualized counselling of pros and cons of vaginal birth vs CD.
- Continuous EFM is advised in labour.
- Consider elective CD if EFW is >4.5kg with appropriate antibiotic and thromboprophylaxis.

💣 Shoulder dystocia is more common at all birth weights than in women without diabetes. Experienced obstetricians should perform instrumental deliveries.

Glycaemic control at delivery

- *Insulin pump:* aim to continue use of the pump unless the mother has problems achieving satisfactory glycaemic control.
- *Basal-bolus insulin:* continue long-acting insulin, variable rate IV insulin infusion (VRIII) may be required if hyperglycaemic.

⚠ Avoid maternal hyperglycaemia as causes fetal hypoglycaemia.

⚠ If steroids are given for threatened preterm labour, monitor glucose closely—hyperglycaemia should be anticipated and VRIII might be required.

Postpartum care

- Encourage breast-feeding.
- 💣 Metformin and insulin are appropriate to use in breast-feeding.
- Baby needs early feeding and glucose monitoring.

Contraception

- Avoid the COCP if breast-feeding or vascular complications.
- Progesterone-based contraception is safe.
- Long-acting reversible contraceptives (LARCs) may be the best choice and should be discussed.
- There are no contraindications to an IUCD.

Postpartum insulin requirements

- Insulin requirements ↓ dramatically after delivery of the placenta.
- Halve the VRIII initially and change back to SC insulin when eating and drinking, starting with the pre-pregnancy dose.
- If pre-pregnancy is not known, use 50% of the dose on at delivery.
- The dose may need to be further ↓ if breast-feeding (by 20–30%).

Gestational diabetes

The WHO now includes gestational impaired glucose tolerance with gestational diabetes. A proportion of women diagnosed in pregnancy will actually have previously unrecognized type 1 or 2 diabetes (20–30%). WHO does not advocate universal screening. Selective screening should be based on risk factors (Box 5.5).

The diagnosis is based on an oral glucose tolerance test (OGTT) (Box 5.6), usually undertaken at 26–28wks gestation. A normal result in early pregnancy does not mean that gestational diabetes will not develop, and an OGTT should be repeated at 24–28wks if normal in early pregnancy.

Management of GDM
- Management by an MDT.
- Measure glucose 4–6×/day (1h post-prandial measurements may be more effective in preventing macrosomia than pre-meal glucose).
- *Diet should be 1st-line treatment:*
  - aim for normoglycaemia and avoid ketosis
  - weight should remain steady if diet followed
  - compliance is often poor—dietitian input may help.
- *Start metformin and/or insulin if:*
  - fasting glucose >5.3mmol/L
  - 1h post-prandial glucose >7.8mmol/L.
  - AC >95th centile despite apparent good control.
- No ↑ risk of miscarriage or congenital anomalies; other fetal and neonatal risks are similar to established diabetes.
- Antenatal and intrapartum care as for established diabetes.
- *Postpartum:*
  - stop metformin, insulin, and glucose infusions
  - check glucose prior to discharge to ensure normal (risk of previously undiagnosed type 2 diabetes)
  - arrange OGTT at 6wks postpartum
  - *education*—50% risk of developing type 2 diabetes mellitus over next 25yrs (this risk can be ↓ by maintaining physical activity and avoiding obesity)
  - 40% of recurrence of GDM in any subsequent pregnancy.

Box 5.5 Risk factors for gestational diabetes

- BMI >30kg/m².
- Previous macrosomic baby weighing ≥4.5kg.
- Previous gestational diabetes.
- 1st-degree relative with diabetes.
- Family origin with a high prevalence of diabetes (South Asian, black Caribbean, and Middle Eastern).

Box 5.6 Oral glucose tolerance test

- Overnight fasting (8h minimum):
  - water only may be consumed during this time
  - no smoking.
- 75g glucose load in 250–300mL water.
- Plasma glucose measured fasting and at 2h.

Results
- Gestational diabetes:
  - Fasting ≥5.6mmol/L (92mg/dL)
  - 2h ≥7.8mmol/L (153mg/dL).

⚠ Only one value needs to be abnormal to make the diagnosis.

Further reading

NICE (2015, updated 2020). Diabetes in pregnancy: management from preconception to the postnatal period.
🔗 https://www.nice.org.uk/guidance/ng3

Hyperthyroidism

Hyperthyroidism occurs in 1:500 pregnancies. The most common cause is Graves' disease (95%), an autoimmune disease characterized by the production of thyroid-stimulating hormone (TSH) receptor stimulating antibodies. Most women have been diagnosed before pregnancy and may be on treatment. Many symptoms and signs occur in normal pregnancy. The most discriminatory features are weight loss, tremor, persistent tachycardia, and eye signs. Diagnosis is made by a low TSH and high free T_4 or free T_3 levels.

▶ Use pregnancy-specific reference ranges for each trimester. See Table 5.2.

Effect of pregnancy on hyperthyroidism

- Usually improves in the 2nd and 3rd trimester.
- Pregnancy is a state of relative immunodeficiency, but with return of normal immunity in the puerperium hyperthyroidism can worsen.

Effect of hyperthyroidism on pregnancy

- Maternal and fetal outcome usually good if disease is controlled.
- Untreated or poorly controlled hyperthyroidism is associated with subfertility (amenorrhoea due to weight loss), ↑ risk of miscarriage, FGR, and premature delivery.
- Neonatal/fetal hyperthyroidism occurs in up to 10% of babies born to women with current or past history of Graves' disease (transplacental passage of thyroid receptor stimulating antibodies).

▶ Check antibody levels in women with a history of Graves' disease.
- If antibodies are present, monitor by FHR, and serial USS for growth and some centres also assess for the presence of a fetal goitre (treatments include antithyroid drugs titrated to FHR, or delivery).

⚠ With the stress of infection, labour, or operative delivery a 'thyroid storm' can occur in women with suboptimal treatment of their hyperthyroidism. This is a medical emergency, characterized by pyrexia, confusion, and cardiac failure.

Treatment

- *Antithyroid drugs:* carbimazole and propylthiouracil (PTU).
- Aim for clinical euthyroid with T_4 at the upper limit of normal with the lowest dose of drug.
- Both drugs cross the placenta and may cause fetal hypothyroidism.
- PTU is preferred for new cases diagnosed in the 1st trimester because of lower teratogenic risk.
- β-Blockers may safely be used for symptom relief.
- *Surgery:* thyroidectomy can be safely done in pregnancy; indications include dysphagia, stridor, suspected carcinoma, and allergies to both antithyroid drugs.

⚠ Radioactive iodine is contraindicated in pregnancy and breast-feeding.

Causes of hyperthyroidism

- Graves' disease.
- Toxic multinodular goitre.
- Toxic adenoma.
- Carcinoma.
- Subacute thyroiditis.
- Amiodarone.
- Lithium.

⚠ Women with hyperemesis or a molar pregnancy may mimic biochemical hyperthyroidism as hCG, at high levels, can stimulate TSH receptors. They usually have no clinical signs of hyperthyroidism and so should not be treated.

Management of Graves' disease in pregnancy

- Graves' disease often improves in pregnancy, but relapses postpartum.
- With treatment the outlook is good for mother and baby.
- Untreated hyperthyroidism is dangerous for mother and baby.
- PTU and carbimazole may be used as treatment; both cross the placenta.
- Check TSH receptor antibodies.
- Monitor thyroid function every 4–6wks in new cases, less frequently in stable cases.
- Monitor fetus by FHR and serial USS for growth and presence of fetal goitre.

Table 5.2 Reference ranges for TFTs by trimester

	Non-pregnant	1st trimester	2nd trimester	3rd trimester
TSH (mU/L)	0.3–4.2	0–5.5	0.5–3.5	0.5–4
Free T$_4$ (pmol/L)	9–26	10–16	9–15.5	8–14.5
Free T$_3$ (pmol/L)	2.6–5.7	3–7	3–5.5	2.5–5.5

Hypothyroidism

Hypothyroidism complicates ~1% of pregnancies. Most cases have been diagnosed and patients are on replacement therapy. New diagnosis in pregnancy is rare. The commonest cause is autoimmune and may be associated with other autoimmune conditions.

- Classical symptoms and signs may be seen in normal pregnancy.
- The most discriminatory features are cold intolerance, bradycardia, and slow relaxation of tendon reflexes.
- Diagnosis is made by a low free T_4.
- TSH is also ↑, but in isolation is not diagnostic.

▶ Use pregnancy-specific reference ranges for each trimester (Table 5.2). Free T_4 levels are normally lower in the 2nd and 3rd trimester, TSH level is most useful.

Effect of pregnancy on hypothyroidism

No effect usually. Most women do not need to alter their dose of levothyroxine. The most common reason for increasing levothyroxine is an inadequate pre-pregnancy dose.

Effect of hypothyroidism on pregnancy

- Untreated hypothyroidism is associated with anovulatory infertility.
- Severe or untreated hypothyroidism is associated with ↑ risk of miscarriage, fetal loss, pre-eclampsia, and low birth weight.
- Hypothyroidism is also associated with gestational diabetes.
- The fetus requires maternal T_4 for normal brain development before 12wks (inadequate replacement may lead to ↓ IQ in the offspring); after this time T_3/T_4/TSH do not cross the placenta.

▶ Aim for optimal control before conception.
- Women on adequate replacement therapy are euthyroid at the onset of pregnancy and have good maternal and fetal outcomes.
- Neonatal/fetal hypothyroidism is very rare and caused by the transplacental transfer of TSH receptor blocking antibodies, which may be seen in atrophic thyroiditis.

Management of hypothyroidism in pregnancy
- Most women should continue their maintenance dose of levothyroxine; the dose should only be ↑ if they are under-replaced (shown by TSH level).
- TSH levels need to be checked before conception and every trimester through pregnancy, unless there has been a dose adjustment, in which case it should be repeated in 4–6wks.
- If the diagnosis is made in pregnancy, in the absence of cardiac disease, consider a starting dose of 25–50 micrograms daily.
- In practice, aim for a TSH level of <2.5–3mU/L in the 1st trimester.
- Levothyroxine can be safely taken during breast-feeding.

Causes of hypothyroidism
- Hashimoto's thyroiditis.
- Atrophic thyroiditis.
- Congenital absence of thyroid.
- Iatrogenic:
  - thyroidectomy
  - radioiodine
  - drugs (amiodarone, lithium, iodine, antithyroid drugs).
- Pituitary cause (rare).

Other thyroid diseases

Postpartum thyroiditis

- An autoimmune condition causing destructive thyroiditis.
- Presents postpartum due to return to normal immunity after the relative immunosuppression of pregnancy.
- Preformed T_4 is released, which may cause transient hyperthyroid symptoms followed by hypothyroidism as the reserve of T_4 is used up.
- Can present for up to 1yr after delivery, but usually occurs 3–4mths postpartum.
- Incidence varies (5–10%) and it may manifest as:
  - transient hypothyroidism (40%)
  - hyperthyroidism (40%)
  - biphasic with 1st hyperthyroidism then hypothyroidism (20%).
- May be a family history of thyroid disease in 25% of cases.
- Many women are asymptomatic and often symptoms are vague and may be attributed to the postpartum state.
- Initiation of treatment should be based on symptoms and not biochemical results.
- Some women may not require any treatment.
- Most recover spontaneously.
- Risk of recurrence in future pregnancy is 70%.
- Risk of permanent hypothyroidism is 5%/yr for antibody-positive women (90% of patients have thyroid peroxidase antibodies).
- The hyperthyroid phase should be treated with β-blockers (not antithyroid drugs).
- ▶▶ *Differential diagnosis:* Graves' disease.
- The hypothyroid state should be treated with thyroxine; treatment should be withdrawn after 6mths to check for recovery.
- ▶▶ *Differential diagnosis:* hypothyroidism or Sheehan's syndrome.
- Long-term follow-up should be with annual TFT.

Thyroid nodules

- Thyroid nodules are common, affecting 5% of women in their reproductive years.
- ⚠ A small proportion of thyroid nodules are malignant.
- Differential diagnosis is a solitary toxic nodule, subacute (de Quervain's) thyroiditis, or a bleed into a cystic lesion.
- *Investigations:*
  - TFT and thyroid antibodies
  - thyroglobulin level: suggests malignancy if >100 micrograms/L
  - USS—cystic nodules are more likely to be benign than solid nodules
  - fine needle aspiration for cytology (cystic lesion)
  - biopsy (solid lesion).
- Malignant lesions can be surgically treated in the 2nd and 3rd trimesters, and postoperatively thyroxine can be safely given to completely suppress TSH in TSH-dependent tumours.

⚠ Radioiodine is contraindicated in pregnancy.

Thyroid nodules: symptoms or signs suggestive of malignancy

- Past history of radiation to neck or chest.
- Fixed lump.
- Lymphadenopathy.
- Rapid growth of painless nodule.
- Voice change.
- Neurological involvement such as Horner's syndrome.

Further reading

De Groot L et al. (2012). Management of thyroid dysfunction during pregnancy and postpartum: an Endocrine Society clinical practice guideline. *J Clin Endocrinol Metab*. 97:2543–2565.
Stagnaro-Green A et al. (2011). Guidelines of the American Thyroid Association for the diagnosis and management of thyroid disease during pregnancy and postpartum. *Thyroid*. 21:1081–1125.

Phaeochromocytoma

This is a tumour of the adrenal medulla that causes excess secretion of catecholamines. They are bilateral in 10% of cases and malignant in 10%. In non-pregnant hypertensive women, the incidence is around 1:1000; it is exceedingly rare in pregnancy. A high index of clinical suspicion is required to make the diagnosis—the condition should be considered in hypertensive women if there are atypical features (Box 5.7).

Untreated, mortality is high: maternal mortality ~17% and fetal mortality ~26%. Maternal mortality can be ↓ to ~4% with treatment.

Box 5.7 Symptoms and signs

- Hypertension.
- Sweating.
- Palpitations.
- Anxiety.
- Headache.
- Vomiting.

⚠ Symptoms may mimic pre-eclampsia and may be paroxysmal.

Investigations

- ↑ 24h urinary catecholamines or their metabolites, such as vanillylmandelic acid (VMA) confirm the diagnosis—a level 2× normal is highly suggestive and 3× normal diagnostic (methyldopa and labetalol can interfere with the results).
- Plasma metanephrines can also be used for screening.
- Imaging is required to localize the tumour (USS, CT, or MRI are all used but MRI is preferable in pregnancy).

Management

- MDT management including endocrine physician and surgeon.
- Main risk from this condition is potentially fatal hypertensive crises that can cause strokes, congestive cardiac failure, and arrhythmias.
- Patients should be commenced on α-blockers (phenoxybenzamine) to control BP, then β-blockers (propranolol) to control tachycardia.

⚠ Do *not* start β-blockers until a few days after α-blockers or a hypertensive crisis may ensue.

- Surgery is the only cure for the condition and should only be undertaken once pharmacological blockade has been achieved (if the diagnosis is made after 24wks, surgery should be delayed until fetal maturity is achieved).
- CS is preferred for delivery as it minimizes potential catecholamine surges (removal of the adrenal tumour can be done at the time of CS or later).
- Anaesthetic experience is vital as the patient may have a catecholamine surge during delivery due to inadequate pharmacological blockade.

Congenital adrenal hyperplasia

This is an autosomal recessive disorder affecting the synthesis of gluco-corticoids and mineralocorticoids. In response to low levels of these hormones, the pituitary gland produces large amounts of ACTH and this results in excessive production of sex steroids. A number of enzyme deficiencies can lead to this condition: the commonest is 21-hydroxylase deficiency. Many different gene mutations exist, which result in variable clinical presentations. Treatment is replacement with corticosteroid ± fludrocortisone.

Affected individuals present in several ways:
- Salt-losing crisis in neonate.
- Masculinization of female fetus (ambiguous genitalia at birth).
- Precocious puberty in boy.

▶ If a couple has an affected child, risk in subsequent pregnancies is 1:4.

Maternal and fetal risks

Pregnancies in women with congenital adrenal hyperplasia (CAH), diagnosed in infancy, are uncommon. Many are subfertile due to anovulation; others have psychosexual and emotional difficulties or anatomical problems related to corrective surgery for virilization.
- ↑ Risk of miscarriage, pre-eclampsia, and FGR.
- ↑ Risk of CD due to android-shaped pelvis.

Management

- Maternal steroid therapy should be continued at same dose throughout pregnancy.
- Genetic counselling should be offered to all couples after the birth of an affected child; antenatal diagnosis can be untaken in subsequent pregnancies, but the female fetus is at risk of virilization before these tests can be undertaken,

▶ Start dexamethasone, 1.5mg/day, as soon as pregnancy confirmed, and before 5wks gestation (dexamethasone crosses placenta and suppresses excessive fetal ACTH production, which prevents masculinization and neuroendocrine effects to female fetus).
- Fetal sexing via non-invasive prenatal diagnosis is now possible at around 10wks gestation.
- Fetal sex can usually be determined by USS at 16wks.
- If the fetus is male, or an unaffected female, stop dexamethasone.
- If the fetus is an affected female, options include continuation of dexamethasone throughout pregnancy or TOP.

▶ Mother needs to be monitored for gestational diabetes and ↑ BP.
- Suppression of virilization with dexamethasone is not always successful and parents should be appropriately counselled.
- During labour, parenteral steroids are required.
- Postnatally, the child needs to be reviewed by a paediatrician and evidence of virilization sought; replacement glucocorticoid and mineralocorticoid therapy should be continued.

Antenatal diagnosis
- NIPT—fetal cells in maternal blood analysed to ascertain fetal sex.
- Amniocentesis (≥16wks):
  - Fetal sex.
  - 17-Hydroxyprogesterone and androgen levels in amniotic fluid.
  - Human leucocyte antigen (HLA) typing of amniotic cells.
- Chorionic villus sampling (≥10wks):
  - fetal sex
  - gene probe for specific mutations of 21-hydroxylase

Further reading
NICE (2019). Intrapartum care for women with existing medical conditions or obstetric complications and their babies. NICE guideline [NG121].
🔗 https://www.nice.org.uk/guidance/ng121

Addison's disease, Conn's and Cushing's syndromes

Addison's disease

Adrenocortical failure with deficiency of glucocorticoids and mineralocorticoids; may be associated with other autoimmune conditions (e.g. pernicious anaemia, diabetes, or thyroid disease). Most common cause in the UK is autoimmune destruction of the adrenals. Worldwide, TB is an important cause. It is rare to make a new diagnosis in pregnancy.

- Diagnosis is based on ↓ cortisol, ↓ ACTH, and poor response to tetracosactide (synthetic ACTH).

▶ Cortisol measurements are normally ↑ in pregnancy; care should be taken in interpreting results.

- Pregnancy does not affect the course of Addison's disease and if the condition is treated there are no adverse fetal effects.
- Patients should continue with their usual steroid doses (hydrocortisone, prednisolone, or fludrocortisone) but an ↑ in glucocorticoid is often required in the 3rd trimester.
- ↑ or IV doses of steroids are required to cover periods of stress, such as infection, hyperemesis, labour, or surgery.
- In the puerperium, physiological diuresis can cause profound hypotension; tail steroids ↓ to maintenance over several days.

Clinical features of Addison's disease
- Weight loss.
- Vomiting.
- Postural hypotension and syncope.
- Weakness.
- Hyperpigmentation (skin folds, scars, mouth).

Conn's syndrome
- Rare cause of hypertension in pregnancy.
- 1° hyperaldosteronism is caused by adrenal aldosterone-secreting adenoma or carcinoma or bilateral adrenal hyperplasia.
- Clinical features are:
  - hypokalaemia (K^+ <3.0mmol/L occurring in ~40%)
  - hypertension.
- Diagnosis is based on:
  - ↓ K^+ (but the absence of this does not exclude the diagnosis)
  - ↑ plasma aldosterone
  - ↓ renin.
- Treat hypertension as usual (but avoid spironolactone which is used outside pregnancy) and give K^+ supplements.

Cushing's syndrome

- A condition of glucocorticoid excess.
- Very rare in pregnancy as anovulation leads to infertility.
- Causes in pregnancy are:
  - excessive pituitary ACTH secretion (44%)
  - adrenal adenoma (44%)
  - adrenal carcinoma (12%).
- Diagnosis based on ↑ cortisol, which fails to suppress with high-dose dexamethasone suppression test (ACTH levels depend on cause).
- Maternal morbidity and mortality are ↑, specifically pre-eclampsia, diabetes, and poor wound healing.
- Fetal loss, prematurity, and perinatal mortality are ↑.
- Adrenal insufficiency can occur in the neonate.
- Surgery is the treatment of choice for adrenal and pituitary causes, and it may be successfully performed in pregnancy.
- Medical treatment includes drugs that suppress cortisol production (metyrapone) or ACTH activity (cyproheptadine).

💣 Limited knowledge of use of drugs in pregnancy.

Clinical features of Cushing's syndrome

- Bruising.
- Myopathy.
- Hypertension.
- Excessive weight gain/oedema.
- Hirsutism.
- Excessive striae.
- Headaches.
- Acne.
- Obesity.
- Impaired glucose tolerance/diabetes.

Prolactinomas

Prolactinomas are the most common pituitary tumours seen in pregnancy. They can be classified according to their size into microprolactinoma (≤1cm) and macroprolactinoma (>1cm). Outside pregnancy, diagnosis is based on a ↑ serum prolactin level in conjunction with imaging of the pituitary fossa by CT or MRI. In pregnancy, there is a 10× physiological ↑ in prolactin levels, so prolactin level is not a useful test in diagnosis or follow-up.

Effect of pregnancy on prolactinoma

- Possibility that prolactinomas will ↑ in size and cause symptoms.
- Highest risk (15%) is in the 3rd trimester with macroprolactinomas.
- Pregnancy should be delayed until tumour shrinkage has occurred with drug therapy—↓ risk of symptomatic tumour expansion to 4%.
- Risk is small for microprolactinomas (1.6%).

Effect of prolactinoma on pregnancy

- Untreated, high prolactin levels lead to infertility.
- With preconception treatment fertility can be restored.
- Most cases have no complications in pregnancy.
- Breast-feeding is not contraindicated.

Management

- Outside pregnancy, dopamine receptor agonists (cabergoline and bromocriptine) ↓ prolactin levels; these could be stopped upon confirmation of pregnancy.
- The woman should report symptoms that might suggest tumour expansion—headache, visual disturbance, thirst, and polyuria; this should be investigated by CT or, preferably, MRI of the pituitary.
- Formal visual field testing is recommended in pregnancy for women with macroprolactinomas.
- Bromocriptine or cabergoline can safely be restarted if there is concern regarding tumour expansion and can be continued during breast-feeding, but may suppress milk production.
- Surgery is reserved for macroprolactinomas that fail to shrink despite drug therapy, but is usually delayed until after delivery.

Clinical features of prolactinoma
- Amenorrhoea.
- Galactorrhoea.
- Headache.
- Visual field defects (bitemporal hemianopia).
- Diabetes insipidus.

Hypopituitarism

This is anterior pituitary failure. The diagnosis is based on ↓ levels of anterior pituitary and target organ hormone levels: thyroxine, TSH, cortisol, ACTH, follicle-stimulating hormone (FSH), luteinizing hormone (LH), and growth hormone. There is also a failed response to an insulin stress test with lack of ↑ in growth hormone, ACTH, and prolactin levels.

⚠ Imaging of the pituitary area, by MRI or CT, should be undertaken to exclude a space-occupying lesion.

- Pregnancy is possible, but may require ovulation induction with gonadotrophins.
- Once pregnancy is achieved, the fetoplacental unit can sustain pregnancy by sufficient production of oestradiol and progesterone.
- Maternal and fetal outcome is normal if the condition is adequately treated.
- Inadequately treated cases are at ↑ risk of adverse outcomes including:
  - maternal hypotension
  - hypoglycaemia
  - mortality
  - miscarriage and stillbirth.
- Treatment involves replacement therapy with levothyroxine and hydrocortisone (additional IV hydrocortisone is required in labour).

Sheehan's syndrome

- Caused by avascular necrosis of the pituitary, as a result of profound hypotension usually 2° to a PPH.
- The pituitary is particularly vulnerable in pregnancy due to its 2–3× ↑ in size.
- Partial or complete pituitary failure can occur.
- Posterior pituitary is unaffected as it has a different blood supply.
- Treatment is as above.
- Pregnancies have been reported following this diagnosis.

Clinical features of Sheehan's syndrome
- Failure of lactation.
- Persistent amenorrhoea.
- Loss of pubic and axillary hair.
- Hypothyroidism.
- Adrenal insufficiency (vomiting, hypotension, hypoglycaemia).

Diabetes insipidus
- Incidence 1:15,000 pregnancies.
- Caused by a lack of antidiuretic hormone (ADH),

Four types
- *Central:* lack of ADH production by the posterior pituitary caused by expanding tumours.
- *Nephrogenic:* ADH resistance in the kidney.
- *Transient:* production of an enzyme by the placenta that results in ↑ breakdown of ADH, occurs in association with pre-eclampsia or AFLP.
- *Psychogenic:* compulsive water drinking.

Clinical features
- Excessive thirst and polyuria.
- Pregnancy may unmask the condition or make it worse (60%).
- Treatment is with desmopressin (intranasal preparation preferred), but this is rarely required in transient diabetes insipidus and should be used with caution in pregnancy.

Causes of hypopituitarism
- Pituitary surgery.
- Radiotherapy.
- Pituitary or hypothalamic tumours.
- Postpartum pituitary infarction (Sheehan's syndrome).
- Autoimmune lymphocytic hypophysitis.

Obesity in pregnancy: maternal risks

- Obesity is an ↑ problem in the developed world.
- The WHO definition of normal weight is a BMI between 18.5 and 24.9kg/m²:
  - overweight is BMI between 25.0 and 29.9kg/m²
  - obese is BMI ≥30kg/m².
- 1/5 pregnant women in the UK are now obese.
- The MBRRACE-UK 2021 rapid report identified that obesity carries an ↑ risk of maternal death and adverse perinatal outcome.

Maternal risks associated with obesity

Hypertension and pre-eclampsia
- Over twice as likely to develop gestational hypertension.
- BMI >30kg/m² significantly ↑ risk of pre-eclampsia.
- Excessive weight gain in pregnancy is associated with ↑ rates of pre-eclampsia in already overweight women.

Gestational diabetes
Over 3× more likely to develop GDM compared with women with a normal BMI.

Thromboembolism
Incidence of thromboembolic disease during pregnancy is doubled in obese women.

Antenatal requirements for obese women

- 5mg folic acid pre-conception and until 12wks.
- Vitamin D supplementation.
- VTE risk assessment.
- Referral for consultant care.
- Anaesthetic referral.
- GTT at 24–28wks.

⚠ It may be difficult to palpate the uterus in obese women, leading to:
- Missed diagnosis of breech presentation.
- Missed diagnosis of FGR or macrosomia.
- Unsuccessful ECV attempts.

⚠ USS is also technically difficult and may be inaccurate.

Postnatal complications associated with obesity

- ↑ rates of postoperative complications also occur, including:
  - wound infection and endometritis
  - lower respiratory tract infection
  - PPH.
- Also associated with a ↓ in breast-feeding frequency.

Peripartum risks of obesity
- Difficulty in siting regional anaesthesia due to body habitus.
- If a general anaesthesia (GA) is needed:
  - intubation is technically more difficult
  - ↑ risk of aspiration.
- Difficulty monitoring both the fetus and uterine contractions.
- Higher rate of:
  - induction of labour
  - failed induction
  - CD.
- If vaginal delivery, there is an ↑ rate of:
  - instrumental deliveries
  - shoulder dystocia
  - 3rd- and 4th-degree perineal tears.
- High pre-pregnancy BMI and weight gain in the inter-pregnancy interval has been shown to ↓ the success of VBAC by 50%.

Strategies for managing pregnancy in obese women
- Counselling regarding weight loss and lifestyle changes pre-pregnancy is ideal.
- ↑ vigilance for pre-eclampsia:
  - regular antenatal checks with urine dipstick analysis (low threshold for quantifying proteinuria)
  - measure arm circumference to ensure the correct size BP cuff.
- ↑ vigilance for diabetes:
  - consider random blood sugar at booking
  - urine dipstick analysis at each visit for glycosuria
  - GTT at 24–28wks (NICE).
- ↑ vigilance for both macrosomia and FGR: may need serial USS to monitor growth as SFH measurement may not be accurate.
- May require USS at 36wks gestation for presentation (to prevent an undiagnosed breech) if unable to palpate the fetus accurately.
- Women should aim for a weight neutral pregnancy.

Further reading

NICE (2010). Weight management before, during and after pregnancy. Public health guideline [PH27].
⌂ www.nice.org.uk/guidance/ph27

RCOG (2018). Care of women with obesity in pregnancy. Green-top guideline no. 72.
⌂ https://obgyn.onlinelibrary.wiley.com/doi/epdf/10.1111/1471-0528.15386

Obesity in pregnancy: fetal risks

Miscarriage

↑ rate of early miscarriage (both spontaneous and IVF pregnancies); this is thought to be related to ↓ insulin sensitivity.

Congenital abnormalities

⚫ Conflicting evidence regarding congenital abnormality risk.

Some groups have reported an ↑ rate of neural tube defects, heart, and intestinal abnormalities, with ↑ serum insulin, triglycerides, uric acid, and oestrogens; in addition to ↑ insulin resistance, hypoxia and hypercapnia have been proposed as mechanisms for these effects.

Stillbirth

- Risk of stillbirth ↑ consistently with ↑ pre-pregnancy BMI.
- Morbidly obese women are 3× more likely to have a stillbirth than women with normal BMI.

Macrosomia

- ↑ risk, independent of maternal diabetes and carries ↑ risk of:
  - Instrumental delivery
  - CD
  - 3rd-degree perineal tears
  - PPH.

Long-term risks for fetus

- Maternal weight is independent determinant of childhood obesity.
- Macrosomic fetuses have an ↑ risk of adolescent and adult obesity related to an ↑ incidence of the metabolic syndrome.

Chapter 6

Labour and delivery

Labour: overview

Labour is the process by which the fetus is delivered after the 24th wk of gestation. The onset of labour is defined as the point when uterine contractions become regular and cervical effacement and dilatation becomes progressive. Hence, it is difficult to define the precise time of the onset. For clinical management, the duration of observed labour is considered and not the duration the mother had painful contractions at home. Show and rupture of membranes may or may not be associated with labour, and these characteristics in themselves do not suggest onset of labour.

Labour is characterized by:
- Onset of uterine contractions, which ↑ in frequency, duration, and strength over time.
- Cervical effacement and dilatation.
- Rupture of membranes with leakage of amniotic fluid.
- Descent of the presenting part through the birth canal.
- Birth of the baby.
- Delivery of the placenta and membranes.

The mechanism of labour

The head usually engages in the transverse position and the passage of the head and body follows a well-defined pattern through the pelvis (Fig. 6.1). Not all the diameters of the fetal head can pass through a normal pelvis (➋ Diameters of the female pelvis, p. 12). The process of labour therefore involves the adaptation of the fetal head to the various segments of the pelvis.

Sequence for the passage through the pelvis for a normal vertex delivery

- *Engagement and descent*: the head enters the pelvis in the occipito-transverse position with flexion ↑ as it descends.
- *Internal rotation to occipito-anterior*: occurs at the level of the ischial spines due to the forward and downward sloping of the levator ani muscles.
- *Crowning*: the head extends, distending the perineum until it is delivered. The head does not recede between contractions.
- *Restitution*: the head rotates so that the occiput is in line with the fetal spine.
- *External rotation*: the shoulders rotate when they reach the levator muscles until the biacromial diameter is anteroposterior (the head externally rotates by the same amount).
- *Delivery of the anterior shoulder*: occurs by lateral flexion of the trunk posteriorly.
- *Delivery of the posterior shoulder*: occurs by lateral flexion of the trunk anteriorly and the rest of the body follows.

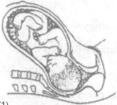

(1)
First stage of labour. The cervix dilates. After full dilation the head flexes futher and descends further into the pelvis.

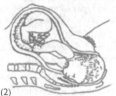

(2)
During the early second stage the head rotates at the levels of the ischial spine so the occiput lies in the anterior part of the pelvis. In late second stage the head broaches the vulval ring (crowning) and the perineum stretches over the head.

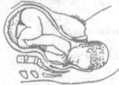

(3)
The head is born. The shoulders still lie transversely in the midpelvis.

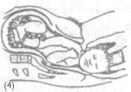

(4)
Birth of the anterior shoulder. The shoulders rotate to lie in the anteroposterior diameter of the pelvic outlet. The head rotates externally, 'restitutes', to its direction at onset of labour. Downward and backward traction of the head by the birth attendant aids delivery of the anterior shoulder

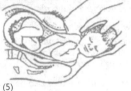

(5)
Birth of the posterior shoulder is aided by lifting the head upwards whilst maintaining traction.

Fig. 6.1 Mechanism of labour and delivery. Reproduced from Collier J, Longmore M, Brinsden M. (2003). *Oxford Handbook of Clinical Specialties*, 6th edn. Oxford: OUP. By permission of Oxford University Press.

Labour: 1st stage

The continuum of labour is divided into three stages.

1st stage is from onset of labour to full dilatation and is divided into two phases:
• *Latent phase:* the period taken for the cervix to completely efface and dilate up to 4cm (NICE, 2020).
• *Active phase:* there should be regular painful contractions when the cervix dilates from 4 to 5cm to full dilatation (10cm).
⚫ Recently, the WHO suggested that the active phase starts from 5cm.

Braxton Hicks contractions

Mild, often irregular, non-progressive contractions that may occur from 30wks gestation (more common after 36wks) and may often be confused with labour. However, contractions in labour are painful, with a gradual ↑ in frequency, amplitude, and duration.

▶ Intervention should not be offered or performed if the progress of labour is normal and there is no concern for the mother or the fetus.

Slow progress

• There is <2cm dilatation in 4h (on a 4h action line partogram the plotted progress falls to the right of the action line).
• Slowing in progress in parous women.

▶ Consideration should also be given to effacement of cervix and descent of the head.
• If labour is slow from onset, it is 1° *dysfunctional labour.*
• If there was previous adequate progress followed by slow or no progress then it is 2° *arrest.*

▶ These patterns observed on the partogram do not indicate the cause for the poor progress.

Some causes of poor progress in the 1st stage

• Inefficient uterine activity (*power*—most common cause).
• Malpositions, malpresentation, or large baby (*passenger*).
• Inadequate pelvis due to bony problems (e.g. previous fracture of pelvis) or other physical cause like fibroids (*passage*).
• A combination of ≥2 of the above.

Monitoring in labour (recorded on the partogram)
See Fig. 6.2.
• The FHR should be monitored every 15min (or continuously).
• The contractions should be assessed every 30min.
• Maternal pulse should be checked hourly.
• BP and temperature should be checked 4-hourly.
• VE should be offered every 4h to assess progress.
• Maternal urine is tested 4-hourly for ketones and protein.

Poor progress in the 1st stage

Assessment

- Review the history.
- Abdominal palpation, frequency, and duration of contractions.
- Review fetal condition, FHR, and colour/quantity of amniotic fluid.
- Review maternal condition including hydration and analgesia.
- Vaginal assessment; cervical effacement, dilatation, caput, moulding, position, and station of the head.

Management

- Amniotomy (artificial rupture of membranes (ARM)) and reassess in 2–4h.
- Amniotomy + oxytocin infusion and reassess in 2–4h of adequate uterine contractions: this should always be considered in nulliparous women.
- Lower segment CD (if there is fetal distress).

⚠ For multiparous women and those with a previous CD, an experienced obstetrician should review before starting oxytocin.

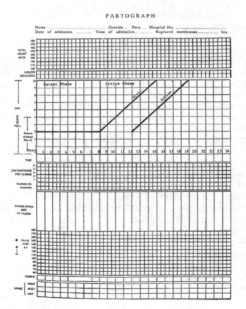

PARTOGRAPH

Fig. 6.2 Example of a partogram.

Further reading

NICE. Intrapartum care overview.
⅋ http://pathways.nice.org.uk/pathways/intrapartum-care

Labour: 2nd stage

2nd stage is the time from full cervical dilatation until the baby is born.

▶ If the woman has an epidural and the CTG is reassuring, 1h is usually allowed for passive descent before active pushing is commenced.
- During this hour it is important to ensure that contractions are of adequate frequency (3–5 in 10min) and duration (>40s).
- If already on oxytocin there is a possibility of hyperstimulation and the dose may need to be ↓.
- If contractions are inadequate, oxytocin may be considered if the FHR is not pathological and there is no obvious cephalopelvic disproportion.

▶ Birth should take place within 3h of the start of 2nd stage for nulliparous women and within 2h for multiparous women.

Description of a normal 2nd stage
- Active 2nd stage commences when the mother starts expulsive efforts using her abdominal muscles with the Valsalva manoeuvre to 'bear down'.
- Women may choose many different positions to deliver:
  - squatting, standing, on all fours, or supine
  - lithotomy may be required for instrumental deliveries.
- As the head comes down, it distends the perineum and anus: a pad may be used to support the perineum and cover the anus, while the other hand is used to maintain flexion and prevent sudden deflexion and to control the rate of delivery of the head (this helps to slow perineal distension, ↓ tears by preventing rapid delivery).
- An episiotomy may be performed if there is concern that the perineum is tearing towards the anal sphincter: episiotomy should not be used routinely.
- With the next contraction gentle traction guides the head towards the perineum until the anterior shoulder is delivered under the subpubic arch.
- Gentle traction upwards and anteriorly helps to deliver the posterior shoulder and the trunk over the perineum.
- The cord is double-clamped and cut:
  - delaying cord clamping for 2–3min results in ↑ blood volume and haematocrit levels in the neonate and provides short- and long-term benefits.
- As long as it is born in good condition, the baby should be handed to the mother as soon as possible.
- The condition of the baby is assessed at 1, 5, and 10min using the Apgar scoring system.

Delay in the 2nd stage of labour

Nulliparous women
- Suspected if delivery is not imminent after 1h of active pushing:
  - VE should be offered and amniotomy recommended if membranes are intact.
- If not delivered in 2h:
  - requires review by obstetrician to consider instrumental delivery or CD.

Multiparous women
- If delivery is not imminent after 1h of active pushing:
  - requires review by obstetrician to consider instrumental delivery or CD.

⚠ Delay in the 2nd stage in a multiparous woman must always raise suspicions of malposition or disproportion.

Labour: 3rd stage

3rd stage is the duration from delivery of the baby to delivery of the placenta and membranes.

Active management of the 3rd stage

Consists of:
- Use of uterotonics.
- Clamping and cutting of the cord.
- Controlled cord traction.

Benefits
- ↓ rates of PPH >1000mL.
- ↓ mean blood loss and postnatal anaemia.
- ↓ length of the 3rd stage.
- ↓ need for blood transfusions.

Adverse effects
- Nausea and vomiting.
- Headache.

Physiological management of the 3rd stage

Consists of:
- No Syntometrine® or oxytocin is given.
- Cord is allowed to stop pulsating before it is clamped and cut.

▶ NICE (2020) recommends that the cord should not be clamped for 1min, unless the baby's heart rate is <60 beats/min and not picking up.
- Currently equipment is available that can be kept by the side of the mother to help resuscitation with the cord intact.
- Cord should be clamped before the end of 5min.
- The placenta is delivered by maternal effort alone.

⚠ The cord must not be pulled and the uterus not pushed on in any direction to help to expel the placenta.

A planned physiological 3rd stage should be changed to active management in the event of:
- Haemorrhage.
- Failure to deliver the placenta within 1h.
- Maternal desire to shorten the 3rd stage.

Description of an actively managed 3rd stage

- Syntometrine® IM (ergometrine 0.5mg + oxytocin 5IU) or oxytocin 10IU IM or carbetocin 100 micrograms is given as the anterior shoulder of the baby is born.
- A dish is placed at the introitus to collect the placenta and any blood loss, and the left hand is placed on the abdomen over the uterine fundus.
- As the uterus contracts to 20wk size, the placenta separates from the uterus through the spongy layer of the decidua basalis.
- The uterus will then feel firmer, the cord will lengthen, and there is often a trickle of fresh blood (separation bleeding).
- Controlled cord traction is applied with the right hand, while supporting the fundus with the left hand (Brandt–Andrew's technique). RCTs have shown that controlled cord traction is not an essential component of active management of 3rd stage.

⚠ Multiple pregnancy must be excluded before uterotonics are given.

▶ NICE recommends the use of oxytocin 10IU rather than Syntometrine® as it has similar efficacy but with fewer side effects.

▶ Cochrane network meta-analysis indicates that combination of oxytocin and misoprostol, or oxytocin and ergometrine, or heat-stable carbetocin alone are superior to oxytocin only. Carbetocin has fewer side effects than the combination of drugs.

Care immediately after delivery

- Most complications occur in the first 2h after delivery, including:
  - PPH
  - uterine inversion
  - haematoma formation.
- Usually, women are kept in the delivery unit during this time to observe: pulse, BP, temperature, uterine size and contractions, bleeding, or painful swelling of the vulva, vagina, or perineum.
- Where there is an ↑ risk of PPH (e.g. multiple pregnancy), an oxytocin infusion may be given prophylactically for 3–4h.
- Encouragement should be given for skin-to-skin contact as soon as possible and the mother and baby should not be separated for the 1st hour.
- Support should be provided for breast-feeding, which should be initiated in the 1st hour.
- If there are no complications during these 2h, the mother may then be transferred to the postnatal ward:
  - some women may then go home after a further 3–4h of observation.

Induction of labour: indications

- 10–20% of all pregnancies are induced.
- Overall success rate is ~60–80% at term.
- Chance of achieving vaginal birth after induction of labour (IOL) <34wks is <35%.
- Indication may be obstetric or medical.

⚠ IOL on maternal request should be avoided as it is associated with risks for both mother and fetus.

Obstetric indications
- Uteroplacental insufficiency (one of the most common indications).
- Prolonged pregnancy (41–42wks).
- FGR.
- Oligo- or anhydramnios.
- Abnormal uterine or umbilical artery Dopplers.
- Non-reassuring CTG.
- Prelabour rupture of membranes (PROM).
- Severe pre-eclampsia or eclampsia after maternal stabilization.
- IUD of the fetus.
- Unexplained APH at term.
- Chorioamnionitis.

💣 There is inadequate evidence for induction for suspected fetal macrosomia. Some advocate IOL around 40–41wks with an aim of preventing further intrauterine growth and associated risks like shoulder dystocia and birth trauma.

Medical indications
- With underlying maternal medical conditions, planned early IOL may potentially limit the maternal risks associated with pregnancy.
- Careful timing is required to balance the best interests of the mother with any potential risks of prematurity.
- Such situations may include:
  - severe hypertension
  - uncontrolled diabetes mellitus
  - renal disease with deteriorating renal function
  - malignancies (to facilitate definitive therapy).

Cervical ripening

Predictors for successful induction of labour

- ↑ Gestational age at induction.
- ↑ Parity.
- Modified Bishop's score of the cervix (Table 6.1):
  - Indicates 'ripeness' of the cervix (↑ score, ↑ success).

Mechanical methods of cervical ripening

Separation of the membranes from the cervix leads to the local release of prostaglandins.

- A common method is artificial separation ('stretch and sweep'):
  - requires that the cervical os admits a finger and involves digitally separating the membranes from the cervix
  - uncomfortable and may lead to some bleeding
  - 30% will go into spontaneous labour in <7 days
  - in the majority it results in a more favourable cervix.
- Balloon catheters have similar success rates as prostaglandin E2 (PGE2 = dinoprostone) but without the risk of hyperstimulation:
  - catheter (a Foley is often used) is inserted through the cervix, the balloon is inflated, and is pulled down against the internal os
  - no risk of hyperstimulation so this can be safely performed as an outpatient
  - when the cervix is 2cm dilated, the balloon will fall out.

Pharmacological methods

Prostaglandins (PGE2)

- Usually given intravaginally into the posterior fornix.
- The gel form is absorbed well.
- Tablets are easier to remove if hyperstimulation occurs (5–7%).
- Vaginal prostaglandins (3mg tablets, 2mg gel) ↑ vaginal delivery rates within 24h with no ↑ in operative delivery rates.
- PGE2 slow release is available as a Propess® pessary—shaped like a small flat tampon with a tail for easy removal. It is left *in situ* for 24h. Results suggest ↓ induction to delivery intervals and slightly ↓ instrumental vaginal delivery rates, but no difference in CD rates.
- WHO recommends the use of 25 micrograms misoprostol orally every 2h or vaginally every 6h.

🅜 Misoprostol appears to have ↑ success rate in vaginal delivery but has ↑ of hyperstimulation and passage of meconium by the fetus.

🅜 Misoprostol is not licensed for induction in all countries and is contra-indicated in women with a Caesarean scar.

Oxytocin infusion

- Has been shown to ↑ cervical prostaglandin levels.
- As most receptors are located in the myometrium, it is more suitable for initiating uterine contractions.
- Best used where membranes have ruptured, whether spontaneously or after amniotomy.

Table 6.1 Modified Bishop's score: to assess the favourability for induction of labour. A total score of >8 indicates a favourable cervix

Score	0	1	2
Position of cervix	Posterior	Axial	Anterior
Length of cervix	2cm	1cm	<0.5cm
Consistency of cervix	Firm	Soft	Soft and stretchy
Dilatation of cervix	0	1cm	>2cm
Station of the presenting part (distance in cm in relation to the ischial spines)	−2	−1	0

Data from Kennedy JH, et al. (1982). Induction of labor with a stable-based prostaglandin E2 vaginal tablet. *Eur J Obstet Gynecol Reprod Biol.* 13(4):203–208.

Suggested alternative methods for cervical ripening

▶ Although often suggested to pregnant women, there is no evidence that any of the following are effective in cervical ripening or IOL:
- Sexual intercourse.
- Herbal remedies (raspberry leaf tea).
- Nipple stimulation.
- Acupuncture.
- Castor oil.

Induction of labour: methods

Amniotomy

- ARM or amniotomy releases local prostaglandins causing cervical ripening and myometrial contractions.
- If regular, painful contractions have not started or there are no cervical changes after 2h, oxytocin infusion should be commenced.
- Starting oxytocin at the time of amniotomy has been shown to ↓ the induction–delivery interval, thereby ↓ both the fetal and maternal risk of sepsis.
- ARM alone is not recommended for IOL.

Prostaglandins for induction of labour

- A CTG should be performed 30min before, as well as after insertion of prostaglandins to confirm fetal well-being and to detect possible hyperstimulation.
- VE after 6h:
  - if the cervix is not favourable, another dose may be administered (>2 doses need to be reviewed by a senior obstetrician)
  - multiparous women seldom require >1 dose.
- Oxytocin should not be started for 6h to ↓ the risk of uterine hyperstimulation.

Synthetic oxytocin for induction or augmentation of labour

- Should be started on a low dose (1–4mU/min).
- Is ↑ (usually doubled) every 30min to achieve optimal contractions (3–4 every 10min, moderate to strong on palpation, each lasting 40–60s).
- Continuous CTG monitoring should be used:
  - the sensitivity of the myometrium to oxytocin ↑ during labour and it may be necessary to ↓ the rate of infusion as labour advances
  - infusion pumps should be used to carefully control the amount given and ↓ the risk of uterine hyperstimulation.

⚫ Women should be advised that the use of oxytocin will ↓ the length of labour but benefits in ↓ operative births due to dystocia and impact on neonatal outcomes need further study.

Risks and complications of IOL

Prematurity
- Iatrogenic (e.g. in severe pre-eclampsia).
- Unintentional (failure to correctly assess the gestational age).

Cord prolapse
- With rupture of membranes if the presenting part is not engaged.

Side effects of pharmacological agents used
- Pain or discomfort.
- Uterine hyperstimulation.
- Fetal distress.
- Uterine rupture (rare but ↑ in grand multipara or a scarred uterus).
- Prostaglandins rarely cause non-selective stimulation of other smooth muscle leading to:
  - nausea and vomiting
  - diarrhoea
  - bronchoconstriction (caution in asthmatics)
  - maternal pyrexia may result owing to the effect on thermoregulation in the hypothalamus.

Caesarean delivery
- Due to failed induction.

Postpartum haemorrhage
- Mostly due to atony.

Intrauterine infection
- With prolonged induction.

⚠ Oxytocin has the properties of ADH, and U&E should be checked if it has been used for >12h as it may very rarely cause dilutional hyponatraemia.

⚠ WHO advises proper counselling of women scheduled for IOL. Should they not deliver after a course of prostaglandin, then do not consider these cases as failed IOL but counsel the woman to have deferred induction in a few days using the same or a different method.

Induction of labour: special circumstances

Prelabour rupture of membranes
Prostaglandins may be used before starting oxytocin for IOL if the cervix is unfavourable.

Stabilizing induction
This is carried out when the presenting part is not engaged or when there is an unstable lie, to avoid the risk of cord prolapse.
- The head is 'stabilized' by an assistant holding it suprapubically and, if possible, pushing the head into the pelvic brim.
- Amniotomy is performed after excluding cord presentation.
- Once cord prolapse is excluded, oxytocin infusion is started.

▶ Usually performed in a delivery unit with the theatre team available should an emergency of cord prolapse occur.

Grand multipara (≥para 5)
⚠ Risk of uterine rupture is ↑ and hence caution should be exercised.

💣 Prostaglandin gel should not be used.

- Onset of labour is awaited for up to 4h after ARM.
- In the absence of contractions, oxytocin infusion can be started and titrated to get 3–4 contractions every 10min, which are moderate to strong on palpation.
- Once contractions are established, it should be possible to stop the oxytocin as most will continue to labour and deliver normally.

⚠ Malpresentation (obstructed labour) must be excluded before starting oxytocin.

Induction for intrauterine death at term
The WHO and RCOG guidelines recommend misoprostol 25 micrograms orally every 2–4h:
- As this strength is not available in the UK 200-microgram tablets can be dissolved in 40mL water and 5mL aliquots administered.
- Although uniformity of strength cannot be guaranteed, it is potentially safer than administering a higher dose.

IOL with previous Caesarean delivery

⚠ The risk of scar dehiscence with previous uterine surgery is:
- 5:1000 with spontaneous labour.
- 8:1000 with use of oxytocin.
- 24:1000 with prostaglandins.

▶ Women should be counselled regarding these risks and have continuous CTG monitoring throughout the whole of the induction process when contractions are present.

▶ Facilities should be available for immediate CD should there be a scar rupture and fetal bradycardia.

Further reading

NICE (2021). Inducing labour. NICE guideline [NG207].
🔗 https://www.nice.org.uk/guidance/ng207

RCOG (2010). Late intrauterine fetal death and stillbirth. Green-top guideline no. 55.
🔗 https://www.rcog.org.uk/media/0fefdrk4/gtg_55.pdf

WHO (2018). WHO recommendations: induction of labour at or beyond term.
🔗 https://apps.who.int/iris/bitstream/handle/10665/277233/9789241550413-eng.pdf

Fetal surveillance in labour: overview

- It is estimated that 10% of CP is due to intrapartum hypoxia (the rest may be attributed to antenatal events).
- Blood supply to the placenta is restricted with contractions on the fetal side by cord compression or ↓ blood flow on the maternal side (especially in the 2nd stage because of more frequent and longer duration of contractions), placing a physiological strain on the fetus.
- Ability to withstand the stress is dependent on fetal reserve:
  - ↓ reserve is seen with FGR and prolonged pregnancy
  - a fetus that was coping in the antenatal period but has no extra reserve may decompensate in labour.

Intrapartum surveillance

- Intermittent auscultation.
- Continuous CTG, also known as electronic fetal monitoring (EFM).
- Routine CTG is not advised for low-risk women in suspected or established labour (NICE, 2017).
- CTG should be performed if there is difficulty or some abnormality of the FHR on auscultation:
  - if CTG is then normal for 20min, it could be discontinued.

Assessment for surveillance

- On admission in labour, an assessment should be made to identify fetal and maternal risk factors (Box 6.1 and Box 6.2).
- FHR should be auscultated for 1min and entered as a single rate.
- Graphic display Dopplers can identify features of fetal well-being (accelerations) or compromise (↓ variability or decelerations).
- Maternal heart rate should be palpated simultaneously to ensure the FHR is distinctly different.
- If the woman has no risk factors she should be offered intermittent auscultation performed for a full minute after a contraction:
  - at least every 15min in the 1st stage
  - every 5min or after every other contraction in the 2nd stage.
  - any accelerations or decelerations that are auscultated should be recorded
  - if fetal death is suspected, a USS should be performed.

Box 6.1 Intrapartum risks requiring EFM

- Oxytocin augmentation.
- Epidural analgesia.
- Intrapartum vaginal bleeding.
- Pyrexia >37.5°C.
- Fresh meconium staining of liquor.
- Abnormal FHR on intermittent auscultation.
- Prolonged labour.

Electronic fetal monitoring

- Results in:
  - ↑ intervention and operative delivery rates
  - no marked ↓ in CP.
- Most likely because:
  - CTG is not specific enough to detect fetal hypoxia
  - failure to consider the clinical situation
  - poor interpretation
  - delay in taking action
  - intrapartum hypoxia as a cause of CP is rare.
- Additional tests, such as fetal scalp blood sampling (FBS) in labour, are required to ↑ specificity.
- Decisions to intervene should not be based purely on CTG.

💧 Some centres use fetal ECG ST waveform analysis (STAN) to improve the positive predictive value of the CTG.

💧 Cochrane review suggested that with STAN there is ↓ of FBS and total operative delivery, but not CD and there is no ↓ in poor outcome of the neonate.

Box 6.2 Antenatal risk factors that should prompt EFM in labour

Maternal
- Previous CD.
- Cardiac problems.
- Pre-eclampsia.
- Prolonged pregnancy (>42wks).
- PROM (>24h).
- IOL.
- Diabetes.
- APH.
- Other significant maternal medical conditions.

Fetal
- FGR.
- Prematurity.
- Oligohydramnios.
- Abnormal Doppler velocimetry.
- Multiple pregnancy.
- Meconium-stained liquor.
- Breech presentation.

Fetal surveillance: cardiotocography

Definitions of terms used in EFM

- *Baseline rate:* mean level of the FHR when stable, assessed over 10min, and after exclusion of accelerations and decelerations.
- *Baseline variability:* degree to which the baseline varies, i.e. bandwidth of baseline after exclusion of accelerations and decelerations. Variability of 5–25 beats/min is defined as normal, 0–5 beats/min as ↓, and >25 beats/min as saltatory.
- *Acceleration:* a transient rise in FHR from a steady baseline rate by at least 15 beats over the baseline lasting for ≥15s (Fig. 6.3).
- *Deceleration:* a reduction in the baseline of ≥15 beats for >15s.

Baseline rate and variability

- Reassuring features in assessing fetal well-being are:
  - normal variability of >5 beats/min as this is a reflection of a fully functioning autonomic nervous system
  - 'cycling' alternating periods of quiescence and activity
  - presence of accelerations (somatic nervous system).

⚠ *Always be concerned about a CTG if you cannot identify the baseline rate.*

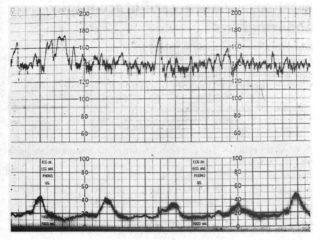

Fig. 6.3 Cardiotocographic trace, showing baseline rate of 140 beats/min, several accelerations and normal baseline variability, and no decelerations with contractions suggestive of a non-hypoxic fetus.

Causes of ↓ baseline variability

- Fetal hypoxia.
- Fetal sleep cycle (should be for <50min).
- Fetal malformation (CNS or cardiac) or arrhythmias.
- Administration of drugs including:
  - pethidine
  - methyldopa
  - MgSO₄
  - opiate analgesics
  - corticosteroids
  - tranquillizers
  - barbiturates
  - general anaesthesia.
- Severe prematurity.
- Fetal heart block.
- Fetal anomalies.
- Fetal infection/chorioamnionitis.
- Fetal brain haemorrhage.
- Fetal anaemia (associated with a sinusoidal pattern).

Fetal surveillance: cardiotocography abnormalities

Abnormalities in baseline rate

Bradycardia

- Baseline FHR of <110 beats/min.
- 100–110 beats/min is moderate bradycardia and on its own is not considered to be associated with fetal compromise if the variability is normal and accelerations are present.
- A baseline <100 beats/min should raise the possibility of hypoxia or other pathology.

⚠ When the FHR is <110 beats/min, beware of maternal heart rate being recorded as the FHR.

Tachycardia

- Baseline FHR of >160 beats/min and is associated with maternal pyrexia and tachycardia, prematurity, and fetal acidosis especially if associated with decelerations.
- 160–180 beats/min is moderate baseline tachycardia and on its own is probably not indicative of hypoxia if the variability is normal and accelerations are present.
- A baseline >180 beats/min should always raise suspicion of underlying pathology.

Other abnormalities

Sinusoidal pattern

- Relatively rare, consists of an undulating pattern (sine wave) with little, or no, baseline variability.
- Can indicate significant fetal anaemia, but in short spells (<10min) may be a result of fetal behaviour (thumb-sucking).

⚠ A sinusoidal pattern should always be taken seriously. Blood group antibodies, Kleihauer test, and a scan for MCA velocity to detect fetal anaemia may be indicated.

Maternal factors that may contribute to an abnormal CTG

- The woman's position: advise her to adopt left lateral.
- Hypotension.
- Vaginal examination.
- Emptying bladder or bowels.
- Vomiting.
- Vasovagal episodes.
- Siting and topping up of regional anaesthesia.

Fetal blood sampling

- FBS is used to improve the specificity of CTG in the detection of fetal hypoxia.
- It should be obtained if the trace is pathological, unless obvious immediate delivery may be required (e.g. bradycardia of <80 beats/ min for >3min without signs of recovery).
- The woman should be in the left lateral position.

Interpretation of the FBS results
- *Normal* (pH ≥7.25):
  - repeat FBS within 1h if CTG remains pathological.
- *Borderline* (pH 7.21–7.24):
  - repeat FBS within 30min if CTG remains pathological.
- *Abnormal* (pH ≤7.20):
  - immediate delivery.

💣 There have been calls challenging the validity and usefulness of FBS, but NICE recommends continued use of FBS.

💣 Newer technology of computer-assisted CTG interpretation has not proven to be useful (e.g. INFANT study of 45,000 cases).

Decelerations

Early decelerations

- Peak coincides with the peak of the contraction.
- The onset and recovery to baseline follows the onset and offset of the contraction (Fig. 6.4).

▶ This is related to head compression and, therefore, should only be seen in late 1st stage or 2nd stage of labour.

Late decelerations

- Have at least a 20s time lag between the peak of the contraction and the nadir of the deceleration (Fig. 6.5).

⚠ They may be suggestive of acidosis, especially if accompanied with tachycardia and ↓ baseline variability.

⚠ Shallow, late decelerations in the presence of ↓ baseline variability on a non-reactive trace should be of particular concern and may even be preterminal, especially if there are associated clinical risks including FGR, absent FM, bleeding, infection, prolonged pregnancy, or severe pre-eclampsia.

Variable decelerations

- Variable pattern in timing, size, and shape and are associated with cord compression (Fig. 6.6):

Non-concerning characteristics (or 'typical')

- U or V shaped.
- Quick to drop and to recover.
- Often have 'shouldering'.
- Not usually associated with hypoxia if:
  - the decline of the FHR is with the onset of the contractions and returns to baseline with the offset of the contraction
  - the inter-deceleration intervals are longer than the duration of the deceleration
  - there is no rise in baseline rate and the variability is normal.

Concerning characteristics (or 'atypical')

- Duration of >60s.
- A loss >60 beats/min from the baseline.
- Slow recovery.
- A combined variable.
- A late deceleration component, i.e. the recovery of the deceleration to the baseline rate is after the offset of the contraction.
- With progressive hypoxia the decelerations become:
  - deeper and wider with ↓ of inter-deceleration interval
  - rising baseline rate.

💊 Such pattern with ↓ of baseline variability for 1–2h suggests possible fetal acidosis.

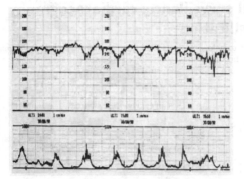

Fig. 6.4 Cardiotocograph trace with early decelerations.

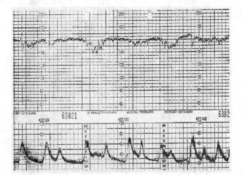

Fig. 6.5 Cardiotocograph trace with late decelerations.

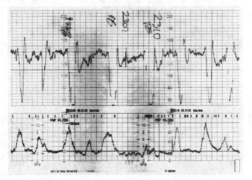

Fig. 6.6 Cardiotocograph trace with variable decelerations.

Fetal surveillance: cardiotocography classification

In order to help with the difficulties encountered when assessing a CTG, a classification scheme was introduced that can be used to define a CTG as normal, suspicious, or abnormal (Table 6.2).

Table 6.2 Fetal heart rate feature classification

Description	Baseline (beats/min)	Variability (beats/min)	Decelerations	Accelerations
Reassuring	110–160	5–25	None Or Early variable with no concerning characteristics for <90min	Present
Non-reassuring	100–110[a] Or 161–180	<5 for ≥30 to 50min Or >25 for 15–25min	Variable decelerations with no concerning characteristics[b] for 90min Or More or variables with concerning characteristics[b] in up to 50% of contractions for ≥30min Or Variable decelerations with concerning characteristics[b] in >50% contractions for <30min Or Late decelerations in >50% of contractions for <30min with no maternal or fetal clinical risk factors such as vaginal bleeding or significant meconium	
Abnormal	<100 >180 Or Sinusoidal pattern	<5 for >50min Or >25 for >25min	Variable decelerations with any concerning characteristics in >50% contractions for ≤30min if any maternal or fetal risk factors (see above) Or Late decelerations for 30min (or less if any maternal or fetal clinical risk factors) Or Acute bradycardia or single prolonged deceleration for ≥3min	

[a] Although baseline 100–109 beats/min is a non-reassuring feature, continue normal care if there is normal baseline variability and no variable or late decelerations.

[b] Regard the following as concerning characteristics of variable decelerations: lasting >60s, reduced baseline variability within the deceleration, failure to return to baseline, biphasic (W) shape, no shouldering.

Management based on CTG classification

Management should be based on using Table 6.2.

Normal

All four features are reassuring:
- Continue CTG unless it was started because of concerns arising from intermittent auscultation and there are no ongoing risk factors.
- Talk to the woman and her birth companion(s) about what is happening.

Suspicious

One non-reassuring and two reassuring features:
- Correct any underlying causes, such as hypotension or uterine hyperstimulation.
- Perform full set of maternal observations.
- Start ≥1 conservative measures.
- Inform an obstetrician or a senior midwife.
- Document a plan for reviewing the whole clinical picture and the CTG findings.
- Talk to the woman and her companion(s) about what is happening and take her preference into account.

Pathological

One abnormal feature or two non-reassuring features:
- Obtain a review by an obstetrician and a senior midwife.
- Exclude acute events (e.g. cord prolapse, suspected placental abruption, or suspected uterine rupture).
- Correct any underlying causes, such as hypotension or uterine hyperstimulation.
- Start ≥1 corrective measures.
- Talk to the woman and her birth companion(s) about what is happening and take her preferences into account.
- If the CTG trace is still pathological after implementing conservative measures—obtain a further review by an obstetrician and senior midwife.
- Offer digital fetal scalp stimulation and document the outcome.
- If the CTG trace is still pathological after digital scalp stimulation, consider FBS or to expedite birth.
- Take the woman's preference into account.

Further reading

NICE. Fetal monitoring during labour: pathway.
🖑 https://pathways.nice.org.uk/pathways/intrapartum-care/fetal-monitoring-during-labour

Meconium-stained liquor

Meconium is made up of water, bile pigment, mucus, and amniotic fluid debris. Detection in amniotic fluid causes anxiety as it is associated with ↑ perinatal morbidity and mortality; it may be aspirated by fetus.

- Meconium-stained amniotic fluid (MSAF) is rare in preterm infants (<5%) and is associated with infection (e.g. *Listeria*) and chorioamnionitis.
- Incidence of MSAF gradually ↑ from 36 to 42wks.
- Passage of meconium signifies the maturation of CNS and gastrointestinal system.
- Sometimes hypoxia causes peristalsis of the bowel and relaxation of anal sphincters resulting in MSAF.
- Use of PGE1 (misoprostol) for IOL is associated with passage of meconium by the fetus.

Meconium aspiration syndrome

- Occurs in 1:1000 births in Europe.
- May happen *in utero* when fetal breathing movements draw amniotic fluid into the airway:
  - fetal gasping *in utero* is thought to be associated with prolonged decelerations (>2min) that cause transient hypoxia.
- Meconium aspiration syndrome can occur in fetuses that are not acidotic in labour.
- Meconium:
  - causes mechanical blockage of the airway
  - acts as a chemical irritant, causing pneumonitis and alveolar collapse
  - predisposes to 2° bacterial infection.

⚠ Suction of the mouth and upper airway immediately after delivery is not currently recommended if the baby is active and crying.

⚠ If the newborn has respiratory difficulty, meconium should be cleared from the oro- and nasopharynx and, if needed, from the trachea by using a laryngoscopy.

▶ This will not help with pre-existing *in utero* aspiration.

Description of MSAF

- It is important to record the presence or absence of meconium.
- Dark green or black meconium-stained fluid that is tenacious or that contains lumps of meconium is considered 'significant'.

Management of meconium-stained liquor

- Major consideration is the colour and quantity of amniotic fluid.
- Light meconium with abundance of liquor is likely to be due to the function of CNS and bowel maturity while thick meconium with scanty fluid or freshly passed meconium in a cephalic presentation may suggest possibility of hypoxia especially if the CTG is pathological.
- Consider IOL if PROM.
- Advise continuous fetal monitoring.
- Consider delivery if there is failure to progress needing oxytocin infusion in the presence of thick meconium, as hyperstimulation and prolonged deceleration may cause aspiration.
- If there is maternal pyrexia or evidence of chorioamnionitis and thick meconium with scanty fluid, infected meconium is likely to cause severe meconium aspiration syndrome.
- Advise delivery in a unit able to provide FBS and advanced neonatal life support at birth:
  - if the baby is born with depressed vital signs, they will require laryngoscopy and suction by a healthcare professional trained in advanced neonatal life support
  - if the baby is born in good condition, they will still require close monitoring for 12h.

Operative vaginal delivery: overview

- CD in the 2nd stage of labour is associated with ↑ morbidity to the mother and ↑ risk of subsequent preterm delivery.
- Instrumental vaginal delivery helps to avoid maternal and perinatal morbidity and mortality and an emergency CD.
- In the UK, the operative vaginal delivery rate is stable at between 10% and 15%.
- It is important to appreciate that forceps and ventouse are complementary to each other and that operator's skill and experience, as well as clinical findings, should help decide which one to use.

▶ If in doubt, senior help must be called.

Indications for instrumental delivery

Maternal
- Exhaustion.
- Prolonged 2nd stage:
  - >1h of passive phase and 1h of active pushing in multiparous women
  - >2h of passive phase and 1h of active pushing in primiparous women.
- Medical indications for avoiding Valsalva manoeuvre, such as:
  - severe cardiac disease
  - hypertensive crisis
  - uncorrected cerebral vascular malformations.
- Pushing is not possible (paraplegia or tetraplegia).

Fetal
- Fetal compromise.
- To control the after-coming head of breech (forceps).

▶ It is important to discuss with the woman why an operative delivery is indicated, the instrument chosen, the likelihood of success, and the alternatives available (emergency CD).

⚠ Consent (verbal or written) must be obtained by explaining the indication and it should be recorded.

Complications of operative vaginal delivery
- Forceps are associated with ↑ maternal trauma (including anal sphincter trauma).
- Rotational forceps may cause spiral tears of the vagina.
- Fetal injuries with forceps are rare but may occur (mostly due to incorrect application of the blades) including:
  - facial nerve palsy
  - skull fractures
  - orbital injury
  - intracranial haemorrhage.
- Ventouse is associated with fetal injuries including:
  - scalp lacerations and avulsions (rarely, alopecia in the long term)
  - cephalohaematoma
  - retinal haemorrhage
  - rarely, subgaleal haemorrhage and/or intracranial haemorrhage.

⚠ The use of sequential instruments (usually forceps after a failed ventouse) is associated with an ↑ risk of fetal trauma when attempted with no significant descent.

▶ It is not uncommon for ventouse to slip when the head is at the introitus, then delivery is completed by a lift-out forceps—hence, the discrepancy in the Cochrane review of more failed ventouse deliveries, but a lower CD rate compared with forceps deliveries.

Operative vaginal delivery: instruments

Forceps

Consist of curved blades that sit around the fetal head allowing traction to be applied along the 'flexion point' of the head (3cm in front of the occiput). This is usually to expedite delivery but may be used to slow rate of delivery of the head in a breech delivery (Fig. 6.7).

Low-cavity forceps (Wrigley)
- Short and light.
- These are also the forceps used to deliver the baby at CD.

Mid-cavity forceps (Neville–Barnes, Haig Ferguson, Simpson)
- Used when the sagittal suture is in the direct anteroposterior position (usually direct occipito-anterior (OA)).
- Malposition (occipito-lateral (OL)) can be corrected manually between contractions and the forceps applied once the head is OA.

Mid-cavity rotational forceps (Keilland)
- ↓ pelvic curve on the blades of the forceps allows rotation about the axis of the handle.
- Helps to correct asynclitism and malposition.
- Must only be attempted by an experienced operator.

Vacuum extraction (ventouse)

Works on the principle of creating 'negative pressure' to allow scalp tissues to be sucked into the cup. This creates artificial caput called a 'chignon'. The cup is held in place by the atmospheric pressure on the cup against the negative pressure created.

⚠ It should not be used at <34wks gestation (Fig. 6.7).

Metal cup
- Available with 60, 50, or 40mm standard anterior cup (for OA positions) or posterior cup (for OL or occipito-posterior (OP) positions).
- Pressure is created by a suction pump.
- Excessive traction is likely to cause fetal trauma.

Soft cup
- Soft and easier to apply (important in women without epidural) for OA positions.
- Moulds around the fetal head covering a greater surface area.
- Causes fewer scalp abrasions.

Kiwi Omni Cup™
- Single-use cup.
- Pressure created with hand pump (quick in an emergency).
- Allows application to flexion point (3cm in front of the occiput on the sagittal suture) in OL and OP position.

Comparison of forceps and vacuum extractor

- Ventouse is more likely to fail.
- Ventouse is more likely to cause fetal trauma such as:
  - cephalohaematoma
  - retinal haemorrhage.
- Ventouse is more likely to be associated with maternal concerns about the baby.
- Forceps are more likely to cause significant maternal genital tract trauma.
- There is:
  - slightly less CD with ventouse (figures may be skewed as forceps are more likely to be selected by the operator if the delivery appears difficult)
  - no difference in low 5min Apgar scores
  - no difference in need for neonatal phototherapy.

▶ Bottom line—ventouse appears safer for mother and forceps may be safer for baby.

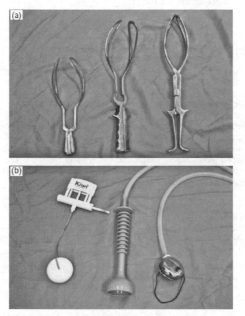

Fig. 6.7 (a) Forceps (left to right: Wrigley's, Neville–Barnes', Keilland's forceps). (b) Ventouse cups (left to right: Kiwi Omni Cup™, silc cup, Bird's cup). With permission of Clinical Innovations Europe Ltd, 2008, and Menox AB, Goteborg, Sweden, 2008.

Operative vaginal delivery: criteria

▶ Currently the training needed for the use of ventouse and forceps are provided by using specifically designed mannequins. Most structured training programmes assess the competency using Objective Structured Assessment of Technical Skills (OSATS) prior to permitting the first few cases under supervision of an experienced operator before unsupervised independent practice.

The following should be satisfied before attempting an operative vaginal delivery. This may be best remembered as '*FORCEPS*'.

* *F*:
  * *Fully* dilated cervix (i.e. confirm 2nd stage).
* *O*:
  * *Obstruction* should be excluded (head ≤1/5 palpable abdominally).
* *R*:
  * *Ruptured* membranes
  * *Review* the procedure (if forceps blades don't lock, or lack of rotation or descent despite traction over three contractions and expulsive effort by the mother).
* *C*:
  * *Consent*
  * *Catheterize* bladder ('in and out' technique, indwelling catheters must be removed)
  * *Check* instrument prior to application.
* *E*:
  * *Explain* the procedure to the patient
  * *Epidural* (or pudendal) analgesia
  * *Examine* the genital tract to exclude genital tract trauma.
* *P*:
  * check *Presentation* and *Position* of the head (must be sure before applying any instrument)
  * *Power*: are the contractions effective? Consider oxytocin infusion if needed (propulsion is better than extraction)
  * correct *Placement* of forceps blades or ventouse cup (ensure no maternal tissues are caught).
* *S*:
  * *Station* of the leading bony presenting part (not above ischial spines)
  * *Senior* help should be called if needed.

See Fig. 6.8.

Further reading

RCOG (2020). Assisted vaginal birth. Green-top guideline no. 26.
🔗 https://obgyn.onlinelibrary.wiley.com/doi/epdf/10.1111/1471-0528.16092

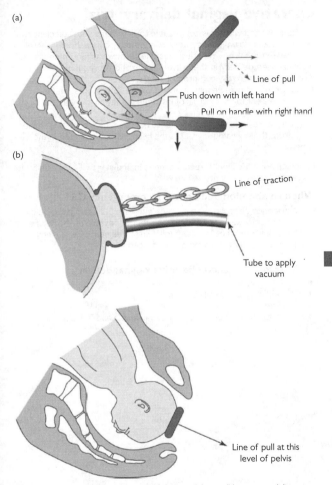

(a)

Line of pull

Push down with left hand

Pull on handle with right hand

(b)

Line of traction

Tube to apply vacuum

Line of pull at this level of pelvis

Fig. 6.8 Assisted delivery techniques: (a) forceps delivery; (b) ventouse delivery. Reproduced from Chamberlain G, Steer P. (1999). ABC of labour care: operative delivery. *Br Med J.* 318:1260–1264. With permission. © BMJ Publishing Group Ltd 1999.

Operative vaginal delivery: trial

This term is used when it is not possible to determine with sufficient confidence that an instrumental delivery will be successful. It should, therefore, take place in theatre, where it is possible to move to an immediate CD, avoiding failed delivery in the delivery room and subsequent delay in performing CD, which may compromise fetal well-being.

- The woman should be fully informed of the likely success and sign a consent form for 'Trial of instrumental vaginal delivery ± emergency CD'.
- If procedure is abandoned, assistance may be required to 'push head up' from the vagina during CD as the head may be impacted in the pelvis.

⚠ Senior obstetric input is recommended in 2nd-stage CD, especially after a failed trial of instrumental delivery.

When to abandon and deliver by emergency CS

- No evidence of progressive descent with each pull (care must be taken with the ventouse to not interpret ↑ caput as descent of the head).
- Where delivery is not imminent following three pulls of a correctly applied instrument by an experienced operator.

Risk factors for failed operative vaginal delivery
- BMI >30kg/m².
- EFW >4000g or clinically big baby.
- OP position.
- Mid-cavity delivery or if head is >1/5 palpable abdominally.

Episiotomy

Of women delivering vaginally in the UK, >85% will sustain some perineal trauma. Episiotomy is a surgical incision to enlarge the vaginal introitus. The decision to perform an episiotomy is made by the birth attendant. The worldwide rates of episiotomy vary (14% in England, 8% in the Netherlands, 50% in the US). There is clear evidence to recommend a *restricted* use of episiotomy.

> **WHO recommends that episiotomy should be considered in the following circumstances**
> * Complicated vaginal delivery:
>   * breech
>   * shoulder dystocia
>   * forceps
>   * ventouse.
> * If there is extensive lower genital tract scarring:
>   * female genital mutilation
>   * poorly healed 3rd- or 4th-degree tears.
> * When there is fetal distress.
> ▶ It is also often recommended if there is an indication that there may be extensive perineal trauma such as the appearance of multiple vaginal/perineal tears or perineal button-holing.

Types of episiotomy

* Mediolateral episiotomy extends from the fourchette laterally (thus ↓ the risk of anal sphincter injury).
* Midline episiotomy extends from the fourchette towards the anus (common in the US, but not recommended in the UK).

▶ Every effort should be made to anaesthetize the perineum early to provide sufficient time for effect.

▶ It will cause bleeding so must not be done too early and should be repaired as soon as possible.

⚠ Always check for any extension or other tears (including a PR examination to ensure no trauma to the anal sphincter).

⚠ Women who have undergone female genital mutilation (FGM) should be seen antenatally and de-infibulation discussed. However, if they present in labour the episiotomy should be anterior and upwards (➔ Female genital mutilation, p. 339).

How to perform an episiotomy

See Fig. 6.9.
- If the woman does not have an effective regional block (epidural) then the perineum should be infiltrated with lidocaine (lignocaine).
- Two fingers should be placed between the baby's head and the perineum (to protect the baby).
- Sharp scissors are used to make a single cut in the perineum about 3–4cm long (ideally this should be at the height of the contraction when the presenting part is not receding in between contractions and the perineum is at its thinnest).

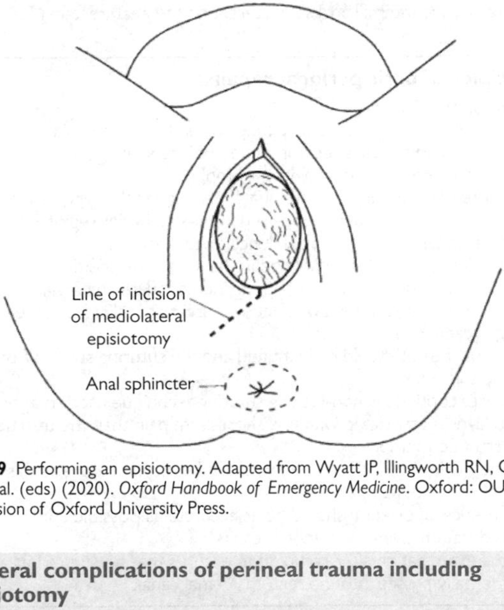

Line of incision of mediolateral episiotomy

Anal sphincter

Fig. 6.9 Performing an episiotomy. Adapted from Wyatt JP, Illingworth RN, Graham CA, et al. (eds) (2020). *Oxford Handbook of Emergency Medicine.* Oxford: OUP. By permission of Oxford University Press.

General complications of perineal trauma including episiotomy

- Bleeding.
- Haematoma.
- Pain.
- Infection.
- Scarring, with potential disruption to the anatomy.
- Dyspareunia.
- Very rarely, fistula formation.

Perineal tears

Classification of perineal tears
- *1st degree:* injury to the skin only.
- *2nd degree:* injury to the perineum involving perineal muscles (includes episiotomy).
- *3rd degree:* injury to the perineum involving the anal sphincter complex:
  - 3a: <50% of the external anal sphincter thickness torn
  - 3b: >50% of the external anal sphincter thickness torn
  - 3c: internal anal sphincter torn.
- *4th degree:* injury to perineum involving the anal sphincter complex (external and internal anal sphincters) and the anal/rectal epithelium.

Principles of basic perineal repair
See Fig. 6.10.
- Suture as soon as possible to ↓ bleeding and infection risk.
- A rectal examination is recommended before starting, to ensure there is no trauma to the anal sphincter complex.
- The attendant should have adequate training for the type of tear: complex trauma should be repaired in theatre under regional or general anaesthesia by an experienced operator.
- The woman should preferably be in the lithotomy position.
- There should be a good light source and adequate analgesia.
- Use of rapid-absorption polyglactin suture material is associated with a significant reduction in pain.
- Apex of the cut should be identified and the suturing started from just above this point.
- A loose, continuous non-locking suturing technique used to appose each layer is associated with less short-term pain than the traditional interrupted method.
- Perineal skin should be sutured with a subcuticular suture as this is associated with less pain.
- Anatomical apposition should be as accurate as possible and consideration given to cosmetic results.
- Rectal examination after completion ensures that no suture has accidentally passed into the rectum or anal canal.

⚠ Needle and swabs must be counted afterwards (lost swabs are a recurring cause of litigation in obstetrics).

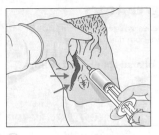

1. Swab the vulva towards the perineum. Infiltrate with 1% lidocaine (→arrows).

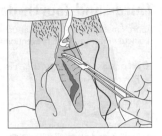

2. Place tampon with attached tape in upper vagina. Insert 1st suture above apex of vaginal cut (not too deep as underlying rectal mucosa nearby).

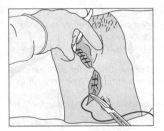

3. Bring together vaginal edges with continuous stitches placed ^{1}cm apart. Knot at introitus under the skin. Appose divided levator ani muscles.

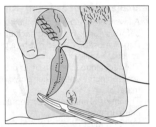

4. Close perineal skin (subcuticular continuous stitch is shown here).

5. When stitching is finished, remove tampon and examine vagina (to check for retained swabs). Do a **PR** to check that apical sutures have not penetrated rectum.

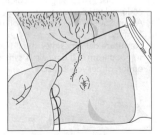

Fig. 6.10 Episiotomy repair. Reproduced from Collier J, Longmore M, Brinsden M. (2006). *Oxford Handbook of Clinical Specialties*, 7th edn. Oxford: OUP. By permission of Oxford University Press.

Third- and fourth-degree tears

Approximately 1–3% of vaginal deliveries will result in injury to the anal sphincter. Prediction and prevention are both difficult.

Factors associated with ↑ risk of anal sphincter trauma

- Forceps delivery.
- Nulliparity.
- Shoulder dystocia.
- 2nd stage >1h.
- Persistent OP position.
- Midline episiotomy.
- Birth weight >4kg.
- Epidural anaesthesia.
- IOL.

Management of 3rd- and 4th-degree tears

- All women sustaining genital tract injury should be carefully examined before suturing is started (including a rectal examination).
- Repair must be carried out by a trained senior clinician in theatre with adequate analgesia.
- The technique used can be end to end or overlapping for the external anal sphincter using either polydioxanone suture (PDS) or vicryl suture material.
- The internal anal sphincter should be repaired with vicryl using interrupted sutures.
- Women must receive broad-spectrum antibiotics and stool softeners.
- They should receive physiotherapy input.
- Ideally, they should be reviewed 6wks later by an obstetrician or gynaecologist.
- Women must be warned of the risk of incontinence of faeces, fluid, and flatus: those experiencing symptoms at 6wks should be referred to a specialist gynaecologist or colorectal surgeon for investigation with endoanal ultrasonography.
- Around 60–80% will have a good result and be asymptomatic at 12mths.
- For future deliveries they should be advised that the result may not be so good from a 2nd repair: if symptomatic they should be given the option of delivery by CD.

Further reading

RCOG (2015). The management of third and fourth degree perineal tears. Green-top guideline no. 29.
🕮 www.rcog.org.uk/globalassets/documents/guidelines/gtg-29.pdf

Female genital mutilation

➔ Female genital mutilation: overview, p. 542 and ➔ Female genital mutilation: management, p. 543.

- Women should be asked about history of FGM at the booking visit and if identified it should be recorded in the notes.
- The impact of FGM on labour and delivery should be discussed with the woman and her partner and documented in the notes.
- Consultant-led care is recommended as complications may arise at delivery unless the woman has had a normal vaginal delivery when she can be under midwifery-led care in labour.
- When identified as a woman with FGM, she should be referred to the designated consultant and midwife who have had suitable training and experience in managing FGM holistically.
- The woman and partner should be informed that de-infibulation would be offered and carried out but not re-infibulation as it is against the UK laws.
- Screening for hepatitis C should be offered at booking or at the time when blood is taken for hepatitis B, syphilis, and HIV.
- Offer psychological assessment and treatment.

De-infibulation

- Inspect the vulva to determine the type of FGM (I–IV: ➔ Female genital mutilation: overview p. 542) and decide whether de-infibulation is necessary:
  - if the urethral meatus is visible and a vaginal examination is possible without discomfort, then a de-infibulation may not be needed
  - it is needed if the two sides of the labia minora are stitched in the midline.
- The practitioner undertaking de-infibulation should be appropriately trained in the procedure.
- Can be performed in the antenatal period under local anaesthesia:
  - the fused labia are cut upwards from the introitus in the midline till the urethral meatus is clearly exposed
  - the fresh edges of the labia are sutured separately with interrupted stitches to achieve haemostasis and keep the labia apart.
- This can be undertaken during labour in the 1st or 2nd stage:
  - if the woman has epidural for pain relief that may ↓ the pain and anxiety.
- If the woman has a CD then the procedure can be done perioperatively:
  - if this is not possible, a follow-up appointment should be made to carry out the de-infibulation before the next pregnancy.
- Labial/perineal tears seen after delivery should be dealt with in the same way as in a woman without FGM.
- On discharge, the midwife should check that all legal and regulatory processes have been completed and recorded.

Further reading

RCOG (2015). Female genital mutilation and its management. Green-top guideline no. 53.
🕮 https://www.rcog.org.uk/media/au0jn5of/gtg-53-fgm.pdf

Caesarean delivery: overview

Background

- CD involves delivery of the fetus through a direct incision in the abdominal wall and the uterus.
- Rates vary in different countries and populations:
- Overall CD rate for nulliparous women in the UK has ↑ to ~24%:
  - for multiparous women who have not previously had a CD the rate is <5%
  - for women who have had at least one previous CD the rate is ↑ to about 67%; most are elective.

Caesarean section

Associated with a higher incidence of:
- Abdominal pain.
- VTE.
- Bladder or ureteric injury.
- Hysterectomy.
- Very rarely maternal death.
  Associated with a lower incidence of:
- Perineal pain.
- Urinary incontinence.
- Uterovaginal prolapse.

⚫ Long-term effect of the last two are debated.

Some interventions to ↓ morbidity from CD

- Preoperative haemoglobin check and correction of anaemia.
- Intraoperative prophylactic antibiotics given just before skin incision.
- Risk assessment and appropriate thromboprophylaxis (graduated stockings, hydration, early mobilization, and LMWH).
- In-dwelling bladder catheterization during the procedure.
- Antacids and H_2 receptor analogues before surgery.
- Antiemetics as appropriate.
- Regional rather than general anaesthesia.
- The risk of hypotension can be ↓ using:
  - IV ephedrine or phenylephrine infusion
  - volume preloading with crystalloid or colloid
  - lateral tilt of 15°.
- General anaesthesia for emergency CD should include preoxygenation and rapid sequence induction to ↓ the risk of aspiration.

Vaginal birth after CD
- Uterine rupture is very rare but is ↑ with VBAC:
  - 50:10,000 with VBAC and spontaneous onset of labour
  - 1:10,000 with repeat CD.
- Intrapartum infant death is rare: 1:1000—the same as for primiparous women.
- EFM is recommended during labour as FHR changes may be the earliest signs of scar rupture.
- Women should deliver in a unit where there is immediate access to CD and on-site blood transfusion.
- With IOL, there is ↑ risk of uterine rupture:
  - 8:1000 if oxytocin infusion is used
  - 24:1000 if prostaglandins are used.
- Women with both previous CD and a previous vaginal birth are more likely to give birth vaginally.

Caesarean delivery: indications

The main indications for CD are:
- Repeat CD.
- Fetal compromise.
- 'Failure to progress' in labour.
- Breech presentation.

🔊 Maternal request accounts for 7% of CD, but is not, on its own, an indication for CD.

Categories to determine the timing of CD

- Immediate threat to the life of the woman or fetus (immediate, 'crash CD').
- Maternal or fetal compromise, which is not immediately life-threatening (urgent).
- No maternal or fetal compromise but needs early delivery (scheduled).
- Delivery timed to suit woman and staff (elective).

⚠ In cases of suspected or confirmed acute fetal compromise, delivery should be as soon as possible. The accepted standard for category 1 (immediate) CD is within 30min.

Indications for category 1 CD
- Placental abruption with abnormal FHR or uterine irritability.
- Cord prolapse.
- Scar rupture.
- Prolonged bradycardia.
- Scalp pH <7.20.

Indications for category 2 CD
- Pathological CTG in the first stage of labour.

Indications for category 3 (scheduled) CD
- Severe pre-eclampsia.
- FGR with poor fetal function tests.
- Failed IOL.

Indications for category 4 (elective) CD
- Term singleton breech (if ECV is contraindicated or has failed).
- Twin pregnancy with non-cephalic 1st twin.
- Maternal HIV.
- 1° genital herpes in the 3rd trimester.
- Placenta praevia.
- Previous hysterotomy or classical CD.

▶ Elective CD is usually carried out after 39wks unless indicated, as the risk of respiratory morbidity (transient tachypnoea of the newborn) is ↑ at lower gestational ages.

Caesarean delivery: types

Skin incision

The two main types of skin incision are:
- *Pfannenstiel incision:* a straight horizontal incision 2cm above the symphysis pubis—superior cosmetic result.
- *Joel–Cohen incision:* a straight horizontal incision, but higher, about 3cm below the level of the anterior superior iliac spines—allows quicker entry to the abdomen.

Transverse uterine incision

- A transverse incision in the uterine lower segment is used in >90% of CD as it is associated with:
  - ↓ adhesion formation.
  - ↓ blood loss.
  - ↓ incidence of scar dehiscence in subsequent pregnancies.
- If the lower segment is poorly developed, a low transverse incision carries a risk of lateral extension into the uterine vessels and haemorrhage.
- Following delivery of the fetus and completion of the 3rd stage, the lower uterine segment is closed preferably in two layers.

Vertical 'classical' uterine incision

- This involves a vertical incision into the upper uterine segment. It is rarely performed, but indications may include:
  - structural abnormality of the uterus
  - difficult access to the lower uterine segment due to fibroids or severe adhesions over the lower segment
  - postmortem CD delivery (if the fetus is viable)
  - anterior placenta praevia with abnormally vascular lower uterine segment or suspicion of PAS
  - contraction ring
  - very preterm fetus (especially breech presentation) where the lower segment is poorly formed
  - elective Caesarean hysterectomy
  - transverse lie of the fetus with ruptured membranes.
- Allows rapid delivery and has a lower risk of bladder injury.
- Closure is more complicated and time-consuming and there is a higher incidence of infection and adhesion formation.

⚠ There is a greater risk of uterine rupture in subsequent pregnancies with a greater risk of the fetus being expelled into the peritoneal cavity. For these reasons, a classical incision is an absolute contraindication to a trial of a VBAC.

Caesarean delivery: complications

Intraoperative complications

Major complications are most common with an emergency CD.

Anaesthesia-related maternal deaths occur in women undergoing CD with general anaesthesia.

Intraoperative complications occur in 12–15% of CDs and include:
- Uterine or uterocervical lacerations (5–10%).
- Blood loss >1L (7–9%).
- Bladder laceration (0.5–0.8%).
- Blood transfusion (2–3%).
- Hysterectomy (0.2%).
- Bowel lacerations (0.05%).
- Ureteral injury (0.03–0.09%.).

Risk factors predisposing to uterocervical lacerations include:
- Low station of the presenting part and full dilatation.
- Birth weight >4000g.
- ↑ Maternal age.
- Category 1 CD.

Risk factors predisposing to intraoperative haemorrhage include:
- Placenta praevia or abruption.
- Extremes of fetal birth weight.
- BMI >25kg/m².

Postoperative complications

▶ Postoperative complications occur in up to 1/3 of CDs and include:
- Endometritis (5%).
- Wound infections (3–27%).
- Pulmonary atelectasis.
- VTE.
- UTIs.

Risk factors independently associated with infection are:
- Preoperative remote infection.
- Chorioamnionitis.
- Maternal severe systemic disease.
- Pre-eclampsia.
- High BMI.
- Nulliparity.
- ↑ Surgical blood loss.

Long-term effects of CD

In subsequent pregnancies there is a higher risk of:
- Uterine rupture (1:200 with spontaneous labour).
- Placenta praevia (17% ↑ of background risk).
- PAS.
- Antepartum stillbirth: absolute risk doubles with a previous CD.
  Women undergoing multiple CD (≥3) are at higher risk of:
- Excessive blood loss (8%).
- Difficult delivery of the neonate (5%).
- Dense adhesions (46%).
- Risk of any major complication is higher (9%).
- Complications are ↑ with ↑ number of CD:
  - 4% for 2nd
  - 8% for 3rd
  - 13% for 4th.

Prelabour rupture of membranes at term

> **Definition**
> PROM at term is defined as leakage of amniotic fluid in the absence of uterine activity after 37 completed wks of gestation.

Incidence
8% of term pregnancies (2–3% before 37wks).

Aetiology
- Unknown.
- Clinical or subclinical infection.
- Polyhydramnios.
- Multiple pregnancy.
- Malpresentations.

Clinical assessment
It is important to establish a correct diagnosis to plan further management. If unnecessary interventions are undertaken, there is a risk of ↑ maternal and fetal morbidity.

History
Women give a history of a sudden gush of fluid leaking from the vagina, recurrent dampness, or constant leaking.

Examination
- There is no need to carry out a speculum examination with certain history of ruptured membranes at term with liquor seen on the pad or undergarments.
- If the history is uncertain, a speculum examination should be offered (liquor should be seen pooling in the upper vagina or trickling through the cervical os):
  - coughing or straining (Valsalva manoeuvre) may help to demonstrate leaking fluid
  - note the colour of the liquor (?blood or meconium stained).
- Temperature, pulse, and BP.
- Obstetric examination of abdomen (including lie and presentation).
- CTG.

▶ If conservative management is planned, avoid digital examination as it ↑ the incidence of chorioamnionitis, postpartum endometritis, and neonatal infection.

⚠ Any concern regarding fetal well-being is an indication to deliver.

⚠ Signs of chorioamnionitis should prompt treatment with antibiotics and rapid delivery.

Clinical features of chorioamnionitis
- Fetal tachycardia.
- Maternal tachycardia.
- Maternal pyrexia.
- Rising leucocyte count.
- Rising CRP.
- Irritable or ↑ tender uterus.

Prelabour rupture of membranes: management

If there are no contraindications to waiting, women should be offered the choice between immediate induction and expectant management.

Expectant management versus immediate induction

- 60% of women will labour spontaneously within 24h.
- No evidence of a difference in the mode of delivery for either.
- 1% risk of serious neonatal infection (compared with 0.5% for women with intact membranes).

With expectant management

- Women are more likely to develop chorioamnionitis and endometritis with expectant management of >24h.
- Baby is more likely to be admitted to the special care baby unit: no evidence of a difference in eventual neonatal outcome (morbidity/mortality) with expectant management of <24h.

▶ The NICE guidelines recommend induction after 24h.

Conservative management advice

If the woman opts for this she should be advised to:

- Record her temperature every 4h (during waking hours).
- Urgently report any change in colour or offensive smell.
- Avoid sexual intercourse (showering and bathing is okay).
- Report any ↓ in fetal movements.
- Deliver in a unit with neonatal services and remain in hospital for >12h after delivery to allow close observation of the baby.
- Consider induction if not in labour by 24h.
- Seek medical advice if any concerns regarding the baby's well-being in the 1st 5 days of life (especially in the first 12h).

💧 Use of antibiotics is controversial. NICE does not recommend prophylactic antibiotics for either mother or baby in the absence of symptoms, even if her membranes have been ruptured for >24h.

▶ In labour, regular maternal observations are essential to pick up signs of infection early. FHR monitoring should be carried out as it may be tachycardic in the presence of infection.

⚠ If there is clinical evidence of infection a full course of broad-spectrum IV antibiotic therapy should be started after blood cultures have been sent.

PROM in known group B *Streptococcus* carriers
(➲ Group B *Streptococcus*, p. 196.)

GBS carriers (high risk)

- Mothers should be regarded as high-risk carriers and offered intrapartum antibiotic prophylaxis (IAP) in labour if they:
  - had a previous baby affected by early- or late-onset GBS disease
  - had GBS bacteriuria in the current pregnancy.
- Standard IAP is benzylpenicillin from the time admitted in labour until delivery.
  - cephalosporins can be used as an alternative
  - if allergic to penicillin, vancomycin is recommended.
- Birth in a pool is not contraindicated if the mother is a carrier but IAP should be given.

⚠ Women with pyrexia >38°C should be given broad-spectrum antibiotics that will cover GBS.

<34wks

- Cases with ROM <34wks may be managed conservatively as risks of prematurity may be greater:
  - erythromycin should be given for 7–10 days.
- IAP should be given to those in preterm labour with unknown carrier status.

≥34wks

- Immediate induction should be encouraged.
- Method of induction according to local protocol:
  - whether prostaglandin gel ↑ infection risk remains uncertain.

Neonates

- Should be screened soon after birth and should be examined at 1h, 2h, and every 2h for 12h for signs of sepsis.
- Signs of infection include high or low temperature, rapid heartbeat, rapid breathing, intolerance to feed, floppiness, change in skin colour.
- Antibiotics are not given as a routine unless there is evidence of infection.
- If there are signs of early-onset GBS disease—treatment should be commenced within 1h with penicillin and gentamycin.

Further reading

RCOG (2019). Care of women presenting with suspected preterm prelabour rupture of membranes from 24+0 wks of gestation. Green-top guideline no. 73.
🔗 https://obgyn.onlinelibrary.wiley.com/doi/10.1111/1471-0528.15803

RCOG (2017). Prevention of early onset Group B streptococcal disease. Green-top guideline no. 36.
🔗 https://obgyn.onlinelibrary.wiley.com/doi/full/10.1111/1471-0528.14821

Abnormal lie: transverse and oblique

Transverse and oblique lie occur in 1:300 pregnancies and result in a shoulder, limb, or cord presentation. If this persists, vaginal delivery is not feasible (➔ Fig. 2.4, p. 85).

Diagnosis

- The maternal abdomen is unusually wide and the fundus is lower than expected for the gestation.
- Neither fetal pole is palpable entering the pelvis.
- Fetal head is identifiable at one side.
- On vaginal examination the pelvis is empty.
- A limb or cord may prolapse through the cervix.

Management

When this presents in labour, fetal well-being should be established and a USS performed to try to identify the cause.

⚠ *Exclude placenta praevia before attempting vaginal examination.*

- CD is indicated in almost all cases.
- An unstable lie at term due to multiparity alone may warrant a gentle attempt at ECV if the following criteria are met:
  - membranes must be intact
  - labour not advanced
  - fetus must have no signs of compromise.
- If ECV is successful, cord presentation or prolapse should be excluded before labour is allowed to establish.
- CD for transverse lie, especially with placenta praevia or fibroids, requires an experienced obstetrician and cross-matched blood.
- Vertical or 'J'-shaped uterine incision on the uterus or acute tocolysis with a transverse incision may be necessary for safe delivery of fetus.

Malpresentations in labour: overview

- >95% of fetuses at term present with vertex (area subtended by two parietal eminences, anterior, and posterior fontanelle), hence vertex is called normal presentation.
- Malpresentation describes any presentation other than vertex lying near internal os of the cervix and includes:
  - breech (most common malpresentation with an incidence of 3–4% at term; ➔ Breech presentation: delivery, p. 82)
  - brow
  - face
  - shoulder
  - arm
  - cord.

Some causes of malpresentation

Maternal
- Multiparity.
- Pelvic tumours.
- Congenital uterine anomalies.
- Contracted pelvis.

Fetal
- Prematurity.
- Multiple pregnancy.
- IUD.
- Macrosomia.
- Fetal abnormality including:
  - hydrocephalus
  - anencephaly
  - cystic hygroma.

Placental
- Placenta praevia.
- Polyhydramnios.
- Amniotic bands.

Malpresentations: brow and face

Brow presentation

Incidence ranges between 1:1000 and 1:3500 deliveries. The head occupies a position midway between full flexion (vertex) and full extension (face). It can revert to a face or vertex presentation, but if it persists vaginal delivery is not usually possible (Fig. 6.11a).

Diagnosis

- Often diagnosed in advanced labour (may be suspected on abdominal palpation when both occiput and chin are palpable).
- The head does not descend below the ischial spines.
- Vaginal examination is diagnostic as the frontal sutures, anterior fontanelle, orbital ridges, eyes, and the root of nose are palpable.

Management

- Watch and wait: may become a vertex or face presentation.
- If progress is slow or if the brow persists then CD is indicated.

Face presentation

Incidence of face presentation is between 1:600 and 1:1500 deliveries. It is due to hyperextension of the fetal neck (Fig. 6.11b).

Diagnosis

- Face presentation is diagnosed in labour on vaginal examination.
- The orbital ridges, nose, malar eminences, mentum, gums, and mouth can be distinguished.

▶ It may be mistaken for a breech, but presence of gum margins will help to differentiate between a mouth and an anus.

Management

- 90% are mentoanterior (MA) and head can flex to allow vaginal delivery.
- Expectant management should be considered with mentoposterior (MP) as about 20–30% will rotate on reaching the pelvic floor.
- Persistent MP face presentations cannot deliver vaginally as it would require the head to descend through the narrow space in the anterior aspect of the pelvis.
- If there is poor progress or failure to rotate, CD is indicated.
- Fetal monitoring should be external and FBS is contraindicated.
- The use of ventouse is absolutely contraindicated but forceps delivery is possible with an MA position well below spines.

⚠ Attempts to convert face presentations manually into vertex or use of forceps to rotate persistent MP positions can lead to complications of cord prolapse and fetal cervical cord injury.

⤷ Fig. 1.6, p. 15 and Fig. 1.7, p. 17.

Cord presentation

This occurs when one or more loops of cord lie below the presenting part and the membranes are still intact. It is associated with malpresentation, abnormal lie, and a high head. The risk is of cord prolapse when the membranes rupture. This is an obstetric emergency (Cord prolapse, p. 437).

Diagnosis
- The diagnosis of cord presentation is often made on USS, but may be found on VE in labour.
- It can be suspected clinically when persistent prolonged variable fetal heart decelerations occur especially early in labour.
- ARM is contraindicated as it will cause cord prolapse.

(a) Brow presentation   (b) Face presentation

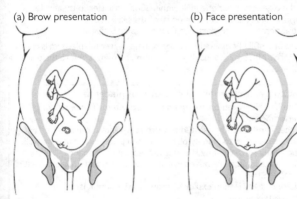

Fig. 6.11 Malpresentations: (a) brow presentation; (b) face presentation.

Retained placenta

Retained placenta should be suspected if it is not delivered within 30min of the baby in an actively managed 3rd stage and 1h in a physiological 3rd stage.

⚠ Care must be taken as blood can gather behind placenta → significant occult blood loss—beware of high uterus full of blood!

Management of retained placenta

- IV access, FBC, and cross-match.
- If it was physiological management, revert to active management:
  - give Syntometrine® or oxytocin
  - try controlled cord traction.
- If the oxytocin is not effective within 30min, transfer to theatre for regional block and manual removal of the placenta.
- Intraoperative prophylactic antibiotics should be given.

✦ Use of a 40IU IV oxytocin infusion to help deliver the placenta is controversial. The NICE guidelines do not recommend using it before the placenta is delivered.

How to perform manual removal of placenta

- One hand is placed on abdomen to steady uterus (↓ the risk of perforation).
- Other hand is gently inserted through cervix into uterus.
- Fingers are used to identify plane between placenta and uterine wall, and gently separate it by shearing movement of the hand.
- Placenta should be removed in one piece and inspected to ensure it is complete.
- Uterine cavity is then explored again to make sure it is completely empty.
- Oxytocin infusion is continued for 4h prophylactically.
- IV antibiotics are given.
- Mother is observed for bleeding or infection by observing vaginal bleeding, fundal height, change in pulse, BP, temperature, urinary output, and Hb.

Postpartum haemorrhage

- 1° *PPH*: defined as blood loss of ≥500mL from the genital tract occurring within 24h of delivery.
- 2° *PPH*: defined as 'excessive' loss occurring between 24h and 6wks after delivery.

- Major cause of maternal morbidity and mortality: globally >75,000 women die of PPH each year.
- Major cause of maternal deaths in the UK (often after CD).
- Incidence is 2–11% in the UK.
- With a low BMI and/or low Hb, <500mL loss may cause haemodynamic disturbance requiring prompt and appropriate management.

Causes of 1° PPH (four Ts: tone, tears, tissue, thrombin)

Tone—uterine atony (80%)
- Caused by failure of uterus to contract effectively after delivery.
- May be due to many factors:
  - overdistended uterus with twins or polyhydramnios
  - prolonged labour
  - infection
  - failure to actively manage 3rd stage of labour
  - rarely, due to placental abruption (diffuse bleeding into uterine muscle preventing contraction).

Trauma—genital tract trauma (15%)
- Tears, episiotomy, and lacerations of the cervix.
- Uterine inversion and/or rupture (➋ Massive obstetric haemorrhage: management, p. 416.)

Tissue
- Retained placenta/placental tissue, membranes.
- Placenta praevia.
- PAS (➋ Placenta accreta spectrum: diagnosis and management p. 142).

Thrombin—coagulation disorders
- Severe PET.
- Placental abruption.
- Sepsis.
- Autoimmune disease.
- Liver disease.
- Inherited or acquired coagulation disorders.
- Iatrogenic (anticoagulant administration).

Causes of 1° PPH
- Uterine atony.
- Genital tract trauma.
- Coagulation disorders.
- Large placenta.
- Abnormal placental site.
- Retained placenta.
- Uterine inversion.
- Uterine rupture.

Antenatal risk factors for PPH
- Previous PPH.
- Previously retained placenta.
- Maternal Hb ≤8.5g/dL at onset of labour.
- ↑ BMI.
- Para 4 or more.
- APH.
- Overdistention of uterus (multiple pregnancy or polyhydramnios).
- Uterine abnormalities/fibroids.
- Low-lying placenta.
- Maternal age >35yrs.

⚠ The presence of any risk factors for PPH should lead to the woman being advised to deliver in an obstetric unit (facilities for blood transfusion and surgical management of PPH).

Intrapartum risk factors for PPH
- IOL.
- Prolonged 1st, 2nd, or 3rd stage.
- Use of oxytocin.
- Precipitate labour.
- Vaginal operative delivery.
- CD.

Home birth: overview

Home birth can be safe for women screened as low risk, and emotionally satisfying for the mother and her family. For women identified as having risk factors, hospital delivery is safer. Debates about the safety of home births focus on risk of preventable perinatal morbidity and mortality, and on issues of screening and referral.

The numbers

- Proportion of births at home fell from 80% in 1930 to 1% in 1990.
- As a result of UK Government committee recommendation (1993), stating that a full choice including home births should be offered, followed by 'Maternity matters', a Government white paper (2007), the UK home birth rate has ↑ and is now ~2–3%.
- Studies suggest that 10–14% of women would choose home birth if given the opportunity.
- In some regions where there is difficulty in geographical accessibility to a hospital, the home birth rate could be ~10%.
- In women booked for home births:
  - change to hospital care is nearly 29%
  - transfer in labour is ~15% in multiparae and ~30% in nulliparae
  - most of these transfers are for failure to progress or pain relief.
- Risk of intrapartum fetal death in appropriately selected low-risk women is 1:1000.
- It is difficult to compare directly the perinatal mortality rates for home and hospital, as more complex deliveries occur in hospital.
- Recent prospective study suggests a slight ↑ in perinatal mortality with home births.

Discussion points when considering home birth

- In the presence of obvious risk factors (hypertension, diabetes, placenta praevia), the advice must be to deliver in hospital.
- If mother is low risk and wishes to have a home birth, she should be counselled appropriately with full information about the very slight ↑ in perinatal mortality and possibility of transfer in labour.
- If a risk arises before birth, the booking should be changed.
- If risk is minimal, the lead professional in charge should offer the woman and her partner the opportunity to review their choice and respect their decision.

Reasons for women to choose home birth

- Wish for a familiar setting where they feel relaxed and in control.
- Fear of hospital setting.
- To have a continuing relationship with a known midwife.
- To be with more family members who provide support.
- Previous home birth.
- To avoid intervention.

Home birth: risks and GP involvement

The potential risks of home birth are rare but should be discussed with the woman as part of her decision. These include:

- Should a complication occur, transfer to hospital may be required.
- Should there be a delay in transfer, response to acute complications, such as intrapartum fetal hypoxia or PPH, may be delayed, potentially → a worse outcome although such complications are rare.
- The facilities for neonatal resuscitation will be limited but the midwife should be well trained in basic neonatal resuscitation.
- Inadequate lighting and analgesia may make diagnosis of the extent of perineal tears difficult, necessitating transfer to hospital.

Discussion of the risks and other factors, including type of pain relief available, will help the woman to make an informed choice. Clear documentation of these discussions in the antenatal period is essential for the mother not to regret her choice and for medico-legal reasons.

The role of the GP

- The GP should be fully informed about the local options for place of birth and will then be able to provide the options to the woman in a clear, understandable, and balanced manner.
- GPs who do not wish to provide care for home births should refer women to the community midwife or a GP who provides this care.
- In case of any unfortunate event occurring with intrapartum care of a woman being looked after by her GP and if the case proceeds to a litigation, the GP would not be judged by the standards of a consultant obstetrician, but by those of a GP with similar skills and standing (the Bolam test).
- The GP does not have to attend a home birth even when the woman has been accepted by the GP for full maternity care, unless asked to do so by the midwife.
- The GP should provide support to the woman and midwife, help identify any deviations from normal course of labour, and arrange for hospital care.
- Where the midwife feels that the GP is supportive, the likelihood of transfer to hospital is ↓.
- In current practice, very few GPs offer care in labour and delivery services.

Further reading

Bandolier. The GP's guide to home birth.
🕮 www.bandolier.org.uk/band32/b32-8.html

Home birth: the evidence

Meta-analysis of several methodologically sound observational studies comparing the outcomes of planned home births (irrespective of the eventual place of birth) with planned hospital births for women with similar characteristics showed that there was no ↑ in maternal mortality. The rate is unlikely to be different as the maternal mortality is generally low, and good midwifery and ambulance services help to avoid such deaths, although occasional cases have been described.

Home birth study in the UK showed:
• Slightly ↑ perinatal mortality, but when all studies in literature are considered there is little statistically significant difference. This is partly due to the complexity of such studies, some being retrospective or prospective descriptive.
• In the home births group there were significantly fewer medical interventions (including in women transferred to hospital).
• Fewer babies had low Apgar scores, neonatal respiratory problems, and instances of birth trauma with home births.

Further RCTs are needed to resolve this controversy over relative safety of home and hospital births. Because maternal and perinatal mortality and morbidity are so low in low-risk pregnancies, to observe differences in these 1° outcome measures large numbers need to be studied.

Home birth: general points
GPs and midwives have the responsibility for creating the right circumstances for safe and satisfying home births.

This means:
• Selecting women without risk factors.
• Establishing an infrastructure for safe obstetric care including:
  • hygiene during delivery
  • keeping the baby warm
  • care of the eyes.
• Providing support and care during labour, delivery, and in immediate postnatal period.
• Arrangements for transfer to hospital in the event of any unforeseen complication.
• Care should be provided based on a prearranged protocol that provides guidance as to conduct of labour and what action needs to be taken should the woman need help.

Chapter 7

Obstetric anaesthesia

Pain relief in labour

Uterine contractions in labour are associated with pain. Professionals can help to reduce women's fears by giving precise, accurate, and relevant information antenatally including the types of analgesia available in their unit.

Ideal pain relief in labour

Should

- Provide good analgesia.
- Be safe for the mother and baby.
- Be predictable and constant in its effects.
- Be reversible if necessary.
- Be easy to administer.

Should not

- Interfere with uterine contractions.
- Interfere with mobility.

Non-pharmacological methods

- Education regarding what to expect may help reduce fear and the sense of loss of control.
- A trusted companion present throughout labour and birth reduces the need for pain relief.
- Warm bath, acupuncture, hypnosis, and homeopathy are also helpful.
- Transcutaneous electrical nerve stimulation (TENS):
  - may help with short labour and postpone the need for stronger analgesia, but may not be adequate as labour advances.

Pharmacological methods

Nitrous oxide (Entonox®)

Entonox® is premixed nitrous oxide and oxygen as a 50:50 mixture. It is self-administered and has quick onset of action and a short half-life. Side effects can include feeling faint, nausea, and vomiting.

Narcotic agents

- *Pethidine:* administered at a dose of 50–150mg IM; onset of action is 15–20min. It lasts about 3–4h and can be repeated. It is usually given with an antiemetic. If given within 2h of delivery, it can cause neonatal respiratory depression and naloxone may be needed.
- *Diamorphine:* may also be used at a dose of 2.5–5mg IM. There is controversy about the extent and timing of neonatal respiratory depression, but it may be up to 3–4h after the last dose.
- *Meptazinol:* is an opioid that may cause less respiratory depression. The onset of action starts in 15min and lasts for about 2–7h.

Intracutaneous sterile water for back pain in labour
- Severe constant lower back pain occurs in ~30% of labouring women.
- It is believed to be associated with the stretching of the lumbosacral nerve plexus and compression of the viscera.
- It is often associated with an OP position.

▶ The painful stimuli is not actually occurring in the lower back but is instead 'referred' there due to intercommunication in the dorsal horns of the spinal segments between the afferent fibres from the lumbosacral plexus and viscera, and the Aδ afferent fibres of the dermatomes of the lower back.

- Where epidural analgesia is not available, the pain can lead to an extremely distressing, potentially traumatic, birth experience.
- Intracutaneous sterile water, administered into the skin bordering the Michaelis rhomboid has been demonstrated to be effective in reducing this back pain.

Pudendal nerve block and local perineal infiltration
- Pudendal nerve block is used for operative vaginal delivery and is performed by the obstetrician:
  - lidocaine (lignocaine) is injected 1–2cm medially, and below the right and left ischial spines
  - this is done transvaginally with a specially designed pudendal needle.
- Local anaesthetic such as lidocaine is infiltrated in the perineum before performing an episiotomy at the time of delivery, or before suturing tears and episiotomies.

Epidural analgesia: overview

Safe and effective analgesia for labour is still something that is not available for the vast majority of women in the world today. Although the provision of epidural analgesia during labour has been one of the greatest advances in the care of women during this difficult and distressing time, it still carries a small, but definite complication rate.

Consent for analgesia in labour

Women in labour present a particular group of patients in whom obtaining fully informed consent may be difficult because of a variety of factors such as pain, fatigue, or the effects of narcotic analgesia administered previously.

Ideally, anaesthetists should try to explain the risks and benefits of epidural analgesia to women in the antenatal period.

Anatomy

- The epidural space lies between the spinal dura and the vertebral canal (Fig. 7.1).
- The superior margin is the foramen magnum, inferiorly the sacrococcygeal membrane.
- Posteriorly lie the ligamentum flavum and the anterior surfaces of the laminae, anteriorly the posterior longitudinal ligament.
- Within the epidural space lie the spinal nerve roots as well as the spinal arteries and extradural veins.
- The usual distance between skin and the epidural space in the lumbar region in adults is ~4–5cm.

▶ It is important to realize that the epidural space is continuous the whole way down the back. The lumbar region is chosen for the provision of labour analgesia as this is where the nerve roots involved in the production of pain during labour are found.

- The pain of the first stage of labour is caused by uterine contractions and is referred by afferent Aδ and C fibres mainly to dermatomes T10–L1, and by distension of the perineum during the second stage of labour to S2–S4.

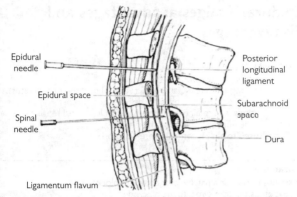

Fig. 7.1 Subarachnoid and epidural spaces. Reproduced from Allman KG, McIndoe A, Wilson I. (2011). *Oxford Handbook of Anaesthesia*, 3rd edn. With permission from Oxford University Press.

Epidural analgesia: advantages and disadvantages

Advantages
- Effective analgesia in labour.
- Reduced maternal catecholamine secretion (thought to benefit fetus).
- Can be topped up for an operative delivery or any other complications, e.g. retained placenta or difficult perineal repair.
- Can provide effective postoperative analgesia.
- Can be used to aid BP control in pre-eclampsia.

Disadvantages
- Failure to site, or a patchy, or incomplete block.
- Hypotension from sympathetic blockade.
- ↓ mobility.
- Tenderness over the insertion site.

Complications
- *Inadvertent dural puncture:*
  - incidence <1:200
  - may develop a post-dural puncture headache, worse when sitting up or standing
  - may need treatment with an epidural blood patch.
- *Respiratory depression:*
  - from the catheter migrating into the subarachnoid space followed by bolus of local anaesthetic (total spinal)
  - from accumulation of epidurally administered opiates.
- *Extremely rare complications resulting in neurological deficits:*
  - epidural abscess formation
  - epidural haematoma
  - damage to individual nerves or the spinal cord itself.
- ↑ risk of operative delivery.

An alternative to epidural: fentanyl or remifentanil patient-controlled analgesia

There are a few women in whom epidural analgesia is contraindicated and who are not able to obtain adequate analgesia from more conventional methods such as nitrous oxide. Fentanyl or remifentanil are both powerful opiates which may be used via a patient-controlled IV system (patient-controlled analgesia).

Contraindications to epidural analgesia
- Septicaemia.
- Infection at site of insertion.
- Coagulopathy/thrombocytopaenia (platelet count <70 × 10⁹)

⚠ Beware of a falling count over the past few days—always check the platelet count if this has occurred. If the platelet count is between 70 and 100 × 10⁹, clotting studies should be performed before proceeding with the epidural.

- Raised intracranial pressure.
- Haemorrhage and cardiovascular instability/hypovolaemia.
- Known allergy to amide (lidocaine-type) local anaesthetic solutions or opioids.
- Fixed cardiac output states, e.g. severe aortic stenosis, hypertrophic obstructive cardiomyopathy (HOCM).

Technique for siting an epidural
- The procedure should be explained and consent sought.
- There should be no clotting abnormalities.
- Establish wide-bore IV access.
- Position the woman either on her side or sitting, with the back curved to open intervertebral spaces.
- Full aseptic technique must be followed.
- A suitable interspace, usually L3/L4, is identified and lidocaine 1% injected.
- The epidural space is identified by a loss of resistance technique, usually to saline 0.9%.
- Once the space is identified, a catheter is threaded in and the needle withdrawn and the catheter firmly fixed to the skin.
- A test dose of local anaesthetic, usually bupivacaine, can be given to check that the epidural catheter has not inadvertently entered the subarachnoid space.
- Various regimens exist for the delivery of local anaesthetic to the epidural space either involving bolus administration or infusions.
- Careful monitoring is mandatory following epidural top-up doses including BP reading every 5min for 20min following the administration of a top-up dose.
- Block height and degree of motor block should be recorded.
- Continuous electronic fetal monitoring is required if an epidural has been sited.

Further reading
How to perform epidural spinal anesthesia.
🔗 https://www.youtube.com/watch?v=rM1aQC-HAX0

North Bristol NHS Trust. Epidural—patient information.
🔗 https://www.nbt.nhs.uk/maternity-services/pain-management-opti ons/epidural-anaesthesia

Anaesthetic techniques for Caesarean delivery: spinal

Regional anaesthetic techniques are ideal for the majority of obstetric operative deliveries and most anaesthetists would counsel women having a CD to opt for a neuraxial technique. However, the choice of anaesthetic technique may be influenced by the urgency of the CD and the medical history of the patient. Facilities for conversion to general anaesthesia (GA), such as drugs and endotracheal tubes, must always be available, as conversion to GA may be required if the block wears off during surgery, or is too high, or if the woman requests it due to pain or discomfort.

Spinal anaesthesia

- Accounts for the majority anaesthesia for CD performed in the UK.
- Fasting and antacid precautions are ideal, as GA may be required if the block is unsatisfactory.
- Good IV access is essential to provide fluids rapidly to counteract hypotension that may occur. Vasopressor drugs, such as phenylephrine or ephedrine, should also be available.
- Hyperbaric bupivacaine 0.5% in a dose of 12.5–15mg is usually used, together with an opiate such as fentanyl (15 micrograms) or diamorphine (around 300 micrograms).

Advantages and disadvantages

Advantages
- Technically relatively easier than epidurals to perform.
- Enable mother to bond immediately with baby.
- The most reliable option for establishing a dense, bilateral block.

Disadvantages
- May cause severe hypotension.
- May wear off if surgery is unexpectedly prolonged.

⚠ Hypotension is common due to sympathetic blockade and inadequate tilt → aortocaval pressure, and must be prevented using fluids, adequate left lateral tilt, and vasopressors if appropriate.

▶ Patients must be warned of the risk of intraoperative pain and the small chance of conversion to GA.

▶ The full extent of the block must be tested and recorded by the anaesthetist, prior to the commencement of surgery.

Anaesthetic techniques for Caesarean delivery: epidural

Conversion of a functioning epidural from analgesia to anaesthesia is the choice if a woman requires an operative or instrumental delivery, provided there is sufficient time (it takes ~20min or longer).

Advantages and disadvantages

Advantages
- Can be topped up, should the surgery be extended.
- Can be used for good postoperative analgesia.

Disadvantages
- More likely than spinal anaesthesia to produce patchy or unilateral blockade.
- Takes longer to establish an adequate block.
- Can be technically difficult, with a higher incidence of headache in the event of inadvertent dural puncture.
- The catheter can migrate into the subarachnoid or subdural space, resulting in unpredictable and possibly fatal complications if large doses of local anaesthetic are administered.
- Larger doses of local anaesthetic agents are required, → the possibility of toxicity if the catheter has migrated intravenously.

Anaesthetic techniques for Caesarean delivery: combined spinal epidural

These are usually performed by inserting a spinal needle through an epidural needle, although two separate injections may be performed.

▶ Combined spinal epidural anaesthesia combines the advantages of spinal anaesthesia, i.e. speed of onset and dense block, with the ability to prolong the period of anaesthesia and analgesia via the epidural route.

Advantages and disadvantages

Advantages
- The epidural component can be used to top up the block.
- A smaller volume of local anaesthetic can be used intrathecally and the block extended gradually with the epidural component (this may cause less cardiovascular instability and be useful in women with cardiac disease).
- The epidural component can provide postoperative analgesia.

Disadvantages
- There is a higher risk of failure of the intrathecal component.
- The epidural component of the technique is untested and any local anaesthetic agents must be given in small boluses in case the catheter is in the subarachnoid space.

Anaesthetic techniques for Caesarean delivery: general anaesthesia

There has been a general trend throughout the developed world away from using GA for CD. However, it is still necessary in the presence of contra-indications to regional anaesthesia or when there is urgent time pressure to quickly provide an effective anaesthesia.

Problems with GA

- *Potential airway difficulties:* incidence of failed intubation in pregnant women is ~1:300 compared with 1:3000 in the general surgical population.
- Pulmonary aspiration of gastric contents.
- *Awareness:* rare with modern anaesthetic techniques, but may occur if inadequate levels of inhalational agents are used; this can be a particular problem in the obstetric populous.

Technique for GA in pregnancy

- Adequate assessment of the airway is essential, as well as questioning about relevant medical, obstetric, and drug treatment, and allergies.
- Antacid prophylaxis must be administered.
- Left lateral tilt maintained at all times to prevent aortocaval compression.
- Adequate preoxygenation must precede induction of GA, regardless of the obstetric indications for the CD.
- ECG, pulse oximetry, and capnographic monitoring must be available.
- For full discussion of GA for CD, readers are advised to consult a specialist anaesthetic text.

⚠ Emergency GA is associated with ↑ maternal morbidity and mortality.

▶ There are few absolute indications for GA for CD.

Chapter 8

Neonatal resuscitation

Overview

Most babies establish normal respiration and circulation without help after delivery. However, all babies should be assessed at delivery. Newborn infants who are born at term, have clear liquor, and are breathing and crying with good tone will only require drying and keeping warm. <1% of babies need resuscitation. Anticipation of problems before delivery is the key to success.

It is prudent, where possible, to call for specialist skilled personnel to attend deliveries where need for additional support may be anticipated.

These situations include:
- Preterm deliveries.
- Emergency CDs.
- Vaginal breech birth.
- Thick meconium-stained liquor.
- Major fetal abnormality.
- Other concerns (multiples, signs of significant fetal compromise).

All trained personnel attending a delivery have a responsibility for initiating resuscitation at birth and should possess the appropriate knowledge and skills to approach the management of the newborn infant during the first 10–20min in a competent manner. The environment should be warm, draught free, and well lit, with a flat surface available for resuscitation. Equipment should be checked on a daily basis and before each delivery.

Some of the important items are:
- A warmed flat surface (resuscitaire with radiant warmer) (Fig. 8.1).
- Source of air and oxygen with pressure-limited gas delivery.
- Appropriate size face masks, oropharyngeal airways, and endotracheal tubes (ETTs).
- Suction device with different size suction catheters.
- Stethoscope.
- Laryngoscope with straight laryngeal blades.
- Instruments for clamping and cutting the umbilical cord.
- Emergency resuscitation box for advanced resuscitation.
- Clock or stopwatch.

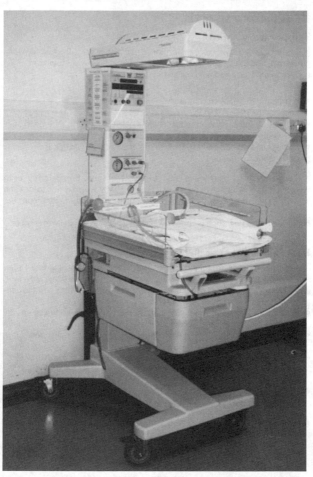

Fig. 8.1 Neonatal radiant warmer (Resuscitaire®). Reproduced with permission of Dräeger Medical UK, 2008.

Practical aspects

Temperature control

Hypothermia can lower oxygen tension, ↑ metabolic acidosis, lead to hypo-glycaemia, and inhibit the production of surfactant. Low temperature is associated with poor neonatal outcome.

Heat loss should be prevented by:
• Protecting the baby from draught.
• Keeping the delivery room warm.
• Drying the term baby immediately after delivery, covering the head and body with warm towels to prevent further heat loss.
• Placing the baby on a warm surface under a radiant warmer, if resuscitation is needed.

▶ For a preterm baby born before 28wks of gestation (<~1kg birth weight), the most effective way of keeping the baby warm is not to dry and wrap it in warm towels, but to cover the head and body (apart from the face) with a plastic bag before placing under a radiant heater.
▶ Plastic wrapping should therefore be available at all deliveries of extremely preterm infants.

Initial assessment at delivery

The immediate assessment includes colour, tone, breathing, and heart rate. Apgar scoring is often used for the initial assessment of the baby. However, it is a retrospective, highly subjective tool and was never intended to identify babies needing immediate resuscitation.
• *Colour:* baby may be centrally pink, cyanosed, or pale (peripheral cyanosis is common and does not by itself indicate hypoxaemia).
• *Tone:* a very floppy baby is likely to be unconscious, and may need respiratory support.
• *Breathing:* the rate, depth, and symmetry of respiration together with any abnormal breathing pattern such as grunting and gasping should be noted.
• *Heart rate:* best evaluated by auscultating with a stethoscope (palpating the umbilical cord is often effective, but can be misleading).

After the initial assessment, infants can be generally classified into one of four groups and further management guided by this (Table 8.1).

Further reading

About the Apgar score.
🔖 https://www.youtube.com/watch?v=98ikG8a9JKs

Table 8.1 Classification of babies at birth with appropriate action

	Assessment	Clinical condition	Action
Group 1	Healthy	• Vigorous baby • Crying • Becoming pink • Good tone • Heart rate >100 beats/min	• Dry and warm • Hand to mother for skin-to-skin contact
Group 2	Primary apnoea	• Apnoeic or inadequate breathing • Remaining blue ↓ tone • Heart rate >100 beats/min	• Dry and warm • Tactile stimulation • Facial oxygen • Consider mask ventilation if not improving
Group 3	Terminal apnoea	• Apnoeic • Blue or pale • Floppy • Heart rate <100 beats/min	• Dry and warm • Mask ventilation • If no improvement may need intubation, ventilation, and chest compressions if heart rate not improving
Group 4	Fresh stillbirth	• Apnoeic • Pale floppy • No heart rate	• Full cardiopulmonary resuscitation

Airway, breathing, and circulation (ABC)

⚠ *Call for skilled help as soon as a problem is identified.*

Airway

The head should be placed in neutral position. This is different from the head position for adult resuscitation because of the relatively large occiput of babies. Overextension of the neck can occlude the airway. A jaw thrust may be helpful, but care must be taken not to compress the airway under the chin. Use of an appropriately sized Guedel airway can be considered, particularly in infants with micrognathia. Suction of the airway is only required if there is blood or particulate material in the oropharynx. Aggressive pharyngeal suction should be avoided and suction should always be done under direct vision with a laryngoscope.

⚠ Blind suction is not helpful; even in the presence of meconium-stained liquor. It may lead to trauma and induce bradycardia or laryngospasm.

Breathing

Mask ventilation may be necessary if the infant is apnoeic, has irregular breathing, or is bradycardic. The aim is to achieve adequate lung inflation and to deliver oxygen. In most cases mask ventilation is as effective as intubation in the initial resuscitation scenario.

It is essential to use the correct-sized mask. The mask should cover the nose and mouth, but should not extend beyond the chin or over the orbits. Mask ventilation can be performed using a bag and mask, or via a constant flow T-piece system (Fig. 8.2).

The lungs of newborn infants are fluid-filled immediately after birth and the first five breaths given should sustain an inflation pressure of approximately 30cm of water (for a term infant) for 2–3s (inflation breaths). These long breaths aim to displace the lung fluid and expand the lungs. If effective, chest wall movement and improvement of heart rate should be seen. If the heart rate rises, but baby is still not breathing, continue to ventilate at 30–40 breaths/min (maintain the inflation for ~1s for each breath).

⚠ If there is no improvement, the airway should be checked again. Help should be sought and early additional assistance will be beneficial if there is no improvement.

Circulation

⚠ *Chest compressions are effective only if the lungs have been successfully inflated.*

Chest compressions aim to deliver oxygenated blood to the heart allowing the circulation to recover. Chest compressions should be commenced if the infant remains bradycardic despite adequate ventilation.

How to perform chest compressions in the neonate

- Both thumbs should be placed over the lower 1/3 of the sternum, encircling the chest with both hands; other fingers lie behind the baby supporting the back.
- For effective chest compressions, the chest is compressed to a depth of 1/3 the anteroposterior diameter allowing the chest wall to return to its relaxed position between compressions.
- 3:1 ratio of compression and ventilation is used, i.e. 90 compressions and 30 breaths/min, each breath lasting for 1s.
- The quality of compressions and ventilation are more important than the rate.
- Recheck the heart rate after 30s and every 30s after that.

(See video teaching basic neonatal resuscitation to midwifery students: www.youtube.com/watch?v=TWaZBcjmxu8)

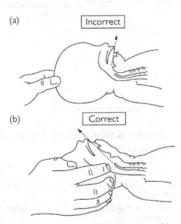

Fig. 8.2 Neonatal resuscitation. (a) Incorrect head position. Neonates have a prominent occiput and in the prone position will naturally adopt flexed head posture, compromising the airway. (b) Correct 'neutral' head position. Neutral position is neither extended nor flexed, but opens the airway to allow effective inflation breaths.

Drugs

Drugs are rarely indicated in neonatal resuscitation. They should be considered only if adequate ventilation and effective chest compression have failed to ↑ the heart rate to >60 beats/min.

▶ In the resuscitation situation, drugs should be given via an umbilical venous catheter.

Drugs used in neonatal resuscitation

- *Adrenaline*: 1:10,000, dose 0.1–0.3mL/kg equivalent to 10–30 micrograms/kg; route through umbilical venous catheter or IV.

▶ Adrenaline should not be given down the ETT.

- *Sodium bicarbonate (NaHCO₃)*: dose 1–2mmol/kg (2–4mL/kg of 4.2% $NaHCO_3$); route through IV or umbilical venous catheter. Reversing the intracardiac acidosis may help bump-start the heart.

▶ Repeated doses of $NaHCO_3$ should be avoided without proper evidence of metabolic acidosis from blood gas analysis.

Glucose 10%: dose 2mL/kg/dose (200mg/kg/dose), route through IV or umbilical venous catheter. Glucose should be given if there is hypoglycaemia.

- *Volume replacement*: crystalloid (0.9% saline, 10mL/kg/dose) is the preferred fluid if the infant appears to be in shock. Blood should be given if there is evidence of hypovolaemia and evidence of acute blood loss.

- *Naloxone*: is no longer kept in the resuscitation trolley.

Actions in the event of a poor response to resuscitation

Check for a technical problem

- Is the gas flow connected?
- Is there a leak in the circuit? Check the tubing.
- Is the ETT in the trachea? If in doubt, remove ETT, give breaths by mask, and replace ETT if necessary.
- Is the ETT blocked? If in doubt, remove ETT, give breaths by mask, and replace ETT if necessary.
- Check the blow-off valve pressure (30cm of water for term infant).

Does the baby have other pathology?

- Pneumothorax.
- Congenital lung problem, e.g. diaphragmatic hernia.
- Lung hypoplasia.
- Hydrops fetalis.
- Perinatal asphyxia.

Recent advances

Delayed cord clamping

For uncompromised babies, a delay in cord clamping of at least 1min from complete delivery of the infant is now recommended.

Infants with meconium-stained liquor

There is now evidence that suctioning of the meconium from the infant's airway after delivery of the head but before delivery of the shoulder is not beneficial and so it is no longer recommended.

▶ No suctioning should be performed if the infant is active, vigorous, and crying.
▶ If an infant is born through thick meconium and is floppy and depressed after birth, it is reasonable for a skilled person to inspect the larynx directly with a laryngoscope and suction the oropharynx and trachea. There is no role for bronchial lavage.

Preterm infants

It is easier to maintain the preterm infant's temperature by placing it into a food-grade plastic wrap or bag (while wet, leaving the face uncovered) and then under a radiant heater. This is more effective than drying and wrapping for infants <28wks gestation. For these infants the delivery room temperature should be at least 26°C.

Also, preterm infants usually require less pressure to inflate their lungs and therefore the blow-off valve on the resuscitaire should be initially set at *20–25cm* of water (rather than 30cm of water for term infants). Initial respiratory support of spontaneously breathing preterm infants with respiratory distress may be provided by CPAP rather than intubation.

Use of air versus oxygen in resuscitation

There is evidence that using air for the resuscitation of near-term and term babies is as effective as using oxygen, although there is still active debate. It is therefore reasonable to resuscitate infants in air, with supplemental oxygen available if needed and its use guided by pulse oximetry.

Confirmation of tracheal tube placement

Detection of exhaled carbon dioxide in addition to clinical assessment is recommended as the most reliable method to confirm placement of a tracheal tube in neonates with spontaneous circulation.

Therapeutic hypothermia

Newly born infants born at term or near term with evolving moderate to severe hypoxic ischaemic encephalopathy should, where possible, be offered therapeutic hypothermia. This does not affect immediate resuscitation, but is important for post-resuscitation care.

Communication with parents

Resuscitation decisions

If resuscitation is required, parents should be fully informed of the procedure undertaken and the purpose.

The decision to resuscitate an extremely preterm infant should be a combined decision of parents, and paediatric and obstetric staff. This is a difficult conversation, but one that is best had early. The obstetricians caring for any woman who has a strong probability of delivering very prematurely must raise the issue early and actively involve their paediatric colleagues. The decision taken about resuscitation should also influence the level of fetal monitoring in labour. The British Association of Perinatal Medicine (BAPM) has published a Framework for Practice outlining an approach to assist clinicians in decision-making relating to perinatal care and preterm delivery at ≤27+6 weeks gestation in the UK.

▶ The decision to discontinue resuscitation should involve senior paediatric staff. Proper birth plans should be in place in cases of severe congenital malformations. All communication with parents should be documented in the mother's notes and later in the baby's notes after delivery.

Stopping resuscitation

- If there are no signs of life after 10min of continuous and effective resuscitation, it is appropriate to consider stopping ongoing attempts as the outcome is universally poor.
- The decision should be made by the resuscitation team and the most senior staff available.
- Local and national guidelines are very helpful in making such decisions.

Further reading

BAPM (2019). Perinatal management of extreme preterm birth: a framework for practice.
🖰 www.bapm.org/resources/80-perinatal-management-of-extreme-preterm-birth-before-27-weeks-of-gestation-2019
European Resuscitation Council (2015). European Resuscitation Council guidelines for resuscitation 2015. Section 7: Resuscitation and support of transition of babies at birth.
🖰 https://ercguidelines.elsevierresource.com/european-resuscitation-council-guidelines-resuscitation-2015-section-7-resuscitation-and-support

Postnatal care

Normal changes in the puerperium

The puerperium begins after delivery of placenta and lasts until the reproductive organs have returned to their pre-pregnant state—usually about 6wks.

Hormones

- *Human placental lactogen and βhCG:* levels ↓ rapidly; by 10 days neither should be detectable.
- Oestrogen and progesterone: non-pregnant levels are achieved by 7 days postpartum.

Genital tract

- *Uterus:* undergoes rapid involution. Weight of the uterus falls from 1000g post delivery to about 500g at the end of a week. By 2wks, it returns to pelvis and is no longer palpable abdominally.
- *Vagina:* initially vaginal wall is swollen, but rapidly regains tone, although remains fragile for 1–2wks. Gradually, vascularity and oedema ↓, and by 4wks rugae reappear, but are less prominent than in a nullipara.
- *Cervix:* cervical os gradually closes after delivery. It admits 2–3 fingers for the first 4–6 days and by the end of 10–14 days is dilated to barely >1cm.

Perineum

Perineal oedema persists for some days. It may take longer if there was a prolonged 2nd stage, especially with a long period of pushing, operative vaginal delivery, or perineal tears that needed repair.

Lochia

Lochia consists of sloughed-off necrotic decidual layer mixed with blood. It is initially red (lochia rubra), becomes paler as bleeding ↓ (lochia serosa), and finally becomes a yellowish white (lochia alba). The flow of lochia may last for 3–6wks.

Breasts

Between 2nd and 4th days, breasts become engorged, vascularity ↑, and areolar pigmentation ↑. Enlargement of lobules results from an ↑ in number and size of the alveoli.

Cardiovascular system

After the 3rd stage of labour, cardiac output initially ↑ due to return of blood from the contracted uterus. Plasma volume, which expanded by 40% during pregnancy, rapidly ↓ as a result of diuresis and returns to normal by 2–3wks postpartum. Heart rate ↓ and returns to pre-pregnancy rate, and is partly responsible for ↓ cardiac output. Blood loss at delivery, excretion of extracellular fluid, and ↓ of plasma volume due to changes in hormonal status are responsible for alterations in the blood volume.

Major postnatal problems

The three major causes of morbidity in the postnatal period are:
- 2° PPH (Box 9.1; ➔ Postpartum haemorrhage, p. 356; ➔ Massive obstetric haemorrhage: causes, p. 414).
- VTE (Box 9.2; ➔ Venous thromboembolism: overview, p. 424).
- Puerperal pyrexia.

Puerperal pyrexia is defined as the presence of fever in a mother ≥38°C in the first 14 days after giving birth.

Box 9.1 2° PPH

- Any 'abnormal' bleeding occurring 24h to 6wks postnatally.
- In developed countries, 2% of postnatal women are admitted to hospital with this: 50% undergo surgical evacuation.
- In developing countries, it is a major cause of maternal death.
- Caused by retained products, endometritis, or a tear.
- Management depends on the cause (➔ Postpartum haemorrhage, p. 356; ➔ Massive obstetric haemorrhage: causes, p. 414).

Box 9.2 VTE

⚠ 2nd major cause of direct maternal death in the UK (➔ Venous thromboembolism: overview, p. 424). May be asymptomatic until it presents with a PE, but signs and symptoms may include:

Deep vein thrombosis (DVT)
- Leg pain or discomfort (especially in the left leg).
- Swelling.
- Tenderness.
- Erythema, ↑ skin temperature and oedema.
- Lower abdominal pain (high DVT).
- Elevated white cell count.

Pulmonary thromboembolism
- Dyspnoea.
- Collapse.
- Chest pain.
- Haemoptysis.
- Faintness.
- Raised jugular venous pressure (JVP).
- Focal signs in chest.
- Symptoms and signs associated with DVT.

⚠ In the postnatal period there should be a high level of suspicion for women presenting with any of the above-listed symptoms, and urgent investigation is warranted starting with pulse oximetry, ECG, and CXR.

Puerperal sepsis: overview

Puerperal sepsis was the most common cause of maternal mortality before the mid-1930s, accounting for >40% of all maternal deaths.

The ↓ of sepsis and maternal deaths was achieved by hand washing and following aseptic and antiseptic procedures. Further control and cure of puerperal infection began in 1935 with introduction of the first sulphonamides. Resurgence of puerperal infection as the leading cause of direct maternal deaths was reported in the last UK Confidential Enquiry into Maternal Deaths (in the 2006–2008 as well as the 2009–2012 reports). ➲ Care of women with sepsis, p. 460.

- With puerperal sepsis, early identification, and rapid and appropriate management saves lives.
- Young, healthy mothers maintain vital parameters slightly altered and suddenly decompensate; regular and frequent monitoring of pulse, BP, respiratory rate, and temperature on a 'modified early obstetric warning chart' would help in early identification of a worsening condition.

Think 'sepsis'

- Think 'sepsis' in an unwell pregnant woman or who was recently pregnant, especially if she presents a few times as unwell.
- Early diagnosis, rapid broad-spectrum antibiotics, review by senior doctors and midwives, and implementation of the 'sepsis care bundle' can make the difference between life and death.
- Consultant-to-consultant referral and advice from a microbiologist when the first drug is not effective is essential.

Definition of sepsis

Sepsis is defined as life-threatening organ dysfunction caused by a dysregulated host response to infection (see The UK Sepsis Trust: ℰ https://sepsistrust.org/).

'Red Flag Sepsis'

The Sepsis-3 international consensus recommends the use of an ↑ in a patient's Sequential (or Sepsis-related) Organ Failure Assessment Score (SOFA) of 2 points as the 'official' definition of sepsis, as this score is the most appropriate measure available at present to formally identify organ dysfunction. However, this is a complex scoring system for the bedside.

'Red Flag Sepsis' was developed by the UK Sepsis Trust in collaboration with NHS England and the Royal Colleges as a pragmatic, operational solution for use at the bedside (Fig. 9.1).

Further reading

RCOG (2012). Sepsis in pregnancy, bacterial. Green-top guideline no. 64a
ℰ www.rcog.org.uk/en/guidelines-research-services/guidelines/gtg64a/
The UK Sepsis Trust.
ℰ https://sepsistrust.org/

Sepsis red flag symptoms

- Objective evidence of new or altered mental state.
- Systolic BP ≤90mmHg (or drop of >40mmHg from normal).
- Heart rate ≥130 beats/min.
- Respiratory rate ≥25 breaths/min.
- Needs O_2 to keep SpO_2 ≥92%.
- Non-blanching rash/mottled/ashen/cyanotic.
- Lactate ≥2 mmol/L.*
- Not passed urine in 18h (<0.5mL/kg/h if catheterized).

If there are any red flag symptoms in the presence of a likely diagnosis of infection, the 'Sepsis Six' must be started within 1h.
*Lactate may be raised in and immediately after normal delivery.

The 'Sepsis Six' (The UK Sepsis Trust)

The Sepsis Six care bundle needs institution within 1h of diagnosis:

1. Ensure senior clinician attends

- Not all patients with red flags will need the 'Sepsis Six' urgently.
- A senior decision maker may seek alternative diagnoses/de-escalate care.

2. Oxygen if required

- Start if O_2 saturations less than 92%.
- Aim for O_2 saturations of 94–98%.
- If at risk of hypercarbia aim for saturations of 88–92%.

3. Obtain IV access, take bloods

- Blood cultures.
- Blood glucose.
- Lactate.
- FBC, U&Es, CRP, and clotting.
- Lumbar puncture if indicated.

4. Give IV antibiotics

- Maximum dose broad-spectrum therapy (consider: local policy/allergy status/antivirals).

5. Give IV fluids

- Give fluid bolus of 20mL/kg if age <16, 500mL if 16+.
- NICE recommends using lactate to guide further fluid therapy.

6. Monitor

- Use a modified early obstetric warning system chart.
- Measure urinary output: this may require a urinary catheter.
- Repeat lactate at least once per hour if initial lactate elevated or if clinical condition changes.

The UK Sepsis Trust:
꿈 https://sepsistrust.org/

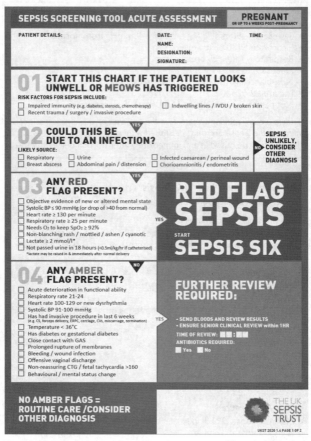

Fig. 9.1 Example of a pregnancy-specific sepsis screening tool from the UK Sepsis Trust (available to download at https://sepsistrust.org/).

SEPSIS SCREENING TOOL - THE SEPSIS SIX

PREGNANT
OR UP TO 6 WEEKS POST-PREGNANCY

PATIENT DETAILS:

DATE:
NAME:
DESIGNATION:
SIGNATURE:

TIME:

COMPLETE ALL ACTIONS WITHIN ONE HOUR

01 ENSURE SENIOR CLINICIAN ATTENDS
NOT ALL PATIENTS WITH RED FLAGS WILL NEED THE 'SEPSIS 6' URGENTLY. A SENIOR DECISION MAKER MAY SEEK ALTERNATIVE DIAGNOSES/ DE-ESCALATE CARE. RECORD DECISIONS BELOW
NAME: GRADE:

TIME
☐☐:☐☐

02 OXYGEN IF REQUIRED
START IF O₂ SATURATIONS LESS THAN 92% - AIM FOR O₂ SATURATIONS OF 94-98%
IF AT RISK OF HYPERCARBIA AIM FOR SATURATIONS OF 88-92%

TIME
☐☐:☐☐

03 OBTAIN IV ACCESS, TAKE BLOODS
BLOOD CULTURES, BLOOD GLUCOSE, LACTATE, FBC, U&Es, CRP AND CLOTTING
LUMBAR PUNCTURE IF INDICATED

TIME
☐☐:☐☐

04 GIVE IV ANTIBIOTICS
MAXIMUM DOSE BROAD SPECTRUM THERAPY
CONSIDER: LOCAL POLICY / ALLERGY STATUS / ANTIVIRALS

TIME
☐☐:☐☐

05 GIVE IV FLUIDS
GIVE FLUID BOLUS OF 20 ml/kg if age <16, 500ml if 16+
NICE RECOMMENDS USING LACTATE TO GUIDE FURTHER FLUID THERAPY

TIME
☐☐:☐☐

06 MONITOR
USE MEOWS. MEASURE URINARY OUTPUT: THIS MAY REQUIRE A URINARY CATHETER REPEAT LACTATE
AT LEAST ONCE PER HOUR IF INITIAL LACTATE ELEVATED OR IF CLINICAL CONDITION CHANGES

TIME
☐☐:☐☐

RED FLAGS AFTER ONE HOUR – ESCALATE TO CONSULTANT NOW

RECORD ADDITIONAL NOTES HERE:
e.g. allergy status, arrival of specialist teams, de-escalation of care, delayed antimicrobial decision making, variance

THE UK
SEPSIS
TRUST

UKST 2020 1.4 PAGE 2 OF 2

Fig. 9.1 (continued)

Puerperal infection: genital causes

Uterine infection (endometritis)

Predisposing factors

- CD—more with failure to use prophylactic antibiotics.
- PROM—incidence ↑ with the latency to onset of labour.
- Intrapartum chorioamnionitis.
- Prolonged labour.
- Multiple pelvic examinations.
- Internal fetal monitoring—use of scalp electrodes/intrauterine pressure catheters.
- Other risk factors, e.g. anaemia, low socioeconomic status.

Signs and symptoms

- Fever usually in proportion to the extent of infection.
- Foul smelling, profuse, and bloody discharge.
- Subinvolution of uterus.
- Tender bulky uterus on abdominal examination.

Perineal wound infection

- Includes infection of episiotomy wounds and repaired lacerations.
- Perineum becomes painful and erythematous.
- May cause breakdown of wound.

Complications of pelvic infection

- Wound dehiscence.
- Adnexal infections.
- Pelvic abscess.
- Septic thrombophlebitis.
- Septicaemia.
- Subsequent subfertility.

Factors predisposing to puerperal pyrexia

Antepartum

- Anaemia.
- Duration of membrane rupture.

Intrapartum

- Duration of labour.
- Bacterial contamination during vaginal examination.
- Instrumentation.
- Trauma, e.g. episiotomy, vaginal tears, CD.
- Haematoma.

Puerperal infection: non-genital causes

Breast causes (mastitis, breast abscess)
- ~15% of women develop fever from breast engorgement.
- Fever may be as high as 39°C.
- Associated with a painful and hard breast.
- Antibiotics may be needed in the presence of infection.
- Breast-feeding should be continued.
- Abscess may need surgical drainage.

Urinary tract infection
- ~2–4% of women develop a UTI postpartum.
- Hypotonic bladder may result in stasis and reflux of urine.
- Catheterization, birth trauma, pelvic examinations during labour.
- *Presenting symptoms:* ↑ frequency of micturition, dysuria, and/or urgency. High fever, rigors, loin pain, and tenderness may be present in pyelonephritis.
- Most common organisms involved: *Escherichia coli*, *Proteus*, and *Klebsiella*.

Thrombophlebitis
- Superficial or DVT of legs may cause pyrexia.
- Caused by venous stasis.
- Diagnosis made by the observation of a painful, swollen leg, usually accompanied by calf tenderness.

⚠ High risk of postpartum DVT and PE—be vigilant and carry out appropriate investigations urgently.

Respiratory complications
- Usually seen within the first 24h after delivery.
- Almost invariably in women who underwent CD.
- Complications due to atelectasis, aspiration, and/or bacterial pneumonia.

Abdominal wound infection
- Incidence following CD is ~6%.
- With prophylactic antibiotics, the rate of infection could be <2%.
- Recent guidelines recommend antibiotics prior to skin incision (e.g. cefuroxime 1.5g IV; if sensitive then clindamycin 900mg IV. Co-amoxiclav is best avoided for fear of necrotizing enterocolitis in the neonate).
- Risk factors include:
  - obesity
  - diabetes
  - corticosteroid therapy
  - poor haemostasis at surgery with subsequent haematoma.

⚠ VTE can also cause low-grade pyrexia and must always be considered in the differential diagnosis.

Puerperal infection: management

Investigations

Investigations should be aimed at identifying the most likely source of infection, causative organism, and antibiotic sensitivity, and include:
- FBC.
- Blood cultures.
- MSU.
- Swabs from cervix and lochia for *Chlamydia* and bacterial culture.
- Wound swabs.
- Throat swabs.
- Sputum culture and CXR.

Management

Supportive
- Analgesics and anti-inflammatory drugs (NSAIDs).
- Wound care in cases of wound infection.
- Ice packs for pain from perineum or mastitis.

Antibiotics
- A regimen with activity against the *Bacteroides fragilis* group and other penicillin-resistant anaerobic bacteria is better than one without.
- There is no evidence that any one regimen is associated with fewer side effects, except that cephalosporins are associated with less diarrhoea.
- No specific recommendations can be made for the treatment of women who develop endometritis after receiving antibiotic prophylaxis for CD.
- Combination of clindamycin and an aminoglycoside (such as gentamicin) is appropriate for the treatment of endometritis.
- Tetracyclines should be avoided in breast-feeding women.
- Involvement of microbiologists is indicated in women who fail to respond to antibiotics.

Surgical
- Incision and drainage of breast abscess.
- Secondary repair of wound dehiscence.
- Drainage of pelvic haematomas and abscesses.

Prevention

- Women with suspected UTI during the antenatal period should be investigated and any infection treated vigorously.
- Advice should be offered regarding breast-feeding and care of breasts during the antenatal period.
- Prevention and treatment of pre-existing anaemia (especially important in women from developing countries).
- Rigid antiseptic measures taken during labour and delivery also help to eliminate infection, including:
  - hand washing and use of alcohol hand gel by midwives and doctor before examining the patient
  - examining in a sterile environment and using sterile instruments
  - use of antiseptic creams and lotions
  - catheterizing only when it is indicated and using all sterile precautions while introducing the catheter.
- Prophylactic antibiotic administration at CD.
- Treatment with broad-spectrum antibiotics while waiting for the culture results.

Further reading

Cochrane (2015). Antibiotic regimens for postpartum endometritis.
🔊 www.cochrane.org/CD001067/PREG_antibiotic-regimens-postpartum-endometritis

Other postnatal problems

Pain

- 'After-pains' due to uterine contractions cause lower central abdominal pain mainly during the first 3–4 days.
- Perineal pain could be severe, especially after instrumental delivery, episiotomy, or vaginal tears:
  - ↑ pain may suggest haematoma or infection
  - haematoma is managed conservatively or by surgery depending on its site, size, symptoms, and signs
  - if infected, antibiotics are prescribed according to local policy.

▶ RCTs of oral analgesia for perineal pain show that paracetamol and NSAIDs are as effective as oral narcotic medications. Some may find topical application of local anaesthetic (e.g. 1% lidocaine gel) helpful.

Bladder problems

Urinary retention

- Occurs commonly with an epidural as bladder sensation and the desire to void is masked.
- Instrumental delivery or extensive tears (especially peri-urethral), perineal pain, and oedema can cause retention.
- Reassurance along with analgesics is helpful in most situations.
- Occasionally, catheterization is required to protect from over-distention—leave indwelling for 24–48h.

⚠ An indwelling catheter should be used after a spinal, until full sensation returns to protect the bladder.

UTI

- Low threshold for suspicion; confirm with MSU and treat with appropriate antibiotics and plenty of oral fluids.

Bowel problems

- Lack of fluid and food, and dehydration during labour lead to constipation, which may continue into the puerperium.
- Pain and fear of wound disruption following perineal tears could further exacerbate the problem, as can opiate analgesia.
- Advice should be offered to ↑ the intake of fibre and fluids.
- Osmotic laxatives such as lactulose may be helpful.
- Women with 3rd- or 4th-degree tears should be prescribed stool softeners and laxatives (➜ Third- and fourth-degree tears, p. 338).

Symphysis pubis discomfort

- Symptoms include severe pubic and groin pain exacerbated by weight bearing.
- Most cases resolve by 6–8wks.
- Conservative approach includes rest, a belt that wraps around the femoral trochanters to discourage separation, weight-bearing assistance, and analgesics.
- Rarely, surgical assistance may be needed.

Maternal obstetric paralysis

- This is very rare but manifests as intrapartum foot drop due to lumbosacral trunk compression by the fetal head at the pelvic brim.
- Placing the legs in lithotomy without protection at the region of the head of the fibula can compress the peroneal nerve and cause palsy.
- The primary pathology is predominantly demyelination, and recovery is usually complete in up to 5mths.
- Referral for neurological assessment and input is recommended.

Identifying mental health problems

- Lack of social and psychological support during puerperium is a common problem and may occur in 7–30% of women in developed countries.
- Psychological well-being of women should be carefully and continually assessed in the postnatal period.
- Enquiry should be made of every mother about past mental health.
- Close liaison between midwives, GPs, and obstetricians is essential to provide appropriate care.

⚠ Mental illness is one of the leading causes of maternal death in the UK. In the 2015–2017 period, it contributed to 10% of maternal deaths.
- The majority of these deaths are the result of suicide, which is itself most strongly associated with perinatal depression.
- Over half of suicides occur between 6wks prenatally and 12wks postnatally and are sudden and of a violent nature and hence the need to provide appropriate treatment to avoid such occurrences (➔ Postnatal psychosis, p. 522).

Other postnatal care issues

Lifestyle

Both care and information provided should be culturally appropriate. The cultural practices of women from ethnic minority groups should be incorporated into their postnatal care. Advice should be given regarding diet, exercise, breast-feeding, weight and shape, rest, and support for coping with changes.

Postpartum contraception

- Discussion of contraception should be a routine part of postpartum care.
- WHO recommends LARCs such as postpartum IUDs or implants as the category 1 choice for postpartum women according to the medical eligibility criteria.
- Contraception is not needed in the first 3wks.
- Breast-feeding (lactational amenorrhoea) may be used as contraception (⟴ Breast-feeding: benefits, p. 400).
- Breast-feeding women can start POP without the need for additional contraceptive protection.
- The COCP should be avoided in lactating women as it can affect milk composition and ↑ the incidence of breast-feeding failure.
- Bottle-feeding women can start COCP 21 days postpartum.

▶ There may be an ↑ risk of VTE with earlier commencement of COCP.

Maternal immunization

Rubella

- Women found to be seronegative on antenatal screening for rubella should receive rubella vaccination after delivery, before discharge from the maternity unit.
- Breast-feeding is not a contraindication for rubella immunization.
- Women should be warned to avoid conceiving in the following 3mths, although the risk is theoretical.

Anti-D

- The RCOG recommends the administration of anti-D immunoglobulin 500IU to every non-sensitized RhD −ve woman within 72h after the delivery of an RhD +ve infant.
- ➔ Rhesus isoimmunization (immune hydrops), p. 130.

Hepatitis B

- There are no specific recommendations for postpartum vaccination against HBV.
- It could be offered to individuals who are at ↑ risk because of their lifestyle or occupation.
- Neither pregnancy nor lactation should be considered a contraindication for hepatitis B vaccination of susceptible women.
- Neonatal vaccination is recommended for the babies of women at risk or who already have the virus.
- Babies of mothers who are surface s antigen +ve should receive active immunization; those whose mothers are core e antigen +ve should receive active and passive immunization.

Breast-feeding: overview

Breast-feeding confers several advantages to the newborn and is supported by healthcare institutions. WHO and UNICEF launched the Baby-Friendly Hospital Initiative (BFHI) in 1992, to strengthen maternity practices to support breast-feeding. The foundation for the BFHI are the ten steps to successful breast-feeding described in *Protecting, Promoting and Supporting Breast-feeding: A Joint WHO/UNICEF Statement*. Breastmilk provides enormous medical and physical benefits to the infant.

The aggregate breast-feeding rate for England for quarter 3 of 2019/2020 was 48.2%.

Colostrum

- Thick yellow fluid produced from around 20wks gestation.
- It has a high concentration of secretory IgA.
- It is rich in proteins that play an important part in gut maturation and immunity for the infant.
- It is produced in small quantities following the birth of the baby.

Human milk

- The amount of milk produced rapidly ↑ to ~500mL at 5 days postpartum.
- It has 57–65kcal/dL (2.4–2.7mJ/L) and is more energy efficient than formula milk.

Initiation and frequency

Initiation

- Skin-to-skin contact should start as soon as possible after delivery and is provided as 'Kangaroo care' from birth.
- Early contact ↑ breast-feeding within the first 2h after birth and ↑ duration of breast-feeding when compared with delay of ≥4h.

Frequency

- Varies widely.
- Demand feeding should be encouraged because of its benefits of less weight loss in the immediate postpartum period and ↑ duration of breast-feeding subsequently.
- Frequent feeding is associated with less hyperbilirubinaemia during the early neonatal period.
- For mothers, demand feeding helps to prevent engorgement, and breast-feeding is established more easily.

Demand feeding: facts and figures
- Exclusively breast-fed term infants feed a median of eight times/day—six times during the day, and twice in the night.
- Feeds tend to be infrequent in the first 24–48h and could be as few as three feeds in the first 24h (this should not cause concern in an otherwise well baby).
- The frequency ↑ gradually and reaches a peak around the 5th day of life.
- WHO recommends exclusive breast-feeding for 4–6mths, with introduction of appropriate complementary foods after this period.

Further reading

WHO (2011). Exclusive breast feeding for six months best for babies everywhere.
⌖ https://www.who.int/news/item/15-01-2011-exclusive-breastfeeding-for-six-months-best-for-babies-everywhere

Breast-feeding: benefits

Human breastmilk contains numerous protective factors against infectious disease and may influence immune system development.

Includes effect of colostrum on immunity, fewer diarrhoeal diseases, benefits of omega-3 fatty acids on visual developments in small infants, improved bonding, and ↓ risk of breast disease for mother.

For the infant

Gastrointestinal illness

Infants who are exclusively breast-fed for 6mths experience less morbidity from gastrointestinal infection than those who are mixed breast-fed at 3–4mths.

UTIs

Breast milk is a part of the natural defence against UTIs.

Respiratory infection

Exclusive breast-feeding protects against chest infections.

Atopic illness

Breast-fed babies are less likely to have atopic illnesses, such as eczema and asthma.

Leukaemias

Breast-feeding is associated with a ↓ risk of childhood acute leukaemia, acute lymphoblastic leukaemia, Hodgkin's disease, and neuroblastoma in childhood.

Giardiasis

Children born to non-immune mothers are at higher risk of acquiring *Giardia* infection and developing giardiasis with more severe symptoms compared with breast-fed children of immune mothers.

Intelligence

It remains unclear whether the child's intelligence is affected by breast-feeding, although it remains an unequalled way of providing ideal nutrition.

For the mother

Uterine involution

Breast-feeding helps in uterine involution and ↓ risk of postpartum haemorrhage.

Amenorrhoea and contraception

- Lactational amenorrhoea, and full breast-feeding for up to 6mths is nearly 99% effective as contraception.
- At 12mths the effectiveness during amenorrhoea dropped to 97%.
- Amenorrhoea can be helpful for anaemia in developing countries.

Other benefits

Breast-feeding protects the mother against premenopausal breast cancer, ovarian cancer, and osteoporosis.

Breast-feeding: potential problems

Inadequate milk supply

- <1% of women are physiologically unable to produce an adequate milk supply.
- Treatment for insufficient milk includes adequate fluids, nutrition, secure and private environment, dopamine antagonists, thyrotropin-releasing hormone, and oxytocin.

Problems with milk flow

Breast engorgement, mastitis, and breast abscess
- Limitations on feeding frequency and duration.
- Problems with positioning the baby at the breast.
- Allowing the baby unrestricted access to the breast is the most effective method of treating.

See Box 9.3.

Sore or cracked nipples
- It could be because of incorrect attachment of the baby to the breast.
- It may be necessary to rest the breast and express the breastmilk manually until the crack has healed.

Lactation after breast cancer
- There will be little or no enlargement of the treated breast during pregnancy.
- The ability to lactate and breast-feed from an untreated breast remains normal.
- Tamoxifen inhibits milk production.

Drugs that may ↓ milk production
- Progestins.
- Oestrogens.
- Ethanol.
- Bromocriptine.
- Ergotamine.
- Cabergoline.
- Pseudoephedrine.

Box 9.3 Breast problems

Mastitis (non-infective)

- Results from obstruction of milk drainage from one section of the breast, which may be due to:
  - restriction of feeding
  - a badly positioned baby
  - blocked ducts
  - compression from fingers holding the breast or from wearing too small a bra.
- Characterized by swollen, red, and painful area on breast, tachycardia, pyrexia, and an aching, flu-like feeling, often accompanied by shivering and rigors.
- Resolves with relieving the obstruction by continuing to breast-feed with correct positioning of the baby.

Mastitis (infective)

- If non-infective mastitis is not managed appropriately, it may become infected.
- *Staphylococcus aureus* is the most common organism involved.
- The antibiotics that should be used include penicillinase-resistant penicillins (e.g. cloxacillin, flucloxacillin, co-amoxiclav) or cephalosporins (cefalexin, cefradine, cefaclor).
- Breast-feeding should be continued.

Breast abscess

- Possible complication of inappropriately managed infective mastitis.
- It may need surgical drainage under anaesthetic.
- In severe cases, breast-feeding may have to cease on the affected side.

Drugs and breast-feeding

Almost all drugs, to some extent, pass in breastmilk. The effect of the drug depends on the degree of passage into milk, amount of milk ingested by the infant, absorption of the drug, and whether the drug affects the infant. There are limited human studies to advise on which drugs are contraindicated in pregnancy.

▶ Prescribe medication only when absolutely indicated. Choose ones with shorter half-lives, less toxicity, those commonly used in infants, and those with ↓ bioavailability. Only a few medications are unsafe.

Medications with poor bioavailability and low risk
- Heparin.
- Insulin.
- Aminoglycoside antibiotics.
- 3rd-generation cephalosporins.
- Omeprazole and lansoprazole.
- Inhaled steroids and β-agonists.

Drugs generally contraindicated in breast-feeding mothers
- Amiodarone.
- Antineoplastic.
- Chloramphenicol.
- Ergotamine.
- Cabergoline.
- Ergot alkaloids.
- Iodides.
- Methotrexate.
- Lithium.
- Tetracycline.
- Pseudoephedrine.

Drugs to avoid in breast-feeding mothers
- Acebutolol.
- ACEIs (except captopril).
- Alcohol.
- Caffeine.
- Cocaine.
- Marijuana.
- Fluoxetine.
- Iodine.
- Sulphonamides.

Viruses and breast-feeding

HIV
HIV can be transmitted through breastmilk. Risk factors are:
• Maternal viral load.
• Duration of breast-feeding.
• Oral lesions in infant and maternal breast lesions.

⚠ In developed countries, breast-feeding by HIV-infected mothers should be avoided.

Human lymphotropic virus type 1 (HTLV-1)
Breast-fed babies of HTLV-1-infected mothers are likely to become infected, especially with prolonged breast-feeding.

⚠ HTLV-1 seropositive women are advised not to breast-feed.

Hepatitis B virus
Infants born to HBV +ve mothers, already exposed to maternal blood, amniotic fluid, and vaginal secretions during delivery, may be breast-fed. Babies of all mothers +ve for HBV surface antigen should be immunized at birth. Babies of mothers +ve for HBV e antigen are also given immunoglobulins as additional protection.

▶ Breast-feeding does not appear to ↑ the rate of infection among infants.

Herpes simplex virus
If there are no breast lesions, breast-feeding should be encouraged.

Chickenpox/varicella
If the mother contracts chickenpox while breast-feeding, she should continue to breast-feed, because the antibodies in her milk confer immunity against chickenpox to her baby. This passive immunization may even spare the baby from symptoms of chickenpox.

Cytomegalovirus
CMV is possibly the most commonly detectable virus in human milk. No serious illness or clinical symptoms in neonates 2° to breast-feeding has been reported.

Rubella
Can be passed on to the infant if the mother has active infection. However, the infant does not become ill as transmission of maternal antibodies serves as a natural vaccine. If the mother is immunized to rubella postpartum, the breast-feeding infant will not show symptoms of the illness.

Chapter 10

Obstetric emergencies

Sudden maternal collapse

⚠ **Immediate maternal resuscitation is vital, this requires help so call for it immediately**

- *Airway:* open airway with head tilt and chin lift; jaw thrust may be required (care must be taken if a cervical spine injury is suspected).
- *Breathing:* assess for chest movements (feel for breathing) and listen for breath sounds for up to 10s; if no breathing, put out cardiac arrest call and start cardiopulmonary resuscitation (CPR).

▶ *If CPR required at >20wks, CS (at the location of the arrest) within 5min of arrest is essential for maternal resuscitation.*

- *Circulation:* capillary refill, pulse rate, and BP; optimize circulation by aggressive IV fluids and blood transfusion if indicated.
- *Drugs:* to maintain circulation, combat infection, antidotes if drug overdose, anticoagulants in cases of massive embolism.
- *Environment:* avoid injury (eclampsia), ensure safety of patient and staff.
- *Fetus:* if CPR is required at >20wks, unless there is immediate reversal, immediate CS must be performed. If CPR is not required, assess fetal well-being and plan delivery as appropriate once maternal condition is stable.

General investigations

- *History:* from the patient or her relatives.
- *Observations:* BP, pulse, respiration, oxygen saturation, temperature, and urine output every 15min.
- *Bloods:* FBC, coagulation profile, U&Es, LFTs, uric acid, group and save or cross-match, and blood glucose.

Specific investigations

- If a cardiorespiratory cause is suspected: ECG, CXR, ABG.
- If PE is suspected: Doppler ultrasound of calf veins, ventilation (Q) scan or ventilation/perfusion (V/Q) scan, or CT pulmonary angiogram (CTPA).
- If intracranial pathology is suspected: cerebral imaging (CT/MRI).

Treatment

- Specific treatment depends on the cause.
- Important to ensure MDT input early to optimize outcome.
- Anaesthetic and ICU assistance urgently required.
- If focal neurological signs are present, early neurosurgical input may save lives.

Some causes of sudden maternal collapse

Obstetric
- Massive obstetric haemorrhage (⚠ may be concealed):
  - placenta praevia
  - placental abruption
  - PPH
  - uterine rupture
  - supralevator haematoma following genital tract trauma.
- Severe pre-eclampsia with intracranial bleeding.
- Eclampsia.
- Amniotic fluid embolism.
- Neurogenic shock due to uterine inversion.
- Surgical complications:
  - bleeding after CD
  - pelvic/broad ligament haematoma.
- Severe sepsis, e.g. chorioamnionitis.
- Cardiac failure, e.g. peripartum cardiomyopathy.

Medical/surgical
- Massive PE.
- Cardiac failure:
  - pre-existing cardiac disease
  - myocardial infarction.
- Shock:
  - anaphylactic
  - septic.
- Intra-abdominal bleeding:
  - hepatic
  - splenic
  - aortic rupture.
- Intracerebral haemorrhage.
- Overdosage or substance abuse.
- Metabolic/endocrine: diabetic coma.
- Cerebral infection:
  - encephalitis
  - cerebral malaria.

Shoulder dystocia: overview

Defined as any delivery that requires additional obstetric manoeuvres after gentle traction on the head has failed to deliver shoulders.

Complicates ~1:200 deliveries, and has potential for serious fetal complications.

Complications of shoulder dystocia

Fetal
- Hypoxia and neurological injury (CP).
- Brachial plexus palsy.
- Fracture of clavicle or humerus.
- Intracranial haemorrhage.
- Cervical spine injury.
- Rarely, fetal death.

Maternal
- PPH.
- Genital tract trauma including 3rd- and 4th-degree perineal tears.

Mechanism

- Usually the anterior shoulder is impacted against the symphysis pubis, often due to the failure of internal rotation of the shoulders.
- Rarely, the posterior shoulder may be impacted against the sacral promontory, resulting in bilateral impaction, causing problems at delivery.
- Fetal deterioration is rapid, often without cord acidosis, largely due to cord compression and trauma.

Risk factors

Although there are well-known risk factors, these have poor predictive value for shoulder dystocia. It is estimated that only 50% of shoulder dystocia is associated with a birth weight of >4kg. However, it is important to be aware of antepartum and intrapartum risk factors, so that some shoulder dystocias may be anticipated allowing senior input to be available.

Shoulder dystocia can often be anticipated by limited or slow delivery of the head and McRoberts' manoeuvre is often used prophylactically.

Attempts at delivery, however, should not occur before the next contraction.

Risk factors for shoulder dystocia

Antenatal
- Fetal macrosomia.
- Maternal obesity.
- Excessive weight gain in pregnancy.
- Diabetes.
- Prolonged pregnancy.
- Advanced maternal age.
- Previous history of shoulder dystocia.
- Previous big baby.
- *In utero* death.

Intrapartum
- Lack of progress in late 1st or 2nd stage of labour.
- Instrumental vaginal delivery (especially rotational deliveries).

Shoulder dystocia: management

- Prompt, skilful, and well-rehearsed manoeuvres may improve outcome.
- Main objectives are to facilitate the entry of anterior (or posterior) shoulder into pelvis and to ensure rotation of shoulders to larger oblique or transverse diameter of the pelvis.

Management of shoulder dystocia

- Avoid prophylactic manoeuvres, i.e. do not diagnose or attempt manoeuvres until 1st contraction after delivery of head.
- *Diagnosis*: gentle axial traction (not downwards) fails to deliver the baby.
- Call for help (including additional midwife, senior obstetrician, neonatologist, anaesthetist).
- Legs into McRoberts' position (hyperflexed at hips with thighs abducted).
- Suprapubic pressure applied to posterior aspect of anterior shoulder to dislodge it and move to wider oblique diameter.
- By 1min, if failure: attempt internal manoeuvres.
- Evaluate if an episiotomy as it may aid access.
- Enter pelvis for internal manoeuvres, with entire hand behind the head—these manoeuvres include:
  - delivering the posterior arm by finding the hand which is often at the level of the fetal chest and bringing the entire arm out of the vagina—flexing the elbow may allow the hand to come within reach
  - pressure on the anterior and posterior shoulder/s (Rubin II, wood screw, etc.), trying to rotate the shoulders to the larger oblique diameter.
- Roll over to 'all fours' may help aid delivery by the changes brought about in the pelvic dimensions (Gaskin manoeuvre).
- Re-attempt manoeuvres or try posterior axillary traction/sling.

In practice, 80% of babies will deliver with suprapubic pressure and McRoberts' manoeuvre. If these fail, delivery of posterior arm is probably the best next manoeuvre.

Last-resort manoeuvres

These should be vanishingly rare if management has been appropriate.
- *Symphysiotomy:* may be performed to 'open up' pelvic girdle, provided pelvis is supported to not over-open. Urethral injury should be avoided by displacing urethra with a metal catheter at time of symphysiotomy.
- *Zavanelli:* replacement of head into the vagina by reversing the mechanism of labour (i.e. flexion and 'de-restitution') then performing a CS is the last resort. Tocolysis may be required to facilitate this procedure.

Other considerations in the event of a shoulder dystocia

- Traction should be gentle, axial not downward.
- Time-keeping is essential and it is good practice to allocate a member of the team to document the timeline of events (a 'scribe')
- Paediatric team must be called urgently as a need for neonatal resuscitation should be anticipated.
- PPH should also be anticipated and prophylactic measures considered, such as a 40IU oxytocin infusion.
- The genital tract should be carefully examined for trauma.
- Carefully document the timing and sequence of events, who was involved, and what each person did, as soon as possible afterwards.
- It is important to explain delivery and discuss outcome with parents after the event.
- An incident report form should be filled for risk management.
- If an injury has occurred, it may become a medico-legal issue, making documentation even more important.

Posterior axillary traction or sling

These techniques aim to deliver the posterior arm and are reported to be helpful when the posterior shoulder is held up on the sacral promontory.

Traction

- The clinician inserts their hand along the sacral hollow, places their finger in the axilla, and delivers the posterior shoulder before the arm.

Sling

- Using a soft catheter looped around the posterior shoulder and under the axilla, an attempt is made to deliver the posterior shoulder using downwards traction.

⚠ Both techniques are associated with a high risk of humeral fracture.

Further reading

PROMPT Maternity Foundation.
Ⓡ www.promptmaternity.org

Massive obstetric haemorrhage: causes

This is an important cause of maternal morbidity and mortality.

Identification of risk factors, institution of preventive measures, and prompt and appropriate management of blood loss are likely to improve outcome. It is also important to remember that all bleeding can be concealed.

⚠ Massive obstetric haemorrhage occurs when ≥1.5L of blood have been lost and, if ongoing, needs urgent management.

⚠ In women with a very low BMI, 1L should be considered as the cut-off for massive haemorrhage.

Causes of massive obstetric haemorrhage

Antepartum
- Placental abruption.
- Placenta praevia.
- Severe chorioamnionitis or septicaemia.
- Severe pre-eclampsia (including hepatic rupture).
- Retained dead fetus.

Intrapartum
- Intrapartum abruption.
- Uterine rupture.
- Amniotic fluid embolism.
- Complications of CD; angular or broad ligament tears.
- Morbidly adherent placenta (accreta/percreta).

Postpartum
- 1° PPH is usually due to:
  - atonic uterus ('tone')
  - genital tract trauma ('trauma')
  - coagulopathy ('thrombin')
  - retained products of conception ('tissue').
- 2° PPH is due to:
  - infection (often associated with retained products of conception)
  - rarely, gestational trophoblastic disease or uterine arteriovenous malformation including a pseudo-aneurysm.

Massive obstetric haemorrhage: pathophysiology

Pregnancy is associated with an ↑ in blood volume (→ Physiology of pregnancy: haemodynamics, p. 26). The blood flow to the pregnant uterus at term is ~500–800mL/min with the placental circulation accounting for ~400mL/min. It is therefore easy for a large proportion of the circulating volume to be lost in a short time.

Poor organ perfusion from hypovolaemia and severe anaemia causes the anoxic uterus to becomes atonic. This and the ensuing coagulopathy worsen the situation.

A loss of about 500–1000mL (10–15% of blood volume) is usually well tolerated by a fit, healthy young woman, as she is able to maintain her cardiovascular parameters by effective compensatory mechanisms until about 30–40% of the blood volume is lost (Table 10.1).

Pulse rate, rather than BP, is more useful in assessing the degree of blood loss, especially with occult loss such as concealed abruption or scar rupture. In these situations, the degree of haemodynamic instability may be out of proportion to the visually estimated blood loss (EBL).

If ante- or intrapartum, however, the fetus will rapidly become hypoxic and die either because of maternal redistribution away from non-essential organs (including the uterus) or because of the cause, e.g. placental abruption.

Table 10.1 Blood loss and cardiovascular parameters

Blood loss	Heart rate	Systolic BP	Tissue perfusion
10–15%	↑	Normal	Postural hypotension
15–30%	↑+	Normal	Peripheral vasoconstriction
30–40%	↑++	70–80mmHg	Pallor, oliguria, confusion, restlessness
40%+	↑+++	<60mmHg	Collapse, anuria, dyspnoea

Massive obstetric haemorrhage: management

Massive obstetric haemorrhage is a life-threatening emergency requiring swift and appropriate treatment. Most units will have a local guideline for its management, with a detailed protocol and hospital alert system once blood loss continues beyond 1500mL.

This massive obstetric haemorrhage protocol should, in a single call, lead to laboratory alerts, summing key staff, and the arrival of blood and blood products.

In the ante- or intrapartum period, CTG is essential but massive blood loss will rapidly cause fetal demise if the baby is not delivered by the fastest route possible. Unless the mother's cervix is fully dilated and the prerequisites for vaginal birth are met, this should be by CD.

Principles of management of obstetric haemorrhage
- Immediate resuscitation with restoration of circulating volume.
- Blood and fresh frozen plasma (FFP) if patient unstable or EBL >1500mL and continuing, to maintain oxygen-carrying capacity and prevent DIC.
- Deliver baby if fetal distress or EBL >1500mL.
- Rapid treatment of the underlying cause.
- Supportive therapy and monitoring.
- Give 1g IV tranexamic acid.

Consequences of massive obstetric haemorrhage
- Acute hypovolaemia.
- Sudden and rapid cardiovascular decompensation.
- If antenatal, fetal distress or death.
- DIC.
- Iatrogenic complications associated with fluid replacement and multiple blood transfusions.
- Pulmonary oedema.
- Adult respiratory distress syndrome.
- Sheehan's syndrome (hypopituitarism).

Disseminated intravascular coagulopathy

The main cause of DIC is massive blood loss, but it can occur with other conditions such as amniotic fluid embolism. It occurs due to the depletion of fibrinogen, platelets, and coagulation factors that are consumed or lost with the blood. Infusions of replacement fluids further dilute the remaining coagulation factors and combined with hypotension-mediated endothelial injury may trigger DIC.

The most useful tests to diagnose DIC are fibrinogen, partial thromboplastin time (PTT), and activated PTT (APTT). Early involvement of a senior haematologist is vital to advise on appropriate replacement of blood products.

Blood products
- *FFP*: contains all the clotting factors required. Ideally, 1U of FFP should be given with each unit of rapidly transfused blood.
- *Cryoprecipitate*: contains more fibrinogen but lacks antithrombin III which is often depleted in massive obstetric haemorrhages.
- *Platelet concentrate*: rarely indicated, but may be required if surgical intervention is planned.
- *Recombinant activated factor VII*: used successfully in severe coagulopathy but is expensive and not always readily available.

Adjuvant therapy
- Consider tranexamic acid 1g IV.

Prevention of massive obstetric haemorrhage
- Risk stratification.
- Routine prophylaxis:
  - Vaginal birth: Syntometrine® (oxytocin and ergometrine) or oxytocin (if hypertensive or cardiac disease)
  - Caesarean birth: oxytocin 5IU IV and consider repeating.
- Recognition and early and appropriate treatment of more minor haemorrhage.

Massive obstetric haemorrhage: resuscitation

The most common situation is postnatal. In the ante- or intrapartum situation, the principles are the same but delivery of the fetus once the mother is stable is required.

Resuscitative measures may need to occur at the same time as stopping the bleeding.

If EBL <1000mL and no clinical signs of shock

- Call for assistance.
- Insert large IV cannular, take blood for group and save, FBC, clotting.
- Give IV crystalloid.
- Monitor pulse, BP, respiratory rate every 15min.

If EBL >1000mL or clinical signs of shock

As above plus
- Call anaesthetist.
- Lie flat and keep warm.
- Administer oxygen.
- Check fibrinogen.
- Give IV crystalloid (maximum 3.5L).

If EBL >1500mL and continuing: massive obstetric haemorrhage

As above plus
- Activate massive obstetric haemorrhage protocol, which includes:
  - 4U of blood and 4U of FFP
  - summon anaesthetic and obstetric consultant
  - porter on site for blood samples
  - scribe for timeline
  - alert to haematologist.
- Administer blood and FFP in ratio of 1:1.
- Avoid relying on HemoCue™ or point-of-care Hb estimations.
- Give cryoprecipitate if >6U given or fibrinogen <2g/L.
- Give platelets if level <75 × 10⁹.

General interventions in the management of massive obstetric haemorrhage

- Clearly communicate with other staff, particularly anaesthetist.
- Resuscitation including replacement of blood volume with blood and clotting products.
- Empty uterus:
  - deliver fetus
  - remove placenta or retained tissue.
- Apply bimanual compression or squeeze uterus from above.
- Give drugs to ↑ uterine contraction:
  - oxytocin 40IU infusion
  - ergometrine 500 micrograms IV or IM
  - misoprostol 800–1000 micrograms
  - carboprost 250 micrograms IM or into myometrium.
- Repair any genital tract injuries (including cervical tears).
- Uterine tamponade with a Rusch/Bakri balloon.
- Laparotomy:
  - if bleeding from placental bed, may need oversewing and insertion of a Rusch/Bakri balloon
  - if uterus is atonic, not responding to drug treatment but the bleeding is ↓ with compression, a B-Lynch or vertical compression suture should be placed
  - uterine artery embolization may be helpful but is not always an option in emergency situations
  - total or subtotal hysterectomy.

▶ Compression of the aorta (external or internal) may be used to gain temporary control while a definitive treatment gets under way.

Life-saving aortic compression: how to do it

External

Place the operator's right fist firmly into the abdomen in the midline, just above the umbilicus with the palmar aspect of the hand directed caudad. Here the aorta can be easily palpated and compressed by firm pressure backwards against the spinal column.

Internal

The operator can compress the aorta against the spinal column using a gloved hand, entering the hemithorax from the left of the patient.

⚠ Only an experienced surgeon should clamp the aorta as the inferior vena cava is very easily damaged and very difficult to repair.

Massive obstetric haemorrhage: stopping the bleeding

General measures

- Appropriate resuscitation will treat coagulopathy ('thrombin') and help prevent further bleeding.
- Tranexamic acid 1g IV should be given.
- Consider the cause: the four Ts.
- Uterine pressure or bimanual compression and oxytocics should be used routinely postnatally because atony is so common.

The four Ts

- *Tone:* uterine atony.
- *Tissue:* retained placenta or placental parts.
- *Trauma:* intra-abdominal or genital tract.
- *Thrombin:* coagulopathy.

Causes of massive obstetric haemorrhage

'Tissue'

- Retained whole or part of placenta.
- Bleeding from placental bed.
- Placenta accreta/abnormally invasive placenta.

'Trauma'

- Episiotomy/tear.
- Paravaginal haematoma (severe postnatal rectal pain).
- Uterine rupture.
- Uterine/cervical damage at CD.
- Cervical tear at vaginal birth (rare).
- Broad ligament haematoma (chronic bleed, no pain).

Uterine atony

- General:
  - previous PPH
  - raised BMI.
- Distended uterus:
  - multiple pregnancy
  - polyhydramnios.
- Infection.
- Anatomical distortion, e.g. fibroids.
- Functional problems:
  - rapid labour
  - dystocic labour.
- Uterine relaxants, e.g. magnesium, tocolytics.
- Maternal blood loss and coagulopathy.

Management of uterine atony

⚠ Should be accompanied by physical attempts to contract uterus, such as rubbing up contractions and bimanual compression. This is very rapid and effective.

- 500 micrograms of ergometrine are given IV (may be given IM if difficulties with IV access).
- Start oxytocin infusion (40IU).
- If the bleeding does not stop, 10U of oxytocin may be given IV.
- If the bleeding still persists (or ergometrine is contraindicated) then 800 micrograms of misoprostol (tablets) is given rectally.
- If the atony continues, carboprost 250 micrograms IM is given:
  - this is best directly into the myometrium if at CD
  - repeat at 15min intervals up to a total of four doses.
- If all these measures fail, examination under anaesthesia with possible further surgical management is indicated without delay.

Massive obstetric haemorrhage: surgical management

Examination under anaesthesia

Initially examine vaginally and inside uterine cavity.
- *Trauma—vaginal:*
  - inspect/feel for high vaginal tears
  - inspect cervix and suture tears
  - inspect/feel for paravaginal haematoma.
- *Tissue:*
  - feel around inside of uterus and ensure empty.

Surgical management of obstetric haemorrhage: laparotomy

⚠ Laparotomy will be required if ongoing bleeding despite empty uterus and no vaginal trauma. Consider early if CS delivery or previous CS delivery.
- Assess uterine tone and give uterotonics.
- Ensure that the uterine cavity is definitely empty as even very small pieces of retained tissue can cause atony.
- Inspect uterus for rupture including posterior aspect.
- Look for an inadequately closed uterus at CS (usually angles).
- Inspect abdominal wall and peritoneum for bleeding sites.
- If bleeding point not identified: consider rarities, e.g. splenic artery aneurysm, dissected aorta, ruptured liver capsule.
- If the bleeding is from the placental bed then oversewing the bed ± insertion of a Rusch/Bakri balloon may control the bleeding.
- If the bleeding is from uterine atony unresponsive to drug treatment, but which ↓ with manual compression, a B-Lynch or vertical compression suture should be attempted (this provides continuous compression and ↓ the blood flow into the uterus).
- Systematic pelvic devascularization by ligation of uterine, tubal branch of the ovarian, or anterior division of internal iliac arteries:
  - ligation of uterine artery and utero-ovarian artery anastomosis will not control the bleeding from the vaginal branch of the internal iliac artery which supplies the lower segment
  - internal iliac artery ligation will help in controlling both the uterine artery and the vaginal branch bleeding (bilateral ligation results in 85% ↓ in the pulse pressure and 50% ↓ in blood flow, and bleeding is ↓ by 50%).
- Hysterectomy is the last option:
  - subtotal hysterectomy is safer and quicker to perform for atony
  - if the bleeding is from the lower segment (placenta praevia, accreta, or tears) then total hysterectomy is carried out.
- Consider arterial embolization.

⚠ The decision to carry out hysterectomy should not be unduly delayed as this can result in the death of the mother.

Paravaginal haematoma
- Severe rectal/vaginal post vaginal birth.
- Forceps/episiotomy common but can occur with spontaneous delivery.
- Often not visible on inspection: do vaginal examination.
- Examine under anaesthetic.
- Evacuate haematoma, oversew vaginal wall only.
- Insert vaginal pack and consider drain.
- Blood loss greater than is visible: consider calling massive obstetric haemorrhage.

Arterial embolization for massive obstetric haemorrhage

Advantages
- Less invasive than laparotomy.
- Helps to preserve fertility.
- Can target individual bleeding vessels.

Disadvantages
- Only available in a few centres.
- It may not be possible to get the required equipment to the obstetric theatres or to transfer a woman to the radiology department.
- Appropriately trained interventional radiologists must be available.

Method
- A catheter is inserted through the femoral artery and advanced above the bifurcation of the aorta and a contrast dye is injected to identify the bleeding vessels.
- The catheter is then directed to the bleeding vessel and embolized with gelatin sponge, which is usually reabsorbed in about 10 days.

▶ If excessive bleeding is anticipated (e.g. major placenta praevia with accreta), prophylactic interventional radiology can be a planned procedure where balloons are placed in the internal iliac or uterine vessels in advance if embolization is required.

Venous thromboembolism: overview

Background

VTE is a leading cause of maternal morbidity and mortality in developed countries. Thromboembolic events include DVT of the leg, calf, or pelvis, and PE.

- Incidence of pregnancy-associated VTE is 1–2:1000 pregnancies.
- Incidence of DVT is 3× higher than that of PE.
- Emergency CD is associated with a higher incidence of DVT than elective CD or vaginal delivery.
- Thromboembolic disease can occur at any point in pregnancy.
- DVT leads to PE in ~16% of untreated patients.

Women with past history of VTE

⚠ The risk of VTE in pregnancy is ↑ in women with past history of VTE.

- For a single previous thrombosis with no known thrombophilia, the risk of VTE in pregnancy is ↑ from about 0.1% to 3%.
- The risk is higher if the woman has thrombophilia or if the previous VTE was in an unusual site or unprovoked.
- Women with previous VTE should be screened for thrombophilia before pregnancy.

Inherent pregnancy-associated risk factors for VTE

Pregnancy itself is a risk factor for VTE, due to:
- Venous stasis in the lower limbs.
- Possible trauma to the pelvic veins at the time of delivery.
- Changes in the coagulation system including:
  - ↑ in procoagulant factors (factors X, VIII, and fibrinogen)
  - ↓ in endogenous anticoagulant activity
  - suppression of fibrinolysis
  - significant ↓ in protein S activity.

▶ All pregnant women are at risk of thrombosis from early in the 1st trimester until at least 6wks postpartum. Some women are at even higher risk during pregnancy because they have one or more additional risk factors.

Other risk factors for VTE

Pre-existing risk factors
- Previous VTE.
- Congenital thrombophilia:
  - antithrombin deficiency
  - protein C deficiency
  - protein S deficiency
  - factor V Leiden
  - prothrombin gene variant.
- Acquired thrombophilia (antiphospholipid syndrome):
  - lupus anticoagulant
  - anticardiolipin antibodies.
- Age >35yrs.
- Obesity (BMI >30kg/m²) either before pregnancy or in early pregnancy.
- Parity >4.
- Gross varicose veins.
- Paraplegia.
- Sickle cell disease.
- Inflammatory disorders, e.g. inflammatory bowel disease.
- Medical disorders, e.g. nephrotic syndrome, cardiac diseases.
- Myeloproliferative disorders, e.g. essential thrombocythaemia, polycythaemia vera.

New-onset or transient risk factors
- Ovarian hyperstimulation syndrome.
- Hyperemesis.
- Dehydration.
- Long-haul travel.
- Severe infection, e.g. pyelonephritis.
- Immobility (>4 days' bed rest).
- Pre-eclampsia.
- Prolonged labour.
- Mid-cavity instrumental delivery.
- Excessive blood loss.
- Surgical procedure in pregnancy or puerperium, e.g. evacuation of retained products of conception, postpartum sterilization.
- Immobility after delivery.

Further reading

RCOG (2015). Reducing the risk of venous thromboembolism during pregnancy and the puerperium. Green-top guideline no. 37a.
⅏ www.rcog.org.uk/globalassets/documents/guidelines/gtg-37a.pdf

Venous thromboembolism: prevention

- LMWHs are the agents of choice for antenatal thromboprophylaxis.
- They are as effective as unfractionated heparin in pregnancy, safer, and easier to monitor.
- Monitoring anti-Xa levels is not usually required when using LMWH for thromboprophylaxis.

▶ Women should be reassessed before, during, and after labour for risk factors for VTE using mandatory, often electronic, 'scoresheets'.

▶ An individual's score will guide management.
See Fig. 10.1 for an example of an antenatal assessment tool.
See Fig. 10.2, p. 429, for an example of a postnatal assessment tool.

Thromboprophylaxis: other considerations

- All women should undergo an assessment of risk factors for VTE in early pregnancy.
- Repeat if they develop any other problems and after delivery.
- Women with previous VTE should be screened for inherited and acquired thrombophilia, ideally before pregnancy.
- Immobilization and dehydration should be avoided.
- Antenatal thromboprophylaxis should begin as early as practical.
- Postpartum prophylaxis should begin as soon as possible after delivery (with precautions after use of regional anaesthesia).
- Excess blood loss and blood transfusion are risk factors for VTE, so thromboprophylaxis should be commenced or reinstituted as soon as the immediate risk of haemorrhage is ↓.

Further reading

RCOG (2015). Reducing the risk of venous thromboembolism during pregnancy and the puerperium. Green-top guideline no. 37a.
🕮 www.rcog.org.uk/globalassets/documents/guidelines/gtg-37a.pdf

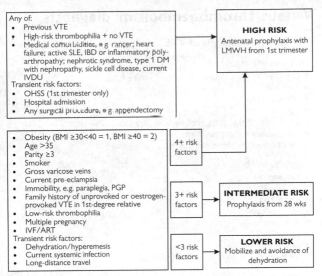

Any of:
- Previous VTE
- High-risk thrombophilia + no VTE
- Medical comorbidities, e.g. cancer; heart failure; active SLE, IBD or inflammatory polyarthropathy; nephrotic syndrome, type 1 DM with nephropathy, sickle cell disease, current IVDU

Transient risk factors:
- OHSS (1st trimester only)
- Hospital admission
- Any surgical procedure, e.g. appendectomy

HIGH RISK
Antenatal prophylaxis with LMWH from 1st trimester

- Obesity (BMI ≥30<40 = 1, BMI ≥40 = 2)
- Age >35
- Parity ≥3
- Smoker
- Gross varicose veins
- Current pre-eclampsia
- Immobility, e.g. paraplegia, PGP
- Family history of unprovoked or oestrogen-provoked VTE in 1st-degree relative
- Low-risk thrombophilia
- Multiple pregnancy
- IVF/ART

Transient risk factors:
- Dehydration/hyperemesis
- Current systemic infection
- Long-distance travel

4+ risk factors

3+ risk factors

INTERMEDIATE RISK
Prophylaxis from 28 wks

<3 risk factors

LOWER RISK
Mobilize and avoidance of dehydration

Fig. 10.1 Antenatal assessment and management for thromboprophylaxis. ART, assisted reproductive technology; DM, diabetes mellitus; IVDU, intravenous drug user; OHSS, ovarian hyperstimulation syndrome; PGP, pelvic girdle pain.

Venous thromboembolism: diagnosis

Symptoms and signs of VTE

Deep vein thrombosis
- Leg pain or discomfort (especially in the left leg).
- Swelling.
- Tenderness.
- Pyrexia.
- Erythema, ↑ skin temperature, and oedema.
- Lower abdominal pain (high DVT).
- Elevated white blood cell count.

Pulmonary embolism
- Dyspnoea.
- Collapse.
- Chest pain.
- Haemoptysis.
- Faintness.
- Raised JVP.
- Focal signs in chest.
- Symptoms and signs associated with DVT.

⚠ In pregnancy there should be a high level of suspicion for women presenting with any of the above-listed symptoms and urgent investigation undertaken. If VTE is suspected, treatment should be commenced while diagnostic tests are awaited.

Investigations
- Thrombophilia screen.
- FBC, U&E, LFTs.
- Coagulation screen.
- ECG.

Imaging
- USS of upper leg/pelvis.
- Contrast venography with shielding of the uterus.

▶ If PE suspected:
- CXR.
- ABG.
- Cardiac echo may be helpful: right-sided strain/failure.
- Ventilation/perfusion lung scanning (V/Q or Q scan).
- Spiral CT.
- Bilateral duplex USS leg examinations.

▶ See Fig. 10.3, p. 431, and Fig. 10.4, p. 433, for guidance on diagnosis and management.

⚠ Among women with clinically suspected VTE, <50% have the diagnosis confirmed as some of the symptoms and signs are commonly found in normal pregnancy.

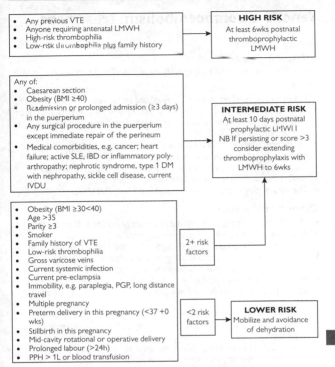

Fig. 10.2 Postnatal assessment and management to be assessed at delivery.
DM, diabetes mellitus; IBD, inflammatory bowel disease; IVDU, intravenous drug user; PGP, pelvic girdle pain.

Venous thromboembolism: treatment

Anticoagulation

Unfractionated heparin

Unfractionated heparin is now virtually never used in the treatment of VTE.

LMWH

- LMWHs are as effective as unfractionated heparin for treatment of PE.
- A bd dosage regimen for LMWHs is recommended in the treatment of VTE in pregnancy (enoxaparin 1mg/kg bd; dalteparin 100U/kg bd up to a maximum of 18,000U/24h).
- Long-term users of LMWHs have a lower risk of osteoporosis and bone fractures than unfractionated heparin users.
- The peak anti-Xa activity (3h post injection) should be measured to ensure the woman is appropriately anticoagulated.
- The target range for the anti-Xa level is 0.35–0.70IU/mL.

Other considerations

- Therapeutic anticoagulation should be continued for at least 6mths.
- After delivery, treatment should continue for at least 6wks.
- Warfarin can be used postnatally and is safe for breast-feeding.
- The leg should be elevated and a graduated elastic compression stocking applied to reduce oedema; mobilization is recommended.
- Inferior vena caval filter may be considered for recurrent PEs, despite adequate anticoagulation or if anticoagulation is contraindicated but is seldom used.
- In life-threatening massive PE thrombolytic therapy, percutaneous catheter thrombus fragmentation or surgical embolectomy may be required.
- Where DVT threatens leg viability, surgical embolectomy or thrombolytic therapy may be considered.

▶ See Fig. 10.3 and Fig. 10.4, p. 433, for guidance on diagnosis and management.

Further reading

RCOG (2015). Reducing the risk of venous thromboembolism during pregnancy and the puerperium. Green-top guideline no. 37a.
℧ www.rcog.org.uk/globalassets/documents/guidelines/gtg-37a.pdf

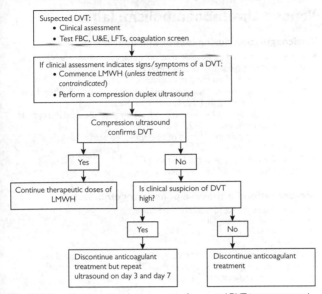

Fig. 10.3 Investigation and initial management of suspected DVT in pregnancy and the puerperium.

Venous thromboembolism: labour

Anticoagulation during labour and delivery

- The woman should be advised that once she thinks that she is in labour, she should not inject any further LMWH.
- To avoid the risk of epidural haematoma:
  - regional anaesthesia should be avoided until at least 12h after the last dose of LMWH (24h if she is on a therapeutic dose)
  - LMWH should not be given for at least 4h after the epidural catheter has been removed
  - the epidural catheter should not be removed within 10–12h of a LMWH injection.
- ↑ risk of wound haematoma following CD.
- Wound drains should be considered.

Resuscitation for massive pulmonary embolism

- Resuscitation for cardiac arrest if required.
- Call on call medical team.
- Early (<1h) cardiac echo or CTPA.
- IV heparin.
- Consider thrombolysis if haemodynamic compromise or ischaemic complications (recent birth including CD not contraindications).
- Consider embolectomy if *in extremis*.

Further reading

RCOG (2015). Reducing the risk of venous thromboembolism during pregnancy and the puerperium. Green-top guideline no. 37a.
ℐ www.rcog.org.uk/globalassets/documents/guidelines/gtg-37a.pdf

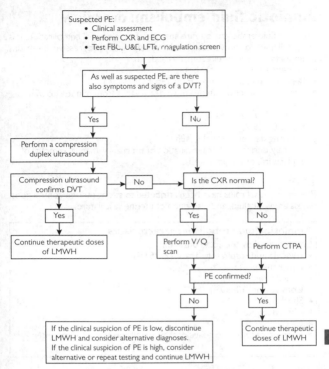

Fig. 10.4 Investigation and initial management of suspected PE in pregnancy and the puerperium.

Amniotic fluid embolism: overview

Amniotic fluid embolism is a rare and often fatal maternal complication. It is not predictable or preventable, and is usually rapidly progressive. It remains an important cause of direct maternal death.

- Incidence 1:8000–30,000 births.
- Reported mortality ranges from 13% to 80%.
- Time from onset of symptoms to death varies from minutes to 32h.
- Can occur:
  - with SROM or ARM (70%)
  - at CD (19%)
  - during delivery or within 48h (11%)
  - rarely during or after termination of pregnancy, manual removal of placenta, or amniocentesis.

Causes

Presumed causal roles have been attributed to strong uterine contractions, excess amniotic fluid, and disruption of uterine vasculature.

Amniotic fluid embolism characteristics

Characterized by the acute onset of:
- Hypoxia and respiratory arrest (27–51%).
- Hypotension (13–27%).
- Fetal distress (17%).
- Convulsions (10–30%).
- Shock.
- Altered mental status.
- Cardiac arrest.
- Haemorrhage due to coagulopathy, usually presents <30min after the event.

Risk factors for amniotic fluid embolism
- Multiple pregnancy.
- Older maternal age.
- CD or instrumental vaginal delivery.
- Eclampsia.
- Polyhydramnios.
- Placenta praevia.
- Placental abruption.
- Cervical laceration.
- Uterine rupture.
- Medical induction of labour.

Amniotic fluid embolism: diagnosis and management

Diagnosis

Diagnosis is clinical and essentially a diagnosis of exclusion.

Differential diagnosis should include:

* PE.
* Anaphylaxis.
* Sepsis.
* Eclampsia.
* Myocardial infarction.

⚠ In some patients, severe haemorrhage with DIC may be the 1st sign. Clinical diagnosis is supported by retrieval of fetal elements in pulmonary artery aspirate and maternal sputum. However, diagnosis is only definitively confirmed by the presence of fetal squamous cells and debris in the pulmonary vasculature at a postmortem examination.

Investigations

* ABG.
* Electrolytes including calcium and magnesium levels.
* FBC (↑ white blood cell count).
* Coagulation profile.
* CXR (pulmonary oedema).
* ECG (ischaemia and infarction).

Management of amniotic fluid embolism

* Rapid maternal CPR and admission to ICU under MDT care with input from obstetrics, anaesthetics, and haematology.
* Pulmonary artery wedge pressure monitoring will assist in the haemodynamic management—blood aspirated via the catheter can be examined to aid with the diagnosis.
* Oxygen to maintain saturation close to 100% (helps to prevent neurological impairment from hypoxia).
* Fluid resuscitation is imperative to counteract hypotension and haemodynamic instability.
* For refractory hypotension, direct-acting vasopressors, such as phenylephrine, are required to optimize perfusion pressure.
* Inotropic support may be needed.
* DIC should be managed with the help of a haematologist (➡ Massive obstetric haemorrhage: management, p. 416).
* Plasma exchange techniques may be helpful in clearing fibrin degradation products from the circulation.
* If not yet delivered, continuous fetal monitoring is indicated: delivery by CS within 1min of cardiac arrest is recommended to facilitate CPR of mother.

Uterine inversion

Uterine inversion can cause serious maternal morbidity or death. The incidence is about 1:2000–3000 deliveries. Maternal mortality can be as high as 15%.

Risk factors for uterine inversion
- Strong traction on umbilical cord with excessive fundal pressure.
- Abnormal adherence of the placenta.
- Uterine anomalies.
- Fundal implantation of the placenta.
- Short cord.
- Previous uterine inversion.

Signs and symptoms
- Haemorrhage (present in 94% of cases).
- Severe lower abdominal pain in the 3rd stage.
- Shock out of proportion to the blood loss (neurogenic, due to ↑ vagal tone).
- Uterine fundus not palpable abdominally (or inversion may be just felt as a dimple at the fundus).
- Mass in the vagina on VE.

Management of uterine inversion
- Immediate replacement by pushing up the fundus through the cervix with the palm of the hand (the Johnson manoeuvre).
- Call for help (including a senior obstetrician and anaesthetist). If this fails:
- IV access with two large-bore cannulae.
- Bloods for FBC, coagulation studies, and cross-match 4–6U.
- Immediate fluid replacement.
- Continuous monitoring of vital signs.
- Transfer to theatre and arrange appropriate analgesia.
- If the placenta is still attached to the uterus, it is left *in situ* to minimize the bleeding, and removal attempted only after replacement.
- Tocolytic drugs, such as terbutaline, or volatile anaesthetic agents may be tried to make replacement easier.
- If manual reduction fails then hydrostatic repositioning (O'Sullivan's technique) may be tried:
  * warm saline is infused into the vagina with one hand, sealing the labia (a silicone ventouse cup may be used to improve seal)
  * uterine rupture should be excluded 1st.
- Sometimes both manual and hydrostatic methods fail and a laparotomy is needed for correction (Haultain's or Huntingdon's procedure).

Cord prolapse

In cord prolapse, the umbilical cord protrudes below the presenting part after ROM. This may cause compression of the umbilical vessels by the presenting part and vasospasm from exposure of the cord. These acutely compromise fetal circulation and if delivery is not immediate may lead to neurological sequelae or fetal death.

Predisposing factors for cord prolapse
- Abnormal lie or presentation (transverse lie, breech).
- Multiple pregnancy.
- Polyhydramnios.
- Prematurity.
- High head.
- Unusually long umbilical cord.

Prevention
When the presenting part is high or if there is polyhydramnios, a stabilizing induction (➔ Induction of labour: indications, p. 306) may be performed. During ARM, if cord presentation is detected (i.e. presence of cord below presenting part with intact membranes), the procedure should be abandoned and senior help summoned.

Management of cord prolapse
⚠ The fetus should be delivered as rapidly as possible; this may be by instrumental delivery or category 1 CD.
- Prevent further cord compression during transfer for CD by:
  - knee-to-chest position
  - fill the bladder with about 500mL of warm normal saline to displace the presenting part upwards (remember to unclamp the catheter before entering the peritoneal cavity at CD)
  - a hand in the vagina to push up the presenting part (may not always be practical).
- Prevent spasm by avoiding exposure of cord.
  - replace cord into vagina to maintain body temperature and insert a warm saline swab to prevent cord coming back out.

⚠ It is important to avoid handling the cord as much as possible, as this provokes further spasms.

- Tocolytics (terbutaline 250 micrograms SC) may be administered to abolish uterine contractions and improve oxygenation to the fetus: may cause PPH at CD due to uterine atony; tackle with oxytocics but propranolol 1mg IV may be given if needed.
- Neonatal team must be present at delivery.

Fetal distress of second twin

➲ Multiple pregnancy: labour, p. 76.

Common causes of distress in the 2nd twin
- Placental abruption (indicated by profuse bleeding).
- Cord prolapse.
- Excessive uterine contractions.

⚠ Fetal distress of the 2nd twin can be iatrogenic (e.g. too much oxytocin, too hurried a delivery, too early amniotomy, or aortocaval compression).

⚠ Failure to adequately monitor a 2nd twin is a common cause of problems. Electronic fetal monitoring is wise, if necessarily aided by ultrasound location of the best place to monitor, or a fetal scalp electrode.

▶ The 2nd twin must be delivered by the fastest safe route.
- If it is *cephalic* and if the presenting part is at or below the ischial spines, an instrumental vaginal delivery may be attempted: with preterm babies (before 34wks), a ventouse delivery should be avoided.
- With a *breech* presentation, a 'breech extraction' may be attempted by an experienced clinician:
  - this involves grasping the feet of the fetus and gently pulling them through the vagina, aided by maternal effort
  - the arms will often become nuchal and Løvset's manoeuvre will then be required
  - in modern obstetric practice, a 2nd twin with fetal distress is the only acceptable indication for breech extraction.
- With a *transverse* lie, internal podalic version with breech extraction may be attempted.
- If vaginal delivery is not possible, immediate CD (category 1) should be performed.
- This also applies if the operator does not have the experience to perform a breech extraction.

Chapter 11

Maternal and perinatal mortality

Maternal mortality: an overview

- Maternal mortality refers to deaths due to complications from pregnancy or childbirth.
- Between 2000 and 2017, the global maternal mortality rate ↓ by 38%— from 342 to 211 deaths per 100,000 live births.

International Classification of Diseases for Maternal Mortality (ICD-MM)

Maternal deaths are classified internationally using the ICD-MM, which is based upon the ICD-10 coding rules and was developed to facilitate consistent collection, analysis, and interpretation of information relating to maternal deaths.

Definitions: maternal mortality indicators

- *Maternal mortality rate:* the number of maternal deaths per 100,000 live births.
- *Pregnancy-related death:* the death of a woman while pregnant or within 42 days of termination or pregnancy, irrespective of the cause of death.
- *Maternal death:* the death of a woman while pregnant, or within 42 days of termination of pregnancy, from any cause related to or aggravated by the pregnancy, but not from accidental or incidental causes.
- Maternal deaths are subdivided into three 'types' of death:
  - *direct obstetric deaths:* deaths resulting from obstetric complications or pregnancy, interventions, omissions, or incorrect treatment, or a chain of events resulting from the above
  - *indirect obstetric deaths:* deaths resulting from a pre-existing disease, or disease that developed during pregnancy that was not due to direct obstetric causes but was aggravated by physiological effects of pregnancy
  - *unspecified deaths:* deaths where the cause was not determined.
- Maternal deaths are also subdivided into one of the following 'groups'—irrespective of type:
  1. pregnancy with abortive outcome
  2. hypertensive disorders
  3. obstetric haemorrhage
  4. pregnancy-related infection
  5. other obstetric complications
  6. unanticipated complications of managements
  7. non-obstetric complications
  8. unknown causes of death
  9. coincidental causes of death.

Further reading

WHO (2012). The WHO application of ICD-10 to deaths during pregnancy, childbirth and puerperium: ICD MM.
🔗 https://apps.who.int/iris/handle/10665/70929

UK confidential enquiry: maternal deaths and morbidity

Background

The UK's national Confidential Enquiry into Maternal Deaths was introduced in 1952 but has origins that stretch back to the mid-19th century.

Reports were published initially on a 3-yearly basis, reflecting the relatively small number of maternal deaths. Analysis using 3yrs worth of surveillance data is needed to identify trends as the basis for 'lessons learned', while simultaneously protecting the anonymity and confidentiality of those affected by the tragic loss.

Since 2014, the Mothers and Babies: Reducing Risk through Audits and Confidential Enquiry across the UK (MBRRACE-UK) collaboration has been responsible for implementing an updated version of the confidential enquiry process. MBRRACE-UK publishes an annual report containing surveillance data and analysis of trends over 3yrs with subgroup of chapters focusing on individual causes of death to emphasize the lessons to be learned for future care.

Maternal deaths are reported to MBRRACE-UK by the staff caring for women who died. To ensure that notification is complete, the team cross reference reported cases with those notified by coroners, procurators fiscal, and media reports, and by cross-checking with data held by the Office for National Statistics.

Methodology

- Full medical records are obtained from each death and anonymized before review.
- A cause of death is established by a pathologist and obstetrician or physician.
- Notes are reviewed subsequently by between 10 and 15 expert reviewers and assessed by comparison to current standards and guidelines.
- The care provided to each woman is classified as either:
    1. good care
    2. improvements to care identified which would have made no difference to outcome, or
    3. improvements in care which may have made a difference to outcome.
- A multidisciplinary writing group meets to identify common themes among deaths and lessons to be learned.
- Chapters aim to include recommendations for care that are embedded within national guidance and are presented with appropriate linkage.
- See Fig. 11.1 for a summary of these methods.

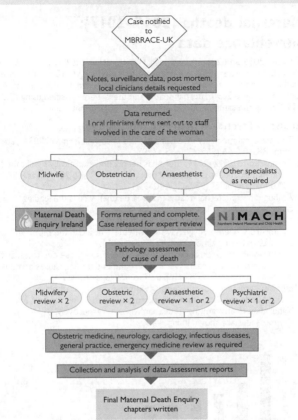

Fig. 11.1 Flowchart summarizing the methodology used by MBRRACE-UK to investigate and report maternal mortality in the UK. Reproduced with permission of MBRRACE-UK

Maternal deaths (2015–2017): surveillance data

Between 2015 and 2017 the maternal death rate in the UK was 9.16 per 100,000 maternities (95% confidence interval (CI) 7.96–10.5). Two hundred and thirty-six women died and 27 were classified as coincidental. As such, there were 209 maternal deaths and these were classified using ICD-MM. During the same period, there were 2,280,451 maternities.

Analysis of trends in maternal mortality

- The maternal mortality rate has ↓ by 1/3 in comparison to 2003—rate ratio (RR) = 0.66 (95% CI 0.55–0.79).
- Compared to 2012–2014, there has been a non-statistically significant ↑ in the maternal deaths. Maternal mortality rate (2012–2014) was 8.54/ 100,000 maternities (95% CI 7.40–9.81).
- Among direct maternal deaths (42% of deaths), VTE is the leading cause—and this has been the case for >20yrs.
- Maternal suicide was the 2nd leading cause.
- Deaths from haemorrhage have ↓, with the ↑ noted in the report in 2014–2016 having almost reversed; see Fig. 11.2.
- Among indirect maternal deaths (58% of deaths)—those due to cardiac and neurological disorders were the 1st and 2nd leading causes and this remains unchanged when compared to previous reports.
- Ethnicity—maternal deaths among women from black ethnic backgrounds and Asian ethnic backgrounds were 5× higher, and 2× higher than deaths among Caucasian women, respectively.
- Key messages are shown in Fig. 11.3.

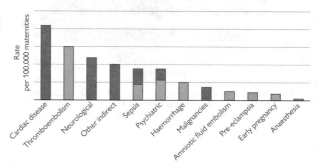

Fig. 11.2 Breakdown of maternal deaths classified using ICD-MM (2015–2017). Reproduced with permission of MBRRACE-UK.

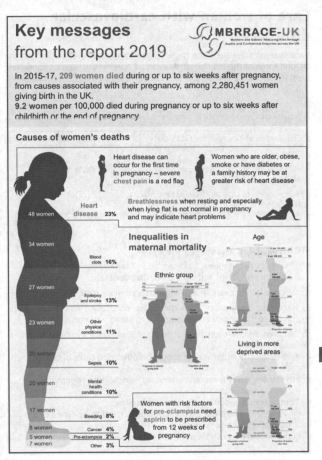

Fig. 11.3 Maternal Deaths in 2015–2017: key messages from MBRRACE-UK (2019). Reproduced with permission of MBRRACE-UK.

Care of women with cardiovascular disorders

Cardiovascular disease is the single leading cause of maternal death in the UK and some of this may be attributed to ↑ numbers of women conceiving later in life, with a greater burden of cardiovascular risk. See Table 11.1 and Fig. 11.4.

Table 11.1 Deaths caused by cardiovascular disorders

Classification of care received (2015–2017)	Women who died, n (%)
Good care	35 (43)
Improvements in care which would have made no difference to outcome.	17 (21)
Improvements to care which would have made a difference to outcome	22 (27)

MBRRACE-UK messages for care

- Chest pain, orthopnoea, tachycardia, and raised respiratory rates are important symptoms and signs of cardiac disease.

⚠ Syncope during exercise also suggests a cardiac cause.

⚠ Recurrent presentation with chest pain, particularly that requiring opiates, is a 'red flag' and needs assessment to identify the case.

⚠ Women who are unable to care for their baby represent a similar 'red flag'.

- A 12-lead ECG and troponin should be offered in cases of unexplained chest pain.
- Echocardiography is recommended with unexplained symptoms suggesting cardiac origin.
- Contraception and pre-pregnancy counselling:
  - women with high-risk cardiac conditions need to be aware of the risks of unplanned pregnancy
  - this should be available at the transition between paediatric and adult cardiac services.

Aortic dissection

The majority of cases in women of reproductive age occur in association with pregnancy (50% in 3rd trimester and 33% postpartum) and presents with sudden-onset, severe pain in the chest, back, neck, or abdomen.

⚠ Severe pain and new-onset neurological symptoms should always prompt consideration of aortic dissection.

▶ Recommendation 1: reaching a positive diagnosis

- Recurrent presentations require clinicians to reach a diagnosis to justify such presentations.
- Excluding diagnoses alone is not sufficient.

(See MBRRACE-UK (2019): ⌖ www.npeu.ox.ac.uk/)

▶ Recommendation 2: cardiac arrest out of hospital

- Ambulance staff *must not* attempt to stabilize at the scene; instead, a *time critical transfer* to the nearest emergency department is vital with obstetric team alerted in advance.
- Resuscitative CD (also known as perimortem caesarean) is an essential part of resuscitating women ≥20wks.
- The baby should be delivered by 5min if there is no return of cardiac output—this is primarily to aid maternal resuscitation.

(See MBRRACE-UK (2019): ⌖ www.npeu.ox.ac.uk/)

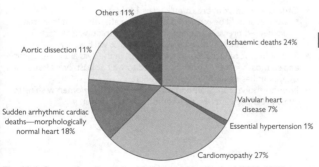

Fig. 11.4 Causes of cardiovascular deaths in the UK and Ireland (2015–2017). Reproduced with permission of MBRRACE-UK.

Care of women with breast cancer

- Pregnancy-associated breast cancer is defined as a breast cancer diagnosed during or up to 1yr after pregnancy.
- 1/3 of diagnoses are made during pregnancy, and 2/3 after when there is a transient ↑ in risk.
- See Table 11.2.

Table 11.2 Deaths associated with breast cancer

Classification of care received (2015–2017)	Women who died, n (%)
Good care	10 (33)
Improvements in care which would have made no difference to outcome.	18 (60)
Improvements to care which would have made a difference to outcome	2 (7)

MBRRACE-UK messages for care

⚠ Women with suspected breast cancer should be referred for specialist review using a cancer pathway—i.e. NHS 2 week wait.

- For women diagnosed in the 3rd trimester, the risk:benefit profile is likely to favour mother and baby if the woman receives at least two cycles of chemotherapy before delivery at term:
  - as such, delivery to avoid delays should not be routinely recommended.
- Drug clearance from breast milk takes 14 days:
  - women should be reassured that feeding after this time from the unaffected breast is safe but should stop if treatment restarts.
- Pregnancy planning should be individualized to each woman.
- Risk of breast cancer recurrence is highest in the 2yrs after treatment and so most women should be advised to wait at least 2yrs after treatment has passed before conception.
- Non-hormonal contraception is recommended for women wishing to avoid pregnancy after being treated for breast cancer.

► **Recommendation 3: radiological investigation**

With few exceptions, radiation exposure through radiography, CT, or nuclear medicine imaging techniques is at a dose much lower than the exposure associated with fetal harm.

⚠ If these techniques are necessary in addition to ultrasonography or MRI, or are more readily available for the diagnosis in question, they should not be withheld from a pregnant patient.

(See ACOG (2017). Committee opinion no. 723: guidelines for diagnostic imaging during pregnancy and lactation. ℘ https://pubmed.ncbi.nlm.nih.gov/28937575/)

► **Recommendation 4: thromboprophylaxis and cancer in pregnancy**

Cancer is a recognized risk factor for thromboembolic disease and women should be prescribed thromboprophylaxis in accordance with RCOG guidelines.

(See RCOG (2015). Reducing the risk of thrombosis and embolism during pregnancy and the puerperium. Green-top guideline no. 37a.

℘ www.rcog.org.uk/globalassets/documents/guidelines/gtg-37a.pdf)

Care of women with hypertensive disorders

- Between 2015 and 2017, six women died as a result of hypertensive disorders of pregnancy (Table 11.3).
- Two deaths were in women with fulminant liver failure as part of HELLP and three women died of cerebral or subarachnoid haemorrhage.
- There were no deaths as a result of eclampsia.

Table 11.3 Deaths caused by hypertensive disorders of pregnancy

Classification of care received (2014–2016)	Women who died, n (%)
Good care	0
Improvements in care which would have made no difference to outcome.	2 (33)
Improvements to care which would have made a difference to outcome	4 (67)

MBRRACE-UK messages for care

- Low-dose aspirin in high-risk women ↓ the risk of pre-eclampsia and improves newborn outcomes; ↓ the number of preterm births and babies who are SGA.
- Hypertension:
  - ≥140/90mmHg requires pharmacological treatment aiming for a BP <135/85mmHg.
  - ⚠ *Severe hypertension (≥160/110mmHg) requires immediate action.*
  - BP should be measured at least every 30min until <160/110mmHg.
- Women with gestational hypertension who have given birth should have their BP measured:
  - daily for the first 2 days
  - at least once between days 3 and 5
  - as clinically indicated if antihypertensive treatment is adjusted.
- Women who have given birth should be advised:
  - to continue antihypertensive treatment if it was required before birth
  - the duration of treatment postnatally will be similar to that of their antenatal treatment (but may be longer)
  - to ↓ antihypertensive medication if their BP is <130/80mmHg.

Further reading

NICE (2019). Hypertension in pregnancy: diagnosis and management.
℘ www.nice.org.uk/guidance/ng133

▶ Recommendation 5: aspirin in pregnancy

- Advise women at high or moderate risk of pre-eclampsia to take 75–150mg of aspirin daily from 12wks until birth.
- Women are considered *high risk* if they have ≥1 of the following:
  - hypertensive disease during a previous pregnancy
  - chronic kidney disease
  - autoimmune disease such as SLE or antiphospholipid syndrome
  - type 1 or 2 diabetes
  - chronic hypertension.
- Women are considered at *moderate risk* if they have ≥2 of the following:
  - 1st pregnancy
  - age ≥40yrs
  - pregnancy interval >10yrs
  - BMI ≥35kg/m² at first visit
  - family history of pre-eclampsia
  - multifetal pregnancy.

(See NICE (2019). Hypertension in pregnancy: diagnosis and management. www.nice.org.uk/guidance/ng133)

Care of women with major obstetric haemorrhage

- Rates of PPH are ↑ in high-income settings.
- In the UK, the provision of specialist services to diagnose and manage PAS since 2013–2015 is associated with a reduction of deaths from this cause in the 2015–2017 report.
- See Table 11.4.

Table 11.4 Deaths caused by haemorrhage

Classification of care received (2012–2013)	Women who died, n (%)
Good care	4 (12)
Improvements in care which would have made no difference to outcome.	5 (15)
Improvements to care which would have made a difference to outcome	25 (74)

MBRRACE-UK messages for care

- CD in advanced labour is associated with a risk of uterine angle extensions:
  - these can be difficult to control and can cause concealed intra-abdominal bleeding postoperatively
  - these procedures should be attended by consultant obstetricians until doctors from other grades have assessed as competent.
- PPH (>1000mL) should always be attended by senior team members, who should consider and exclude each of the four Ts to identify cause:
  - *Tone*
  - *Tissue*
  - *Trauma*
  - *Thrombin*.
- A consultant obstetrician should attend in person to assess women with blood loss ≥1500mL.

► **Recommendation 6: tamponade test**

⚠ If pharmacological measures fail to control the haemorrhage, initiate surgical haemostasis sooner rather than later.

- Intrauterine balloon tamponade is an appropriate first-line 'surgical' intervention for most women where uterine atony is the only or main cause of haemorrhage.
- A 'positive test' (control of PPH following inflation of the balloon) indicates that laparotomy is not required, whereas a 'negative test' (continued PPH following inflation of the balloon) is an indication to proceed to laparotomy.

⚠ *Hysterectomy should not be delayed until the woman is in extremis.*

(See RCOG (2011). Prevention and management of postpartum haemorrhage. Green-top guideline no. 52. ℅ www.rcog.org.uk/en/guidelines-research-services/guidelines/gtg52/)

► **Recommendation 7: placenta accreta spectrum**

- Women with a previous CD and a low placenta are at ↑ risk of PAS.
- All women with a previous CD *and* placenta covering the cervical os at 20wks require imaging by an expert in PAS.
- Women who have had a previous CD who also have either placenta praevia or an anterior placenta underlying the old CS scar at 32wks are at ↑ risk of PAS and should be reviewed by an expert in PAS.
- Any woman with suspected PAS should be managed by an experienced MDT in a centre of excellence in order to:
  - discuss different risks and treatment options
  - plan surgery with anticipated skin and uterine incisions and whether conservative management of the placenta or proceeding straight to hysterectomy is preferred in the situation where PAS is confirmed
  - discuss interventions such as cell salvage and interventional radiology
  - a care bundle for PAS should be applied in all cases where there is a placenta praevia and a previous CS or an anterior placenta underlying the old CS scar
  - any woman going to theatre electively with suspected PAS should be attended by an experienced MDT
  - if the delivery is unexpected, out-of-hours consultant obstetric and anaesthetic staff should be alerted and attend immediately.

(See RCOG (2018). Placenta previa and accreta. Green-top guideline no. 27a. ℅ www.rcog.org.uk/en/guidelines-research-services/guidelines/gtg27a/)

Care of women with venous thromboembolism

- VTE remains the leading direct cause of maternal death, which has been the case for >20yrs.
- There were 39 deaths from VTE between 2014 and 2016 and 35 of these were from PE.
- Evidence suggests that doctors and midwives find existing risk scoring systems difficult to apply and a tool to make risk assessment simpler and more reproducible is needed as a priority.
- See Table 11.5.

Table 11.5 Deaths caused by VTE

Classification of care received (2014–2016)	Women who died, n (%)
Good care	6 (16)
Improvements in care which would have made no difference to outcome.	6 (16)
Improvements to care which would have made a difference to outcome	25 (68)

MBRRACE-UK messages for care

- All women should have a documented risk assessment for VTE in early pregnancy and this should be repeated in the following cases:
  - admission for hospital care is needed
  - she develops problems that ↑ her risk of VTE
  - after miscarriage or ectopic pregnancy, when risk assessment is as important as reassessing after delivery.
- Some women will need thromboprophylaxis as soon as they become pregnant.

⚠ There should be clear pathways for accessing prescriptions.

- Antenatal admission places a woman at intermediate risk for VTE and so she should be considered for antenatal thromboprophylaxis.
- Women with a BMI >30kg/m² should be counselled about the symptoms of VTE.
- Women with BMI ≥40kg/m² score 2 points within the RCOG scoring system and require postnatal thromboprophylaxis irrespective of mode of birth or other risk factors.

Further reading

RCOG (2015). Reducing the risk of thrombosis and embolism during pregnancy and the puerperium. Green-top guideline no. 37a.
🔗 www.rcog.org.uk/globalassets/documents/guidelines/gtg-37a.pdf

► **Recommendation 8: management of acute, life-threatening PE in pregnancy**

⚠ Collapsed, shocked women who are pregnant or in the puerperium should be assessed by a team of experienced clinicians including the on-call consultant obstetrician.

- Women should be managed on an individual basis regarding IV unfractionated heparin, thrombolytic therapy, or thoracotomy and surgical embolectomy.
- Management should involve an MDT including senior physicians, obstetricians, and radiologists.
- IV unfractionated heparin is the preferred, initial treatment in massive PE with cardiovascular compromise.
- Maternity units should develop guidelines for the administration of IV unfractionated heparin.
- The on-call medical team should be contacted immediately.
- An urgent portable echocardiogram or CTPA within 1h of presentation should be arranged.
- If massive PE is confirmed, or in extreme circumstances prior to confirmation, immediate thrombolysis should be considered—this should not be delayed by pregnancy-related factors such as proximity to delivery.

(See RCOG (2015). Reducing the risk of thrombosis and embolism during pregnancy and the puerperium. Green-top guideline no. 37a. ℘ www.rcog.org.uk/globalassets/documents/guidelines/gtg-37a.pdf)

Care of women with mental health problems

- In 2014–2016, 71 women died by suicide during pregnancy (Table 11.6).
- When women whose deaths were related to alcohol and substance misuse were included, 114 women died from mental health-related causes, with a mortality rate of 4.57 per 100,000 maternities (95% CI 3.77–4.58).

There are large gaps in the provision of mental health services across the UK despite an estimated 10% of pregnant women experiencing a mental health problem during or after pregnancy (➲ Chapter 13, p. 499).

Table 11.6 Deaths caused by suicide

Classification of care received (2014–2016)	Women who died, n (%)[a]
Good care	10 (15)
Improvements in care which would have made no difference to outcome.	21 (31)
Improvements to care which would have made a difference to outcome	37 (54)

[a] Records for three women not available.

MBRRACE-UK messages for care

- Most women who died by suicide had a history of mental illness.
- Recurrent depressive disorder was the most common coexisting diagnosis.
- Previous psychotic disorder was rare among women who died by suicide; whether bipolar, postpartum, or non-affective.

> ▶ **Recommendation 9: mental health risk assessment**
>
> ⚠ Women with the following 'red flags' require urgent psychiatric review:
> - Recent significant change in mental state, or emergence of new symptoms.
> - New thoughts or acts of violent self-harm.
> - New and persistent expressions of incompetency as a mother or estrangement for her infant.
> - Women with the following 'amber flags' require close monitoring and referral if there is a change in mental state:
>   - history of bipolar disorder or postpartum psychosis
>   - *any post-psychotic disorder.*
>
> (See MBRRACE-UK (2018). ℗ www.npeu.ox.ac.uk/)

▶ **Recommendation 10: admission to mother and baby units**
- Consider admission where there are any of the following:
  - rapidly changing mental state
  - suicidal ideation (particularly of a violent nature), pervasive guilt, or hopelessness
  - significant estrangement from the infant, new or persistent beliefs of inadequacy as a mother
  - evidence of psychosis.

(See MBRRACE-UK (2018). ✎ www.npeu.ox.ac.uk/)

▶ **Recommendation 11: information sharing between care providers**
- Health professionals have a duty of care to pass on relevant information which may affect the care during pregnancy.
- GPs should inform maternity services of relevant past psychiatric history and maternity services should communicate with GPs about a woman's pregnancy and care planning.
- All booking questionnaires must include questions to identify:
  - women at high risk of early postpartum serious mental illness
  - women with current mental health problems.

(See RCOG (2009). Good practice statement no. 14: management of women with mental health issues during pregnancy and the postnatal period.
✎ www.rcog.org.uk/globalassets/documents/guidelines/management womenmentalhealthgoodpractice14.pdf)

▶ **Recommendation 12: assessing mental capacity**
- Healthcare staff have a duty to ensure patients have mental capacity.
- The Mental Capacity Act sets out a two-stage test of capacity:
  - does the person have an impairment of their mind or brain, whether as a result of an illness, or external factors such as alcohol or drug use?
  - does the impairment mean the person is unable to make a specific decision when they need to?
- If someone lacks capacity to make a decision, and the decision needs to be made for them, the MCA states that the decision must be made in their best interests.

(See NHS Digital (2021). Making decisions for someone else. Mental Capacity Act. ✎ www.nhs.uk/conditions/social-care-and-support-guide/making-decisions-for-someone-else/mental-capacity-act/)

Care of women with neurological disorders

- Epilepsy is the most common neurological disorder of pregnancy and improving care in pregnancy is a national priority.
- Stroke is the other main neurological cause of maternal death.
- See Table 11.7.

Table 11.7 Deaths from neurological causes

Classification of care received (2014–2016)	Women who died, n (%)
Good care	14 (48)
Improvements in care which would have made no difference to outcome.	3 (10)
Improvements to care which would have made a difference to outcome	12 (42)

MBRRACE-UK messages for care

Epilepsy

- Women should be provided with information about the risks of pregnancy and offered contraception until their control is optimized.

⚠ *Fetal exposure to sodium valproate is associated with birth defects; valproate must not be used without effective contraception.*

- Pregnant women with epilepsy should be managed by specialist MDTs, with access to senior neurologists or obstetric physicians and epilepsy specialist nurses.
- Women should be counselled about antenatal screening and the risks associated with discontinuing medication, and the effects of both medications and seizures upon the fetus.

Stroke

⚠ Headache with the following 'red flag' symptoms should prompt consideration of imaging investigations and referral for neurological opinion:
  - sudden onset—described as the 'worst ever'
  - associated with additional features not usually experienced—such as neck stiffness, fever, weakness, double vision, drowsiness
  - one or more seizures
  - repeated episodes of vomiting
  - duration longer than usual or persisting >48h.
- Doctors assessing pregnant women should be competent to perform a neurological examination, including assessing for neck stiffness and performing fundoscopy.

▶ **Recommendation 13: caring for pregnant women with epilepsy**

- GPs, 2° care providers, and commissioners should work together to ensure that women with epilepsy have access to appropriately specialized care, before, during, and after pregnancy.
- Preconception counselling for women with epilepsy is widely advised, but is not always delivered effectively and should be robustly offered in all care settings on an opportunistic basis.
- All antenatal services should identify a liaison epilepsy nurse to integrate into their routine antenatal service.
- All women with a possible new diagnosis of epilepsy should be seen promptly by a specialist in epilepsy and the care of pregnant women with epilepsy should be shared between an epilepsy specialist or obstetric physician and an obstetrician.
- The diagnosis of epilepsy *per se* is not an indication for planned CD or induction of labour.
- Postpartum safety advice and strategies should be part of the antenatal and postnatal discussions with the mother alongside breastfeeding, seizure deterioration, and antiseizure medication intake.

(See RCOG (2016). Epilepsy in pregnancy. Green-top guideline no. 68. ℘ www.rcog.org.uk/en/guidelines-research-services/guidelines/gtg68/)

Care of women with sepsis

➔ Puerperal sepsis: overview p. 386.
- Sepsis deaths include those with sepsis originating from the genital tract, influenza, and sepsis from other causes (such as pneumonia).
- This group of related conditions was responsible for 20 deaths in 2015–2017 and 19 deaths in 2014–2016.
- Although there was a significant and sustained ↓ in influenza-related sepsis between 2011–2013 and 2012–2014, deaths from non-influenza related sepsis have continued to ↑.
- See Table 11.8.

Table 11.8 Deaths from sepsis

Classification of care received (2013–2015)	Women who died, n (%)
Good care	5 (26)
Improvements in care which would have made no difference to outcome.	5 (26)
Improvements to care which would have made a difference to outcome	9 (47)

MBRRACE-UK messages for care

- Toolkits provided by The UK Sepsis Trust can be used to identify and manage sepsis in pregnant and postpartum women.
- The maternity-inpatient sepsis tool kit includes the following actions when sepsis is confirmed:
  - lactate measurement using venous blood gas analysis
  - microbiological sampling
  - early IV antimicrobial treatment.
- Maternity units should have a local guideline that outlines their sepsis pathway, with information on antimicrobials and how to access advice from clinical microbiologists and critical care services.
- Source control is essential—meaning that clinicians should not delay imaging as the basis for surgical or radiology-guided drainage of collections; removal of the source of infection may be required to improve the clinical situation of a woman with sepsis.
- Prompt source control might include termination of pregnancy (in women who are preterm with chorioamnionitis), or induction of labour or CS once the baby has reached viability.

Further reading

RCOG (2012). Sepsis in pregnancy, bacterial. Green-top guideline no. 64a
✍ www.rcog.org.uk/en/guidelines-research-services/guidelines/gtg64a/

The UK Sepsis Trust
✍ https://sepsistrust.org/

> **Recommendation 14: managing women with seasonal or pandemic influenza**

- The Department of Health/RCOG guideline on the investigation and management of pregnant women with seasonal or pandemic flu should be followed.
- Early neuraminidase inhibitor treatment should be instigated for women with symptoms consistent with influenza, in line with national guidance.
- The benefits of influenza vaccination to pregnant women should be promoted and pregnant women at any stage of pregnancy should be offered vaccination against seasonal and pandemic influenza with inactivated vaccine.

(See UK Government. An nual flu programme. ♫ www.gov.uk/governm ent/collections/annual-flu-programme)

Perinatal mortality: an overview

- *Perinatal mortality* refers to fetal deaths while pregnant (stillbirths after 24wks gestation) and those in the first 7 days of life (early neonatal mortality, UK).
- *Neonatal deaths* include liveborn infants who die before 28 completed days after birth, and so include both early and late neonatal deaths.
- UK surveillance, therefore, also reports an extended perinatal mortality rate comprising all stillbirths and neonatal deaths.
- Since 1986, perinatal morality has ↓ from 9.6 per 1000 births to 5.4 per 1000 in 2017 when there were 3686 perinatal deaths.
- The Still-Birth (Definition) Act 1992 modified the definition of a stillbirth by reducing the gestational age for babies included from 28 to 24wks.

Perinatal mortality: definitions

- *Late fetal loss:* a baby delivered between 22+0 and 23+6wks showing no signs of life, irrespective of when the death occurred.
- *Stillbirth*[a]: a baby delivered at or after 24+0wks showing no signs of life, irrespective of when the death occurred.
- *Neonatal death*[b]: a liveborn baby (born at 20+0wks or later, or with a birthweight ≥400g where an accurate estimate of gestation is not available), who died before 28 completed days after birth.
- *Perinatal death:* a stillbirth or early neonatal death.
- *Extended perinatal death:* a stillbirth or neonatal death.
- *Termination of pregnancy:* the deliberate ending of a pregnancy, normally carried out before the embryo or fetus is capable of independent life.
- *Perinatal mortality rate:* stillbirths + early neonatal deaths per 1000 total births.
- *Extended perinatal mortality rate:* stillbirths + neonatal deaths per 1000 total births.

[a] Stillbirths can be antepartum (birth before onset of care in labour) or intrapartum (birth after the onset of care in labour).
[b] Early neonatal death (death before 7 completed days after birth) or late neonatal death (death after 7 but before 28 completed days after birth).

UK confidential enquiry: perinatal deaths

From 2013, the programme has been managed by the MBRRACE-UK consortium who publish reports once a year.

Methodology

- MBRRACE-UK collects information on all late fetal losses, stillbirths, and neonatal deaths using an online data collection system.
- Individual level information is also collected from all births in the UK to provide the denominator for calculating mortality rates.
- Maps and tables are used to compare outcomes at a national level within the UK, as well at the level of healthcare providers and commissioners.
- Crude mortality rates describe 'what happened' at the level of individual units of comparison, such as different regions or healthcare providers. However, individual 'units of comparison' are likely to serve populations where (1) the number of deaths is small in comparison to the UK as a whole, and (2) the distribution of risk within any population or subgroups will influence outcomes, irrespective of the quality of healthcare provided (e.g. due to areas of high socioeconomic deprivation).
- See Fig. 11.5.

Outcomes reported

- 'Stabilized' and 'stabilized and adjusted' rates are also reported to enable 'fair comparisons'.
- A stabilized rate allows for the effects of chance variation due to small numbers. A stabilized mortality rate will better reflect the 'average' mortality rate than the crude mortality rate.
- Stabilized rates are then adjusted for important characteristics which are known to influence mortality rates, such as a baby's ethnicity or sex, as well as gestational age at birth (for neonatal deaths).
- Adjustment of stabilized rates is used to ensure that mortality estimates consider key characteristics that are known to ↑ perinatal mortality rates. These data must be available at the individual level for all births within a population and are restricted to maternal age, maternal sociodemographic status (using her residence), the baby's sex and ethnicity, their gestational age at birth, and lastly, whether they were from a multiple pregnancy. The adjustment process is unable to adjust for whether the mother smokes or her BMI.
- Stabilized and adjusted rates provide important information on perinatal outcomes but cannot be considered as definitive measures of care quality within populations and between subgroups within a population.
- This chapter summarizes the points highlighted by assessors in the 2019 report and the outputs from confidential enquiries into antepartum and intrapartum stillbirths.

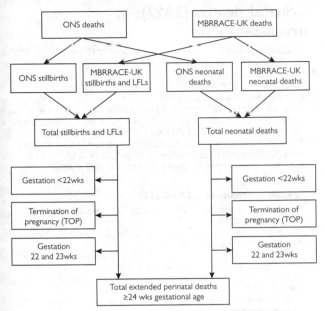

Fig. 11.5 Flowchart summarizing the methodology used by MBRRACE-UK to investigate and report perinatal mortality in the UK. LFLs, late fetal losses; ONS, Office for National Statistics. In Scotland, these data are provided by National Records Scotland (NRS).

Perinatal deaths (2017): surveillance data

The extended perinatal mortality rate in the UK in 2017 was 5.40 per 1000 births compared to 5.64 per 1000 births in 2016.

- Black babies were >2× as likely to be stillborn (compared to white babies), RR = 2.0 (95% CI 1.83–2.36), and 60% more likely to die during the neonatal period, RR 1.67 (95% CI 1.35–2.06).
- Asian babies were ~60% more likely to be stillborn (compared to white babies), RR = 1.59 (95% CI 1.44–1.75); and >70% more likely to die in the neonatal period, RR 1.73 (95% CI 1.50–1.98).
- Babies born to mothers from the most deprived socioeconomic group were >70% more likely to be stillborn, RR = 1.72 (95% CI 1.6–1.86); and ~60% more likely to die during the neonatal period, RR 1.57 (95% CI 1.4–1.76).

Singleton pregnancies (2013–2017)

- The extended perinatal mortality rate ↓ by 12%—equivalent to 500 fewer deaths in 2017.
- The stillbirth rate ↓ from 4.20 per 1000 births to 3.73 per 1000 and so there were 350 fewer stillbirths in 2017.
- The neonatal mortality rate ↓ from 1.84 to 1.67 deaths per 1000 live births—representing 150 fewer neonatal deaths.
- Intrapartum stillbirths ↓ substantially—from 189 (5.8%) in 2014 to 51 (1.4%) in 2017.
- Causes of stillbirths in singleton pregnancies—placental cause in ~33% although unknown cause reported in 35%.

Multiple pregnancies (2013–2017)

- Stillbirths ↓ by a quarter—9.03/1000 to 6.99 /1000 total births.
- Neonatal deaths ↓ by a third—8.01/1000 to 5.45/1000 live births.
- Among twin pregnancies, when compared to singleton pregnancies:
  - stillbirth risk is 1.93× higher
  - neonatal mortality risk 3.53× higher
  - stillbirth and neonatal mortality risks ↑ as maternal age ↓, as maternal social deprivation ↑; both risks are ↑ in female versus male twins
  - stillbirth risk is lower in preterm twins for all gestational ages
  - neonatal mortality risk in twins is 56% at 28+0 to 31+6wks
- Causes of stillbirths in twins—placental cause in ~40% and congenital anomaly in ~10%.

Key messages are shown in Fig. 11.6.

Further reading

Frøen JF et al. (2009). Causes of death and associated causes (CODAC)—a classification system for perinatal deaths. *BMC Pregnancy Childbirth*. 9:22.
🔗 https://bmcpregnancychildbirth.biomedcentral.com/articles/10.1186/1471-2393-9-22

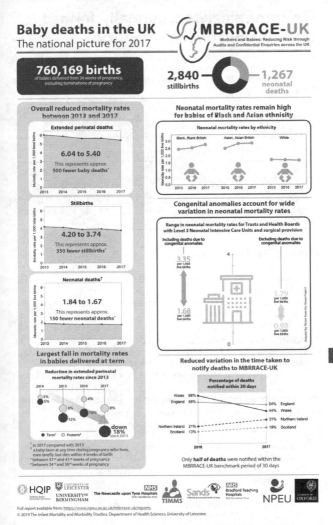

Fig. 11.6 Perinatal deaths in 2017: key messages from MBRRACE-UK (2019).

The term, singleton, normally formed, antepartum stillbirth enquiry

A confidential enquiry examining 85 cases of antepartum stillbirth at term in babies without congenital abnormalities was undertaken to examine why the stillbirth rate in the UK was higher than elsewhere in Europe (Table 11.9).

Table 11.9 Term singleton intrapartum stillbirths—classification of care received (2013)

	Baby, n (%)	Woman, n (%)
Good care	18 (21)	11 (13)
Improvements in care which would have made no difference to outcome.	16 (19)	19 (22)
Improvements to care which would have made a difference to outcome.	51 (60)	55 (65)

Messages for future care

- Gestational diabetes: missed opportunities for screening were frequently identified. ≥1 risk factor in >50% of women with only ~33% of women screened.
- Fetal growth: national recommendations for growth monitoring not followed in nearly 2/3 of cases and 1/3 of stillbirths were in growth-restricted babies.

↓ fetal movements reported to maternity units by women in ~50% of cases. Women should be aware of the importance of reporting ↓ fetal movements because of its association with stillbirth.

Organizations should provide care in accordance with national guidance.

▶ **Recommendation 15: screening for gestational diabetes**

- Offer women with GDM in a previous pregnancy either:
  - early self-monitoring of blood glucose, or
  - 75g OGTT.
- This should be performed as soon as possible after booking and repeated at 24–28wks if negative.
- Offer women with ≥1 of the following an OGTT at 24–28wks:
  - BMI >30kg/m²
  - previous baby weighing ≥4.5kg
  - family history of diabetes (1st-degree relative)
  - ethnic origin with a high prevalence of diabetes.

(See NICE (2015, updated 2020). Diabetes in pregnancy. ℘ www.nice.org.uk/guidance/ng3; NICE (2021). Antenatal care. NICE guideline [NG201]. ℘ www.nice.org.uk/guidance/ng201)

▶ **Recommendation 16: risk assessment and surveillance of fetal growth**

- There is strong evidence suggesting that fetal growth restriction (FGR) is the biggest risk factor in stillbirth and is linked to placental dysfunction.
- All women should have a risk assessment at booking to determine their risk of placental dysfunction and this should be used by clinicians to determine which growth surveillance pathway is appropriate.
- There are challenges associated with diagnosing FGR—both in previous and current pregnancies.
- FGR in a previous pregnancy includes ≥1 of the following:
  - birthweight <3rd centile
  - early-onset placental dysfunction requiring delivery <34wks
  - birthweight <10th centile with evidence of placental dysfunction during the pregnancy.
- FGR in current pregnancy includes ≥1 of the following:
  - estimated fetal weight (EFW) or abdominal circumference <3rd centile.
- EFW or abdominal circumference <10th centile with either:
  - abnormal uterine artery Doppler (mean pulsatility index >95th centile) at 20–24wks, or
  - abnormal umbilical artery Doppler (absent or reversed end-diastolic flow or pulsatility index >95th centile).

Further reading

NHS England. Saving babies' lives version two.
🔗 www.england.nhs.uk/wp-content/uploads/2019/07/saving-babies-lives-care-bundle-version-two-v5.pdf

RCOG (2013). Small-for-gestational-age fetus, investigation and management. Green-top guideline no. 31.
🔗 www.rcog.org.uk/en/guidelines-research-services/guidelines/gtg31/

The intrapartum stillbirth and intrapartum-related death at term enquiry

Between 1993 and 2015 the intrapartum mortality rate ↓ by >50% from 0.62 per 1000 births to 0.28 per 1000 births. This means that there were ~220 fewer deaths per year in 2015.

Based on the premise that a baby that was alive at the onset of labour should be expected to be a healthy newborn, the intrapartum confidential enquiry was established to identify areas upon which improvements could be expected to deliver better outcomes.

- Confidential enquiry panels discussed 78 cases..
- Improvements in care were identified in nearly 80% of cases which may have made a difference to the outcome of the baby.

Messages for future care

Antenatal care

- More women with complex needs are becoming pregnant and so more complex care packages must be devised.
- Fetal growth surveillance using national guidelines did not happen in 1/3 of cases.
- Smoking in pregnancy not screened for in 2/3 of cases.

Care during induction or labour and once labour established

- Capacity issues within maternity units was a problem in 1/4 of cases—mostly on delivery suite.
- Induction of labour and problems → delays in starting the process or monitoring the baby were present in 1/3 of cases.
- Fetal monitoring and interpretation was inappropriate or incorrect in 20% of cases.
- There was a significant delay in decisions to expedite delivery and then to achieve delivery in 1/3 of cases.
- Failure to recognize the evolution of a problem was a common theme and rarely due to a single issue.
- A systemic failure of situational awareness was identified repeatedly.

▶ A series of actions were suggested by reviewers in response to this enquiry and these are summarized in Fig. 11.7.

When babies die at term as a result of something that happened during labour

MBRRACE-UK
Mothers and Babies: Reducing Risk through
Audits and Confidential Enquiries across the UK

1 in 20 stillbirths and deaths of babies within 4 weeks of birth is labour-related

In 80% of cases different care might have prevented the baby's death

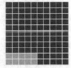

In 1 in 4 deaths there were problems with adequate staffing and resources

What needs to be done to prevent future labour-related deaths

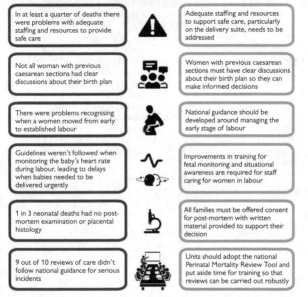

In at least a quarter of deaths there were problems with adequate staffing and resources to provide safe care

Adequate staffing and resources to support safe care, particularly on the delivery suite, needs to be addressed

Not all woman with previous caesarean sections had clear discussions about their birth plan

Women with previous caesarean sections must have clear discussions about their birth plan so they can make informed decisions

There were problems recognising when a women moved from early to established labour

National guidance should be developed around managing the early stage of labour

Guidelines weren't followed when monitoring the baby's heart rate during labour, leading to delays when babies needed to be delivered urgently

Improvements in training for fetal monitoring and situational awareness are required for staff caring for women in labour

1 in 3 neonatal deaths had no post-mortem examination or placental histology

All families must be offered consent for post-mortem with written material provided to support their decision

9 out of 10 reviews of care didn't follow national guidance for serious incidents

Units should adopt the national Perinatal Mortality Review Tool and put aside time for training so that reviews can be carried out robustly

Awareness by Luis Prado, Business Presentation by Gan Khoon Lay, Error by Creative Stall, Group Discussion by Drishya, Microscope by Pedro Santos, Monitor by Astonish and Pregnant Woman by Robiul Alam, all from the Noun Project.
© 2017 The Infant Mortality and Morbidity Studies, Department of Health Sciences, University of Leicester.

Fig. 11.7 Summary of intrapartum stillbirth confidential enquiry and recommended actions.

Perinatal Mortality Review Tool (PMRT)

The UK national PMRT was launched in January 2018 by the MBRRACE-UK collaboration to provide bereaved parents with answers about why their baby died.

Using a robust, standardized process, the tool is used at individual hospital level and was developed to better support local and national learning to improve care and prevent future deaths.

Purpose and scope for PMRT

- To facilitate multidisciplinary, high-quality reviews of the circumstances and care leading up to and surrounding each stillbirth and neonatal deaths.
- To support active communication with parents to ensure they are told that a review of their care and that of their baby will be carried out and how they can contribute to the process.
- Provides a structured process of review, learning, reporting, and actions to improve future care.
- Reaches a clear understanding of why each baby died, accepting that this may not always be possible even when full clinical investigations have been undertaken; this will involve a grading of the care provided.
- A clinical report is produced for inclusion in the medical notes.
- A report for parents is also provided, which includes a meaningful, plain English explanation of why their baby died and whether, with different actions, the death of their baby might have been prevented.
- Supports organizations to identify themes across a number of deaths. Data are assembled into a national report, the first of which is summarized in Fig. 11.8.

Further reading

National Perinatal Epidemiology Unit (2018). Finding the root cause.
https://www.youtube.com/watch?v=PE6b1IcpF2w&feature=youtu.be

National Perinatal Epidemiology Unit (2018). Perinatal mortality review—journey of improvement.
https://www.youtube.com/watch?v=-_TN5Ja8pe0&feature=youtu.be

National Perinatal Epidemiology Unit (2020). PMRT implementation support.
www.npeu.ox.ac.uk/pmrt/implementation-support

National Perinatal Epidemiology Unit (2021). PMRT annual report.
www.npeu.ox.ac.uk/pmrt

National Perinatal Epidemiology Unit (2022). PMRT programme details.
https://www.npeu.ox.ac.uk/pmrt/programme

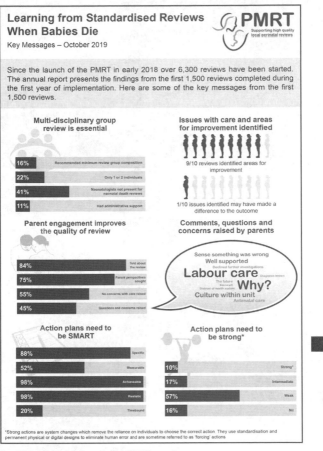

Fig. 11.8 Infographic from the first PMRT annual report.

Chapter 12

Benign and malignant tumours in pregnancy

Fibroids

- Fibroids (leiomyomas) are the most common pelvic tumour encountered in pregnancy.
- Prevalence 10.7% in the 1st trimester:
  - ↑ with advancing maternal age.
- Most frequently in women of African-Caribbean origin.

Effect of pregnancy on fibroids

- Evidence regarding change in size is conflicting.
- An ↑ in size is most common in the 1st trimester.
- >70% will experience regression in the 1st 3–6mths postpartum.

Effect of fibroids on pregnancy

Preconception

- 5–10% of women experience subfertility.
- Exact mechanism is unclear, the following have all been suggested:
  - distortion of the fallopian tube impairing gamete transfer
  - distortion of the endometrial cavity impairing implantation
  - hyperoestrogenic environment.
- Removal of submucosal fibroids ↑ conception rates.
- Subserosal fibroids do not appear to affect fertility.
- The role of intramural fibroids is less clear.

Antenatal

- Pain is the most common complication and may be severe enough to require opioid analgesia.
- Treatment with NSAIDs should be avoided in the 3rd trimester.
- Pain may be due to:
  - red degeneration (necrobiosis)
  - torsion of a pedunculated fibroid
  - pressure symptoms.
- ↑ risk of spontaneous 1st trimester miscarriage:
  - preconceptual myomectomy may ↑ successful pregnancy in recurrent 1st trimester pregnancy loss.
- ↑ risk of preterm labour.
- Large fibroids may exert pressure on the fetus causing limb reduction defects, congenital torticollis, and head deformities (fetal compression syndrome), and FGR.
- Placentation over a fibroid is a strong risk factor for abruption.
- Rare complications include:
  - malignant transformation—⚠ beware rapidly enlarging fibroids
  - uterine incarceration
  - acute kidney injury
  - urinary retention.
- The presence of fibroids is not a contraindication to ECV.

Delivery considerations with fibroids

- ↑ risk of CD (over 3× more likely) due to:
  - malpresentation
  - malposition
  - obstructed labour.
- ↑ risk of PPH:
  - affect uterine contractility by mechanically interfering with restoration of muscle fibres.
- ↑ risk of retained placenta, particularly if in lower segment.
- The presence of asymptomatic fibroids should not dictate timing of birth.

⚠ Myomectomy at CD should be avoided as it carries a high morbidity from haemorrhage; rarely it may be necessary to remove a fibroid to gain access to the fetus or to facilitate uterine repair.

Postnatal complications

Rare but may include:
- Pyomyoma:
  - life-threatening complication resulting from infarction and infection of a fibroid
  - presents with abdominal pain, fever, and sepsis (commonly *Clostridium*).
- Rupture of a degenerated fibroid:
  - presents with acute abdominal pain
  - a large hyperechoic uterine wall mass and free fluid are seen on USS.

Pregnancy after fibroid treatment

Myomectomy

- Women attempting vaginal birth should be treated in the same way as women attempting VBAC.

💣 Risk of uterine rupture following myomectomy is reported as being between 0.4% and 6.8%, but there is a lack of robust data to guide decision-making regarding mode of birth.

- Women with a previous myomectomy and a breach of the endometrial cavity are often advised to give birth by CD.

💣 It is unclear whether it is disruption of the endometrium or the myometrium which is the major factor in ↑ risk of rupture.

- The size of the defect and the interval between myomectomy and pregnancy may also be important (>6mths is recommended).
- Some studies have suggested that the rupture risk is higher following laparoscopic than open myomectomy.

Uterine artery embolization

- Pregnancy following uterine artery embolization has been shown to be associated with higher rates of miscarriage, CD, and PPH.
- Abnormal placentation is also more common, with up to 11% of women developing PAS following uterine artery embolization.

Benign adnexal masses

- Adnexal masses in pregnancy are common:
  - prevalence of 0.19–8.8%
  - often an incidental finding on routine pregnancy scans
  - usually benign.
- Ovarian cysts ≥6cm occur in 0.5–2:1000 pregnancies.

Imaging

→ Benign ovarian tumours: imaging, p. 784.

Ultrasound

- Features of malignancy are the same as in non-pregnant women.
- Greyscale USS for diagnosis of ovarian malignancy:
  - sensitivity: 86–95% and specificity: 68–90%
  - 1st-line modality for evaluating adnexal masses
  - comparable to both CT and MRI.
- The role of colour Doppler in pregnancy is less clear.

MRI

- Valuable for indeterminate masses due to its ability to:
  - characterize tissue composition
  - assess for metastasis.
- Safe and preferable to CT as it avoids radiation exposure.

💣 The safety of gadolinium, which enhances the vascularity of malignant tissue on MRI, remains uncertain.

Serum tumour markers

May be of limited value as normal pregnancy can affect levels.
- Cancer antigen (CA)-125:
  - >80% with epithelial ovarian cancer will have ↑ Ca-125 levels
  - also produced by the decidua, making interpretation challenging.
- LDH:
  - ↑ serum levels may be associated with dysgerminoma
  - pregnancy does not alter LDH, therefore it remains a useful marker.
- AFP and hCG:
  - in the non-pregnant women may be ↑ with germ cell tumours
  - both are ↑ in normal pregnancy.

Screening tools in pregnancy

Risk of Malignancy Index (RMI)

- Limited use in pregnancy due to reliance on the serum tumour marker CA-125.

International Ovarian Tumour Analysis (IOTA) tool

- Uses standardized terminology to categorize ovarian masses on USS.

◈ Has not been evaluated in pregnancy.

➲ Benign ovarian tumours: imaging, p. 784.

Clinically significant benign adnexal masses in pregnancy

Gynaecological

- Functional ovarian cysts including:
  - corpus luteal cysts
  - follicular cysts
  - haemorrhagic cysts.
- Benign cystic teratoma.
- Serous cystadenoma.
- Mucinous cystadenoma.
- Endometrioma.
- Paraovarian cyst.
- Hydrosalpinx.
- Tubo-ovarian abscess.
- Ectopic pregnancy.
- Hyperstimulated ovaries.

Non-gynaecological

- Appendix mass.
- Mesenteric cyst.
- Diverticular mass.
- Pelvic kidney.

Management of ovarian cysts

- Around 75% of adnexal masses seen in pregnancy are simple ovarian cysts <5cm in diameter.
- Often functional cysts which will resolve by the early 2nd trimester.
- If cysts persists, the decision between conservative management and intervention is based on:
  - size
  - morphology
  - likely diagnosis.

Conservative management

- Simple cysts <5cm do not require follow-up.
- Simple cysts >5cm or complex cysts (dermoid, endometrioma, cystadenoma):
  - should be monitored with serial USS
  - inform of the risk of ovarian torsion.

Surgical management

- Ultrasound-guided aspiration may be considered with large simple ovarian cysts to relieve acute pain and ↓ the risk of torsion or rupture.
  - high rate of recurrence (33–40%).

💣 Avoid aspiration if features of malignancy as intraperitoneal spillage ↑ the staging of a cancer and worsens prognosis.
- Surgical management should be considered if:
  - acute abdomen
  - suspicion of malignancy
  - rapidly growing masses (↑ of >20%) as higher risk of malignancy
  - cysts >10cm, which could cause obstruction in labour.

⚠ Acute complications should be managed as an acute surgical abdomen and treated surgically, regardless of the gestation.
- Elective surgery should be at 16–20wks:
  - ↓ risk of miscarriage
  - easier access to the pedicle.

💣 Laparoscopic approach is associated with ↑ maternal outcomes with no ↑ risk to the fetus.

Laparoscopy versus laparotomy
- Choice depends on:
  - skills of the surgeon
  - urgency of the procedure
  - risk of malignancy
  - size of the cyst.

💣 Size is controversial but risk of rupture ↑ if cyst >7cm:

➲ Benign ovarian tumours: management, p. 788.

- Indeterminate masses or those with malignant features warrant:
  - further assessed with MRI
  - input from a specialist MDT in gynaecological oncology.

➲ Ovarian cancer, p. 495.

Complications of ovarian cysts in pregnancy

These are the same as in the non-pregnant state.

Torsion

- Incidence in pregnancy is 1–5:10,000 pregnancies.
- May be as high as 16% in women with ovarian hyperstimulation.
- Most common in the 1st and early 2nd trimester.
- May occur in the absence of an adnexal mass (i.e. in a normal-sized ovary).
- Clinical presentation is similar to non-pregnant women.
- Pregnant women are twice as likely to have recurrence.

Cyst haemorrhage

- May occur as a result of ↑ vascularity.

Malpresentation

- Very large cysts may prevent engagement of the fetal head and predispose to malpresentation.
- Very rarely may cause obstructed labour.

Further reading

RCOG (2011). Management of suspected ovarian masses in premenopausal women. Green-top guideline no. 62

ℛ www.rcog.org.uk/globalassets/documents/guidelines/gtg_62.pdf

Malignancy in pregnancy: overview

- Rare, occurring in ~1:1000 pregnancies annually.
- During the 2014–2016 triennium:
  - 104 women died during or up to 1yr after pregnancy from malignant disease in the UK and Ireland
  - 26 women died during or up to 6wks after the end of pregnancy
  - mortality rate of 1.04 per 100,000 maternities.
- Most common malignancies in pregnancy are:
  - breast cancer
  - malignant melanoma
  - cervical cancer
  - lymphomas
  - leukaemias.

Diagnosis

- Delays in diagnosis are not uncommon:
  - signs and symptoms may be attributed to normal physiological changes seen in pregnancy
  - may also be a reluctance to perform the necessary investigations due to concerns about their effects on the fetus.

Treatment

- MDT input is essential to plan investigation and treatment which must be individualized taking into account:
  - gestation
  - tumour histology
  - staging
  - patient wishes.

💣 Surgery should not be delayed if it is clinically indicated.

Radiotherapy

- Radiotherapy is not routinely recommended during pregnancy and should be postponed until after birth where possible.
- Oncological emergencies such as spinal cord compression and CNS metastases may justify its use during pregnancy:
  - at later gestations, delivery may be deemed more appropriate.

Chemotherapy

- Should ideally follow standard protocols for non-pregnant patients.
- Cytotoxic chemotherapy should be avoided in the 1st trimester if possible.
- If there is an urgent need to commence treatment in the 1st trimester then TOP should be offered.
- Exposure in the 2nd and 3rd trimesters has been associated with FGR and serial growth scans are recommended.

Key points

⚠ Repeated presentation with pain requiring opioid analgesia should be considered a 'red flag' and warrants a thorough assessment to establish the cause.

⚠ If a cancer diagnosis is suspected, investigations and treatment should proceed in the same manner and on the same timescale as for a non-pregnant woman.

⚠ Malignancy diagnosed within 6mths of becoming pregnant is an independent risk factor for VTE. Thrombosis, particularly if migratory or in an unusual location, should be fully investigated as it may be a presenting sign of cancer.

➲ Care of women with breast cancer, p. 448.

Further reading

MBRRACE-UK (2018). Saving lives, improving mothers' care.
ℬ www.npeu.ox.ac.uk/assets/downloads/mbrrace-uk/reports/MBRRACE-UK%20Maternal%20
Report%202018%20-%20Web%20Version.pdf

Breast cancer

Breast cancer is the most common malignancy seen in pregnancy, estimated to occur in 1:3000–10,000 pregnancies.

Presentation

- Usually presents as a painless lump or thickening of the breast tissue.
- Occasionally presents as a unilateral bloody nipple discharge.
- Rare cases with erythema and breast induration:
  - ± a *peau d'orange* appearance of the skin.

Diagnosis

- Should be referred for assessment using standard cancer referral pathways.
- Investigations should follow the usual diagnostic protocols and not be withheld or delayed on account of the pregnancy.

Prognosis

- Pregnancy associated with a poorer prognosis, possibly due to:
  - delays in diagnosis
  - less aggressive therapy due to potential risks to the fetus
  - physiological changes which worsen outcomes
  - or a combination of all three.
- No evidence that TOP improves prognosis.
- ➔ Care of women with breast cancer, p. 448.

Further reading

NICE (2015, updated 2021). Suspected cancer: recognition and referral. NICE guideline [NG12]. ℘ www.nice.org.uk/guidance/ng12

Management of breast cancer in pregnancy

- Should be managed by an experienced MDT.

Treatments

Surgery

- Surgery can be performed in all trimesters.
- Reconstructive surgery should be delayed until after pregnancy:
  - prevents asymmetry resulting from pregnancy-related changes
  - avoids prolonged anaesthesia.
- Sentinel node assessment using radioisotopes does not cause significant uterine radiation and can be performed if required.

Radiotherapy

- Radiotherapy delayed until after delivery unless to prevent either life-threatening or organ-threatening complications, e.g. spinal cord compression.
- It can be performed with fetal shielding.

Chemotherapy

⚠ Systemic therapy is contraindicated in the 1st trimester.
- Can be performed from the 2nd trimester onwards.
- Not associated with late miscarriage, growth restriction, or organ dysfunction in the fetus.
- Anthracycline regimens can be used.
- Taxanes lack safety data in pregnancy and are therefore reserved for high-risk (node +ve) or metastatic disease.

Hormone/targeted therapy

⚠ Trastuzumab (Herceptin®) and tamoxifen are contraindicated in pregnancy and breastfeeding.

Other medications

- Antiemetics, e.g. dexamethasone and ondansetron, can be used.
- Granulocyte colony-stimulating factor can be used in chemotherapy-related neutropenia.
- VTE prophylaxis should be prescribed to all women with malignancy in pregnancy unless contraindications present.

Delivery timing

- At least 2wks after the last cycle of chemotherapy is advisable, to avoid issues with neutropenia at delivery.
- Administration of steroids for fetal lung maturation as normal if preterm delivery is anticipated.
- Granulocyte colony-stimulating factor may be useful prior to delivery.

Lactation

- No evidence that breastfeeding ↑ chance of recurrence.
- Lactation be more difficult depending on the surgical intervention that may have been performed.
- In women with a recent diagnosis of breast cancer, chemotherapy plans will determine whether breastfeeding is advisable.

Cervical cancer

- Most common cancer of the genital tract presenting in pregnancy.
- Estimated incidence 1–10:10,000 pregnancies.
- Most cases diagnosed in the 1st two trimesters are early (≤stage IB).
- NHS Cervical Screening Programme has significantly ↓:
  - incidence of invasive carcinoma of the cervix
  - mortality from cervical cancer.

➔ Cervical screening, p. 804.

Presentation

⚠ *Recurrent or unexpected bleeding in pregnancy should always be investigated with a speculum examination.*
- Pregnancy may result in significant morphological changes to the cervix including:
  - ↑ in cervical volume
  - ↑ in vascularity → a blueish tint
  - ectropion
  - inflammatory changes.

Diagnosis

- Where clinically indicated, urgent referral should be made for colposcopic examination by an operator experienced in pregnancy.
- Cervical smears are not recommended in pregnancy as decidual cells may be mistaken for atypia.
- Visible lesions should be sampled via punch biopsy:
  - carries an ↑ risk of bleeding due to the ↑ cervical vascularity
  - does not ↑ the risk of pregnancy loss.
- Cone biopsy and large loop excision of transformation zone (LLETZ) carry significant risks of haemorrhage (up to 25%) and pregnancy loss.
- Staging is performed as in non-pregnant woman:
  - CXR
  - MRI of the abdomen and pelvis.
  - Occasionally examination under anaesthetic (EUA) may be needed.

➔ Cervical cancer: diagnosis, p. 816.

Prognosis

- No evidence that when early-stage disease is diagnosed in pregnancy the prognosis is worse than for non-pregnant women.

Management of cervical cancer in pregnancy

- Should be managed by an experienced MDT.
- Treatment will depend on:
  - gestational age at diagnosis
  - stage
  - size of the lesion
  - wishes for future fertility.

Invasive (stages IA2, IB, and IIA)

- No evidence that pregnancy accelerates the disease.
- Disease-specific survival is independent of the trimester during which the diagnosis is made.
- Careful counselling is required including the option of TOP (<24wks) to facilitate immediate treatment.
- ⚠ Postponement of surgical treatment to enable the fetus to reach a viable age has not been demonstrated to ↑ the risk of recurrence.
- Platinum-based chemotherapy and taxanes can be used after the 1st trimester.
- Radical surgery can be performed immediately after CD.

Invasive (stages IIB, III, and IV)

- Rare in pregnancy.
- Immediate treatment is usually recommended.

Route of delivery

- CD should be performed for all invasive tumours.

Further reading

Amant F et al. (2019). Gynecologic cancers in pregnancy: guidelines based on a third international consensus meeting. *Ann Oncol*. 30(10):1601–1612.
℘ www.annalsofoncology.org/article/S0923-7534(19)60973-7/fulltext

Lymphoma

- Hodgkin's lymphoma is diagnosed in 1:1000–6000 pregnancies and is the 4th most common malignancy seen in pregnancy.
- In contrast, non-Hodgkin's lymphoma is rare.

Presentation

- Same as for non-pregnant patients, i.e. painless lymphadenopathy.
- Common signs and symptoms are:
  - fatigue
  - shortness of breath
  - anaemia
  - thrombocytopenia.

⚠ These overlap the normal symptoms of pregnancy which can result in a delayed diagnosis.

Diagnosis

- Made following lymph node (LN) biopsy and subsequent histological evaluation.
- Staging investigations include:
  - CXR
  - MRI chest, abdomen, and pelvis
  - FBC, creatinine, LFTs, and HIV serology.

Prognosis

- Pregnancy does not appear to have any effect on the prognosis of Hodgkin's lymphoma.

Management of Hodgkin's lymphoma in pregnancy

• Treatment depends on gestation, stage, and preferred regimen.

1st trimester

• Options include TOP, or use of a single agent, i.e. vinblastine, or use of ABVD (doxorubicin, bleomycin, vinblastine, and dacarbazine).

2nd and 3rd trimesters

• In early disease and near term, delivery can be expedited.
• If treatment is required ABVD does not ↑ adverse outcomes.
• Radiotherapy with adequate shielding does not ↑ adverse outcomes, but should only be done before delivery in extremis.

Other therapies

• Antifungals:
  • amphotericin B is considered the safest antifungal in pregnancy and is recommended if treatment is required.
• Prophylaxis for *Pneumocystis jirovecii*:
  • co-trimoxazole (trimethoprim and sulfamethoxazole) can be used in pregnancy (after the 1st trimester).
• Antivirals:
  • not routinely recommended alongside ABVD chemotherapy.
• Blood products:
  • should be CMV −ve and irradiated.
• DVT prophylaxis:
  • should be prescribed to all pregnant women with an active malignancy.

Delivery plans

• Should be individualized and depend on timing of chemotherapy:
  • aiming for delivery at term is reasonable unless clear indications for preterm elective delivery are present
  • delay of >2wks following chemotherapy is best to allow time for the neutrophil count to recover prior to delivery
  • CD is required for obstetric indications only.

Non-Hodgkin's lymphoma

• Less common in pregnancy as it is more likely to occur in older individuals; however, AIDS-related non-Hodgkin's lymphoma is an ↑ problem particularly in low-income countries.
• Treatment principles are similar to that of Hodgkin's lymphoma.

Leukaemia

- Incidence is between 1:75,000 and 1:100,000, but is ↑.
- Acute leukaemias are the most common:
  - acute myeloid leukaemia accounts for 2/3 of cases.

Presentation

- Acute leukaemia usually presents in the 2nd and 3rd trimesters.
- Common symptoms including:
  - fatigue
  - fever and night sweats
  - breathlessness
  - weight loss
  - ↑ bruising or bleeding
  - lymphadenopathy
  - frequent infections.

Diagnosis

- Blood film and bone marrow biopsy.

Management of acute lymphocytic leukaemia in pregnancy

⚠ It is both possible and appropriate to treat acute lymphocytic leukaemia in pregnancy.
- In the 1st trimester, discussion about TOP should be undertaken given the importance of adequate treatment and the high chance of maternal and fetal morbidity if not.
- Very steroid responsive:
  - high-dose steroids for 1–2wks may prolong the pregnancy to a more favourable gestation for delivery.
- There are a variety of chemotherapeutic agents used as part of induction, consolidation, and maintenance regimens.
- Intrathecal therapy is often used (as is methotrexate, but ⚠ contraindicated in pregnancy).

Acute promyelocytic leukaemia

- Type of acute myeloid leukaemia associated with DIC and bleeding complications.
- Treatment with all-trans retinoic acid (ATRA) should be started as soon as possible.

⚠ ATRA not advised in the 1st trimester due to teratogenicity so TOP versus continuation must be discussed.

⚠ If continuing with the pregnancy, an anthracycline should be used and ATRA initiated in the 2nd trimester.

Management of acute myeloid leukaemia in pregnancy
♦⁑ Tyrosine kinase inhibitors for those who are BCR-ABL ('Philadelphia chromosome') +ve, are advised against in pregnancy.

1st trimester
• TOP should be discussed to facilitate the early commencement of optimal treatment.

2nd and 3rd trimesters
• Decision for treatment and delivery needs to be individualized.
• Delivery of a pancytopenic mother is undesirable therefore where possible induction treatment should be commenced with an elective delivery after the mother has recovered.
• A standard induction regimen can be used (daunorubicin and cytarabine '3 + 10' schedule).

Other therapies
• High-dose steroids:
  • no dose adjustment required
  • monitoring for hyperglycaemia should be commenced.
• Antifungals:
  • amphotericin B is considered the safest antifungal in pregnancy and is recommended if treatment is required.
• Prophylaxis for *Pneumocystis jirovecii*:
  • co-trimoxazole (trimethoprim and sulfamethoxazole) can be used in pregnancy (after the 1st trimester).
• Antivirals:
  • aciclovir can be used in pregnancy if indicated.
• Blood products:
  • should be CMV −ve and irradiated.
• DVT prophylaxis:
  • should be prescribed to all pregnant women with an active malignancy.

Delivery considerations
• Timing depends on gestation and chemotherapy plans.
• Delay of >2wks following chemotherapy is best to allow time for the neutrophil count to recover prior to delivery.
• CD is required for obstetric indications only.
• Anaesthetic input is important as regional analgesia and anaesthesia may be contraindicated in the presence of significant neutropenia, thrombocytopenia, or coagulopathy.
• Active management of the 3rd stage is advised due to the ↑ risk of bleeding.
• Paediatric team should be informed and present at delivery.

Further reading
British Society for Haematology (2015). Management of AML in pregnancy.
🕮 https://b-s-h.org.uk/guidelines/guidelines/management-of-aml-in-pregnancy/

Malignant melanoma

- Melanoma is one of the commonest cancers diagnosed in pregnancy.
- Australian studies report an incidence of 45:100,000 pregnancies.

Presentation

- Changes in skin pigmentation during pregnancy may make diagnosis more challenging.
- 2/3 of melanomas occur in pre-existing naevi.

Diagnosis

⚠ *Any suspicious lesions should be biopsied.*
- Excisional biopsy allows histological analysis and may be curative.
- CXR, MRI, and CT may be used to assess for distant metastases, found most commonly in the lung and brain.

Management of melanoma in pregnancy

- No evidence that the development of melanoma in pregnancy is associated with a worse long-term prognosis.
- Surgery can be performed in pregnancy.
- Sentinel node assessment using radioisotopes does not cause significant uterine radiation and can be performed in pregnancy if required.
- Transplacental passage of melanoma can occur, resulting in a risk of metastatic melanoma in the fetus:
  - placenta should be sent for histology
  - paediatricians should be notified for neonatal assessment.

Metastatic disease

- Pregnancy is associated with ↑ lymphangiogenesis which is thought to contribute to ↑ risk of lymphatic melanoma metastases.
- Placental metastasis is rare and is only observed with widespread metastatic disease.
- Associated with a 22% risk of neonatal metastatic melanoma which has a very poor prognosis.
- It may also result in intrauterine death.

Prognosis

- Despite an ↑ incidence of nodal disease there is no evidence that pregnancy adversely affects survival of women with melanoma.

Ovarian cancer

- Despite ovarian cancer being the 2nd most frequent gynaecological cancer in pregnancy, only 2–10:100,000 adnexal masses seen in pregnancy are malignant.
- Histological distribution is similar to the non-pregnant population:
  - germ cell (6–40%)
  - borderline (21–35%)
  - epithelial (28–30%)
  - sex cord stromal (9–16%).

Diagnosis

- Based on removal of the mass, inspection of the abdominal cavity and biopsy of any suspicious lesions.

➔ Benign ovarian tumours: imaging, p. 784, and ➔ Benign adnexal masses, p. 480.

Management of ovarian cancer in pregnancy

Borderline tumours
- Management similar to non-pregnant women.
- Aim for vaginal birth with surgical management in the postpartum period.

Non-epithelial tumours
- Often large and symptomatic.
- Surgery involves unilateral salpingo-oophorectomy with full peritoneal staging.

Epithelial tumours
- Management depends on stage at presentation.
- MDT involvement is essential.
- Treatment for stage I disease is similar to non-pregnant women:
  - adnexectomy with full peritoneal staging.
- Those with high-risk stage I disease should be offered adjuvant chemotherapy.
- Those with advanced disease should be offered neoadjuvant chemotherapy and interval debulking surgery:
  - debulking surgery should take place as soon as possible
  - include the option of TOP
  - if TOP is declined, neoadjuvant chemotherapy should be given in the 2nd and 3rd trimesters, completing cytoreductive surgery after delivery.

➔ Ovarian cancer: treatment, p. 828.

Further reading

RCOG (2011). Management of suspected ovarian masses in premenopausal women. Green-top guideline no. 62.
ℛ www.rcog.org.uk/globalassets/documents/guidelines/gtg_62.pdf

Colorectal cancer

- Occurs in ~1:13,000 pregnancies.

Presentation

- Most cases are diagnosed during the 2nd and 3rd trimesters.
- Common presenting symptoms are bleeding (more frequent with rectal cancer) and abdominal pain.
- 25% of cases present as an emergency with constipation, acute bowel obstruction, and perforation.

Diagnosis

- Delay in diagnosis is common.
- Symptoms can overlap those of pregnancy:
  - change in bowel habit
  - anaemia
  - abdominal distension
  - rectal bleeding (being attributed to haemorrhoids).
- ~50% of women will have metastatic disease at diagnosis.
- Colonoscopy can be performed safely during pregnancy and should not be withheld.

Management of colorectal cancer in pregnancy

- Treatment is influenced by:
  - tumour location and stage
  - gestational age
  - context of the presentation, i.e. a surgical emergency.
- If early stage and gestation, resection may be possible.
- Neoadjuvant chemotherapy is advised for patients diagnosed with advanced disease at non-viable gestations.
- Evidence regarding mode of birth is conflicting:
  - tumours may cause obstruction during labour and delivery by CS is often advocated.

Prognosis

- Often present at a more advanced stage in pregnancy compared with non-pregnant women.
- Patients diagnosed in the 2nd trimester have the worst survival:
  - may be due to delays in investigations and initiation of treatment in an attempt to prolong the pregnancy.
- Outcomes have not improved over time.

Thyroid cancer

- Prevalence: 14.4:100,000 births.
- Papillary thyroid cancer is the most common histological subtype (75–80%).
- The prevalence of thyroid nodules during pregnancy is between 3% and 21%.

Presentation

- A hard, painless thyroid nodule is suspicious of malignancy.

Diagnosis

- USS may reveal characteristic features of malignancy including:
  - irregular or indistinct borders
  - microcalcifications.

⚠ *USS is not diagnostic.*
- Tissue diagnosis using fine-needle aspiration can be safely performed safely in all trimesters.
- MRI is used for staging.
- TFTs are usually normal in women with thyroid cancer.

Management of thyroid cancer in pregnancy

- Surgery is the treatment of choice for differentiated carcinoma.
- Radio-iodine should not be used as it destroys the fetal thyroid.
- Small papillary carcinomas, with no spread to the cervical LNs, may be monitored with USS and surgery delayed until after delivery if there is no change in size or evidence of metastasis.
- Surgery is the 1° treatment modality for advanced disease and/or rapidly growing tumours.
- 2nd trimester is the optimal time for performing surgery.
- Limited data on the optimal management of medullary and anaplastic carcinomas, surgery is the preferred management.
- Risk of maternal hypothyroidism and hypoparathyroidism after thyroidectomy should be anticipated.
- Chemotherapy may be appropriate for distant metastasis.

Prognosis

- Pregnancy does not appear to have any adverse effect on survival.

Chapter 13

Substance misuse and psychiatric disorders

Substance misuse in pregnancy

The prevalence of substance abuse in the perinatal population is uncertain, arguably more so than in other populations. Reasons for under-identification may include reluctance to disclose amid fears of loss of custody.

- Polydrug use is common and must always be considered.
- ↑ Risk of severe adverse outcomes for maternal and infant health.
- Associated with:
  - social adversity including poverty, abuse, and loss of custody
  - tobacco smoking
  - psychiatric and medical comorbidities.

Implications for antenatal care

- Substance misuse services are often separate from maternity services, predisposing to fragmented antenatal care.
- Women often find it difficult to engage with optimal antenatal care, which further ↑ the risks of adverse outcomes.
- Screening for drug and alcohol misuse should be a routine part of antenatal care.

Definitions relating to substance abuse

- Substance misuse disorders are categorized in the International Classification of Diseases, 11th Revision (ICD-11) under 'Disorders due to substance use'.
- Substances identified: alcohol, cannabis and synthetic cannabinoids, opioids, sedatives, cocaine, stimulants (amphetamines, cathinones), caffeine, hallucinogens, nicotine, volatile inhalants, MDMA, dissociative agents (ketamine, phencyclidine).
  The ICD-11 categorizes the pattern and consequences of misuse:
- *Intoxication:* acute psychoactive of substance use.
- *Harmful use:* pattern of use that damages health.
- *Dependence:* disorder of regulation of use; physiological, behavioural, and cognitive features including physiological tolerance and withdrawal, craving, prioritization of use over other daily activities despite harm (usually for >12mths).
- *Withdrawal:* characteristic acute psychological and physical features following cessation or administration of an antagonist.
- *Delirium:* disturbed attention and acute confusion due to acute intoxication or withdrawal.
- *Psychosis:* delusions and hallucinations due to intoxication or withdrawal from the substance.
- *Substance-induced mental disorders:* such as mood or anxiety disorders or dementia.

Morbidity and mortality

Adverse effects of substance misuse
- Risks compounded by association with social deprivation, nutritional deficiency, and poor hygiene.
- Worsens outcomes of comorbid health problems.
- Association with other mental disorders which are a known risk factor for maternal mortality.
- IV drug use is associated with:
  - transmission of blood-borne viruses (prevalence of hepatitis C 50–80% and hepatitis B 30–50% in UK drug users)
  - VTE
  - SC abscess
  - bacterial endocarditis
  - sepsis
  - difficult venous access in emergencies.
- Withdrawal effects may cause direct harm to the fetus and neonate.

Obstetric complications
- Preterm labour.
- Placental abruption.
- Haemorrhage.
- FGR and low birth weight.
- Miscarriage, stillbirth, neonatal death.

Fetal and neonatal complications
- Congenital abnormalities.
- Neonatal adaptation syndrome:
  - irritability
  - hypertonia and hyperreflexia
  - agitation
  - feeding problems
  - poor sleep
  - seizures.

Social impact
- Risks of abuse to and neglect of children must always be considered.
- Formal child protection proceedings are usually required.

Death
- In the UK in 2014–2016, 43 women died due to substance misuse; with a mortality rate of around 1.7 per 100,000.
- This accounted for >1/3 of mental health-related deaths.

General principles of management

Maternal management

Pregnancy presents a unique opportunity for services to engage with substance misusers. The goal of management must be clear. Achieving lifestyle stability and 'clean' drug use may be more desirable and realistic for some (especially opiate users), while complete abstinence should be the goal for others (especially alcohol and stimulant users).

Screening

- All women should be screened at their booking assessment. Use of specific biomarkers is not routine in the UK; identification ultimately relies on:
  - self-reporting
  - index of suspicion in the clinician.
- A detailed history of use of illicit drugs, tobacco, and alcohol should be taken, including:
  - frequency
  - route of administration
  - how use is funded.

Antenatal management

- Multi-agency care is required to address complex medical, psychological, and social problems which includes:
  - maternity services
  - 1° care
  - substance misuse services
  - mental health services
  - social care and 3rd-sector support services (housing, domestic abuse, child protection).
- A lead clinician or care coordinator should be identified.
- Flexible appointments should be offered to facilitate engagement with antenatal care.
- Contraceptive advice should be offered.
- Patient education to ↑ awareness of the associated risks to health.

Labour

- Delivery in an obstetric-led unit is recommended.
- Prior anaesthetic review due to potential difficulties with IV access.

Fetal and neonatal management

- Detailed anomaly USS:
  - consider fetal echo where appropriate.
- Serial USS due to ↑ risk of FGR.
- Neonatal review even if the baby is not admitted to the special care baby unit.

Alcohol misuse and dependency

- Up to 20% of pregnant women may drink more than the recommended limit, and up to 3% are dependent on or misusing alcohol.
- Alcohol is teratogenic.
- Complete abstinence is the 1° goal of management.
- Acute alcohol withdrawal risks serious morbidity and mortality including delirium tremens, seizures, and miscarriage.
- Gradual detoxification using long-acting benzodiazepines such as diazepam or chlordiazepoxide should be offered.
- Detoxification should be under medical supervision in pregnancy due to ↑ risks of complications including seizures.

Screening in pregnancy

- This should be a core component of routine antenatal care.
- T-ACE, AUDIT (or the abbreviated AUDIT-C), and TWEAK have been validated and recommended for use in pregnancy.

Maternal effects of alcohol misuse

- Miscarriage.
- Preterm labour.
- More likely to need induction of labour or CD.
- Associated with poor engagement with antenatal care.

Infant effects

- Low birthweight.
- Neonatal intensive care admission.
- Fetal alcohol syndrome.
- Stillbirth (related to placental dysfunction with heavy intake).

Treatment

- Psychosocial interventions and detoxification to achieve abstinence.
- Motivational interviewing can ↓ consumption in pregnancy.
- Evidence of benefit of engaging with regular antenatal appointments.
- Drugs for maintenance treatment, including. acamprosate and disulfiram, not recommended in pregnancy due to lack of safety data.

Fetal alcohol syndrome
- Spectrum disorder arising in a dose-dependent fashion.
- It is not known how much alcohol causes fetal alcohol syndrome, only complete abstinence guarantees no risk.
- Usually only severe cases are identified.
- Classic triad of symptom clusters:
  - FGR
  - CNS problems: developmental delay, and behavioural, learning problems, soft neurological signs such as motor skill problems
  - craniofacial abnormalities: micro-ophthalmia, short palpebral fissure, short nasal bridge, microcephaly, thin upper lip and small philtrum, oral cleft, maxillary hypoplasia.

Management of pregnancy in women abusing alcohol
- Attempt to ↓ harm by:
  - counselling about risks
  - encourage antenatal attendance by providing supportive, non-judgemental environment
  - facilitating contact with specialist substance misuse services including Alcoholics Anonymous (AA)
  - screening for abuse
  - facilitating access to social services and support agencies.
- Detailed anomaly USS.
- Serial USS to assess growth and fetal health.
- Multidisciplinary management with involvement of maternity, paediatric, social services, and specialist alcohol services.
- May need child protection proceedings.

Drugs of abuse: opiates

Opiate drugs

- All are potentially drugs of misuse.
- Include prescribed (primarily for analgesia) and illicit drugs.
- Natural opiates derived from the opium poppy include codeine and morphine (and its prescribed derivative, oxycodone).
- Synthetic opioids include methadone, fentanyl, and tramadol.
- Act on endogenous opioid receptors.

Routes of administration

- Route depends on the drug and the person's pattern of misuse.
- Can be smoked, taken orally or intranasally, or be injected.

Effects of opiates

- Acute intoxication: euphoria, analgesia, sedation, respiratory depression, nausea and vomiting, hypotension, pupillary constriction.
- *Dependency:* following regular use over a period of wks.
- *Withdrawal:* range from mild (rhinorrhoea, lacrimation, sweating, yawning, myalgia, arthralgia) to severe (diarrhoea, dysphoria, insomnia, agitation, piloerection, and shivering).
- Drugs with a shorter half-life are more prone to misuse and produce a withdrawal syndrome more quickly.
- Heroin withdrawal symptoms arise 4–12h post-dose, peak at 48–72h, and subside after 7–10 days.
- Withdrawal can be distressing but is not life-threatening.

Effects on pregnancy

- ↑ Risk of APH and preterm labour.
- Withdrawal risks miscarriage and premature labour.
- Higher analgesic doses intrapartum and postpartum may be needed.
- Monitoring of opiate toxicity required with ↑ doses.

Effects on infants

Not thought to be teratogenic.

- Opiate misuse often associated with multiple other risk factors.
- ↑ Risk of FGR, stillbirth, and neonatal death.
- Neonatal withdrawal usually occurs within 48h of birth.
- Withdrawal includes irritability, exaggerated startle response, jitteriness and tremors, poor feeding, and hypotonicity.
- Severe withdrawal can be fatal in neonates.
- May require admission to intensive care for IV methadone to prevent acute withdrawal.

Maintenance treatment
- Methadone (opioid receptor agonist) or buprenorphine (opioid receptor partial agonist) available.
- Both have longer half-life than heroin, with more stable plasma levels, allowing once-daily dosing without acute withdrawal.
- Outcomes better for mothers and infants if enrolled in substitute prescribing programme compared to women not in treatment.
- Maternal mortality and morbidity are ↓.
- ↓ Use of illicit or IV opiates.
- ↓ Exposure to impurities with illicit opiates.
- Avoidance of lifestyles associated with illicit drug use.
- ↑ Contact with healthcare services.

Management of pregnancy in women abusing opiates
- Attempt to ↓ harm by:
  - counselling about risks
  - offering substitute prescribing to reduce use of illicit opiates
  - encourage antenatal attendance by providing supportive, non-judgemental environment
  - facilitating contact with specialist substance misuse services including Narcotics Anonymous (NA)
  - screening for abuse
  - facilitating access to social services and support agencies.
- Screening for blood-borne viruses.
- Low threshold for antibiotics with symptoms of sepsis (may be atypical pathogens).
- High index of suspicion for VTE symptoms (may be unusual sites).
- Detailed anomaly USS.
- Serial USS to assess growth and fetal health.
- Multidisciplinary management with involvement of maternity, paediatric, anaesthetics (difficult IV access), social services, and specialist addiction services.
- Will probably need child protection proceedings.
- Advice about breast-feeding will need to factor in other drug use, infection with blood-borne viruses, and lifestyle factors.
- Advice about postnatal contraception.

Drugs of abuse: cocaine

Routes of administration
- Intranasal is the major route.
- IV use (including 'speed-balling' with heroin) has high mortality.
- Crack, the free alkaloid base of cocaine, can be smoked or injected.

Effects of cocaine
- Stimulant effects through monoamine (serotonin, noradrenaline, and dopamine) reuptake inhibition in the CNS.
- Sympathomimetic effects include tachycardia, ↑ BP, vasoconstriction, and sweating.
- Psychoactive effects include euphoria and anorexia.
- Harmful effects arise due to overstimulation of CNS and sympathetic nervous system include stroke, myocardial infarction, arrythmias, psychosis, anxiety, agitation, and anorexia.
- Crack is more addictive with a more intense high, and is associated with more chaotic lifestyles and social adversity than cocaine.

Effects of cocaine on pregnancy
- Harm arises from placental vasoconstriction and teratogenicity.
- Vasoconstriction leads to pre-eclampsia and placental abruption.
- Maternal mortality is ↑ due to cerebrovascular complications (intracranial bleed and emboli), and cardiac arrhythmias.
- Downregulation of myometrial β-adrenoreceptors may cause miscarriage, uterine irritability, and preterm labour.

Effects on infants
- Teratogenicity: especially microcephaly and cardiac defects.
- FGR due to placental dysfunction.
- Neonatal effects:
  - neonatal adaptation syndrome or a limited withdrawal syndrome may occur
  - hypotension and cardiac arrhythmias
  - sudden infant death
  - neurodevelopmental delay.

Management of pregnancy in women abusing cocaine
- Attempt to ↓ harm by:
  - counselling about risks
  - encourage antenatal attendance
  - facilitating contact with specialist substance misuse services
  - facilitating access to social services and support agencies.
- Detailed anomaly USS, serial USS with cardiac USS at 23–24wks.
- May need child protection case conference.
- No substitute prescribing is available for cocaine.

Drugs of abuse: stimulants

General principles

- Drugs include:
  - amphetamines (including methamphetamine, 'crystal meth')
  - MDMA ('ecstasy').
- Stimulant drugs are sympathomimetic.
- Psychoactive effects derived from activation of CNS dopaminergic, serotonergic, and noradrenergic pathways.
- Amphetamines may also be used an appetite suppressant.

Routes of administration

Can be smoked (crystal meth), taken orally, intranasally, or IV.

Effects in pregnancy

- Limited evidence base for effects in pregnancy.
- Misuse associated with other maternal and infant risk factors.
- Unclear relationship with congenital abnormalities.
- Neonates may show hyperactivity and poor feeding.
- May ↑ risk of miscarriage, preterm labour, and FGR.

Drugs of abuse: benzodiazepines

General principles

- Benzodiazepines are effective in a range of neurological and psychiatric conditions such as anxiety, agitation, insomnia, and epilepsy.
- Dependency can arise within wks of regular use.
- Act on γ-aminobutyric acid (GABA)-A receptors and enhance response to GABA, the predominant inhibitory neurotransmitter in the CNS.

Routes of administration

- Illicit or recreational use is predominantly oral.
- Medical use can be oral, IM, IV, or SC.

Effects

- Sedation is the most prominent acute effect.
- Drug half-life dictates its use.
- Lorazepam and midazolam (half-lives <24h) can be used for rapid tranquillization and anaesthetic premedication.
- Diazepam and chlordiazepoxide (half-lives >24h) can be used as an anxiolytic and for alcohol detoxification.
- Tolerance can quickly develop.
- Withdrawal syndrome, as with alcohol, is driven by CNS excitation.
- Withdrawal symptoms include agitation and insomnia, with seizures and delirium tremens in severe cases.

Effects in pregnancy

- Limited research means it is not known how much exposure is required to ↑ the risk of congenital abnormalities.
- Oral cleft from 1st-trimester use found in early studies.
- More recent evidence indicates antenatal benzodiazepine use unlikely to be associated with congenital malformations.
- May be specific associations, e.g. lorazepam and bowel atresia.
- Neonatal withdrawal may arise from late-pregnancy exposure.
- 'Floppy baby syndrome', with feeding and breathing difficulties, may arise from intrapartum use.
- Long-term effects of benzodiazepines on the infant are not known.

Management in pregnancy

- Sudden cessation not advised for regular users, just as with alcohol.
- Short half-life drugs should be switched to diazepam for more stable plasma levels, enabling a more gradual withdrawal.

Drugs of abuse: cannabis

General principles
- The most commonly used illicit drug across the world.
- Usually smoked but can be ingested in food or drinks.

Maternal and infant effects
- Direct effects are difficult to study as the majority of users smoke cannabis with tobacco (often without filters).
- Long-term use, especially in adolescence and early adulthood, is associated with an ↑ risk of developing psychotic disorders including schizophrenia, in those predisposed.
- Possible association with low birth weight and preterm labour.

Management
- There is no replacement therapy.
- Nicotine replacement therapy may constitute a key intervention.
- Harm reduction advice centres on reducing use with tobacco.

Tobacco
- Rates of cigarette smoking are declining but it remains a major cause of maternal and infant morbidity.
- Smoking is associated with a range of adverse outcomes:
  - miscarriage
  - placental abruption
  - low birth weight
  - neonatal death
  - sudden infant death syndrome ('cot death').
- Women should be advised to stop or at least ↓ smoking:
  - specialist smoking cessation advisers should be available
  - nicotine replacement therapy can be used in pregnancy.

Drugs of abuse: other

Hallucinogens

- Common hallucinogens include:
  - psilocybin (active substance in 'magic mushrooms')
  - mescaline (from the peyote cactus)
  - lysergic acid diethylamide (LSD)
  - ketamine.
- Very little data available on their effects in pregnancy.
- Misuse associated with other maternal and infant risk factors.

Volatile substances ('glue sniffing')

- Inhalation of solvents and adhesives, including:
  - toluene
  - acetone
  - petrol
  - cleaning fluids
  - aerosols.
- Often associated multiple other risk factors.
- Can cause sudden death from respiratory depression and arrhythmia.
- Animal studies indicate teratogenic effects in pregnancy.

Perinatal psychiatric disorders

Overview

- Perinatal disorders may be new-onset or pre-existing conditions persisting or recurring in the perinatal period.
- Perinatal illness rates are similar to non-perinatal female populations.
- Key distinguishing features of *perinatal* disorders are greater management complexity and the impact of illness.

Effects on broader health

- ↑ Rates of obstetric illnesses and adverse outcomes are associated with psychiatric morbidity, including persistent hyperemesis, pre-eclampsia, GDM, FGR, preterm labour, and placental abruption.
- Relationships between different conditions are highly individual; the evidence does not support causal relationships.
- Risk of adverse outcomes is further compounded by association with risk factors such as smoking, substance misuse, and poverty.
- Women with multimorbidity have complex health and social needs, requiring integrated care from multiple specialists and services.

Effects on the family

- Risk of adverse child outcomes (physiological, psychological) ↑ with maternal mental illness but most do not suffer harm.
- Maternal mental illness can affect children via biological (e.g. genetics, antenatal nutrition, hypothalamic–pituitary–adrenal axis dysfunction), psychological (e.g. attachment and parenting styles), and social (e.g. family support, socioeconomic resources) mechanisms.
- Parent–infant psychosocial interventions may be required, although the evidence base for these interventions is limited.

Importance of screening

- Universal availability of maternity and universal health services in developed nations enables systematic population-based screening.
- There are a range of validated and practicable screening tools available to detect common mood and anxiety disorders.
- Routine screening should also include a basic history of personal and family mental illness and substance misuse.

Planning pregnancy

- Preconception planning can help identify relapse triggers and early warning signs.
- Rationalizing psychotropic medication can reduce fetal risks.

Further reading

NICE (2014, updated 2020). Antenatal and postnatal mental health: clinical management and service guidance. Clinical guideline [CG192].
⌘ www.nice.org.uk/CG192

Depression

- Prevalence in perinatal population is 10–15% (3% severe).
- Most common complication of pregnancy and the postpartum.
- Clinical features must persist for at least 2wks for a diagnosis:
  - *core symptoms:* low mood, anhedonia, and low energy
  - *somatic symptoms:* impaired sleep, concentration, appetite
  - *cognitive symptoms:* hopelessness, helplessness, poor self-esteem, guilt, suicidality
  - *psychotic symptoms:* in severe cases.
- Depression is categorized by severity (mild, moderate, severe), which is determined by:
  - the number of symptoms
  - degree of functional impairment
  - associated risks (especially suicide).
- Functional impairment may distinguish depression from sadness.
- Associated adverse pregnancy outcomes include:
  - low birth weight
  - preterm delivery.
- Associated adverse infant outcomes include developmental behavioural and emotional disorders.
- Depression is, for the majority of patients, a recurrent illness.
- Early identification of women with antenatal depression may help ↓ the prevalence and impact of postnatal episodes.
- The evidence that postnatal depression represents a separate clinical entity to non-perinatal or antenatal depressive disorder is equivocal.
- It is probably as common antenatally as it is postnatally.
- There does seem to be a pattern of postnatal recurrences in multiparous women with previous postnatal episodes.

Postpartum 'baby blues'

- >50% of women experience brief emotional instability and mood disturbance starting around 3 days after delivery and resolving spontaneously within 10 days.
- It may initially be difficult to distinguish baby blues from depression, but the time course and severity of the conditions differ markedly.
- Severe baby blues is associated with progression to clinical depression.
- Clinical treatment is not usually indicated for baby blues.

Screening for depression

- A history of depression is the most significant risk factor for perinatal depression.
- Asking about psychiatric history is routine for all women at their booking assessment.
- NICE recommends the use of the *Whooley depression screening tool*, which can be administered quickly and can be used at any clinical encounter:
  - during the past month, have you often been bothered by feeling down, depressed, or hopeless?
  - during the past month, have you often been bothered by having little interest or pleasure in doing things?

⚠ Answering yes to either question results in a positive screen.

- Other screening questionnaires like the Edinburgh Postnatal Depression Scale (EPDS) are also helpful in identifying postnatal depression, and are routinely used by health visitors in many services.

Anxiety disorders

- 'Anxiety' is not a diagnosis but an umbrella term that includes disorders, symptoms, and normal emotions.
- Range of disorders that share common symptoms.
- Anxiety symptoms are:
  - *cognitive:* intense fear, worry, ruminating
  - *somatic:* palpitations, shortness of breath, sweating, shaking, agitation; driven by autonomic arousal.
- Prevalence rates are between 1% and 10%, depending on the locality and disorder.
- Highly comorbid with mood disorders.
- Associated with adolescent mental disorders.
- *Generalized anxiety disorder (GAD):*
  - most common anxiety disorder
  - persistent symptoms for at least 6mths.
- *Panic disorder:*
  - symptoms more intense than GAD, with recurrent, brief, acute episodes (there may be no anxiety in between).
- *Phobias:*
  - symptoms arise in the presence or anticipation of a feared stimulus, → functionally impairing avoidance behaviours
  - *tokophobia,* fear of childbirth, may be so significant it may constitute an indication for elective CD
  - *needle phobia* can impact antenatal and intrapartum care, and in severe cases mental capacity legislation may be invoked to administer essential parenteral treatment.
- *Obsessive–compulsive disorder:*
  - repetitive, distressing, irrational thoughts, or acts centring on a fear of something bad happening
  - often exacerbated in pregnancy.
- *Health anxiety disorders (somatoform or somatic symptom disorders):*
  - associated with excessive healthcare-seeking behaviour
  - iatrogenic harm may occur through excessive investigations or treatments.
- *Post-traumatic stress disorder:*
  - can arise from any traumatic experience, including birth trauma
  - may affect future family planning and engagement with antenatal and intrapartum care
  - symptoms include reliving experiences (flashbacks, nightmares), hyperarousal (agitation, irritability, poor concentration, insomnia), and avoidance of reminders of the event.

Screening for anxiety disorder

- NICE recommends routine screening for GAD.
- As with depression screening, this can be administered quickly at any clinical encounter:
- *During the past 2wks:*
  - have you been bothered by feeling nervous, anxious or on edge?
  - have you been bothered by not being able to stop or control worrying?
- Answers score 0–3, depending on persistence of symptoms.
- Scoring ≥3 is usually an acceptable cut-off for diagnostic assessment.

Eating disorders

Eating disorders are often comorbid with other mental disorders:
- Depression.
- Obsessive–compulsive disorder.
- Substance misuse.
- Personality disorder.

Anorexia nervosa
- Characterized by:
  - body image disturbance
  - food avoidance
  - severe low weight.

Bulimia nervosa
- Characterized by:
  - recurrent episodes of binge eating
  - compensatory behaviours such as self-induced vomiting and purging through use of diuretics and laxatives.

Binge eating disorder
- Similar to bulimia nervosa but without the compensatory behaviours (patients are usually overweight).

Risks in pregnancy
- Adverse neonatal outcomes as a result of:
  - ↓ food intake
  - low maternal weight
  - recurrent vomiting and purging.
- Eating disorders are associated with:
  - FGR
  - low birth weight
  - prematurity
  - congenital anomalies.
- Pregnancy may constitute a protective factor against eating disorder *behaviours*, but the inevitable body changes in the perinatal period may be exacerbate eating disorder *cognitions*, which may lead to compensatory behaviours postnatally.
- Close antenatal monitoring is required:
  - monitoring weight and food intake may need careful negotiation with the woman
  - specialist eating disorder services may need to be involved in more severe cases.

Other psychiatric disorders

Bipolar affective disorder

- Relapsing–remitting illness characterized by recurrent episodes of depression and mania (bipolar I) or hypomania (bipolar II).
- Affects ~1% of women of childbearing age.
- *Mania:* severe mood elation or irritability with somatic (↓ sleep, psychomotor agitation, ↑ energy) and cognitive (↑ self-esteem, grandiosity) symptoms and psychosis.
- Mania lasts >1wk, hypomania is milder and shorter lasting.
- Mania and hypomania can lead to reckless and dangerous behaviour.
- Between episodes patients can remain well for substantial periods.
- Childbirth is a significant risk factor for relapse.
- At least 25% may relapse postnatally.
- All pregnant women with bipolar affective disorder should have their treatment plan reviewed by a psychiatrist as early as possible.

Schizophrenia and schizoaffective disorders

- Relapsing–remitting or chronic psychotic illness.
- Not clear how relapse rates are affected in the perinatal period.
- In schizoaffective disorders, psychoses coexist with mood disorders.
- Schizophrenia is associated with ↓ fecundity and fertility.
- Clinical features during child-bearing age are usually dominated by 'positive psychotic symptoms':
  - abnormal beliefs (delusions)
  - abnormal perceptions (hallucinations).
- Important to elicit the place of the baby in the symptoms.
- Perinatal psychoses are associated with difficulties in meeting the baby's needs—child protection proceedings are usually necessary.
- Maintenance treatment with antipsychotics is usually required.
- All women with schizophrenia in the perinatal period should be under psychiatric care.
- Multimorbidity and risk factors for adverse outcomes are common in people with schizophrenia, e.g. smoking, obesity, diabetes.
- The lifetime risk of schizophrenia for a child with one affected parent is in the order of 10%.

Personality disorders and learning disabilities

Personality disorders

- There are several different personality disorders and it remains a contentious diagnosis.
- Diagnosis is determined by the dominant personality traits.
- Features must be evident in formative years, persist, and lead to pervasive intra- and interpersonal and social difficulties.
- Often comorbid with mood, anxiety, and substance misuse disorders.
- Associated with social adversity, especially past or current abuse.

Emotionally unstable personality disorder
- Most common personality disorder in clinical settings (borderline personality disorder is a subtype).
- Twice as common in women as men.
- Population prevalence estimated at ~5%.
- Emotionally unstable personality disorder features include:
  - emotional volatility
  - unstable relationships
  - low self-esteem
  - recurrent threats or acts of self-harm.
- Anxious-avoidant, dependent, and obsessive personality disorders are also common.
- Psychotropic drugs are often prescribed to treat symptoms but the evidence for this is weak; there are no licensed drug treatments.
- Psychological treatments available, with mentalization-based therapy and dialectical behavioural therapy having robust RCT evidence, but access often very limited.

Learning disabilities and autism spectrum disorders

- These are separate diagnostic categories but they often coexist in people with one or other of these conditions, especially severe autism spectrum disorder.
- Patients may have specific communication and behavioural needs.
- Commonalities in management of both conditions.
- Specialist input may be required to facilitate antenatal care.
- Ability to maintain independent living skills, parenting capacity, and mental capacity to consent to interventions (and even sexual intercourse) may need to be assessed (usually by specialist teams).

⚠ Women with these conditions may be vulnerable to exploitation; safe-guarding for the mother and baby must always be prioritized.

Further reading
WHO (2022). International Classification of Diseases, 11th Revision.
🕮 https://www.who.int/classifications/classification-of-diseases

Suicide and self-harm

Suicide in the perinatal period

Evidence of this comes from mainly from the UK Confidential Enquiry into Maternal Deaths reports.

- Latest data show a mortality rate of 4.57 per 100,000 from mental health-related causes (mainly suicide and substance misuse).
- Suicide is the 3rd highest cause of early postnatal and the highest cause of late postnatal death (2018), with 2.9 per 100,000 births.
- Majority of suicides occur postnatally, mostly by hanging or overdoses, while pregnancy appears to be protective.
- Most common psychiatric associations are depressive and substance misuse disorders.
- Unlike mental disorders in general, suicide seems to be more common in socially privileged women.
- Suicide is also associated with:
  - psychosocial adversities (chaotic lives, abuse, emotional instability, pregnancy, or custody loss)
  - inadequate antenatal care.
- Infanticide is extremely rare but such thoughts should be explored in women presenting with severe mood or psychotic illness.

Self-harm in the perinatal period

- Motivation varies between individuals and incidents.
- Self-harm is commonly deployed as a maladaptive coping strategy for distress and a means of regulating unstable and extreme emotions.
- How the patient came to the attention of medical services following self-harm is often highly informative of intent and further risk.
- Incidents are often impulsive.
- Self-harm is often a recurrent behaviour.
- Overdosing and cutting are the most common methods.
- More violent methods such as hanging or jumping from a height may be associated with greater suicidal intent.
- A history of self-harm is common in people who complete suicide.

Postnatal psychosis

⚠ This is a descriptive rather than diagnostic term.

Presentation

- Early postnatal period represents the highest risk period for the onset of severe illness across a woman's life span.
- The highest risk of onset is on day 1 after delivery.
- Episodes usually have prominent mood symptoms; they are usually affective rather than schizophreniform psychoses.
- Content of psychosis will often involve the baby or motherhood.
- Risk to the baby usually arises through neglect or accidental harm; desire or intention to harm the baby is extremely rare.
- Aim to manage the mother with her baby, under close supervision.
- Rapid symptom evolution over hours, while most psychotic illnesses evolve over wks–mths.
- NICE guidelines regard suspected postnatal psychosis as an emergency and recommend that women be assessed within 4h.
- Confusion is often present—delirium is a key differential diagnosis and investigations for organic aetiology should be considered.
- Early warning signs may be non-specific, e.g. severe sleep deprivation, agitation, and severe anxiety.
- The UK Confidential Enquiry into Maternal Deaths highlights 'red flag signs': acute mental state change, pervasive sense of estrangement from baby and family, and thoughts or acts of violent self-harm.

Epidemiology

- Incidence 1–2 per 1000 births.
- Can arise in women without any identifiable risk factors.
- Around 1/2 to 2/3 of women whose index episode was postnatal will have non-perinatal recurrences.
- The only consistent obstetric association is primiparity.
- Counsel about future pregnancies essential: >50% recurrence rate.

Risk factors
- Bipolar affective disorder.
- Previous episode of puerperal psychosis.
- 1st-degree relative with either of the above factors.

Treatment and recovery

Treatment plans must comprise biological, psychological, and social interventions; the timing of each intervention may vary, however.

- Antipsychotic medication will be required.
- The short-term prognosis is good, and most patients recover within a few months.
- Setting for acute treatment depends on the risks presented to the mother and her baby, and the availability of family support.
- Treatment should aim to keep mother and baby together; either at home or in a specialist mother and baby psychiatric hospital.

High-risk patients

⚠ A woman with bipolar affective disorder and a personal or family history of puerperal psychosis requires advance planning to mitigate the risk of postnatal psychosis.

Management options include:
- Prophylactic mood stabilizer (limited evidence for *prevention*).
- Promoting sleep in early postpartum: consider hypnotics, infant feeding strategies, available family support.
- Postnatal pain management,
- Monitoring of mental state in the community.
- Access to urgent assessment if early warning signs present.

Psychiatric medications: principles

Psychotropic medications are increasingly commonly prescribed across the adult population. An estimated 10% of women of child-bearing age in the US are prescribed psychotropics, mostly antidepressants. Prescriptions are lower in Europe but on the increase.

- All women on regular psychotropics should have their medication reviewed as pregnancy will affect the risk:benefit analysis.
- Prescription must be with consent of the women making a fully informed choice.
- Conduct individualized risk:benefit analyses; risks of medication weighed against the risks of undertreated mental disorder (in turn dependent on individual psychiatric history).
- Sudden medication cessation without expert oversight is not advised.
- All prescriptions are off-label; no drug is licensed in pregnancy or breast-feeding.
- For mild non-psychotic disorders, non-pharmacological approaches such as cognitive behavioural therapy should be 1st-line; antidepressant efficacy is not superior to that of placebo.
- Within drug classes there is little difference in absolute risks; drug choice should be guided by what has previously worked for the patient as well as the evidence base.
- Switching medication solely due to purported risk profile risks undertreating mother while exposing the baby to another drug.
- Risks from breastmilk exposure for most drugs likely much lower than antenatal exposure because placental drug levels are on average 5–10× higher than breastmilk.
- More caution is required in prescribing medication for breast-feeding mothers of preterm babies.
- Drug choice, especially postnatally, should factor in sedative effects and practicalities of caring for a newborn baby.

Evidence base for psychiatric medications in pregnancy

- Evidence for safety profiles based on observational studies only.
- Causation therefore cannot be determined, and confounding by indication is difficult to control.
- Majority of research is antenatal.
- Research in breast-feeding limited to small, uncontrolled studies and case reports often confounded by antenatal drug exposure.
- There are few long-term studies.
- Major long-term adverse outcomes are not known to be associated with most psychotropics; absence of evidence, however, does not imply evidence of absence.
- Risk profiles must be put into context of baseline population risks of miscarriage (10–20%) and congenital malformations (2–3%).
- Absolute risks are generally low, while relative risks are more variable—this must be carefully communicated to patients.

Psychiatric medications: antidepressants

1st-line drugs for depressive and anxiety disorders, with consistent evidence of effectiveness in moderate and severe conditions.

Pregnancy

- Overall, the absolute risk ↑ of harm to babies seems small and the clinical significance unclear.
- Selective serotonin reuptake inhibitors (SSRIs) have been most studied.
- Unlikely to be teratogenic:
  - SSRIs (paroxetine, fluoxetine) may affect cardiovascular development.
- Small absolute risk ↑ of persistent pulmonary hypertension of the newborn associated with SSRIs:
  - from ~2/1000 to ~3/1000
  - paroxetine most strongly associated and sertraline least.
- Associated with neonatal abstinence syndrome:
  - evidence base for this is limited
  - seems to be benign and self-limiting for most babies.
- Equivocal evidence of association with autism spectrum disorder:
  - the effect of confounding by indication cannot be ruled out.

Breast-feeding

- Levels of drug in breastmilk can vary.
- Most antidepressants are <10% relative infant dose (RID).

▶ If a mother has been on an effective antidepressant in pregnancy, it is not advisable to switch to an antidepressant with a lower level in breastmilk solely for that reason.

- Imipramine, nortriptyline, sertraline, and paroxetine have particularly low concentrations in breastmilk and are therefore are recommended if an antidepressant needs to be commenced in a breast-feeding mother.

Psychiatric medications: other

Antipsychotics

- Effective in treatment of psychotic disorders including bipolar disorder.
- Not thought to be associated with teratogenicity or major adverse maternal or infant outcomes, though long-term data limited.
- Most data for olanzapine, quetiapine, risperidone, and haloperidol.
- Also associated with neonatal adaptation syndrome.
- Risk profile data confounded by indication (usually prescribed for more severe mental disorders) and substance misuse (especially smoking, often coexisting with severe disorders).
- Associated with weight gain (especially quetiapine and olanzapine) so screening for gestational diabetes is advised.
- Not contraindicated in breast-feeding, except clozapine due to risk of agranulocytosis in infant (case report).

Anticonvulsant mood stabilizers

Most data are derived from epilepsy studies, which require higher doses than psychiatric disorders, and which are also known to be confounded by indication due to high levels of epilepsy-associated morbidity.

Sodium valproate

- Strong evidence of significant teratogenicity.
- ~10% neural tube defects and major congenital malformation.
- Associated with miscarriage, cardiac defects, neurodevelopmental disorders, and craniofacial abnormalities.

⚠ *Contraindicated* in all women of child-bearing potential.

Carbamazepine

- ~3% neural tube defects.
- Low doses much safer.
- Caution with breast-feeding due to high RID.

Lamotrigine

- Relatively newer drug so data more limited.
- Inconsistent data about association with oral cleft.
- Seems less teratogenic than valproate and carbamazepine.
- Caution with breast-feeding due to high RID (skin reaction in infants).

Anxiolytics

- Very limited data available on the safety profile of benzodiazepines, related Z-drug hypnotics, and gabapentinoids.
- There is no clear association with major adverse outcomes.

Lithium

- Effective treatment and prophylaxis of bipolar disorder.
- Narrow therapeutic window, requires regular blood level monitoring.
- Main risk of toxicity is dehydration or blood volume reduction.
- Should be stopped at the onset of labour or the day before an elective delivery date, and restarted postnatally only after specialist advice and once the woman is haemodynamically stable.
- Monitoring should ↑ from monthly to weekly after 36wks due to dilutional effects of blood volume ↑.
- Limited data available on risks to baby.
- Some evidence of association with neonatal thyroid dysfunction, arrhythmias, and nephrogenic diabetes insipidus.
- Highly variable RID in breastmilk—breast-feeding discouraged.
- Early pregnancy exposure risk of Ebstein's anomaly lower than previously estimated at 0.05–0.1% (background risk of 0.0005%).
- Women should deliver in consultant-led obstetric unit.

Further reading

National Library of Medicine (US). Drugs and lactation database.
🖉 https://www.ncbi.nlm.nih.gov/sites/books/NBK547437/

NICE (2014, updated 2020). Antenatal and postnatal mental health: clinical management and service guidance. Clinical guideline [CG192].
🖉 www.nice.org.uk/CG192

UK Teratology Information Service. Bumps (best use of medication in pregnancy).
🖉 www.medicinesinpregnancy.org/

Chapter 14

Gynaecological anatomy and development

Gynaecological history: overview

▶ Always introduce yourself fully and explain what you are going to do; patients are often very apprehensive and nervous.

Personal information

- Name, date of birth, age.
- Relationship status.
- Occupation.
- Partner's details and occupation (relevant in subfertility patients).

Current problem

- Description of the problem.
- Severity, duration, relationship to menstrual cycle.
- Aggravating and relieving factors.
- Any previous investigations or treatment.

Menstrual history

- Date of *1st day* of LMP.
- Age at menarche/menopause.
- Menstrual pattern (number of days bleeding/length of cycle).
- Amount/character of bleeding (flooding, clots, double protection).

⚠ Always ask about intermenstrual (IMB) + postcoital bleeding (PCB).

⚠ Always ask about any postmenopausal bleeding (PMB).

- Any associated pain + pattern (dysmenorrhoea). Has this changed?
- Ask about pain at other times including dyspareunia.
- Current and recent contraception (or not!) and details.
- Current/future pregnancy plans—this may alter/limit therapeutic options, as many treatments are contraceptive.

Past obstetric history

All pregnancies must be recorded, including successful ones, miscarriages, ectopic pregnancies, TOPs, and molar pregnancies.

Outcomes, gestation and mode of delivery, complications, birth weight, and current health of child(ren) should all be documented (➔ Obstetric history: current pregnancy, p. 2).

Past gynaecological history

- History of any other gynaecological problems especially endometriosis, fibroids, polycystic ovaries, and subfertility.
- All previous gynaecological surgery.
- Date of last cervical smear and result. Were they always normal?

Sexual history

- *Dyspareunia*: superficial on penetration or deep pain.
- Sexually transmitted infections or pelvic inflammatory disease (PID).
- Any abnormal vaginal discharge.

Think pregnancy

⚠ Always *think*: is this patient pregnant or at risk of pregnancy?

Every woman you see (10–60yrs old) should be considered potentially pregnant until proved otherwise—this way you will never miss it!

Key things to achieve in a gynaecological history

▶ Most diagnoses are clear from a good history alone.

- A clear understanding of the presenting problem(s) including effect on quality of life.
- A good history will inform your examination and investigative rationale.
- Exclude or confirm current pregnancy or risk of it:
  - offer contraceptive advice to the latter if they do not desire pregnancy.
- Discover what current and near-future pregnancy plans are.
- Identify women at higher risk of malignancy or other serious pathology.

⚠ IMB, PCB, and PMB are all red flag symptoms warranting examination and investigation.

- Allow disclosure of a hidden agenda:
  - many women will disclose other issues regarding sex or abuse or fertility concerns if you establish a good rapport
  - if you sense there is another concern, don't be afraid to ask ('You seem concerned about something. Is there anything else you would like to discuss?').

Gynaecological history: other relevant details

Micturition

If urinary symptoms disclosed then explore:
- Frequency (day and night).
- Pain or burning sensation (dysuria).
- Urgency.
- Urinary incontinence (stress or urge).
- Haematuria.
- Presence of 'something coming down' (prolapse-related symptoms).

Bowel habit

If bowel symptoms are disclosed then explore:
- Regularity.
- Associated bloating, pain, or difficulty defecating.
- Use of laxatives.
- Any rectal bleeding.

Medical and surgical history

- All medical conditions, especially diabetes, hypertension, asthma, thromboembolism. Major effect if surgery is being considered.
- All previous abdominal surgery is important also.

Drugs and allergies

- Details of all medication (doses and duration of use).
- Allergies to medications and severity (anaphylaxis or rash?).
- Use of folic acid in early pregnancy.

▶ Consider the risks for all drugs in relation to pregnancy (➔ Substance misuse in pregnancy, p. 500).
- Possible teratogenesis.
- Altered pharmacodynamics and pharmacokinetics.
- Toxicity in breastmilk where appropriate.

Family history

- Especially diabetes, ↑ BP, and thromboembolism.
- Familial cancers should always be considered, as well as others with a genetic association including:
  - breast
  - ovarian
  - endometrial
  - bowel.

Social history

- Home conditions and relationships.
- Occupation.
- Smoking and alcohol intake.
- Lifestyle issues such as use of recreational drugs.

⚠ **Subtle symptoms of gynaecological malignancy**
- Change of urinary and/or bowel habit.
- Persistent bloating.
- Non-specific discomfort.
- Even upper gastrointestinal dyspepsia type.

⚠ These should always prompt further investigation, particularly in women >50yrs, when persistent.

Box 14.1 How to do a speculum examination
- Cusco's bivalve speculum is more frequently used, but Sim's speculum normally used in examination of pelvic organ prolapse.
- Use a warm and well-lubricated speculum.
- Part labia minora adequately with the left hand.
- Insert speculum upwards and backwards (direction of vagina).
- Advance into vagina fully (until it cannot advance any further).
- Directly visualize as you open blades exposing cervix: only open enough to see cervix fully.
- *If cervix not seen:* close blades, withdraw slightly, change direction (usually more anterior), and open again.
- *Speculum removal:* ensure the blades are open while sliding over cervix, avoiding trapping it—watch what you are doing!
- Blades should be closed at introitus, not trapping any vagina.

Common problems to avoid
- *Obvious non-familiarity with the speculum:* patients spot this a mile off and will automatically tense up.
- Inadequate labial parting leads to inversion and pain (start badly and all patient confidence quickly disappears).
- *The speculum is only partially inserted 'so as not to cause pain':* the cervix will usually not be seen, → repeated insertion.
- *Failure to find cervix 1st time:* likely to be more anterior and closer to the introitus—pull back and move anterior as above.
- Not watching for adequate opening of blades and continuing unnecessary wide opening.
- Not having control of closure and pulling out a still-open speculum.

Gynaecological examination

General examination

- Height and weight.
- BMI (= weight (kg)/[height (m)]²):
  - ⚠ ↑ risks with ↑ BMI
- General, e.g. signs of anaemia, thyroid disease.

Abdominal examination

- *Inspection:* skin quality, abdominal distension, surgical scars (umbilical or Pfannenstiel), any visible masses or distension.
- *Palpation:*
  - superficial palpation for guarding, tenderness, rigidity
  - deep palpation for any masses; if present determine if arising from the pelvis ('can I get below the mass?')
  - pelvic masses are compared to the equivalent sized pregnant uterus (e.g. 20/40 sized, firm, mobile fibroid uterus).
- *Percussion:* dull if the mass is solid, tympanic if distended bowel, shifting dullness and fluid thrill in cases of ascites.
- *Auscultation:* usually used postoperatively to detect bowel sounds.

Good practice for intimate examinations

- Full explanation of procedure and reasons for it should precede examination.
- Verbal consent should be obtained.
- A trained chaperone is mandatory.

⚠ *Do not* use partners, friends, or children as chaperones.

- The patient must be able to undress and dress in privacy and cover herself at all other times.
- Any students or extra personnel present should be introduced and consent obtained for their presence *before* procedure.

Further General Medical Council (GMC) guidance on intimate examinations can be found at: ℘ http://www.gmc-uk.org

Pelvic examination

- All equipment must be ready (speculum, KY jelly, swabs, cytobrush, pipelle, etc.) *before* the patient is exposed.
- Position the woman:
  - dorsal (most common in gynaecological outpatient setting)
  - lithotomy (used for vaginal surgery, the feet suspended from poles)
  - Sim's (examination of pelvic prolapse, type of the left lateral).
- *Inspection:* describe any swelling, inflammation, skin changes, lesions, or ulceration seen anywhere on the vulva.
- Do the same for the vagina and cervix once the speculum is passed.
- *Speculum examination:* ⤴ Box 14.1 p. 533, for description of technique. Describe findings in vagina and on cervix.

▶ Don't forget to take any swabs required such as HVS for vaginal pathogens and flora and endocervical for *Chlamydia* and/or *Gonorrhoea*.
- *Bimanual (VE):* see Box 14.2 for description of technique.

Box 14.2 How to do a bimanual vaginal examination

- The lubricated index and middle fingers of the right hand are introduced into the vagina. The fingers of the left hand are on the abdomen above the symphysis pubis, and the uterus and adnexae are palpated between the two hands ('bimanual palpation').
- *Cervix*:
  - consistency (soft and smooth or irregular and hard)
  - tenderness
  - external os (?open during miscarriage).
- *Uterus*:
  - axis (anteverted, axial, or retroverted)
  - size (equivalent to gestational wks of a gravid uterus)
  - consistency (soft in a gravid uterus, firm, or hard with fibroids)
  - mobility (may be fixed in endometriosis/adhesions).
- *Adnexae*:
  - normal ovaries are usually not palpable
  - any masses (cystic/solid) and describe approximate size.
- Direct digital pressure into the fornices assesses tenderness.
- *Cervical excitation*: is a specific sign elicited by moving the cervix laterally thereby stretching the fallopian tube on the side that you are moving the cervix towards (i.e. by moving the cervix to the right and the uterine fundus will tip to the left, stretching the right fallopian tube.)

▶ Uterine masses usually move with cervix, ovarian masses do not.

▶ Obese patients are usually difficult to palpate—consider ultrasound.

Anatomy: female reproductive organs

Female pelvis, p. 10, for anatomy of the bony pelvis.

Vagina
- Fibromuscular tube, 7–10cm long.
- The cervix enters through the anterior wall.
- In the resting state, the anterior and posterior walls are opposed.

Uterus
- ~8 × 5 × 3cm in size (non-pregnant).
- Composed mainly of smooth muscle.
- Divided into the corpus and cervix uteri.
- Cylindrical and joins the uterine cavity at the internal os and the vagina at the external os.
- Anteverted in 80% of women (the remainder are retroverted or rarely axial).

Uterine (fallopian) tubes
- 10cm long; lie in the upper part of the broad ligament.
- Divided anatomically into:
  - isthmus (medial)—opens into the uterus at the ostia
  - infundibulum (lateral) with fimbrial end closely applied to the ovary
  - ampulla—in between (where fertilization takes place).

Ovaries
- ~3 × 2cm during reproductive years.
- Attached to the posterior surface of the broad ligament by the mesovarium.
- Situated in the ovarian fossa at the division of the common iliac artery (the ureter runs immediately underneath).
- See Fig. 14.1.

Supports of the uterus, vagina, and pelvic floor
- Middle:
  - transverse cervical ligaments (cardinal ligaments)
  - pubocervical ligament
  - uterosacral ligaments.
- Lower:
  - levator ani muscles and coccygeus
  - urogenital diaphragm
  - the superficial and deep perineal muscles with the perineal body.

▶ Defects and weaknesses of these supporting structures due to fascial tearing and denervation during parturition and surgery can cause organ prolapse and problems with urinary incontinence.

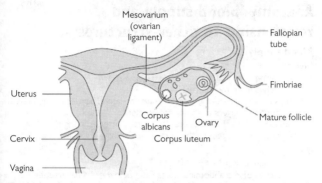

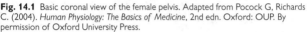

Fig. 14.1 Basic coronal view of the female pelvis. Adapted from Pocock G, Richards C. (2004). *Human Physiology: The Basics of Medicine*, 2nd edn. Oxford: OUP. By permission of Oxford University Press.

Anatomy: blood supply and relationship to other structures

Blood supply

Uterus

- The uterine artery:
  - branches from the internal iliac
  - runs behind the peritoneum to enter the lateral border of the uterus, through two layers of the broad ligament
  - anastomoses with the ovarian and vaginal arteries.
- The venous drainage is to the internal iliac vein.

Ovaries

- The ovarian arteries:
  - branches of the abdominal aorta from below the renal arteries.
- The right ovary drains directly into the inferior vena cava.
- The left ovary drains into the left renal vein.

Vagina

- Supplied by:
  - vaginal artery.
  - inferior vesical artery.
  - clitoral branch of the pudendal artery.

Urinary tract

Ureters

- Retroperitoneal throughout.
- Enter the pelvis in the base of the ovarian fossa.
- Run above the levator ani in the base of the broad ligament.
- Insert into the bladder posterolaterally.

⚠ The ureters are very close to the uterine artery near the lateral fornix and can be injured at hysterectomy.

Bladder

- Lies anterior to the uterus.
- *Three layers:* serous (peritoneal), muscular (detrusor smooth muscle), and mucosa (transitional epithelium).
- Supplied by superior and inferior vesical arteries (internal iliac artery).

Rectum

- Lies posterior to the uterus (separated from it by loops of small bowel lying in the pouch of Douglas). See Fig. 14.2.
- A thin rectovaginal septum separates the vagina and rectum.
- Supplied by superior, middle, and inferior rectal arteries (from the inferior mesenteric, internal iliac, and pudendal arteries respectively).

Lymphatic drainage of the pelvic organs

- *Vulva and lower vagina* → inguinofemoral → external iliac nodes.
- *Cervix* → cardinal ligaments → hypogastric, obturator, internal iliac → common iliac, and para-aortic nodes.
- *Endometrium* → broad ligament → iliac and para-aortic nodes.
- *Ovaries* → infundibulopelvic ligament → para-aortic nodes.

⚠ Knowledge of lymphatic drainage is important when considering metastatic spread from genital tract cancer.

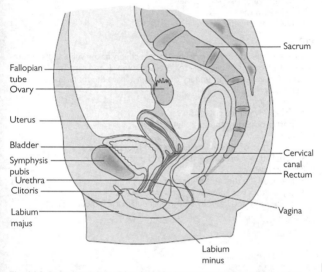

Fig. 14.2 Basic sagittal view of female pelvis demonstrating relationship to other pelvic organs. Adapted from Pocock G, Richards C. (2004). *Human Physiology: The Basics of Medicine*, 2nd edn. Oxford: OUP. By permission of Oxford University Press.

Anatomy: external genitalia

Perineum

- The area inferior to the pelvic diaphragm can be divided into:
  - anterior urogenital triangle (pierced by the vagina and the urethra)
  - posterior anal triangle.
- The superficial and deep perineal fascias are continuous with the labia majora and are attached:
  - anteriorly to the pubic symphysis
  - laterally to the body of the pubis.
- The superficial perineal muscles are:
  - superficial transverse perineus
  - ischiocavernosus
  - bulbocavernosus.

Vulva

The external genital organs are known collectively as the vulva and are composed of the mons pubis, labia majora and minora, and clitoris.

- *Labia majora:* lateral boundary of the vulva from the mons pubis to the perineum.
- *Labia minora:*
  - anteriorly join to cover the clitoris
  - posteriorly form the fourchette.
- *Clitoris:*
  - composed of erectile tissue covered by a prepuce
  - supplied by a branch of the internal pudendal artery.
- *The vestibule:*
  - lies between the labia minora and the hymen
  - the urethra lies anterior in the vestibule
  - posteriorly and laterally lie the vestibular or Bartholin's glands.

See Fig. 14.3.

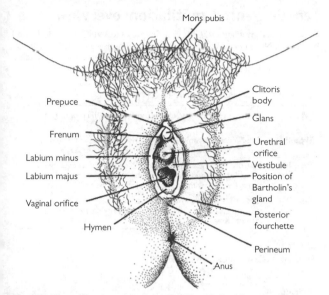

Fig. 14.3 External female genitalia. Reproduced from Collier J, Longmore M, Brinsden M. (2006). *Oxford Handbook of Clinical Specialties*, 7th edn. Oxford: OUP. By permission of Oxford University Press.

Female genital mutilation: overview

Female genital mutilation (FGM) is defined by the WHO and the United Nations (UN) agencies as 'the partial or total removal of the female external genitalia or other injury to the female genital organs for non-medical reasons' (see Table 14.1 for classification and Box 14.3 for complications).

Table 14.1 Classification of FGM (WHO 2007)

Type I	Partial or total removal of the clitoris and/or the prepuce (clitoridectomy)
Type II	Partial or total removal of the clitoris and labia minora, with or without excision of the labia majora (excision)
Type III	Narrowing of the vaginal orifice with creation of a covering seal by cutting and appositioning the labia minora and/or the labia majora, with or without excision of the clitoris (infibulation)
Type IV	Unclassified: all other harmful procedures to the female genitalia for non-medical purposes, e.g. pricking, piercing, incising, scraping and cauterization

Box 14.3 Complications of FGM

Immediate complications
- Death.
- Severe pain and shock.*
- Haemorrhage.*
- Infection including septicaemia.
- Adjacent organ damage and genital swelling.*
- Acute urinary retention.*

Long-term complications affecting pelvic organs
- Failure of wound healing.
- Recurrent UTI and urinary calculus formation.*
- Urethral obstruction and difficulty in passing urine.
- Pelvic infections, BV, and abscess formation.*
- Menstrual difficulties and associated infertility.
- Dyspareunia and sexual dysfunction.*
- Fistulae, mainly urinary and obstetric.

Long-term impact on reproductive health
- AIDS, HIV, and other blood-borne diseases.
- Problems with pregnancy and childbirth.*
- Psychological or psychiatric problems.

* Common complications.

Female genital mutilation: management

The management of girls and women affected by FGM is really determined by the complication that they present with, principally:
- Problems with sexual intercourse, menstrual flow, and/or micturition: de-infibulation under GA.
- Problems during and/or following delivery: obstructed 2nd stage of labour and/or major tears or urethral injury — de-infibulation under local anaesthetic/regional block and/or appropriate repair.
- Individual problems: such as infection, adjacent organ damage, and fistulae can be managed on an individual basis.

De-infibulation
- Obstructing skin/scar divided in the middle.
- Anterior/upward episiotomy in labour.
- Incision extended until external urethral meatus visible.
- Edges of incised surfaces freshened and sutured.
- The urethra needs to be protected to avoid injury.
- Extensive reconstruction may be needed in severe cases.
- De-infibulation should be carried out by practitioners experienced in dealing with this problem.

(➔ Female genital mutilation, p. 339.)

FGM overview
- Deeply rooted cultural tradition in 30 countries, mainly in western, eastern, and north-eastern Africa, and in some countries in Middle East and Asia.
- Highly complex social, religious, and political problem.
- At least 200 million girls and women alive today have been subject to FGM, and >3 million estimated to be at risk for FGM annually.
- Mostly carried out on young girls between infancy and adolescence, and occasionally on adult women.
- May be carried out by a wide range of 'practitioners' mostly untrained with a variety of 'instruments'.
- Complications (➔ Box 14.3, p. 542) are common.
- Management is related to the individual complications/presenting symptoms: usually de-infibulation.
- Prevention of FGM is an ongoing major international human rights issue.

⚠ It is an illegal practice in the UK and most parts of the world including areas where it is commonly practised.

⚠ It is now mandatory to report new FGM in the UK as a criminal offence.

Malformations of the genital tract: overview

These congenital malformations range from asymptomatic minor defects to complete absence of the vagina and uterus. The prevalence is estimated to be as high as 3%.

Aetiology

They arise from failure of the paramesonephric (Müllerian) ducts to form, fuse in the midline, or fuse with the urogenital sinus:

- Complete failure to form: Mayer–Rokitansky–Küster–Hauser (MRKH) syndrome.
- Partial failure to form: unicornuate uterus.
- Failure of the ducts to fuse together properly:
  - longitudinal vaginal septa
  - bicornuate uterus
  - uterus didelphys (complete double system).
- Failure to fuse with the urogenital sinus: transverse vaginal septa.
- Remnants of the mesonephric (Wolffian) ducts may be present as lateral vaginal wall or broad ligament cysts: usually trivial incidental findings and rarely of clinical significance.

⚠ Always look for renal and urinary tract anomalies (up to 40% coexistence).

Clinical features

Presentation often depends on whether it causes obstruction of menstrual flow.

- *MRKH syndrome (vaginal agenesis):* painless 1° amenorrhoea, normal 2° sexual characteristics, blind ending or absent vagina (dimple only).
- *Imperforate hymen:* cyclical pain, 1° amenorrhoea, bluish bulging membrane visible at introitus.
- *Transverse vaginal septum:* cyclical pain, 1° amenorrhoea, possible abdominal mass ± urinary retention due to haematocolpos, endometriosis due to retrograde menstruation, not all obstructed, may present with dyspareunia.
- *Longitudinal vaginal septa and rudimentary uterine horns:* dyspareunia alone if no obstruction, but if one hemi-uterus or hemi-vagina is obstructed then ↑ cyclical pain in the presence of normal menses ± abdominal mass from haematocolpos, and endometriosis.
- *Uterine anomalies* (bicornuate uterus, arcuate uterus, uterine septa): often asymptomatic, incidental finding at CD, may present with 1° infertility, recurrent miscarriage, preterm labour, or abnormal lie in pregnancy (💣 a causal relationship with these conditions is controversial).

Embryology of the female genital tract in a nutshell

- Genetic sex is determined at fertilization.
- Fetal sex becomes apparent in the normal fetus by the 12th wk of development.
- By the 6th wk of development the following structures start to appear either side of the midline:
  - genital ridges (induced by primordial germ cells from the yolk sac)
  - mesonephric (Wolffian) ducts (lateral to the genital ridge)
  - paramesonephric (Müllerian) ducts (lateral to the mesonephric ducts).
- In the female fetus the mesonephric ducts regress.
- The paramesonephric ducts go on to develop into:
  - the fallopian tubes (upper and middle parts)
  - the uterus, cervix, and upper 4/5 of the vagina (this results from the lower part of the ducts fusing together in the midline).
- The lower 1/5 of the vagina develops from the sinovaginal bulbs of the urogenital sinus, which fuses with the paramesonephric ducts.
- The muscles of the vagina and uterus develop from the surrounding mesoderm.

▶ Development of male genitalia is instigated by a single transcription factor encoded on the Y chromosome (*SRY* gene). This leads to the differentiation of the gonad to a testis, and production of testosterone and anti-Müllerian hormone (AMH) with subsequent masculinization. *In the absence of the SRY gene, fetus will develop female phenotype.*

▶ The mesonephric ducts also sprout the ureteric buds (which go on to form the kidneys and ureters) and caudally develop into trigone of the bladder. Hence, there is a close association between genital tract and urinary tract abnormalities.

Malformations of the genital tract: management

Investigations

- A thorough history and examination are required.
- Abdominal and transvaginal (TV) USS are invaluable (but TV may not be appropriate if not sexually active).
- MRI is the gold standard, especially if complex surgery is planned.
- EUA ± vaginoscopy, cystoscopy, and hysteroscopy may be required.
- Karyotyping to exclude 46XY female (androgen insensitivity syndrome) if uterus and upper vagina are absent.

⚠ Renal tract USS ± IV urography should always be undertaken because of high incidence of related renal tract abnormalities.

Aims for the management of genital tract malformations

- Minor anomalies usually need nothing more than reassurance, particularly if an incidental finding, as most are of no clinical significance.
- Management should be a multidisciplinary approach including psychological help for the patient and her parents, as well as arranging correction of anomaly.
- The aim of any treatment should be well defined.

Treatment

- *Imperforate hymen:* easily corrected by a cruciate incision in the obstructive membrane.
- *Vaginal septa:* should be removed surgically:
  - resection of longitudinal septa usually straightforward
  - transverse septa can be more complex, especially if high and thick, requiring surgical vaginoplasty.
- Obstructive uterine anomalies should also be surgically corrected or removed:
  - usually performed laparoscopically
  - technically difficult so should only be performed in centres with expertise in this area.
- *MRKH syndrome:* vaginal dilation is 1st-line treatment for creating a functional vagina. If this fails, surgical vaginoplasty can be performed by several techniques. Timing should be related to when sexual activity is anticipated.
- Patients should be given information regarding their condition; support groups are often very helpful.

Aims for the treatment of genital tract malformations

- Creation of a vagina suitable for penetrative sexual intercourse.
- Relief of menstrual obstruction and associated pain.
- Prevention of long-term sequelae of endometriosis due to obstruction and retrograde menstruation.
- Restoration or optimization of fertility wherever possible.

Disorders of sex development

Sex determination occurs in embryo, with female phenotype being the default setting. Male genitalia require testosterone to develop; the sex determining region gene (SRY) on the Y chromosome is responsible for development of testis, which in turn secretes AMH, causing regression of paramesonephric ducts. If any part of this process fails, resulting offspring may be genetically male, but phenotypically female. In 25% of disorders of sex development (DSDs) there are other congenital malformations or disorders. A full family history including consanguinity may be appropriate.

Causes of DSDs, classified according to karyotype

46XX karyotype
- Virilizing forms of congenital adrenal hyperplasia (CAH).
- Ovo-testicular DSD (previously termed true hermaphroditism).
- Maternal virilizing condition or ingested drugs.
- Placental aromatase deficiency.

46XY karyotype
- Androgen insensitivity syndrome (AIS).
- Defects of testosterone biosynthesis (e.g. 5α-reductase deficiency, 17β-hydroxysteroid dehydrogenase deficiency).
- Swyer's syndrome (pure gonadal dysgenesis).
- Partial gonadal dysgenesis 2° to single gene mutations.
- Leydig cell hypoplasia.

Abnormal karyotype
- Turner's syndrome (45XO): aneuploidy or mosaicism.
- XO/XY mixed gonadal dysgenesis.

Later presentations of DSDs
- DSD is not synonymous with ambiguous genitalia; many conditions will present much later.
- Androgen insensitivity, Swyer's syndrome, and Turner's syndrome often present with 1° amenorrhoea.
- Although often associated with a degree of genital ambiguity, 5α-reductase deficiency and 17β-hydroxysteroid dehydrogenase deficiency may present with virilization at puberty.

Family support

See Box 14.4.

Box 14.4 Coping with a child with ambiguous genitalia

The child with ambiguous genitalia at birth
- Keeping parents informed and psychologically supported at a very difficult time is of prime importance.
- Referral to a dedicated MDT is essential.
- Pressure to decide on sex of rearing should not be allowed to interfere with giving time to allow parents to come to terms with their child's condition or reach the correct diagnosis.
- Parents must be full partners in allocation of sex of rearing.
- Access to relevant support groups is invaluable.

The intersex adult
- Intersex advocates have recently begun to consider 'normalizing' practices such as genital surgeries at birth as undesirable, removing the patient's own bodily autonomy and self-determination, unless the surgery is absolutely medically necessary for the comfort of the child.
- A corollary of repeated surgical interventions during childhood is also associated with missing schooling, which can have negative effects on the patient's education and social development.
- Several different intersex organizations have parental guidance that may be helpful.

Support groups
- Androgen Insensitivity Syndrome Support Group (AISSG):
  ℘ www.aissg.org
- Living with CAH—CAH support group:
  ℘ www.livingwithcah.com
- DSD Families—information and support for families:
  ℘ https://dsdfamilies.org
- InterACT—advocates for intersex youth:
  ℘ https://interactadvocates.org/
- OII-UK–Intersex in the UK. Handbook for parents:
  ℘ https://oiiuk.org/746/handbook-for-parents/

Ambiguous genitalia at birth

Genitalia are said to be ambiguous when their appearance is neither that expected for a girl nor for a boy. Incidence is ~1:4000 births. The extent ranges from mild clitoral enlargement to micropenis with hypospadias.

 Never guess the sex of a baby. It may take wks to determine and requires MDT involvement led by a single clinician, usually a paediatric endocrinologist.

A full family history, drug history, and whether the mother has experienced any virilization during pregnancy should be ascertained.

Examination

- Presence of gonads in labioscrotal folds.
- Fusion of labioscrotal folds.
- Size of phallus and site of urinary meatus.

▶ Findings can be scored using the External Masculinization Score, with investigation warranted by a specialist if the score is <11.

Investigations

△ U&E are essential and must be sent urgently.
- Full assessment of the infant should occur looking for:
  - evidence of life-threatening salt-losing crisis (adrenal insufficiency), including hypovolaemia, hypoglycaemia, and hyperpigmentation
  - features of Turner's syndrome or other congenital anomalies
  - full inspection of genitalia carefully recording the position of orifices.
- Plasma glucose.
- Urgent serum 17-hydroxyprogesterone (raised in CAH).
- AMH (generally higher in boys than girls, originating from the Sertoli cells in testes)
- 24h urine collection for steroid analysis:
  - can be unreliable if taken <36h from birth, may require repeat testing after day 4.
- Karyotyping and genetic sequencing using next-generation sequencing assays/whole-genome and -exome sequencing.
- Ultrasound to locate gonads and presence of a uterus.
- Further investigations as deemed appropriate by MDT.

△ Support for the parents is essential (Box 14.4, p. 549).

Ambiguous genitalia: surgery

Corrective surgery

💧 Timing of surgery is a difficult decision. Traditionally, surgery as an infant was advocated; however, emerging evidence from research and adult patients has led to surgery being deferred until adolescence.

💧 Full disclosure is advocated and parents should be fully informed of the risks of surgery and anaesthesia. These include:

* Surgery as an infant may not be definitive.
* Each episode of surgery ↑ the risk of damage to sensitivity of the genitalia and dissatisfaction with sexual function in adult life.
* Children may one day want to be the opposite sex to that assigned, because of hormonal influences on the fetal brain.

Types of surgery

Aim of surgery is to improve cosmetic appearance of genital area and to provide potentially normal sexual function during adulthood.

Feminizing genitoplasty

* Very complex procedure that requires highly experienced surgeons in a specialized unit.
* Risk of damaging clitoral sensation with surgery consideration must be given to deferring clitoral surgery, especially in mild or moderate clitoromegaly.

Vaginoplasty

* Can be achieved by a variety of techniques, including a 'pull-through' technique, skin flaps, skin grafts, or the use of bowel substitution.
* To avoid postoperative stenosis regular dilator use is required:
  * this is not recommended in children, so delaying surgery may be more appropriate.

Gonadectomy

* Need should be discussed openly with regards to the risk of malignancy, especially for patients with gonadal dysgenesis (~30% lifetime risk) or the presence of a Y fragment.
* In other conditions it may be advocated to prevent further virilization.
* In AIS, it is advised to delay it until after puberty as the malignancy risk is much lower.

▶ In all cases patients and parents must be given time to think.

▶ Children should be given age and developmentally appropriate information regarding their condition at an early stage, with psychological support as required leading up to full disclosure so they can be involved in decisions regarding their care.

Congenital adrenal hyperplasia

- An autosomal recessive condition of enzyme defects in the adrenal steroidogenesis pathways leading to:
  - cortisol deficiency
  - ↑ ACTH secretion with build-up of cortisol precursors
  - ↑ androgen production.
- 90% is due to deficiency of 21-hydroxylase.
- If severe, aldosterone production is also affected → salt wasting.
- Incidence ~1:14,000 births (carrier rate of 1:80).
- The gene responsible is *CYP21*, located on chromosome 6 (but up to 20% cases have no mutation detectable).

Clinical features of CAH (46XX)

CAH is the commonest cause of ambiguous genitalia at birth, responsible for up to 50% of cases (ranges from mild clitoral enlargement to a near-normal male appearance). There is a wide spectrum of presentations including:
- Neonatal salt-wasting crisis and hypoglycaemia.
- Childhood virilization and accelerated growth with early epiphyseal closure and restricted final height.
- Late-onset with hirsutism and oligomenorrhoea.

▶ Diagnosis is by detection of elevated plasma 17-hydroxyprogesterone levels and 24h urinary steroid analysis.

Fertility and CAH

- Menstrual irregularity occurs in:
  - ~30% of non-salt-losers
  - ~50% of salt-losers.
- Natural fertility:
  - ~60% women with non-salt-losing CAH
  - ~10% women with salt-losing CAH.
- Almost all have polycystic ovaries on USS.
- Fertility treatment should be the same as for women without CAH.
- High levels of progesterone in poorly controlled CAH may be contraceptive by blocking implantation.

Management of CAH

- A multidisciplinary approach including:
  - paediatric urologists
  - endocrinologists
  - psychologists
  - gynaecologists.
- Treatment is lifelong and requires replacement glucocorticoid to suppress ACTH and ↓ excess androgen production (whether dexamethasone, hydrocortisone, or prednisolone is used is a balance between risk of iatrogenic Cushing's syndrome and compliance, especially with teenagers).
- Salt-losing CAH requires fludrocortisone to replace aldosterone.
- Antiandrogens may be used to combat the effects of raised androgens with lower doses of glucocorticoids.
- In pregnancy, requirement is ↑ for both mineralocorticoid and glucocorticoid (placental aromatase converts testosterone to oestradiol protecting the fetus from virilization and destroys excess therapeutic hydrocortisone).
- Prenatal diagnosis is available if a previous child has CAH:
  - dexamethasone is started with a +ve pregnancy test (it crosses the placenta and suppresses the fetal adrenal, ↓ the severity of ambiguous genitalia)
  - if CVS then shows the fetus is male or −ve for the gene mutation, dexamethasone can be stopped.

Androgen insensitivity syndrome

- Caused by a mutation in the androgen receptor gene on the X chromosome, causing resistance to androgens in the target tissues:
  - in the embryo the testes develop normally, but the testosterone-dependent Wolffian structures do not
  - AMH is still secreted by the fetal testes, so regression of the Müllerian structures also occurs.
- It has an X-linked recessive pattern in 2/3 of cases.
- Up to 30% *de novo* mutations.
- If the mutation can be identified in a family, then prenatal diagnosis can be offered with CVS.
- Most common form of under-masculinization in an XY individual.
- It can be complete (CAIS) or partial (PAIS).
- Incidence of CAIS is ~1:20,000, that of PAIS is unclear but thought to be at least as common as CAIS.

Clinical features of AIS (46XY but appear female)

- Presentation can be:
  - *prenatally*—fetal karyotype (XY) does not match ultrasound findings
  - *after birth*—inguinal hernias or labial swellings, found to contain testes
  - *at puberty*: 1° amenorrhoea.
- CAIS individuals have:
  - female external genitalia
  - a short blind-ending vagina
  - absent uterus and fallopian tubes
  - normal breast development
  - sparse pubic and axillary hair.
- PAIS includes a broad spectrum of phenotypes and individuals may have predominantly female external genitalia, ambiguous genitalia, or predominantly male genitalia.
- In the mildest form (mild AIS; MAIS), individuals have unambiguously male external genitalia. They usually present at puberty with gynaecomastia with or without under-musculization, or present later with adult male infertility.

Diagnostic tests

- Karyotyping.
- Pelvic USS (to exclude Müllerian structures and locate testes).
- Serum hormone profile (testosterones, LH, and FSH).

Management of AIS

⚠ The lifetime risk for malignancy within the testes is thought to be ~2% and therefore there is no need for immediate gonadectomy.

- If CAIS is diagnosed before puberty the testes may be left in to allow natural puberty without the need for hormone replacement therapy (HRT) in a child.
- After puberty:
  - gonadectomy should be offered because of the difficulty in monitoring intra-abdominal testes
  - HRT with oestrogens should be started following gonadectomy
  - some may require testosterone replacement to feel their best.
- Once sexual activity is anticipated then vaginal lengthening with the use of dilators should be offered.
- If dilators fail then consider surgical vaginoplasty.
- Bone mineral density should be checked periodically through dual-energy X-ray absorptiometry (DXA) scanning as, even with good compliance with HRT, a degree of osteopenia is noted.
- Regular weight-bearing exercises and supplemental calcium and vitamin D are useful to optimize bone health.

▶ Treatment of PAIS in individuals with predominantly female genitalia is similar to treatment of CAIS.

▶ In individuals with PAIS and ambiguous or predominantly male genitalia, parents and healthcare professionals tend to assign sex of rearing after an expert evaluation. This would dictate the surgical and/or hormonal treatment required.

Coping with the diagnosis of AIS

- The patient should be referred to a MDT experienced in the management of DSD.
- Input from a psychologist should be offered with an open-door policy (disclosure may need to be repeated on subsequent visits).
- The clinician should offer to explain the condition to the patient's relatives and/or partner.
- Information should be given regarding her diagnosis and referral to patient support groups offered.

▶ CAIS physical appearance and core gender identity are usually both female.

▶ PAIS patients raised as female have a higher than average dissatisfaction with gender identity (some studies show that >40% request gender reassignment).

Support group

- Androgen Insensitivity Syndrome Support Group (AISSG):
  🖰 http://www.aissg.org

Disorders of growth and puberty

Puberty is the development of 2° sexual characteristics in response to an ↑ in the pulsatile secretion of LH. In girls, breast budding (thelarche) with accelerated growth is usually the 1st sign, followed by development of pubic and axillary hair with menarche occurring ~2yrs after breast budding.

▶ The average age for menarche is 12.7yrs in the UK.

Precocious puberty

This is the onset and progression of signs of puberty before the age of 8yrs or menarche before the age of 10yrs. Precocious puberty leads to early accelerated linear growth with premature epiphyseal closure resulting in restricted final height.

> **Causes of precocious puberty**
> - Central precocious puberty (gonadotropin dependent):
>   - mostly idiopathic (80–90%)
>   - CNS space-occupying lesion
>   - congenital (e.g. CP).
> - Peripheral precocious puberty (gonadotropin independent):
>   - 1° hypothyroidism
>   - hormone-secreting ovarian or adrenal tumours
>   - McCune–Albright syndrome
>   - late-onset CAH (premature pubic hair).

Full history and examination

Document Tanner stage (Box 14.5) and enquire about:
- CP.
- Previous diagnosis of intracranial space-occupying lesion.
- Exposure to sex steroids.

Investigations

- Bone age (X-ray wrist).
- Cranial MRI.
- Pelvic USS.
- FSH/LH/oestradiol/17-hydroxyprogesterone.
- TFTs.
- Gonadotropin-releasing hormone (GnRH) stimulation test.

Treatment

Should be for the underlying cause. If idiopathic central precocious puberty, injectable GnRH analogues are used as they:
- Have minimal side effects in children.
- Enable achievement of normal final height.
- Cause breast, uterine, and ovarian regression (so the child resembles their peers).
- Have no long-term effect on bone mineral density in this age group.
- Are safe to use for 4–5yrs.

Box 14.5 Tanner stages

I   Prepubertal; basal growth rate; no breast or pubic hair development.

II   Accelerated growth; breast budding; sparse, straight, lightly pigmented pubic hair.

III Peak growth velocity; elevation of breast contour; coarser darkened curly pubic hair spreading on to mons pubis, axillary hair.

IV   Growth slowing; areolae form 2° mound; adult pubic hair type, but not spread to inner thigh,

V   No further ↑ in height; adult breast contour; adult pubic hair type and distribution.

▶ Menarche usually occurs in stage III or IV.

Delayed puberty and primary amenorrhoea

Definition

Delayed puberty is the absence of 2° sexual characteristics and menstruation by age 14, or the absence of menstruation with normal 2° sexual characteristics by age 16 (1° amenorrhoea) (➔ Menstrual disorders: amenorrhoea, p. 578).

> ### Causes of delayed puberty
> - Constitutional delay.
> - Chronic systemic disease.
> - Weight loss/excessive exercise.
> - Hypothalamo-pituitary disorders (hypogonadotropic hypogonadism, pituitary tumours, Kallmann's syndrome).
> - Ovarian failure (Turner's syndrome, Swyer's syndrome, iatrogenic).

History

Should include details of:
- Chronic illnesses.
- Anorexia.
- Excessive exercise.
- Anosmia.
- Family history of similar problems.

Examination

Should include assessment of:
- Height and weight.
- Pubertal (Tanner) stage.
- Visual fields (pituitary tumours).
- Hirsutism.
- Any stigmata of chronic disease.
- Signs of Turner's syndrome.

Investigations

- Bone age (X-ray wrist).
- LH/FSH, oestradiol, TFTs, and prolactin.
- Tests to screen for chronic illness, e.g. coeliac, IBD, diabetes.
- Karyotype.
- Pelvic USS or MRI if Müllerian anomaly suspected.
- Cranial MRI if prolactin >1500mU/L or low LH/FSH.

⚠ Urinary or serum hCG—never forget pregnancy as a cause of amenorrhoea, even 1°.

▶ Puberty can be induced with low-dose oestrogen (oral or patches) and growth hormone. This is a specialist area for a paediatric endocrinologist.

Management of delayed puberty
- Referral to an appropriate specialist is critical.
- Input may be required from endocrinologists, psychologists, and neurosurgeons.
- Treatment will depend on diagnosis.

Vaginal discharge: in childhood

Vaginal discharge is the commonest gynaecological symptom in young girls and is often associated with itching or soreness. The history is usually from the carer, but the child should be engaged in the conversation and asked questions about her complaint, which should include:
- Duration, frequency, and quantity of the discharge.
- Colour and odour.
- Blood staining.
- Whether the child wipes 'front to back'.
- Use of bubble baths, soaps, washing powders.
- Previously tried creams or ointments.

Examination should be done carefully with the carer present. Frog-leg position or knee–chest position can be used and often seated in the mother's lap can be most reassuring for the child. A cotton-tipped swab may be used to collect a sample of discharge, for microbiological assessment, from the posterior vulva.

▶ If the discharge is bloodstained, particularly purulent or profuse, then EUA and vaginoscopy (with removal of any foreign body) are appropriate.

Differential diagnosis
- Vulvovaginitis.
- Foreign body (commonly small bits of toilet paper).
- Trauma (including sexual abuse).
- Rare tumours.
- Skin disease.

Vulvovaginitis
- Most common cause of vaginal discharge and soreness.
- Often occurs when girl starts to be responsible for going to toilet.
- Normally no specific organisms are isolated.
- Treatment based on simple measures:
  - wiping front to back
  - avoidance of perfumed soaps, bubble bath, and biological washing powder for underwear
  - loose cotton underwear (avoid tights, leggings, and pants at night)
  - a simple emollient such as nappy cream may be helpful.

⚠ Antifungal, antibiotic, or steroid creams are unhelpful and may cause further irritation.
- If these measures are unhelpful, a short course of oestrogen cream may be beneficial.
- The symptoms always improve at puberty.

Sexual abuse

⚠ Always needs to be considered, but it is an area fraught with difficulty. Seek senior advice if you have any concerns

▶ Many chronically sexually abused girls show no signs on examination.

- Inspection of the hymen can be misleading for inexperienced doctor as irregularities, notches, and hymenal tags can all be normal findings.
- If STI is detected in a young girl it is normally an indicator of abuse, but not always.
- If abuse is suspected, the child should be referred to a lead doctor responsible for child protection.
- The child should be examined by most experienced doctor available; if possible, refer to a local dedicated centre.

If abuse is suspected

⚠ It is your duty to disclose confidential information if there is an issue of child protection.

⚠ If swabs are to be useful medico-legally, set protocols for a chain of evidence need to be followed. Seek senior advice urgently.

Vaginal discharge: in adolescence

Vaginal discharge in adolescents may be:
- Physiological leucorrhoea requiring explanation and reassurance only.
- A foreign body, such as a retained tampon.
- Due to any of the infections that affect adult women (➜ Sexually transmitted infections, p. 628).

The adolescent consultation

The adolescent consultation differs from that of an adult patient as obtaining a history may be more complicated.
- Usually the girl will be accompanied by a parent and unwilling to disclose information in front of them.
- It is important to give her an opportunity to talk to you away from her parent; this may be easily achieved by asking the parent to sit outside for the examination.
- Your manner should be frank and non-judgemental.
- She may need advice regarding contraception, as well as treatment for her presenting symptom.

▶ The girl may be very anxious about the examination and may be much more forthcoming with information once this is completed.

▶ Always explain what you are going to do, as this helps to allay anxiety.

Sexually transmitted infections in adolescents

- The rates of STIs in teenagers are ↑ rapidly.
- Teenagers are likely to have unprotected intercourse and are biologically more susceptible to infections than adults.

⚠ The risk of PID in a sexually active 15yr-old may be up to 10× that of a sexually active 25yr-old.

⚠ Always remember that a teenager having consensual sex may also be the victim of abuse.

Further reading

The BASHH has specific guidelines for the treatment of infections and has a *pro forma* for consultations with the under 16s.
🖱 http://www.bashh.org

Dermatological conditions in children and adolescents

Many dermatological conditions affect children and may well present on the vulva. Children will generally present with itching and soreness, with skin changes being noticed by a carer. Adolescents may be slow to present due to embarrassment and uncertainty of what are normal changes associated with puberty.

Labial adhesions

- The labia minora stick together due to the hypo-oestrogenic state.
- Usually asymptomatic:
  - noticed at nappy changing or bathing by the carer
  - occasionally may be associated with soreness (if an element of vulvovaginitis is present) or dysuria.
- Usually resolves spontaneously at puberty with no long-term problems.
- Treatment is not usually required. A short course of daily topical oestrogen cream can be useful if there is associated dysuria or pain. It may also be reassuring for the carer to see the adhesions disappear; however, they must understand that the adhesions are likely to reappear when treatment is stopped.
- Surgery is not indicated, unless the adhesions persist after puberty.
- USS to check for Müllerian structures can be offered for reassurance if the adhesions are severe.

Lichen sclerosus

- Chronic inflammatory condition.
- Occurs in ~1:900 prepubertal girls.
- Usually presents with severe itching associated with dysuria and surface bleeding, but can be asymptomatic.
- Shiny, white crinkly plaques are classically distributed in a 'butterfly' pattern around the anogenital area. The vagina is spared.
- Diagnosis is usually by inspection alone in children.

➔ Vulval dermatoses: lichen sclerosus, p. 790.

⚠ Rubbing and scratching by the child leads to telangiectasia, purpura, fissures, and bleeding, with possible 2° bacterial infection. This can wrongly lead to suspicions of sexual abuse.

- Can be associated with other autoimmune diseases (careful examination is required for other signs of illness).
- Treatment is symptomatic relief with use of topical corticosteroids.
- Symptoms generally improve at puberty, although the condition will still be present.
- Long-term follow-up is required (association with squamous cell carcinoma in adulthood).

Other common dermatoses found in young people

Molluscum contagiosum

- Caused by *Molluscum contagiosum* virus, a member of the poxviruses.
- Common in nursery and primary school children.
- Lesions are typically 1–5mm, shiny pale pink, domed papules with a central depression, found on the trunk and limbs, but anogenital spread is common.
- Destruction of the papules is painful and can lead to scarring so is not recommended.
- Resolves spontaneously in 6–18mths (but may take up to 3yrs).

Irritant dermatitis

- Trigger factor is dependent on age group:
  - urine and faeces in infants.
  - bubble bath, soap, and sand in toddlers and young girls
  - shampoo and shower gels in adolescents.
- Check no 2° infection with *Candida*.
- Advise avoidance of triggers and use of a simple barrier cream.

Threadworms (pinworms)

- Common in schoolchildren with poor hand hygiene.
- Worms migrate from the anus and cause anogenital itching.
- Skin is excoriated and sore and can have 2° infection.
- Treat with systemic antiparasitic (such as mebendazole) and a local barrier cream.
- Emphasize the need for improved hand washing to prevent reinfection.

Eczema and psoriasis

- May present on the vulva as part of a generalized condition.
- *Vulval ulceration:* differential diagnosis:
  - aphthous ulcers
  - Behçet's disease
  - Lipschütz ulcer
  - herpes simplex (in a young child, consider the possibility of abuse).

Warts

- In sexually active teenagers, human papillomavirus (HPV)-6 and -11 are most common.
- In children, common cutaneous warts (HPV2) are found.
- Most will resolve untreated within 5yrs (destructive treatments may be poorly tolerated in children, but may be useful).

⚠ Sexual abuse should be considered in children with anogenital warts, but vertical transmission can present up to 3yrs of age and transmission can occur from existing warts on the child's fingers.

Gynaecological disorders: in adolescence

Following menarche there is a continuing change in pituitary–ovarian activity. Regular ovulatory cycles usually establish within 2–3yrs. If irregular cycles or menorrhagia persist after this time, then there may be an underlying disorder.

⚠ Vaginal examination should only be performed on sexually active and consenting adolescences, and only if it will add to the assessment.

Menstrual disorders
➔ Chapter 15.

Amenorrhoea
➔ Menstrual disorders: amenorrhoea, p. 578.
- 1°:
  - with no 2° sexual characteristics should be investigated by 14yrs
  - with 2° sexual characteristics by 16yrs.
- 2°:
  - diagnosed after no periods for at least 6mths
  - eating disorders are common in this age group and, if missed, anorexia nervosa can have life-threatening complications.

⚠ *Don't forget pregnancy*—talk to the girl privately.

Oligomenorrhoea
Normal puberty is associated with an ↑ in insulin resistance.
- If associated hirsutism or excessive weight gain, consider polycystic ovary syndrome (PCOS).
- Weight loss should be strongly advised if overweight.
- Long-term risks of insulin resistance and endometrial hyperplasia are harder to get across to adolescents.
- Management can be with the COCP and advice regarding weight ↓.
- Norethisterone can be taken (21 days with 1wk break). It is important to explain this is not licensed as a contraceptive.

Menorrhagia
- Try to get them to quantify loss in terms of pad soakage.
- The COCP is very useful in this age group.
- Tranexamic acid and mefenamic acid are also effective.
- Acquired or congenital bleeding disorders can be present in 15%.

Do not assume that heavy, painful periods, irregular menses, or pelvic pain are a physiological part of adolescence.

Ovarian cysts in childhood and adolescence

Consider all types occurring in adults but with varying frequency (◐ Benign ovarian tumours: diagnosis, p. 782).
- Simple unilateral, unilocular cysts are the most commonly found cysts in children and adolescents (most resolve spontaneously).
- Complex/solid ovarian tumours are most likely to be germ cell in origin, most commonly benign cystic teratomas.

△ 10% of ovarian tumours in children are malignant.

- Epithelial tumours account for <20% of ovarian cysts in children and adolescents.
- 3–5% of ovarian tumours in children are sex-cord tumours.
- Preservation of reproductive function should always be considered in children and adolescents undergoing treatment for ovarian masses whether benign or malignant.

Pelvic pain in adolescence

Acute pelvic pain

◐ Acute pelvic pain, p. 642.
- Adolescents may be more prone to torsion of the ovary or fallopian tube than older women and this should always be considered.
- Consider acute PID.

△ Don't forget to consider pregnancy—?ectopic.

Chronic pelvic pain

- 1° dysmenorrhoea occurs in >80% of adolescents:
  - associated with an early menarche and menorrhagia
  - has a significant effect on schooling, sleep, exercise, and family life
  - treat with NSAIDs and the COCP
  - pain unresponsive to NSAIDs/COCP should be investigated with transabdominal pelvic ultrasound ± diagnostic laparoscopy
  - consider Mirena® intrauterine system (IUS) (may need insertion under GA).
- Endometriosis often presents atypically in adolescents and symptoms may be non-cyclical. Up to 38% of adolescents with chronic pelvic pain have endometriosis.
- Rare Müllerian anomalies (e.g. obstructed rudimentary horn) may present with cyclical pelvic pain of ↑ severity and predispose to endometriosis: if suspected, get an MRI.

△ Chronic pelvic pain is commonly reported in individuals who have suffered sexual abuse. Be aware of any signs of ongoing abuse.

Gynaecological cancers: in childhood

The most common is an ovarian germ cell tumour with the 2nd being a vaginal embryonal rhabdomyosarcoma (sarcoma botryoides).

Ovarian cancer in children

- Incidence 1.7/million in girls <15yrs, 21/million in girls aged 15–19yrs.
- >80% are germ cell tumours (most are dysgerminomas).
- Others include epithelial tumours (especially in the teens) and sex-cord stromal tumours (usually <10yrs).
- Present most commonly with pain, and ovarian mass on pelvic USS.
- Hormone-producing tumours may present with vaginal bleeding and/or precocious puberty.
- Check hormonal profile and tumour markers (➔ Ovarian cancer: presentation and investigation, p. 826, for details of investigations and management).
- In childhood 1° treatment is surgery with chemotherapy if required (as childhood ovarian cancer is so rare the majority will be entered into trials).
- Prognosis is good for germ cell tumours: 5yr survival >85% for all stages.

Non-ovarian cancers in children

- Most common is vaginal embryonal rhabdomyosarcoma, but this is still extremely rare, with incidence of ~0.5/million girls.
- Most present before the age of 5yrs with vaginal bleeding, discharge, and classically a polypoid mass in the vagina.
- EUA, biopsy, cystoscopy, and rectal examination are required for diagnosis.
- Multiagent chemotherapy is the mainstay of treatment.
- 5yr survival is ~82% overall.
- Clear cell adenocarcinomas of the cervix and vagina are now incredibly rare, as diethylstilbestrol (DES) (a synthetic oestrogen) has not been used in pregnancy since the 1970s.

⚠ Extremely rare. All should be managed in a tertiary referral centre with links to the UK Children's Cancer Study Group (UKCCSG).

Fertility implications of childhood cancer

- Childhood cancer has a cumulative risk of ~1:650 by age 15yrs.
- Most common are leukaemias.
- Advances in the treatment means the overall survival has reached 80%, → ↑ numbers of young adults affected by the reproductive consequences.
- Lowest live birth rates are with alkylating agent chemotherapy, and radiotherapy to CNS and/or abdomen and pelvis.

Late effects of cancer therapy

Ovary
- Premature ovarian failure can be caused by radiotherapy or chemotherapy, in particular alkylating agents.
- A prepubertal ovary is more resistant to damage (↑ reserve of primordial follicles).
- Can present as delayed puberty, 2° amenorrhoea, or premature menopause depending on:
    * age at time of treatment
    * dose of radiotherapy
    * chemotherapeutic agents used (some have no effect on ovarian function).
- Can present as precocious puberty, ↑ risk if treatment at <4yrs old, previous acute lymphoblastic leukaemia, and previous CNS tumour survivors.

Uterus
Abdominal, pelvic, or total body irradiation can damage uterine function causing ↓ uterine volume, ↓ elasticity of uterine musculature, and impaired vascularization. Successful pregnancies have been reported following radiotherapy, but there is risk of miscarriage, premature delivery, and FGR. Chemotherapy does not seem to affect uterine function.

Hypothalamus/pituitary
Cranial irradiation or total body irradiation can lead to hypogonadotropic hypogonadism. With high-dose cranial irradiation progressive compromise occurs, 60% having gonadotropin deficiency 4yrs after treatment. Even with low-dose cranial irradiation the presence of regular periods does not equate with fertility.

Early referral to fertility clinic is essential for these women if they present with subfertility as they have a lower outcome from IVF/ intracytoplasmic sperm injection (ICSI).

Further malignancy
Up to 4% of childhood cancer survivors will develop a 2nd 1° malignancy within 25yrs of the initial cancer. This is thought to be the carcinogenic (stochastic) effect of radiotherapy and certain alkylating agents.

Fertility preservation in cancer

⚠ Urgent referral to a specialist-assisted reproduction centre for advice before commencing cancer therapy is essential.

Rapid advances are being made in this field. Current techniques offered are:

- *Oophoropexy:* laparoscopic translocation of the ovaries away from the field of radiation to minimize exposure.
- *Ovarian stimulation and cryopreservation of mature oocytes or embryos:* generally not suitable for paediatric patients.
- *Harvesting and cryopreservation of ovarian tissue prior to treatment:* achieving fertility by *in vitro* maturation of oocytes followed by assisted reproductive techniques.

Normal menstruation and its disorders

Physiology of the menstrual cycle

The menstrual cycle involves the coordinated hormonal control of the endometrium allowing pregnancy or regular shedding (periods).

Peptide hormones from the hypothalamus and pituitary direct the ovary to produce steroid hormones (hypothalamic–pituitary–ovarian (HPO) axis), which in turn control the endometrium (Fig. 15.1). The process is complex and aspects of its initiation, control, and cessation are not fully understood. The average ages of menarche and menopause are 12.8yrs (falling) + 51yrs, respectively. Day 1 of a cycle is the 1st day of fresh bleeding and this should always be clarified on history of LMP.

Follicular phase

- Pulsatile release of hypothalamic GnRH → anterior pituitary to produce FSH.
- FSH promotes ovarian follicular development → recruitment of a dominant follicle containing oocyte.
- Follicular granulosa cells produce oestrogen → endometrial proliferation.
- ↑ Oestrogen levels → –ve feedback on the hypothalamic–pituitary axis (via follicular inhibin) to stop further FSH production.

Ovulation

- ↑ dominant follicle oestrogen (+ve feedback via follicular activin) → altered hypothalamic GnRH pulsatility → pituitary production of LH.
- LH surge 36h before ovulation.

Luteal phase

- The follicle collapses down to become the corpus luteum ('yellow body'), which produces oestrogen and progesterone (from theca cells).
- Progesterone and oestrogen act on an oestrogen-primed endometrium to induce secretory changes → thickening and ↑ vascularity.
- The corpus luteum has a fixed lifespan of 14 days (programmed cell death) before undergoing involution → corpus albicans ('white body').
- If implantation occurs, hCG (luteotropic) 'rescue' of the corpus luteum allows continued production of progesterone to support the endometrium.
- In the absence of pregnancy, corpus luteum degeneration → a rapid fall in progesterone and oestrogen, initiating menstruation.

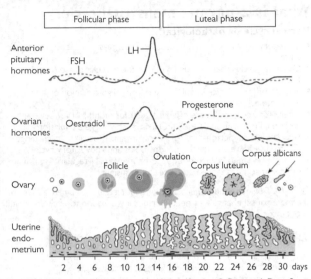

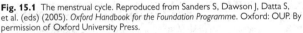

Fig. 15.1 The menstrual cycle. Reproduced from Sanders S, Dawson J, Datta S, et al. (eds) (2005). *Oxford Handbook for the Foundation Programme*. Oxford: OUP. By permission of Oxford University Press.

Menstrual phase

- Rapid ↓ in steroids → shedding of the unused endometrium.
- Inflammatory mediators (prostaglandins (PGs), interleukins, and tumour necrosis factor (TNF)) → vasospasm (~24h) in spiral end arteries → hypoxia and endometrial devitalization.
- Vasodilatation and spiral artery collapse → loss of the layer and bleeding from vessels.
- Endometrium lost down to basalis layer (1/3 of loss reabsorbed).
- Complex vascular changes controlled by above 2° messengers, also → natural haemostatic mechanisms including platelet plugs, coagulation cascade, and fibrinolysis.
- All steroid hormones now at basal level, −ve feedback is lifted, and GnRH–FSH production can begin a new cycle.

What is a normal menstrual cycle?

Normal cycle or pathological?

- Ovulatory cycles vary, but are usually 21–32 days with a basically regular pattern.
- Ovulatory cycles that vary do so due to the follicular phase (luteal phase fixed).
- Shorter or longer cycles usually result from oligo-ovulation or anovulation.
- After menarche, cycles are often irregular for months or for several years until maturation of the HPO axis reliably triggers ovulation.
- Perimenopausal periods are commonly irregular (usually ↑ cycle length) due to ovarian resistance to gonadotropins and anovulatory cycles.
- Nearly all women will experience some menstrual irregularity in timing or flow at some stage—many cases are transient.

⚠ *Do NOT blame erratic, chaotic, or constant bleeding in women >45yrs on 'the menopausal change'—it needs further investigation to exclude genital tract cancer.*

Bleeding and pain: what is normal?

- Bleeding can be for 1–7 days with an average of 3–5 days.
- Reported amount of blood loss is highly variable.
- Periods described as 'heavy' should always be viewed as such.
- Pain is 'normal' (vasospasm and ischaemia), but is highly variable.

▶ Pain interfering with normal functioning needs to be addressed.

⚠ *Bleeding between periods (IMB), after intercourse (PCB), or totally erratic/ constant bleeding is ALWAYS abnormal.*

Menstrual disorders: amenorrhoea

- 1° amenorrhoea is lack of menstruation by age 16 in the presence of 2° sexual characteristics or by age 14 in their absence.
- 2° amenorrhoea is the absence of menstruation for 6 months.

Diagnosis

History

Emphasis on:
- Sexual activity, risk of pregnancy, and type of contraceptive used.
- Galactorrhoea or androgenic symptoms (acne, hirsutism).
- Menopausal symptoms (night sweats, hot flushes).
- Previous genital tract surgery (including LLETZ).
- Issues with eating, stress, or excessive exercise.
- Drug use (especially dopamine antagonists).

Examination

- BMI <17/>30kg/m², hirsutism, 2° sexual characteristics (Tanner staging).
- Stigmata of endocrinopathies (including thyroid) or Turner's syndrome.
- Evidence of virilization (deep voice, clitoromegaly).
- *Abdominal:* for masses due to tumours or genital tract obstruction.
- *Pelvic:* imperforate hymen, blind-ending vaginal septum, absence of cervix and uterus.

Management

Must be guided by the diagnosis and fertility wishes. Options include:
- Treat any underlying causes including attaining normal BMI.
- Cabergoline or surgery for hyperprolactinaemia.
- Cyclical withdrawal bleeds (COCP for PCOS).
- HRT for POF.
- Relief of genital tract obstruction: cervical dilation, hysteroscopic resection, incision of hymen.
- Specific treatment for endocrinopathies and tumours.

▶ Major congenital abnormalities, AIS, etc. should be managed by MDTs in specialist centres.

Common causes of amenorrhoea

Physiological causes

⚠ *Pregnancy must always be excluded.*
- Lactation.
- Menopause.

Iatrogenic causes

- *Progestogenic contraceptives:* Depo-Provera®, Mirena® IUS, Nexplanon®, POP.
- Therapeutic progestogens, continuous COCP use, GnRH analogues, rarely danazol.

Investigations for amenorrhoea

⚠ *Pregnancy test.*
- FSH/LH:
  - ↑ in premature ovarian failure (POF)
  - ↓ hypothalamic causes (not useful in PCOS).
- Testosterone and sex hormone-binding globulin (SHBG) are most useful for PCOS.
- Prolactin should always be tested.
- TFTs.
- Pelvic USS:
  - can define anatomical structures, congenital abnormalities, Asherman's syndrome, haematometra, and PCOS morphology
  - can indicate ovarian activity or endometrial atrophy in POF.
- Karyotype if uterus is absent or suspicion of Turner's syndrome.
- Specific tests for endocrinopathies where clinical suspicion.

Pathological causes of amenorrhoea

- *Hypothalamic:*
  - functional—stress, anorexia, excessive exercise, pseudocyesis
  - non-functional— space-occupying lesion, surgery, radiotherapy, Kallman's syndrome (1° GnRH deficiency).
- *Anterior pituitary:*
  - micro- or macroadenoma (prolactinoma) or other space-occupying lesion
  - surgery
  - Sheehan's syndrome (postpartum pituitary failure).
- *Ovarian:*
  - PCOS
  - POF
  - resistant ovary syndrome
  - ovarian dysgenesis, especially due to Turner's syndrome (45XO).
- *Genital tract outflow obstruction:*
  - imperforate hymen
  - transverse vaginal septum
  - cervical stenosis
  - Asherman's syndrome (iatrogenic intrauterine adhesions).
- *Agenesis of uterus and Müllerian duct structures:*
  - sporadic or associated with AIS (➜ Malformations of the genital tract: overview, p. 544).
- *Endocrinopathies:*
  - hyperprolactinaemia
  - Cushing's syndrome
  - severe hypo/hyperthyroidism
  - CAH.
- *Oestrogen- or androgen-secreting tumours:*
  - usually ovarian or adrenal, e.g. granulosa-thecal cell tumours and gynandroblastoma.

Menstrual disorders: oligomenorrhoea

When cycles are >32 days they usually represent anovulation or intermittent ovulation. Transient oligomenorrhoea is common ('stress' or emotionally related causes are often cited) and usually self-limiting.

Causes of oligomenorrhoea

▶ Similar to many of the causes of 2° amenorrhoea:
- PCOS is the commonest cause (➋ Polycystic ovarian syndrome: overview, p. 652).
- Borderline low BMI.
- Obesity without PCOS.
- Ovarian resistance → anovulation, e.g. incipient POF, is rare, but important.
- Milder degrees of hyperprolactinaemia need to be excluded as well as mild thyroid disease.

Management of oligomenorrhoea

What does the patient want? Regular periods or fertility?
- Provide reassurance.
- Treat any underlying causes as for amenorrhoea.
- It is not uncommon for no cause to be found, but serious pathology must be excluded.
- Attain normal BMI (weight loss or gain as appropriate).
- Provide regular cycles:
  - COCP or cyclical progestogens
  - for PCOS a minimum of 3–4 periods/yr is recommended to ↓ the risk of endometrial hyperplasia due to unopposed oestrogen.
- Full fertility screening should be performed if ovulation induction is required.

Menstrual disorders: dysmenorrhea

⚠ *Dysmenorrhoea:* the pain has no obvious organic cause.

▶ *Dysmenorrhoea:* the pain is due to an underlying condition.

Pain is highly subjective and varies greatly between women. However, if a woman describes her periods as unacceptably painful, then they are!

Diagnosis

History
- Timing and severity of pain (including degree of functional loss):
  - commonly premenstrual pain ↑ in the 1st 1–2 days of bleeding, then eases.
- Pelvic pain and deep dyspareunia (may signify pelvic pathology).
- Previous history of PID or STIs.
- Previous abdominal or genital tract surgery (may cause adhesions).

Examination
- Abdominal exam to exclude pelvic masses.
- Pelvic exam:
  - cervical excitation
  - adnexal tenderness
  - mobility, and masses.

Investigations

- STI screen (including *Chlamydia* swab).
- USS:
  - endometriomata
  - adenomyosis
  - fibroids
  - PID sequelae, e.g. tubo-ovarian abscess
  - congenital abnormalities.
- Laparoscopy is usually reserved for women with USS abnormalities, medical treatment failures, or those with concomitant subfertility.

Trial of hormonal therapy

When no disease is identified then ovulation suppression by tricycling COCP, or GnRH analogues for up to 6–12mths will limit the number of 'periods' and therefore pain. This is an empirical trial of hormonal therapy.

▶ Pain clinic, psychological support, and self-help groups may be of benefit to some women who wish to maintain their fertility, especially when they have other pelvic pain symptoms.

1° dysmenorrhoea

Pain in the menstrual cycle is a feature of ovulatory cycles and is due to uterine vasospasm and ischaemia, nervous sensitization due to PGs and other inflammatory mediators, and uterine contractions. A maternal or sibling history of dysmenorrhoea is very common and the problem usually starts soon after menarche. Theories accounting for 1° dysmenorrhoea include:

* Abnormal PG ratios or sensitivity.
* Neuropathic dysregulation.
* Venous pelvic congestion.
* Psychological causes.

2° dysmenorrhoea

Underlying causes include:
* Endometriosis.
* Adenomyosis.
* PID.
* Pelvic adhesions.
* Fibroids (though not always causal).
* Cervical stenosis (iatrogenic post-LLETZ or instrumentation).
* Asherman's syndrome.
* Congenital abnormalities causing genital tract obstruction, e.g. non-communicating cornua.

Management of dysmenorrhoea

* Appropriate reassurance and analgesia may be all that is required.
* Symptom control:
  * mefenamic acid 500mg tds with each period is effective
  * COCP to abolish ovulation, tricycling will minimize periods
  * Mirena® IUS and other progestogens
  * paracetamol, hot-water bottles, etc., may be helpful for some
  * TENS, vitamin B_1, and magnesium may be of benefit to some women.
* Treat any underlying causes:
  * endometriosis—COCP, progestogens, GnRH analogues
  * antibiotics for PID
  * relief of obstruction (usually surgical).
* *Therapeutic laparoscopy—for above indications:* gold standard for diagnosis + management of endometriosis/adhesions/complicated PID.
* Hysterectomy is now rare for this indication alone.
* Laparoscopic uterine nerve ablation (LUNA) is not currently recommended.

Dysfunctional uterine bleeding: scope of the problem

Dysfunctional uterine bleeding (DUB) is a diagnosis of exclusion and is defined as any abnormal uterine bleeding in the absence of pregnancy, genital tract pathology, or systemic disease.

- Heavy menstrual bleeding (HMB, previously referred to as menorrhagia) is the commonest symptom and DUB will ultimately be the cause in 50–60% of women with this symptom.
- DUB is responsible for 15–20% of gynaecological referrals to hospital and an even higher proportion of GP gynae consultations.

▶ *Objective measures of blood loss >80mL are clinically meaningless and should not be used outside research.*

▶ *If women report their periods are unacceptably heavy, then they are!*

Aetiology

The exact causes of DUB are unknown. Proposed mechanisms at the endometrial level include:
- Abnormal PG ratios (+ other inflammatory mediators) favouring vasodilatation and platelet non-aggregation.
- Excessive fibrinolysis.
- Defects in expression/function of matrix metalloproteinases (MMPs), vascular growth factors, and endothelins.
- Aberrant steroid receptor function.
- Defects in the endomyometrial junctional zone.

The medical treatments tend to reflect the underlying pathologies (⊖ Dysfunctional uterine bleeding: diagnosis and investigations, p. 586).

DUB at a glance

- HMB is the commonest gynaecological symptom you will see, and most of these women will have DUB.
- DUB is an umbrella term and only diagnosed after exclusion of pathology.
- Women with a history of HMB without other related symptoms (IMB, pelvic pain/pressure symptoms) can have pharmacological treatment without physical examination (unless Mirena® IUS is chosen).
- TV USS or hysteroscopy is the 1st line investigation depending on the woman's symptoms.
- In the presence of erratic bleeding or risk factors for endometrial pathology (IMB, infrequent bleeding who are obese/PCOS, taking tamoxifen or if treatment for HMB has failed) offer an outpatient hysteroscopy + endometrial biopsy.
- The majority of women will respond to medical therapy, especially tranexamic ± mefenamic acid.
- The Mirena® IUS is an excellent treatment that significantly ↓ the number of women requiring surgery.
- Surgery should only be used in women who have completed their family and have had failed adequate medical therapy.
- *Endometrial ablation:* microwave endometrial ablation (MEA), balloon ablation, or NovaSure® are easy to perform and should be offered before hysterectomy.
- Hysterectomy (laparoscopic preferred to vaginal/open) has higher morbidity and cost, but is a guaranteed cure, and long-term satisfaction rates are high.

Differential diagnosis for DUB

- Submucous fibroids.
- Adenomyosis.
- Endometrial polyps, hyperplasia, or cancer.
- Very rarely, hypothyroidism or coagulation defects.

Dysfunctional uterine bleeding: diagnosis and investigations

Diagnosis

Symptoms
- Heavy and/or prolonged vaginal bleeding (with clots and flooding): irregular, heavy periods usually occur at the extremes of reproductive life (post-menarche and perimenopausal).
- May be associated with dysmenorrhoea.
- Symptoms of anaemia and disruption of life due to bleeding.
- A smear history and contraceptive use are vital information.

⚠ Totally erratic bleeding, IMB, or PCB should prompt a search for cervical or endometrial pathology.

Clinical signs
- Anaemia.
- Abdominopelvic examination is usually normal:
  - if the uterus is significantly enlarged, fibroids are likely.

Investigations

▶ *Pregnancy should always be considered and excluded.*

⚠ Refer women using 'suspected cancer pathway referral' (seen within 2wks) for endometrial cancer if has PMB.
- FBC (Hb + MCV).
- Ferritin, TFTs, and clotting screens are *not* routine investigations:
  - only consider if clinically indicated.
- Cervical smears not done opportunistically if smear history normal.
- STI screen including *Chlamydia*.
- Start pharmacological treatment for HMB without further investigations if the history ± examination suggests the woman is low risk for fibroids, uterine cavity abnormalities, histological abnormality, or adenomyosis.
- If risk factors for endometrial disease (e.g. IMB, infrequent bleeding in women who are obese, have PCOS, or are taking tamoxifen), or if no clinical response:
  - TV USS: looking for fibroids, polyps, and endometrial thickness (▶ risk of endometrial pathology with a normal TV USS is small, but it may be less accurate during menstruation)
  - hysteroscopy and biopsy (outpatient) may be appropriate as above or if there is no response to initial medical treatment
  - endometrial biopsy should only be taken in context of hysteroscopy, a 'blind' sample is not recommended
  - hysteroscopy is recommended with DUB in a woman if USS reveals focal pathology, e.g. polyp, or is unable to assess the whole endometrium, biopsy is inadequate, or bleeding is persistent or repeated.

Dysfunctional uterine bleeding: medical management

Regular DUB

Includes fibroids <3cm/suspected adenomyosis.

Mirena® IUS

- Releases measured doses of levonorgestrel into the endometrial cavity for 5yrs inducing an atrophic endometrium:
  - blood loss ↓ by up to 90% and ~30% will be amenorrhoeic at 12mths.
- Provides contraception.
- *Side effects:*
  - insertional issues
  - irregular PV bleeding for 1st 4–6mths (usually abates)
  - progestogenic side effects are rare due to minimal systemic absorption.

▶ This IUS has resulted in a major ↓ in number of hysterectomies.

Antifibrinolytics

- Tranexamic acid 1g tds days 1–4 (40% ↓ in loss):
  - safe, non-hormonal, non-contraceptive
  - *side effects*—leg cramps, minor gastrointestinal upset
  - caution in cardiac disease.

NSAIDs

- Mefenamic acid 500mg tds days 1–5 (20–30% ↓ in loss and significant ↓ in dysmenorrhoea):
  - safe, non-hormonal/contraceptive
  - *side effects*—GI upset including ulceration, renal impairment
  - caution if asthmatic, cardiovascular disease, renal impairment, peptic ulcer.

COCP

- 20–30% ↓ loss and improvement in dysmenorrhoea:
  - provides contraception
  - for cautions and side effects ➲ Combined oral contraceptive pill: overview, p. 704.

Oral progestogens

- Are generally of no benefit in regular menorrhagia other than short-term continuous treatment to stop bleeding.

Irregular DUB

- Mirena® IUS: as above.
- Tranexamic and mefenamic acid are useful to ↓ loss during periods.
- COCP will also regulate an irregular cycle (safe up to the menopause if no other cardiovascular risk factors).
- Cyclical (days 5–26) norethisterone 5mg tds or medroxyprogesterone acetate 5–10mg tds:
  - regulates cycle, but little evidence to suggest ↓ in loss
  - *side effects*—bloating, headache
- Where 1st-line therapy has failed, further medical treatment may be used in very anaemic women, bleeding continuously, having their life disrupted, or who have cautions or contraindications to surgery.
- GnRH analogues can achieve amenorrhoea quickly by inducing a medical menopausal state: *side effects*—vasomotor symptoms and use limited to 6–12mths maximum due to bone loss.
- *High-dose progestogens:* medroxyprogesterone acetate 10mg tds continuously will induce amenorrhoea, but may be time-limited due to side effects as before.

▶ Danazol and etamsylate are no longer indicated.

Choice of management for DUB

This will depend on:
- Treatment being directed to symptom relief and improved quality of life.
- A woman's wishes for treatment being of prime importance.
- Her reproductive wishes and contraceptive needs.
- Whether her periods are regular or irregular.

▶ *Many women may just need reassurance that there is no serious cause. Women may continue medical treatments for as long as they are beneficial.*

▶ *Anaemia should be corrected by treating the underlying cause of bleeding and using ferrous sulfate (or equivalent) to replace lost iron stores.*

Further reading

NICE (2018, updated 2021). Heavy menstrual bleeding: assessment and management. NICE guideline [NG88].
♪ www.nice.org.uk/guidance/ng88/

Dysfunctional uterine bleeding: surgical management

* Surgery should be reserved for the minority of women who fail to respond to medical management.
* Appropriate for symptomatic submucosal fibroids.

⚠ Women have to be certain their families are complete before surgery or ablation.

Endometrial ablation

Destruction of the endometrium down to the basalis layer is effective for most women and should be offered to all for consideration.
Methods include:
* Microwave (MEA).
* Thermal balloon (Thermachoice®).
* NovaSure® (electrical impedance).

▶ *Hysteroscopic resection, or rollerball ablation, are now used much less often due to ↑ operative complications.*

⚠ *Endometrial ablation is less effective if the endometrial cavity is >10cm.*

* Typical endometrial ablation results in normal size cavities:
  * 80–90% of women are significantly improved
  * 30% will become amenorrhoeic
  * 20% will need a 2nd procedure by 5yrs.
* The above-listed newer procedures are generally very safe and straightforward; however, there is a small risk of bleeding, infection, uterine perforation, and failed procedure.
* They are generally carried out under GA, but may occasionally be done under cervical block.

Hysteroscopic removal of fibroids/polyps

* Transcervical resection of submucosal fibroid/polyp using electrical energy.

Uterine artery embolization

* Non-surgical way of shrinking fibroids.
* Performed by radiologist.

Myomectomy

* Removal of intramural or subserosal fibroids.
* Performed laparoscopically or open.
* Can maintain fertility.

Ulipristal acetate

* 5mg (up to four courses).
* Shrinks fibroid size.
* Risk of serious liver injury during use.
* Only indicated if patient is not eligible for surgery (risks of surgery outweigh risks of liver damage).

Hysterectomy

- Hysterectomy is the only guaranteed cure for DUB, but RCTs have shown higher morbidity, longer recovery, and financial costs compared to endometrial ablation.
- Complications include:
  - haemorrhage
  - infection
  - bladder, ureteric, or bowel injury (<1%)
  - death is extremely rare

▶ *Long-term satisfaction rates for hysterectomy are generally very high and regardless of method most women report improved sexual function—as one patient put it, 'I actually have sex now I'm not bleeding all the time'.*

Current evidence regarding method of hysterectomy

- When discussing hysterectomy (laparotomy, vaginal, or laparoscopy) and deciding whether a total versus subtotal hysterectomy is performed, an individual assessment and the woman's preferences should be taken into account.
- Ovarian removal at the time of hysterectomy should only be performed after a thorough discussion of the risks and benefits.
- If a subtotal hysterectomy is performed, the woman should be warned that there is a small risk of continuing light menstruation if residual endometrial cells are left and that the woman will require cervical smear tests as per screening guidance.

Premenstrual syndrome: overview

In the general population, 40% of women have premenstrual syndrome (PMS) symptoms, 5–8% severe.

Any definition of PMS should include:

- Distressing psychological, physical, and/or behavioural symptoms:
  - typical psychological symptoms can be depression, anxiety, irritability, loss of confidence, and mood swings
  - typical physical symptoms include bloatedness and mastalgia.
- Occurrence during the luteal phase of the menstrual cycle (or cyclically after hysterectomy with ovarian conservation).
- Significant regression of symptoms with onset of or during the period.

Aetiology

Probable multiple aetiologies, but cyclical ovarian activity is likely to be the central component (ovarian 'trigger', such as ovulation, may initiate a cascade of events). A central ↑ responsiveness to a combination of steroids, chemical messengers (E2/serotonin, progesterone/GABA), and psychological sensitivity may play a part.

Diagnosis

- Most women self-diagnose.
- A detailed history can suggest a diagnosis of PMS, but only prospective assessment with a symptom diary for at least two consecutive menstrual cycles can establish its true nature.
- The Daily Record of Severity of Problems (DRSP) is the most commonly used symptom diary.
- GnRH analogues can be used for 3 months to establish a definitive diagnosis in difficult cases.

▶ It is important to exclude organic disease and significant psychiatric illness.

▶ Perimenopausal women may have ↑ premenstrual symptoms as well as menopausal symptoms.

Classification of PMS

Patient records at least two consecutive menstrual cycles worth of menstrual symptoms:

- *Physiological (mild) premenstrual disorder:*
  - cyclical symptoms relieved by menstruation
  - has a symptom-free wk
  - no influence on quality of life.
- *Core premenstrual disorder:*
  - cyclical symptoms relieved by menstruation
  - has a symptom-free wk
  - affects quality of life.
- *Premenstrual exacerbation:*
  - cyclical symptoms relieved by menstruation
  - no symptom-free wk as has existing non-menstrual condition
  - affects quality of life.
- *Premenstrual disorder with absent menstruation:*
  - as per core premenstrual disorder but no menstruation
  - management is the same.
- *Progestogen-induced premenstrual disorder:*
  - cyclical symptoms relieved by menstruation
  - symptom-free wk
  - affects quality of life
  - taking progesterone treatment.
- *Non-ovulatory premenstrual disorder:*
  - symptoms in the presence of ovarian activity, but without ovulation.
- *Underlying psychological disorder:*
  - non-cyclical symptoms
  - no symptom-free wk
  - constant influence on quality of life.

Further reading

National Association for Premenstrual Syndromes.
℘ www.pms.org.uk

RCOG (2016). Premenstrual syndrome, management. Green-top guideline no. 48
℘ www.rcog.org.uk/en/guidelines-research-services/guidelines/gtg48/

Premenstrual syndrome: management

Hormonal

Progesterone and progestogens

- 2nd-generation progesterone pills (levonorgestrel/norethisterone) can worsen PMS symptoms, hence the majority of COCPs will not help.
- Drospirenone, which is an anti-mineralocorticoid and antiandrogen, has been demonstrated to ↓ severity of symptoms.

Ovulation suppression agents

- *COCP:* Yasmin® contains drospirenone with a better side effect profile, and no pill-free interval may be more therapeutic.
- *Danazol:* benefit reported for PMS, but there are significant masculinizing side effects. Treatment in luteal phase only is effective for breast tenderness.
- *Oestrogen:* transdermal oestrogen or implants at doses sufficient to suppress ovulation are not currently licensed, but they are a well-established and accepted treatment. Estradiol patch 100 micrograms twice weekly with a progestogen (cyclical basis). Implants are generally unsuitable for those who may wish to conceive.
- *GnRH analogues ± add back HRT:* are of proven benefit for moderate to severe PMS, but with a licence for 6mths treatment only due to bone loss. Usually given with add back tibolone (fewer side effects and bone loss). 'GnRH test' useful for those considering hysterectomy and bilateral salpingo-oophorectomy (BSO) for severe symptoms.

Non-hormonal

- *SSRIs/selective noradrenalin reuptake inhibitors:* a meta-analysis confirms benefit for continuous and luteal phase only treatment. No current licence in the UK so careful documentation is required as some women are reluctant to accept antidepressants. Side effects may be problematic, but are ↓ by luteal phase-only dosing.
- *Antidepressants:* tricyclics and anxiolytics have benefits for selected patients as indicated in at least nine studies.
- *Spironolactone:* can be helpful in treating physical symptoms.

Surgery

Trials have confirmed a benefit of removal of the ovarian trigger with the uterus to avoid the need for combined HRT as definitive treatment for severe PMS. However, it is generally recommended that a 'GnRH test' is performed to ensure that a benefit will be realized and/or another indication for hysterectomy is present. Testosterone replacement may be useful as ovaries supply 50%, and low levels can lead to distressing low libido.

Self-help techniques for managing PMS

It is important to acknowledge the 40% placebo response rate while evaluating evidence for certain treatments.

Dietary alteration—possible benefit with less fat, sugar, salt, caffeine, and alcohol, frequent starchy meals, more fibre, fruit, and vegetables, and 4-hourly small snacks.

Dietary supplements

- Vitamin B_6: possible benefit for PMS symptoms. Dose restricted to 10mg daily as high doses can lead to peripheral neuropathy.
- Vitamin E: studies small, but promising.
- Calcium: two studies (1200–1600mg) revealed some improvement in symptoms.
- Magnesium: appears most beneficial in the premenstrual phase.
- Evening primrose oil: of value for mastalgia only.
- Isoflavones: show mixed results and may benefit menstrual migraine.
- Saffron: does show benefit in a small study.

Exercise

Moderate regular aerobic exercise promoting cardiovascular work is beneficial (three controlled studies).

Stress reduction

Relaxation techniques, yoga, meditation, breathing techniques, and encouragement of healthier lifestyle may also help.

Cognitive behavioural therapy

Several studies have indicated a long-term benefit for women with PMS. It should be considered routinely as a treatment option.

Complementary and alternative therapies used in PMS

- Acupuncture: +ve data for dysmenorrhoea.
- Homeopathy: in a pilot study ($n = 20$), improvement in 90% compared to placebo.
- Phytoestrogens: possible benefit for PMS symptoms (may be difficult to incorporate into a Western diet).
- Vitex agnus-castus L.: demonstrates benefit but there is no standardized preparation.
- Ginkgo biloba: some benefit.
- St John's wort: may benefit symptoms, avoid use if on SSRIs.
- Mind–body: aromatherapy, reflexology, photic stimulation, and magnotherapy may show some benefit, but data are sparse.

Further reading

National Association for Premenstrual Syndromes.
ℛ www.pms.org.uk

Chapter 16

Early pregnancy problems

Termination of pregnancy: overview

Around 200,000 TOPs are performed annually in England, Wales, and Scotland; >98% of these are undertaken under clause C—risk of injury to the physical or mental health of the woman (Box 16.1). At least 1/3 of British women will have had a TOP by the time they reach 45yrs of age.

Box 16.1 UK law

Legislation varies throughout the world, with terminations remaining illegal in some countries. The Abortion Act 1967 states that TOP is legal in the UK if two doctors decide in good faith that in relation to a particular pregnancy one or more of the following grounds are met:

- *A:* continuance of the pregnancy would involve risk to life of pregnant woman greater than if pregnancy were terminated.
- *B:* termination is necessary to prevent grave permanent injury to physical or mental health of pregnant woman.
- *C:* pregnancy has not exceeded 24th wk and continuance of the pregnancy would involve risk, greater than if pregnancy were terminated, of injury to physical or mental health of pregnant woman.
- *D:* pregnancy has not exceeded 24th wk and continuance of pregnancy would involve risk, greater than if pregnancy were terminated, of injury to physical or mental health of any existing child(ren) of family of pregnant woman.
- *E:* there is a substantial risk that if the child were born it would suffer from such physical or mental abnormalities as to be seriously handicapped.

▶ Clauses A, B, and E have no time limit.
▶ Clauses C and D have a legal limit of 24wks.

Do doctors have an obligation to participate in TOPs?

According to the GMC:
- Doctors must ensure their personal beliefs do not prejudice patient care.
- Doctors have the right to decline to participate in TOPs on grounds of conscientious objection. If so, they must always refer the patient to another doctor who will help.

What about patients <16yrs?

Patients <16yrs should be encouraged to involve their parents, but provided they are considered to be Fraser competent, they can give their own consent.

Termination of pregnancy: methods

Method of TOP depends on gestation of pregnancy and the woman's choice. Procedures offered also vary from one centre to another (usually determined by local resources).

Surgical

<7wks

- Conventional suction termination should be avoided.
- Vacuum aspiration, either electric or manual, is effective and acceptable.

7–13wks

- Conventional suction termination or vacuum aspiration is appropriate, although, the skill and experience of the practitioner may make medical TOP more appropriate at gestations >12wks.

>13wks

- Dilatation and evacuation following cervical preparation:
  - requires skilled practitioners (with necessary instruments and large enough case load to maintain skills)
  - ↑ gestation, ↑ risk of bleeding, incomplete evacuation, and perforation.
- Cervical preparation is highly beneficial in all cases:
  - it ↓ difficulties with cervical dilation
  - particularly if patient is <18yrs or gestation is >10wks.
- Possible regimens include:
  - misoprostol 400 micrograms PV 3h prior to surgery *or*
  - gemeprost 1mg PV 3h prior to surgery *or*
  - mifepristone 600mg PO 36–48h prior to surgery
  - osmotic dilators—recommended after 14wks.

💣 Outpatient vacuum aspiration under local anaesthesia at some centres is safe in experienced hands, cheaper and avoids the need for GA.

Medical

<9wks

- Using mifepristone priming plus a PG regimen is the most effective method of TOP in gestation.

9–13wks

- Appropriate, safe, and effective alternative to surgery.
- Incomplete procedure rates ↑ after 9wks.

13–24wks

- Appropriate, safe, and effective in this group.
- Feticide should be considered in advanced gestations (>20wks).

Medications used in TOP

Mifepristone
- Antiprogesterone (given 24–48h prior), which results in:
  - uterine contractions
  - bleeding from the placental bed
  - sensitization of uterus to PGs.
- Its use has been shown to ↓ the treatment to delivery interval in medical TOP.

Misoprostol
- PGE1 analogue.
- Used off-licence in medical TOP and for cervical preparation prior to surgical TOP.
- It stimulates uterine contractions.

Gemeprost
- PGE1 analogue.
- It is licensed for softening and dilatation of the cervix before surgical TOP in the 1st trimester and for therapeutic TOP in the 2nd trimester.
- ➲ Box 16.2, p. 603, for side effects.

Termination of pregnancy: management

Considerations before termination of pregnancy

Counselling/support
- Women should receive verbal advice and written information.
- Patients who may require additional support or counselling (evidence of coercion, poor social support, or psychiatric history) should be identified and additional care offered.

Blood tests
- Hb.
- Blood group and antibodies.
- If clinically indicated, HIV, HBV, HCV, haemoglobinopathies.

USS
- Good practice for all TOPs to:
  - give accurate gestation
  - identify already non-viable and ectopic pregnancies (EPs).

Prevention of infection
- Strategy for minimizing risk of post-abortion infection is important.
- May include screening for lower genital tract infections, such as *Chlamydia* (with treatment and contact tracing if +ve).

Prophylactic antibiotic regimens used for TOP
- Metronidazole 1g PR at time of TOP, plus doxycycline 100mg PO bd for 7 days, commencing on day of TOP.
- Metronidazole 1g PR at time of TOP, plus azithromycin 1g PO on day of TOP.

Following TOP
- Anti-D should be given to all Rh –ve women undergoing medical or surgical TOP:
  - 250IU ≤20wks
  - 500IU >20wks.
- Routine histopathological examination of tissue obtained at TOP is not recommended.
- Provide written patient information, which should include:
  - symptoms that may be experienced following TOP
  - symptoms requiring further medical attention
  - contact numbers.
- Follow-up within 2wks of TOP.
- Refer for further counselling if required.
- Discuss and prescribe/provide ongoing contraception.

Box 16.2 Complications of TOP
- Significant bleeding needing transfusion (1–4:1000).
- Genital tract infection (5–10%).
- Uterine perforation (surgical TOP: 1–4:1000).
- Uterine rupture (mid-trimester medical TOP: <1:1000).
- Cervical trauma (surgical TOP: 1:100).
- Failed TOP (surgical: 2.3:1000; medical: 1–14:1000).
- Retained products of conception (1:100).
- Nausea, vomiting, diarrhoea due to PGs:
  - occasional, but transient.
- Psychological sequelae:
  - short-term anxiety and depressed mood.
- Long-term regret and concern about future fertility has been shown to be common.

Further reading
British Pregnancy Advisory Service (BPAS). Abortion care. Tel. 0345 7304030.
🖱 www.bpas.org

Family Planning Association. Tel. 0300 1237123.
🖱 www.fpa.org.uk

Marie Stopes International UK. Tel. 0345 3008090.
🖱 www.mariestopes.org.uk

RCOG (2011). The care of women requesting induced abortion. Green-top guideline no. 7.
🖱 www.rcog.org.uk/guidance/browse-all-guidance/other-guidelines-and-reports/the-care-of-women-requesting-induced-abortion-evidence-based-clinical-guideline-no-7/

Bleeding in early pregnancy and miscarriage

Bleeding in early pregnancy may be associated with:
- Miscarriage.
- EP.
- Gestational trophoblastic disease.
- Rarely gynaecological lower tract pathology (e.g. *Chlamydia*, cervical cancer, or a polyp).

Miscarriage

- Miscarriage is common, occurring in at least 15–20% of pregnancies (Table 16.1).
- Possibly up to 40% of all conceptions.
- Defined as the expulsion of a pregnancy, embryo, or fetus at a stage of pregnancy when it is incapable of independent survival:
  - includes all pregnancy losses before 24wks
  - the vast majority are before 12wks.

Early pregnancy assessment units (EPAUs)

- TVS and serum hCG estimations are invaluable in the diagnosis of early pregnancy problems.
- These should be readily available in dedicated EPAUs.
- TVS provides the definitive diagnosis if a miscarriage is not clinically apparent.
- These units allow for timely assessment, with easy access from the community, improved continuity of care, and fewer admissions.
- Work on the psychological impact of early pregnancy problems demonstrates a major improvement in care with good EPAU care.

Anti-D prophylaxis

Anti-D should be given to all non-sensitized Rh –ve patients in the following circumstances:
- *<12wks:*
  - uterine evacuation (medical and surgical)
  - EPs
  - 250IU IM.
- *>12wks:*
  - all women with bleeding
  - 250IU IM before 20wks and 500IU IM after 20wks.

➔ Rhesus isoimmunization (immune hydrops), p. 130.

Table 16.1 Classification of miscarriage

	Clinical	USS findings	Management
Threatened miscarriage	• PVB ± pain • Closed cervix	• Intrauterine gestation sac • Fetal pole • Fetal heart +ve	• Anti-D if >12wks, heavy PVB or pain • If PVB persists >2wks attend for TVS
Complete miscarriage	• Bleeding and pain cease • Closed cervix	• Empty uterus • Endometrial thickness <15 mm	• Anti-D if >12wks • Serum hCG to exclude EP • Review if PVB persists >2wks and consider endometritis or retained products of conception
Incomplete miscarriage	• Bleeding ± pain • Possible open cervix	• Heterogeneous tissues ± gestation sac • Any endometrial thickness	• Expectant preferable but can be medical/surgical • Anti-D if >12wks, heavy PVB, pain or medical/surgical management
Missed miscarriage/ early fetal demise	• Bleeding ± pain ± loss of pregnancy symptoms • Closed cervix	• Fetal pole >7*mm with no fetal heart • Mean gestation sac diameter >25*mm with no fetal pole or yolk sac	• Seek 2nd opinion on viability or if not available rescan in 7 days • Expectant/medical/surgical • Anti-D if >12wks or medical/surgical management
Inevitable miscarriage	• Bleeding ± pain • Open cervix	• Intrauterine gestation sac ± fetal pole ± fetal heart activity	• Expectant/medical/surgical • Anti-D if >12wks or heavy PVB or pain or medical/surgical management
Pregnancy of uncertain viability	• ± Bleeding ± pain • Closed cervix	• Intrauterine gestation sac <25*mm with no fetal pole or yolk sac • Fetal echo with CRL <7*mm with no fetal heart	• Rescan in 1wk • Anti-D if heavy PVB or pain
Pregnancy of unknown location (PUL)	• ± Bleeding ± pain • Closed cervix	• +ve pregnancy test • Empty uterus • No sign of extrauterine pregnancy	• Serial serum hCG assay (48h apart) + initial serum progesterone level to exclude EP/failing PUL • Anti-D if heavy bleeding

* Until further research establishes definitive, safe parameters these should be used and all patients should have a 2nd scan prior to an evacuation procedure.

Miscarriage: management

Expectant management

- Appropriate 1st-line management for 7–14 days (in those women who are not bleeding heavily and at low risk of haemorrhage, e.g. early 1st trimester or no evidence of infection).
- Highly effective for an incomplete miscarriage.
- With an intact sac, resolution may take several wks and may be less effective.
- A repeat TVS should be offered at 2wks to ensure complete miscarriage:
  - can be repeated after another 2wks if a woman wishes to continue with expectant management.
- Patients should be offered surgical evacuation at a later date if unsuccessful.

Medical management

- PG analogues (usually misoprostol) are used:
  - administered orally or vaginally.
- Bleeding may continue for up to 3wks after medical uterine evacuation, but completion rates up to 80–90% can be expected at <9wks gestation.

⚠ Women should be warned that passage of pregnancy tissue may be associated with pain and heavy bleeding (though unusual) so 24h telephone advice and facilities for admission should be available.

Surgical management of miscarriage (SMM)

- SMM should be performed in patients who:
  - have excessive or persistent bleeding
  - request surgical management.
- Choice of manual vacuum aspiration under local anaesthesia in outpatient setting surgical management in theatre under GA.
- Suction curettage should be used.
- In UK practice, a Human Tissue Act (HTA) form needs to be signed by the patient and a copy sent with the pregnancy tissue to histology, this outlines the patient's wishes regarding disposal of the tissue.

Complications of surgical management of miscarriage

- Infection.
- Haemorrhage.
- Uterine perforation (and rarely intraperitoneal injury).
- Retained products of conception.
- Intrauterine adhesions.
- Cervical tears.
- Intra-abdominal trauma.

▶ Uterine and cervical trauma may be minimized by administering PG (misoprostol or gemeprost) before the procedure.

Psychological sequelae

- Miscarriage is usually very distressing.
- Offer appropriate support and counselling, and written information.

Further reading

Association of Early Pregnancy Units.
🖰 www.earlypregnancy.org.uk

Miscarriage Association.
🖰 www.miscarriageassociation.org.uk

NICE (2019). Ectopic pregnancy and miscarriage. NICE guideline [NG126].
🖰 www.nice.org.uk/guidance/ng126/

Post-miscarriage counselling: patient's FAQs

What did I do to cause it?

Nothing. It was not stress at work, carrying heavy shopping, having sex, or any other reason women commonly worry about. Sadly, miscarriages happen in up to about 40% of pregnancies.

If I had had a scan earlier could you have stopped it happening?

No, we might have found out it was happening sooner, but we could not have stopped it. There is no effective treatment available to stop a 1st-trimester miscarriage.

How bad will the pain be if I opt for expectant management?

It will be like severe period pain, which comes to a peak when tissue is being passed, then settles down shortly afterwards. Ibuprofen, paracetamol, or codeine should help and may be taken. If pain is very bad, contact hospital for advice.

What is heavy bleeding?

Soaking >3 heavy sanitary pads in <1h or passing a clot larger than the palm of your hand. If you bleed heavily, you should seek medical attention urgently.

How long will I bleed for?

It should gradually get less and less but may be up to 3wks after the miscarriage before the bleeding stops completely.

Do I need bed rest afterwards?

No, not necessarily, but obviously it can be physically and emotionally draining so a few days off work may help. You can return to normal activities as soon as you feel ready.

How long will the pregnancy test remain positive?

hCG is excreted by the kidneys and it can take up to 3wks after a miscarriage for it all to be removed from the bloodstream and a pregnancy test to record as –ve.

How long before we can try again?

There is no good evidence that the outcome of a subsequent pregnancy is affected by how soon you conceive after a miscarriage. As long as you have had either a period or a –ve pregnancy test since you miscarried, you can try again as soon as you feel physically and emotionally ready.

Does this make me more likely to have another miscarriage?

There are a very small number of women who will have recurrent miscarriages, but for the vast majority, next time they get pregnant they will face the same odds: 40% risk of miscarriage and 60% chance of a baby.

Ectopic pregnancy: diagnosis

⚠ *ALL women of reproductive age are pregnant until proved otherwise and it is ectopic until demonstrated to be intrauterine.*

- *Definition:* implantation of a conceptus outside the uterine cavity.
- *Incidence:* 11:1000 pregnancies and ↑:
  - 93–95% tubal; the remainder are in CD scars, interstitial, abdominal, ovarian, or cervical
  - ↑ probably due to early presentation, with the advent of EPAUs.
- *Symptoms* (Box 16.3):
  - often asymptomatic, e.g. unsure dates
  - amenorrhoea (usually 6–8wks)
  - pain (lower abdominal, often mild/vague, classically unilateral)
  - vaginal bleeding (usually small amount, often brown)
  - diarrhoea and vomiting should never be ignored
  - dizziness and light-headedness
  - shoulder tip pain (diaphragmatic irritation—haemoperitoneum)
  - collapse (if ruptured).
- *Signs:*
  - often have no specific signs
  - uterus usually normal size
  - cervical excitation and adnexal tenderness occasionally
  - adnexal mass very rarely
  - peritonism (due to intra-abdominal blood if ectopic ruptured).

⚠ There is no evidence that examining patients may lead to rupture of the EP. It is more important to examine them so you do not miss significant abdominal or pelvic tenderness.

Differential diagnosis includes threatened or complete miscarriage, bleeding corpus luteal cyst, ovarian cyst accident, and pelvic inflammation.

- Risk factors are shown in Box 16.4.

Investigations

- *TVS/USS:* establish the location, presence of adnexal masses or free fluid: a good EPAU will positively identify EP on TVS in 90% of cases, rather than the absence of an intrauterine gestation. Up to 20% of EP have a pseudosac.
- *Serum progesterone:* helpful to distinguish whether a pregnancy is failing: <20nmol/L is highly suggestive of this, whether EP or intrauterine pregnancy (IUP).
- *Serum hCG:* repeated 48h later:
  - the rate of rise is important
  - a rise of ≥66% suggests an IUP
  - a suboptimal rise is suspicious, but *not* diagnostic of an EP.
- *Laparoscopy:* gold standard, but should only be necessary for clinical reasons or in a minority where a diagnosis cannot be made (remember TVS/USS should pick up 90%!)

Box 16.3 Symptoms of ectopic pregnancy

- Tend to have a poor +ve predictive value to help discriminate between intra- and extrauterine pregnancy.
- The majority of women with an EP will be clinically well and stable with minimal symptoms and signs.

⚠ All women with a + ve pregnancy test should therefore be considered to have an EP until proved otherwise.

---

hCG values and USS

▶ *At serum hCG ≥1500IU, an IUP should be seen with TV USS.*

⚠ However, there is considerable variation in normal IUPs and this is a guide only—care is needed to avoid harming an early IUP.
▶ The rate of change is more important than any one value.

Box 16.4 Risk factors for ectopic pregnancy

▶ May be present in 25–50% of patients (therefore majority will have *no* obvious risk factors):
- History of infertility or assisted conception.
- History of PID.
- Endometriosis.
- Pelvic or tubal surgery.
- Previous ectopic (recurrence risk 10–20%).
- IUCD, IUS, or progesterone-based contraception.
- Assisted conception, especially IVF.
- Smoking.

Further reading

NICE (2019, updated 2021). Ectopic pregnancy and miscarriage. NICE guideline [NG126]. ℘ www.nice.org.uk/guidance/ng126/

RCOG (2016). Diagnosis and management of ectopic pregnancy. Green-top guideline no. 21. ℘ https://www.rcog.org.uk/en/guidelines-research-services/guidelines/gtg21/

Ectopic pregnancy: management

Expectant and medical management are safe options even with a diagnosed EP if there are strict selection criteria:
- Clinically stable.
- Asymptomatic or minimal symptoms.
- No fetal cardiac activity on TV USS.
- No haemoperitoneum on TV USS.
- Fully understand symptoms and implications of EP.
- Language should not be a barrier to understanding or communicating to a 3rd party (such as phoning an ambulance).
- Live in close proximity to the hospital and have support at home.
- You deem the patient will not default on follow-up.

Expectant
- Initial hCG <1500IU which is falling and fulfilling the above-listed criteria.
- 30% of tubal EPs can be managed expectantly with a 70% success rate.
- EP <30mm.
- Requires serum hCG initially every 48h until repeated fall in level:
  - then weekly until <15IU.
- With a plateauing hCG, as long as they remain clinically well it is perfectly acceptable to wait as the hCG will usually decline if given time as the pregnancy fails—hCG measurement is as above.
- With slow rising hCG in asymptomatic patient, a decision for expectant management should only be made by a senior early pregnancy unit clinician.

Medical
- EP <35mm and initial hCG <5000IU.
- Methotrexate is given IM as a single dose of 50mg/m². hCG levels are measured at 4 and 7 days, and another dose given (up to 25% of cases) if the ↓ in hCG is <15% between days 4–7.
- Measure hCG weekly until <15IU.

⚠ Women should be given clear, written information about adverse effects and the possible need for further treatment. They should use reliable contraception for 3mths after, as methotrexate is teratogenic.

Surgical
- Laparoscopy is preferable to laparotomy as it has shorter operating times and hospital stays, ↓ analgesia requirements, and ↓ blood loss.

⚠ In haemodynamically unstable patients, laparotomy may be more appropriate, if deemed to be quicker.
- Salpingectomy is preferable to salpingotomy when the contralateral tube and ovary appear normal.
  - No difference in subsequent IUP rates, but salpingectomy has lower rates of persistent trophoblast and recurrent EP.
- If visible contralateral tubal disease, laparoscopic salpingotomy is appropriate if safe or possible.

⚠ *Remember anti-D in Rh −ve patients.*

Treatment of the haemodynamically unstable patient

Resuscitation

- Two large-bore IV lines and IV fluids (colloids or crystalloids).
- Cross-match 4U blood.
- Call senior help and anaesthetic assistance urgently.

Surgery

- Laparoscopy or laparotomy with salpingectomy once the patient has been resuscitated.

Expectant management of ectopic pregnancy

All women managed expectantly or medically should be counselled about importance of compliance with follow-up and should be within easy access of the hospital.

⚠ There is no level of hCG at which rupture cannot occur even when it is falling—symptoms and the clinical parameters are always more important than blood tests and scans!

Side effects of methotrexate

- Conjunctivitis.
- Gastrointestinal upset.
- Gastric ulceration.
- Stomatitis.
- Marrow suppression.
- Pulmonary fibrosis, pneumonitis.
- Liver cirrhosis.
- Renal failure.
- Must have reliable contraception due to high risk of fetal defects.

⚠ Some women will experience abdominal pain, which can be difficult to differentiate from the pain of a rupturing ectopic.

Less common sites for ectopic pregnancy

- Cervical, ovarian, CD scar, and interstitial pregnancies need expert input as there are no universally agreed ways to treat them.
- Generally, preference is for conservative or medical treatment, with surgical reserved for clinical need—case series report high rates of success with medical management as long as the patient is asymptomatic and stable.
- Consider referral to a regional EPAU as these units have the best experience of these rare entities.

Pregnancy of unknown location

Definition

Where there is no sign of an IUP, EP, or retained products of conception in the presence of a +ve pregnancy test or serum hCG >5IU/L.

- This is the 1st diagnosis in 10% of EPAU attenders.
- The possible outcomes can be:
  - early IUP
  - failing PUL
  - EP (6–20% of PULs)
  - persisting PUL
  - complete miscarriage
  - very, very rarely another source (hCG secreting tumours).

⚠ Even if the history is highly suggestive of a complete miscarriage having occurred, classify as a PUL until you have evidence of an IUP.

⚠ 5–10% of 'complete miscarriages' diagnosed on history alone with an empty uterus on scan, will in fact be EPs!

Presentation

- Asymptomatic.
- PV bleeding.
- Abdominal pain.

Management

- The symptoms and clinical parameters of the patient are the most important factors as for EP.
- Women with significant pain, tenderness, or a haemoperitoneum usually need laparoscopy.
- If patient is well and stable then take serum progesterone and hCG at the 1st visit, and repeat hCG after 48h.

Interpreting hCG and progesterone results in PUL

If progesterone <10nmol/L
- Likely failing pregnancy.
- Repeat serum hCG or pregnancy test in 14 days.

If hCG >50% fall from 0–48h
- Likely failing pregnancy regardless of location.
- Repeat serum hCG or pregnancy test in 14 days.

If hCG ≥66% rise from 0–48h
- Likely IUP.
- Rescan in 10–14 days.

If rise in serial hCG <66% or fall <50% or plateauing
- Possible EP.
- Close monitoring with serial hCG and TVS until diagnosis made or hCG <15 IU/L.

If hCG plateauing or fluctuating
- Persistent PUL after three consecutive samples with no diagnosis.
- Conservative management if asymptomatic or methotrexate.

If initial hCG >1500IU/L
- Probable EP.
- Consider all management options depending upon clinical need.

⚠ All the same principles and criteria of expectant and medical management of EPs apply equally to PULs.

Further reading
NICE (2019). Ectopic pregnancy and miscarriage. NICE guideline [NG126].
℘ www.nice.org.uk/guidance/ng126/

RCOG (2016). Diagnosis and management of ectopic pregnancy. Green-top guideline no. 21.
℘ https://www.rcog.org.uk/en/guidelines-research-services/guidelines/gtg21/

Understanding βhCG

βhCG is a bi-peptide secreted by the trophoblast. It is almost identical to LH, varying by one amino acid in its β subunit, hence its ability to sustain the corpus luteum. It is detectable very early and modern urinary pregnancy tests detect as little as 25IU.

What is the pattern of hCG in pregnancy?

- In normal IUPs hCG rises quickly and is of main clinical use between 4 and 8wks when it rises in a predictable manner.
- hCG should rise by ≥66% every 48h during this period.
- >8wks it will be raised but is highly variable and fluctuates.

⚠ *There is no absolutely reliable 'discriminatory zone' above which you definitely see an IUP on TVS; 1500IU is a guide only.*

- >90% of ectopics should be visible on TV USS at some point.
- On a single hCG you do not know if the level is ↑ or ↓.
- In an asymptomatic patient there is no rush to act.
- ?Multiple pregnancy (↑ hCG but no IUP seen).

hCGs at different gestations

- hCG levels for any given gestation vary too much to be clinically useful: it is the relative change that matters.
- When hCG levels are very high it is suggestive of molar pregnancy.

⚠ Molar pregnancies are diagnosed with TV USS and confirmed by histology, *not* with hCG levels, but hCG is a vital marker for subsequent monitoring and follow-up especially after chemotherapy in gestational trophoblastic disease.

(➲ Gestational trophoblastic disease: hydatidiform mole, p. 862.)

Interpreting changes in hCG

For PULs

- *hCG ≥66% rise over 48h:* probable early IUP
- *hCG fall >50% over 48h:* indicative of a failing pregnancy regardless of location.
- *<66% hCG rise or <50% fall over 48h:* possible EP.
- *hCG static:* there is still active trophoblast somewhere (production = excretion): consider most probable source given clinical picture.

⚠ Check whether it was actually 48h between tests.

⚠ Remember you are treating the patient *not* the hCG, always use hCG as a part of the whole clinical picture.

⚠ Clinical symptoms are *always* more important than any hCG levels or scan findings.

(➥ Ectopic pregnancy: management, p. 612.)

Serum hCG levels

Valid use

- For aiding diagnosis (ectopic, early intrauterine, failing pregnancy).
- Monitoring of PUL.
- Conservative and medical management of EP and persistent PULs.
- Follow-up of EP post salpingotomy/significant haemoperitoneum to exclude persistent trophoblast.
- Follow-up of women with trophoblastic disease.

▶ Remember, hCG assays are a guide to diagnosis only when a pregnancy cannot be seen on TV USS.

Inappropriate use

- Known IUPs.
- Management in women with significant symptoms—treat them clinically!
- Women who have received hCG support in assisted conception.
- Known multiple pregnancy.

⚠ '*Three strikes and you're out!*' If you do not have a diagnosis and/or management plan after three hCGs you need to ask for advice.

⚠ *Do not* bring them back in 48h for another hCG—*get help!*

Recurrent miscarriage: overview

Definition

Three or more consecutive, spontaneous miscarriages occurring in the 1st trimester with the same biological father, which may or may not follow a successful birth. Incidence is 1–2% and 50% are unexplained.

Risk factors

Advanced maternal age and ↑ number of miscarriages are two independent risk factors.

Causes

Antiphospholipid syndrome (APS)

Most important treatable cause and present in 15% of women with recurrent miscarriages. APS is defined as the presence of anticardiolipin antibodies or lupus anticoagulant antibodies on two separate occasions with any criteria listed below:

- ≥3 consecutive fetal losses before the 10th wk.
- 1 fetal loss 10wks gestation or older.
- 1 or more births of a morphologically normal fetus at <34wks associated with severe pre-eclampsia or placental insufficiency.

Genetic

In 3–5% of couples, one partner carries a balanced reciprocal or Robertsonian translocation. The carrier is phenotypically normal, but 50–75% of their gametes will be unbalanced.

Fetal chromosomal abnormalities

Can be incompatible with life. As number of pregnancies ↑, prevalence of chromosomal abnormality ↓ and chance of recurring maternal cause ↑.

Anatomical abnormalities

Frequency of congenital uterine abnormalities (uterine septa and bicornuate uterus) in the general population is unknown. Minor variations (e.g. arcuate) are 2–3%. In women with recurrent loss, prevalence is estimated to be between 2% and 8%.

Fibroids

Present in up to 30% of women, but their effect on reproductive outcome is controversial. Submucosal and intramural are thought to be more causative, though little data support this assertion.

Thrombophilic disorders

Pregnancy is a hypercoagulable state. Gene mutations in factor V Leiden and factor II prothrombin G20210A have been associated with recurrent miscarriage. Protein C and protein S deficiency similarly have a weak association.

Infection

Inconsistent link to BV with 1st-trimester losses.
Recurrent 2nd-trimester loss has a stronger association.

Endocrine disorders
Well-controlled diabetes and thyroid disease is not a risk factor nor is hypersecretion of LH in PCOS.

Cervical weakness
History of late miscarriage preceded by painless cervical dilatation is a cause of recurrent mid-trimester loss but does not appear to have an association with 1st trimester miscarriage.

Immune dysfunction
Excessive uterine natural killer (NK) cell activity is currently purely hypothetical and no link between peripheral and uterine NK activity has been proven.

Recurrent miscarriage: management

Investigations

- Parental blood for karyotyping.
- Cytogenetic analysis of products of conception (at time of miscarriage).
- Pelvic USS.
- Thrombophilia screening.
- Lupus anticoagulant (dilute Russell Viper Venom Test (dRVVT)/ activated partial thromboplastin time).
- Anticardiolipin antibodies (aCL IgG and IgM).
- Screening for BV during early pregnancy in women with 2nd-trimester miscarriage is inappropriate.
- Cervical weakness is diagnosed on history alone and may be over-diagnosed as there is no objective testing in the non-pregnant state.

▶ There is insufficient evidence for asymptomatic women to be routinely tested for thyroid disease, thyroid antibodies, diabetes, and hyperprolactinaemia.

▶ TORCH (toxoplasmosis, rubella, cytomegalovirus, herpes simplex, and HIV) screening is unhelpful.

▶ NK cell assays should not be taken outside of a research setting.

Management

At least 35% of couples with recurrent miscarriage will have lost pregnancies by chance and fall into the unexplained group. They have 75% chance of a successful pregnancy next time with no therapeutic intervention if offered supportive care alone in the setting of a dedicated EPAU.

- Empirical treatment in the unexplained miscarriage group is unnecessary and should be avoided.
- A patient with recurrent miscarriage should be seen in a dedicated clinic and be offered supportive care in early pregnancy.
- Surgical intervention for intrauterine abnormalities (uterine septum) or uterine fibroids may be beneficial in highly selective cases—a full discussion of the potential risks and benefits is vital.
- In women with APS, future live birth rate is significantly improved from 40% with low-dose aspirin (75mg) alone to 70% with combination therapy of aspirin and heparin:
  - these should be commenced as soon as the viability of fetus is confirmed in 1st trimester up to late 3rd trimester.
- Cervical cerclage may be offered to an extremely select group after meticulous consideration of the diagnosis.
- Genetic referral for parental karyotype abnormalities or fetal chromosomal abnormality.
- Proven BV in mid-trimester loss in previous pregnancy may indicate regular vaginal swabs along with rotating prophylactic antibiotics like clindamycin and amoxicillin up to 3rd trimester.

Other strategies that have been tried for recurrent miscarriage

Lifestyle factors that have not been proven to affect the outcome of a pregnancy include:
- Bed rest.
- Smoking cessation.
- Reducing alcohol intake.
- Losing weight.

▶ Steroids do not ↑ the live birth rate of women with recurrent miscarriage associated with APS or proposed immune dysfunction and may ↑ significant maternal and fetal morbidity.

⚠ They should not be used without another indication.

Other treatments that have been suggested for recurrent miscarriage, but which are not backed by clinical evidence, include:
- Oestrogen or progesterone supplementation.
- Paternal white cell immunization.
- IV immunoglobulin.
- Trophoblastic membrane infusion.
- hCG.
- Vitamin supplementation.

Hyperemesis gravidarum

Vomiting in pregnancy is common (>50% of women). Hyperemesis gravidarum is excessive vomiting and is rare, with an incidence of 1:1000. Women with multiple or molar pregnancies may be at ↑ risk, due to ↑ hCG; however, the vast majority will have a normal singleton pregnancy.

Symptoms and signs

- 1st-trimester intractable vomiting (inability to keep food or fluid down) with triad of:
  - >5% weight loss
  - dehydration
  - electrolyte imbalance.
- Other symptoms and signs may include:
  - muscle wasting
  - ptyalism (inability to swallow saliva)
  - hypovolaemia
  - behaviour disorders
  - haematemesis (Mallory–Weiss tears).

Treatment

- In the community or ambulatory day care unit if PUQE score <13 (Pregnancy-Unique Quantification of Emesis).
- Admit if not tolerating oral fluid.
- IV fluids (NaCl or Hartmann's):
  - avoid glucose-containing fluids as they can precipitate Wernicke's encephalopathy.
- Daily U&E:
  - replace K+ if necessary.
- Keep nil by mouth for 24h, then introduce light diet as tolerated.

Antiemetics

- If no response to IV fluid and electrolyte replacement, consider cyclizine 50mg/8h PO/IM/IV or promethazine as 1st line.
- *Prochlorperazine:* 12.5mg IM/IV tds or 5–10mg PO tds and/or metoclopramide 10mg/8h PO/IM/IV are usually used as 2nd line.
- *Ondansetron:* no longer to be used in the 1st trimester as suspected to cause orofacial malformations including cleft lip and cleft palate.
- *Doxylamine/pyridoxine* (Xonvea®): licensed for cases of treatment failure with conservative management.
- *Thiamine:* thiamine hydrochloride 25–50mg PO tds or thiamine 100mg IV infusion weekly.
- If vomiting remains unresponsive consider a trial of corticosteroids (prednisolone 40–50mg PO daily in divided doses or hydrocortisone 100mg/12h IV).

💣 Data on steroids for this are slight and probably biased by the fact that they are used when things are usually settling spontaneously.

- In the event of intractable hyperemesis gravidarum, TOP may be the only last option or indeed, requested by woman and/or partner.

Complications of hyperemesis

Maternal risks

• Liver and renal failure in severe cases.

⚠ Hyponatraemia and rapid reversal of hyponatraemia → central pontine myelinolysis.

⚠ Thiamine deficiency may lead to Wernicke's encephalopathy.

Fetal risks

• FGR is theoretically possible though most fetal outcome is normal.
• Fetal death may ensue in cases with Wernicke's encephalopathy.

Investigations for suspected hyperemesis gravidarum

• Urinalysis to detect ketones in urine.
• MSU to exclude UTI.
• FBC (↑ haematocrit).
• U&E (↓ K⁺, ↓ Na⁺, metabolic hypochloraemic alkalosis).
• LFT (↑ transaminases, ↓ albumin).
• USS for reassurance and to exclude multiple and molar pregnancies.

▶ There is no role for TFTs as they are often transiently abnormal.

Further reading

RCOG (2016). The management of nausea and vomiting of pregnancy and hyperemesis gravidarum. Green-top guideline no. 69.

🔗 www.rcog.org.uk/globalassets/documents/guidelines/green-top-guidelines/gtg69-hyperemesis.pdf

Genital tract infections and pelvic pain

Vaginal discharge

Normal (physiological) discharge occurs in women of reproductive age and varies with the menstrual cycle and hormonal changes.

Causes of ↑ vaginal discharge

Physiological

- Oestrogen related: puberty, pregnancy, COCP.
- Cycle related: maximal mid-cycle and premenstrual.
- Sexual excitement and intercourse.

Pathological

Infection

- Non-sexually transmitted (BV, candida).
- Sexually transmitted (trichomoniasis, chlamydia, gonorrhoea).

Non-infective

- Foreign body (retained tampon, condom, or postpartum swab).
- Malignancy (any part of the genital tract).
- Atrophic vaginitis (often blood-stained).
- Cervical ectropion or endocervical polyp.
- Fistulae (urinary or faecal).
- Allergic reactions.

History

- Characteristics (onset, duration, odour, colour) (Table 17.1).
- Associated symptoms (itching, burning, dysuria, superficial dyspareunia).
- Relationship of discharge to menstrual cycle.
- Precipitating factors (pregnancy, COCP, sexual excitement).
- Sexual history (risk factors for STIs).
- Medical history (diabetes, immunocompromised).
- Non-infectious causes (foreign body, ectopy, malignancy, dermatological conditions).
- Hygiene practices (douches, bath products, talcum powder).
- Allergies.

Examination

- External genital inspection for vulvitis, obvious discharge, ulcers, or other lesions.
- Speculum: appearance of vagina, cervix, foreign bodies, amount, colour, and consistency of discharge.
- Bimanual examination (masses, adnexal tenderness, cervical motion tenderness).

Investigations
- Endocervical or vulvovaginal swabs for gonorrhoea and chlamydia.
- HVS (Amies transport medium),
- Vaginal pH measurement.
- Saline wet mount and Gram staining (readily available in a GUM clinic, but not usually in gynaecology outpatients).
- Microscopy of vaginal discharge for BV or candida:
  - microscopy of urethral slide if urethral symptoms.
- Urethral swab is only recommended if a culture is being taken for gonorrhoea in a woman who has had a hysterectomy.
- Colposcopy (if abnormal cervical appearance).

Table 17.1 Typical characteristics of vaginal discharge

	Colour	Consistency	Odour	Vulval itching	Treatment
Physiological	Clear/white	Mucoid	None	None	Reassure
Candidal infection	White	Curd-like	None	Itching	Antifungal
Trichomonal infection	Green/grey	Frothy	Offensive	Itching	Metronidazole
Gonococcal infection	Greenish	Watery	None	None	Antibiotics
Bacterial vaginosis (BV)	White/grey	Watery	Offensive	None	Metronidazole
Malignancy	Bloody	Watery	Offensive	None	According to disease
Foreign body	Grey or bloody	Purulent	Offensive	None	Remove object
Atrophic vaginitis	Clear/blood-stained	Watery	None	None	Topical oestrogen
Cervical ectropion	Clear	Watery	None	None	Cryotherapy

Source: data from Clinical Effectiveness Unit (2012). Management of vaginal discharge in non-genitourinary medicine settings. ℞ http://www.bashh.org/documents/4264

Sexually transmitted infections

- Impact disproportionately on adolescents and young adults.
- Partner notification and treatment vital.
- Best treated at specialist GUM clinic to provide counselling and support, as well as assistance with contact tracing.
- Confidentiality paramount:
  - GUM notes are kept separately from hospital notes
  - the patient's GP is not routinely informed of the attendance.

▶ This is a requirement defined by statute in the Venereal Diseases Act of 1917.

▶ Assessment of competency should be undertaken if <16yrs old (Fraser competence).

Risk factors for STIs
- Multiple partners (two or more in the last year).
- Concurrent partners.
- Recent partner change (in past 3mths).
- Non-use of barrier protection.
- STI in partner.
- Other STI.
- Younger age (particularly aged ≤25yrs).
- Involvement in the commercial sex industry.

History
- *Symptoms:* lumps, bumps, ulcers, rash, itching, IMB or PCB, low abdominal pain, dyspareunia, sudden/distinct change in discharge.
- Past history of STIs/GUM clinic attendance/last HIV −ve test.
- All sexual partners in past 12mths.
- Contraception use and risk of pregnancy.
- Safeguarding concerns including intimate partner violence and FGM.
- Risk factors for blood-borne viruses:
  - patient or partner from area of high HIV prevalence
  - IV drug use
  - bisexual male partners.

Testing for STIs—incubation
- Tests should be done at the time of presentation.
- Incubation period before tests for STIs become +ve can give false negative after a single episode of sex:
  - for bacterial STIs this is 10–14 days
  - for HIV and syphilis it may be up to 3mths.

Chlamydia

Epidemiology
- *Chlamydia trachomatis*: obligate intracellular parasite.
- Most common bacterial STI in the UK.
- In 2020, 161,672 new diagnoses were reported in England.
- Estimated infection rates of 1.5%; 10% are seen in young people aged between 15 and 24yrs

Symptoms
Dysuria, vaginal discharge, painful sex, or irregular bleeding (IMB or PCB), but 70% of cases are asymptomatic.

Complications of chlamydia infection
- PID (10–40% of infections result in PID).
- Perihepatitis (Fitz-Hugh–Curtis syndrome).
- Reiter's syndrome (more common in men):
  - arthritis
  - urethritis
  - conjunctivitis.
- Tubal infertility.
- Risk of EP.
- Chronic pelvic pain (CPP).
- Anxiety and psychological stress.

Diagnosis
Vulvovaginal (which can be self-taken) or endocervical swab for nucleic acid amplification test (NAAT). Requires specific medium.

Treatment
- Azithromycin 1g single dose or doxycycline 100mg bd for 7 days:
  - both have similar efficacy of >95%.
- Contact tracing and treatment of partners.

Screening for chlamydia
- In 2020, 954,636 chlamydia tests were undertaken in those aged 15–24yrs, a 31% ↓ compared to 2019 but test positivity remained stable at 9.8%

Implications in pregnancy
- Preterm ROM and premature delivery.
- The risks to the baby are of:
  - neonatal conjunctivitis (30% within the first 2wks)
  - neonatal pneumonia (15% within the first 4mths).

▶ Treat pregnant woman with erythromycin 500mg bd for 10–14 days (73–95% effective).

Gonorrhoea

Epidemiology

- *Neisseria gonorrhoeae*: intracellular Gram −ve diplococcus.
- 3rd most common STI in the UK.
- 56,259 cases of gonorrhoea reported in 2018, a 26% ↑ since 2017.
  - three cases of extensively drug-resistant *N. gonorrhoeae*.
- 1° site of infection: columnar epithelium of urethra, endocervix, rectum, pharynx, and conjunctiva.
- Transmission by direct inoculation.
- >35% of strains are resistant to ciprofloxacin, 70% to tetracyclines.

Symptoms

- Usually asymptomatic, often diagnosed when screening on contact tracing.
- Can present with mucopurulent vaginal discharge (50%), low abdominal pain, IMB or PCB.
- Co-infections with *Trichomonas*, *Mycoplasma*, *Candida* is not uncommon.

Diagnosis

- Endocervical or vulvovaginal swab with NAAT:
  - urethral, pharyngeal, and rectal swabs if contact with gonorrhoea
  - if diagnosed on NAAT, culture for sensitivity testing should be taken from all sites prior to antibiotic treatment.

Treatment

- If antibiotic sensitivity unknown: ceftriaxone 1g IM stat.
- If sensitivity known: ciprofloxacin 500mg orally stat dose (resistance 36% in 2017).
- Penicillin allergy: stat PO cefixime 400mg and azithromycin 2g.
- Contact tracing and treatment of partners.
- Abstain until all contacts are completely treated.
- In pregnancy use ceftriaxone 1g IM or spectinomycin 2g IM or azithromycin 2g PO stat dose.
- All patients need to return after completion of therapy for test of cure (NAAT).

Implications in pregnancy

- Associated with:
  - preterm ROM and premature delivery
  - chorioamnionitis.
- The risks to the baby are of *ophthalmia neonatorum* (40–50%).

Further reading

British Association for Sexual Health and HIV.
℞ www.bashh.org/

Complications of gonococcus infection
- PID (~10% of infections result in PID).
- Bartholin's or Skene's abscess
- Disseminated gonorrhoea may cause:
  - fever
  - pustular rash
  - migratory polyarthralgia
  - septic arthritis.
- Tubal infertility.
- ↑ risk of EP.

Herpes simplex

Epidemiology

- *DNA virus:* herpes simplex type 1 (orolabial/genital) and type 2 (genital only).
- 4th most common STI in 2018.
- Comprised 33,867 (8%) of new STI diagnosis made at sexual health services in England in 2018.
- An ↑ of 3% when compared to 2017 figures.

Symptoms

- 1° HSV infection is usually the most severe and often results in:
  - prodrome (tingling/itching of skin in affected area)
  - flu-like illness ± inguinal lymphadenopathy
  - vulvitis and pain (may cause urinary retention)
  - small, characteristic vesicles on the vulva, but can be atypical with fissures, erosions, erythema of skin.

Recurrent attacks are thought to result from reactivation of latent virus in the sacral ganglia and are normally shorter and less severe. They can be triggered by many factors including:
- Stress.
- Sexual intercourse.
- Menstruation.

> ### Complications of HSV infection (usually of 1° infection)
> - Meningitis.
> - Sacral radiculopathy—causing urinary retention and constipation.
> - Transverse myelitis.
> - Disseminated infection.

Diagnosis

- Usually from appearance of the typical rash.
- PCR testing of vesicular fluid (most sensitive—gold standard).
- Culture of vesicular fluid.
- Serum antibody tests are of no use for diagnosing 1° herpes.

Treatment

- No cure for genital herpes. Symptomatic relief with simple analgesia, saline bathing, ice packs, topical anaesthetic.
- Oral aciclovir (200mg 5× day for 5 days or similar), double dose/length if immunosuppressed.
- Topical aciclovir is not beneficial.
- Condoms/abstinence while prodromal/symptomatic (unless history of HSV in both partners) may ↓ transmission rates.
- Suppressive antiviral treatment—considered if >6 recurrences/yr.

Implications in pregnancy

➲ Herpes simplex, p. 168.

Syphilis

Epidemiology

- *Treponema pallidum*: spirochaete.
- Transmission rate 10–60%.
- Sexual and vertical (high risk in early pregnancy) transmission.
- Relatively rare STI in the UK but 126% ↑ from 3344 cases in 2013 to 7541 in 2018.

Symptoms

1° syphilis

- Incubation period 21 days (9–90 days).
- Painless, single genital papule with inguinal lymphadenopathy later → ulcer (chancre)—may pass unnoticed on the cervix.

2° syphilis

- Occurs within the first 2yrs of infection (typically 3mths).
- Mucocutaneous polymorphic rash affecting palms and soles.
- Generalized lymphadenopathy.
- Genital condyloma lata.
- Anterior uveitis.

3° syphilis

- Presents in about 1/3 of people infected for at least 2yrs, but may take 20–40yrs to develop.
- *Neurosyphilis (7%):* tabes dorsalis and dementia.
- *Cardiovascular syphilis (10%):* commonly affecting the aortic root.
- *Gummata (15%):* inflammatory plaques or nodules.

Diagnosis

- Specific treponemal enzyme immunoassay for IgG + IgM.
- 1° lesion smear may show spirochaetes on dark field microscopy.
- Quantitative cardiolipin (non-treponemal) tests, i.e. rapid plasma regain (RPR)/VDRL are useful in assessing response to treatment.
- Testing for *Treponema pallidum* with NAAT if available.

Treatment

- Depends on penicillin allergy:
  - benzathine benzylpenicillin 2.4 million units single dose IM (used in pregnancy—repeat dose 8 days later if in 3rd trimester)
  - doxycycline 100mg bd PO for 14 days (contraindicated in pregnancy)
  - azithromycin 2g PO stat (contraindicated in pregnancy)
  - erythromycin 500mg qds PO for 14 days (used in pregnancy).
- Treatment courses are longer in tertiary syphilis.
- Contact tracing (potentially over several years).

Implications in pregnancy

- Preterm delivery.
- Stillbirth.
- Congenital syphilis.
- Miscarriage.

→ Syphilis, p. 200.

Trichomoniasis

Epidemiology

- *Trichomonas vaginalis:* flagellated protozoan.
- Relatively rare in the UK: ~6000 cases reported each year, compared with >200,000 chlamydia cases.
- Found in vaginal, urethral, and para-urethral glands.
- Cervix may have a 'strawberry' appearance from punctate haemorrhages (2%).

Symptoms

Asymptomatic in 10–50%, but may present with:
- Frothy, yellow, offensive-smelling vaginal discharge.
- Vulval itching and soreness due to vulvitis and vaginitis.
- Dysuria.

Diagnosis

- Swab from posterior fornix/self-administered vaginal swab.
- Direct observation of the mobile organism by a wet smear (normal saline) or acridine orange-stained slide from the posterior vaginal fornix (sensitivity 45–60% of cases).
- *Trichomonas* rapid test has shown higher sensitivity and specificity than microscopy.
- Culture media are available and will diagnose up to 80% of cases.
- NAATs are becoming the current gold standard with sensitivities and specificities approaching 100%.

Complications

Trichomonas vaginalis infection may enhance HIV transmission.

Treatment

- Metronidazole 2g PO stat dose.
- Metronidazole 400–500mg bd for 5–7 days.
- Alternative—tinidazole 2g PO stat dose.
- Contact tracing and treatment of partners and avoid sexual intercourse for at least 1wk.

Implications in pregnancy

- Some evidence that trichomonal infection may ↑ the risk of preterm birth, but routine screening is not currently recommended.
- Trichomoniasis may be acquired perinatally, occurring in 5% of babies born to infected mothers.

Human papillomavirus

Epidemiology

- DNA virus, many subtypes.
- Subtypes 6 and 11 cause genital warts (condylomata acuminata).
- 25% of people presenting with warts have other concurrent STIs.
- Most common viral STI in England.
- 193 cases of genital warts in 15–17yr-old girls in 2018: 56% ↓ relative to 2017, and 100 cases of genital warts in same aged heterosexual boys, a 46% ↓ relative to 2017, continuation of the steep decline observed since 2014 and is largely due to the high coverage of the national HPV immunization programme.

Symptoms

Majority asymptomatic. Painless lumps anywhere in the genito-anal area. Perianal warts are common even in the absence of anal intercourse.

Diagnosis

Identified by clinical appearance. Non-wart HPV infection diagnosed by characteristic appearance on cervical cytology (smear tests) or colposcopy (whitening on topical application of acetic acid).

Complications

HPV types 16 and 18 associated with high-grade cervical intraepithelial neoplasia (CIN) and cervical neoplasia. Smoking and immunosuppression both affect viral clearance thereby ↑ the risk.

Treatment for genital warts

Removal of the visible wart. High rate of recurrence due to the latent virus in the surrounding epithelial cells.

▶ Consistent condom use ↓ the risk of HPV acquisition.

Clinic treatment

- Cryotherapy.
- Podophyllotoxin and trichloroacetic acid.
- Electrosurgery/scissors excision/curettage/laser.

Home treatment (both contraindicated if pregnancy risk)

- Podophyllotoxin cream (0.15%) or solution (0.5%): this is self-applied and must be used for about 4–5wks. (Avoid in pregnancy.)
- *Imiquimod cream (5%)*: this is also a self-applied immune response modifier. It may need to be used for up to 16wks.

Implications in pregnancy

- Genital warts tend to grow rapidly in pregnancy, but usually regress after delivery.
- Very rarely, babies exposed perinatally may develop laryngeal or genital warts, but it is not an indication for CD.

Routine vaccination

A quadrivalent HPV (types 6, 11, 16, 18) preventive vaccination was introduced in 2012 for pre-exposure protection.

Bacterial vaginosis

Epidemiology

- Most common cause of abnormal vaginal discharge.
- BV is caused by an overgrowth of mixed anaerobes, including *Gardnerella*, *Prevotella* spp., *Atopobium vaginalis*, and *Mycoplasma hominis*, which replace the usually dominant vaginal lactobacilli causing ↑ of the vaginal pH level from <4.5 to >4.5 up to 6.0.
- Prevalence: 5–15% white women, 45–55% black women.
- Not sexually transmitted.
- ~12% of women will experience BV at some point in their lives, but what triggers it remains unclear.

Symptoms

- Many asymptomatic (50%), but usually presents with a profuse, thin, whitish grey, offensive fishy-smelling vaginal discharge.
- The characteristic 'fishy' smell is due to the presence of amines released by bacterial proteolysis and is often distressing.
- Not usually associated with symptoms and signs of inflammation.

Diagnosis

Amsel criteria—3 out of 4 required for diagnosis:
- Thin, homogeneous grey-white discharge.
- ↑ vaginal pH >5.5.
- Characteristic fishy smell on adding alkali (10% KOH).
- 'Clue cells' present on microscopy (squamous epithelial cells with bacteria adherent on their walls).

   Hay/Ison criteria: species seen with Gram stain of vaginal smear.

Complications

↑ risk of endometritis/PID following TOP.

Treatment

- Indicated in symptomatic women or women undergoing surgical procedure.
- May resolve spontaneously and if successfully treated has a high recurrence rate. However, most women prefer it to be treated:
  - metronidazole 400mg PO bd for 5–7 days (avoid alcohol) *or*
  - metronidazole 2g (single dose) *or*
  - clindamycin 2% vaginally nocte 7 days (weakens condoms).
- Lifestyle factors: avoid vaginal douching/over-washing.
- Probiotic lactobacilli/lactic acid preparations not currently recommended.

Implications in pregnancy

Conflicting evidence on preterm birth and BV. Recommend:
- Symptomatic pregnant women treated with same regimen.
- Treat BV in women with additional risk factors for preterm birth.
- Prefer vaginal route for lactating women (metronidazole alters breast milk taste)

Candidiasis (thrush)

Epidemiology

- Yeast-like fungus (90% *Candida albicans*, remainder other species, e.g. *C. glabrata*, *C. tropicalis*, *C. krusei*, *C. parapsilosis*).
- ~75% of women will experience at least one episode, and 10–20% are asymptomatic chronic carriers (40% during pregnancy).
- Predisposing factors are those that alter the vaginal micro-flora and include:
  - diabetes mellitus
  - immunosuppression
  - antibiotics
  - oestrogen (e.g. pregnancy, HRT).

Symptoms

May be asymptomatic, but usually presents with:
- Vulval itching and soreness.
- Non-offensive thick, curd-like, white vaginal discharge.
- Superficial dyspareunia.
- Dysuria.

Diagnosis

- Characteristic appearance of:
  - vulval and vaginal erythema
  - vulval fissuring
  - typical white plaques adherent to the vaginal wall.
- Microscopic detection of spores and pseudohyphae on wet slides.
- HVS for culture only in recurrent or resistant infections.

Complications

Unlikely to cause any significant complications unless the woman is severely immunocompromised.

Treatment

- As so many women are chronic carriers, candidiasis should only be treated if it is symptomatic:
  - avoiding irritants, e.g. soap and bath salts (use emollient)
  - avoid non-breathable underwear.
  - fluconazole 150mg (single dose)—contraindicated in pregnancy
  - clotrimazole 500mg pessary ± topical clotrimazole cream.

Implications in pregnancy

- It is very common in pregnancy with no apparent adverse effects.
- Topical imidazoles are not systemically absorbed and are therefore safe at all gestations.
- Clotrimazole 500mg vaginal pessary for up to 7 consecutive nights.

Pelvic inflammatory disease: overview

Definition
PID is infection of the *upper* genital tract.

Incidence
Exact prevalence is hard to ascertain as many cases may go undetected, but is thought to be in the region of 1–3% of sexually active young women.

Causes
- Most commonly caused by ascending infection from the endocervix, but may also occur from descending infection from organs such as the appendix.
- There are multiple causative organisms:
  - 25% of cases caused by *Chlamydia trachomatis* and *Neisseria gonorrhoeae*
  - anaerobes and endogenous agents, either aerobic or facultative, may be responsible for the remainder.

History and examination
- A full gynaecological history including sexual history.
- An abdominal examination to elicit the site and severity of the pain.
- Speculum and vaginal examination to assess for adnexal masses, vaginal discharge, or cervical excitation.

Risk factors for PID
- Age <25yrs.
- Previous STIs.
- New sexual partner/multiple sexual partners.
- Uterine instrumentation such as surgical TOP and IUCDs.
- Postpartum endometritis.

Protective factors
- Barrier contraception.
- Levonorgestrel IUCD (Mirena® IUS).
- COCP.

Pelvic inflammatory disease: diagnosis and treatment

Symptoms

PID may be relatively asymptomatic, the diagnosis only being made retrospectively during investigation of subfertility.

Symptoms may include some or all of the following:
- Pelvic pain (may be unilateral): constant or intermittent.
- Deep dyspareunia.
- Vaginal discharge (usually due to concurrent vaginal infection).
- Irregular and/or more painful menses.
- IMB/PCB.
- Fever (unusual in mild/chronic PID).

Signs

At least one of which should be present when making a PID diagnosis:
- Cervical motion pain (cervical excitation).
- Adnexal tenderness (commonly bilateral, but may be unilateral).
- Elevated temperature (unusual in mild/chronic infection).

Investigations

- Tests for gonorrhoea and chlamydia.
- WCC and CRP may be elevated.
- USS may be indicated if a tubo-ovarian abscess is suspected.
- Laparoscopy is the gold standard test; however, it is invasive and only used where diagnosis is uncertain.

Complications of PID
- Tubo-ovarian abscess.
- Fitz-Hugh–Curtis syndrome.
- Recurrent PID.
- EP.
- Infertility.

Treatment

Early empirical treatment is recommended. Multiple antibiotic regimens are required to cover all potential causative organisms.
- Most patients can be treated in an outpatient setting.
- Review after 72h to ensure adequate response.
- Contact tracing and treatment of partners is essential.
- Inpatient treatment may be required if symptoms are severe, fail to respond, or abscess is suspected.
- If there is USS evidence of a tubo-ovarian abscess, drainage may be required either by ultrasound-guided aspiration or at laparoscopy.

Outpatient management of PID

- IM ceftriaxone 500mg stat plus oral doxycycline 100mg bd 14 days plus oral metronidazole 400mg bd 14 days;

Or

- Ofloxacin orally 400mg bd 14 days plus metronidazole 400mg bd 14 days (avoid if high risk of gonococcal disease).

▶ Doxycycline and metronidazole are commonly used in clinical practice, but there are no clinical trials to support their effectiveness.

Inpatient management of PID

- IV ceftriaxone 2g od plus IV doxycycline 100mg bd, followed by oral doxycycline 100mg bd 14 days plus oral metronidazole 400mg bd 14 days.

Or

- IV clindamycin 900mg tds + IV gentamicin 2mg/kg loading dose followed by 1.5mg/kg tds, followed by either oral clindamycin 450mg qds for a total of 14 days or oral doxycycline 100mg bd + oral metronidazole 400mg bd for a total of 14 days.

Or

- IV ofloxacin 400mg bd + IV metronidazole 500mg tds for a total of 14 days.

Further reading

RCOG (2008). Management of acute pelvic inflammatory disease. Green-top guideline no. 32. ✒ www.rcog.org.uk/en/guidelines-research-services/guidelines/gtg32/

Acute pelvic pain

⚠ *Acute pelvic pain in a woman of reproductive age with a +ve pregnancy test is an EP until proven otherwise.*

History

- *Pain:*
  - site
  - nature
  - radiation
  - aggravating/relieving factors.
- LMP.
- Contraception.
- Recent unprotected sexual intercourse (UPSI).
- Risk factors for an EP (● Ectopic pregnancy: diagnosis, p. 610).
- Vaginal discharge or bleeding.
- Bowel symptoms like diarrhoea.
- Urinary symptoms.
- Precipitating factors (physical and psychological).

Examination

- *Is she haemodynamically stable?* Risk of bleeding from EP.
- *Abdomen:* does she have an acute abdomen? Masses?
- *Pelvic:* are discharge, cervical excitation, adnexal tenderness, masses present?

Investigations

- Urinary/serum hCG.
- MSU.
- Triple swabs (high vaginal, cervical, and endocervical for *Chlamydia*).
- FBC, group and save (cross-match if ectopic suspected), CRP.
- Pelvic USS—TV or abdominal as appropriate.
- Abdominal X-ray (± contrast), CT, MRI as appropriate.
- Diagnostic laparoscopy.

Treatment

- Resuscitate if necessary.
- Analgesia.
- Specific treatment will depend on cause of pain.
- Avoid unnecessary laparoscopy, especially in a woman with a history of chronic pain.

Gynaecological causes of acute pelvic pain

- *Early pregnancy complications:*
  - EP (⮕ Ectopic pregnancy: diagnosis, p. 610)
  - miscarriage (⮕ Miscarriage: management, p. 606)
  - ovarian hyperstimulation syndrome (⮕ Ovarian hyperstimulation syndrome, p. 686).
- PID (⮕ Pelvic inflammatory disease: overview p. 638).
- *Ovarian cyst accident:*
  - torsion
  - haemorrhage
  - rupture.
- *Adnexal pathology:*
  - torsion of fallopian tube/parafimbrial cyst
  - salpingo-ovarian abscess.
- Endometriosis.
- Endometritis.
- Torsion or degeneration or prolapse of a uterine leiomyoma.
- Mittelschmerz (German: Mittel = middle, Schmerz = pain).
- Pregnancy complications (⮕ Abdominal pain in pregnancy: pregnancy related (<24wks), p. 86):
  - fibroid degeneration
  - ovarian cyst accident
  - ligament stretch.
- 1° dysmenorrhoea (⮕ Menstrual disorders: dysmenorrhea, p. 582).
- Haematometra/haematocolpos.
- Non-gynaecological causes.
- Acute exacerbation of CPP.

Non-gynaecological causes of acute pelvic pain

Gastrointestinal
- Appendicitis.
- Irritable bowel syndrome.
- IBD.
- Mesenteric adenitis.
- Diverticulitis.
- Strangulation of a hernia.

Urological
- UTI.
- Renal/bladder calculi.

Musculoskeletal pain
- From pelvic floor or back muscle dysfunction.

Chronic pelvic pain: gynaecological causes

Definition

Intermittent or constant pelvic pain in the lower abdomen or pelvis of at least 6mths duration, not occurring exclusively with menstruation or intercourse and not associated with pregnancy. It is severe enough to cause functional disability or require treatment.

CPP is a symptom, not a diagnosis.

Prevalence

- Annual prevalence in women aged 15–73yrs is 38/1000 (asthma: 37/1000, back pain: 41/1000).
- Many women do not receive a diagnosis even after many years and multiple investigations.

Causes

Its aetiology is multifactorial, involving social, psychological, and biological factors.

- Endometriosis:
  - ♦ Endometriosis: overview, p. 664.
- Adenomyosis:
  - characterized by the presence of ectopic endometrial tissue in the myometrium
  - often occurs after pregnancy, particularly after CD or TOP (breaches the integrity of the endometrial/myometrial junction)
  - initially causes cyclical pelvic pain and menorrhagia, but can worsen until pain is present daily.
- Adhesions.
- Trapped ovary syndrome:
  - after hysterectomy the ovary becomes trapped within dense adhesions at the pelvic side wall
  - postoperative peritoneal cysts.
- Pelvic venous congestion:
  - dilated pelvic veins, believed to cause a cyclical dragging pain
  - worst premenstrually and after prolonged periods of standing and walking
  - dyspareunia is also often present.
- Chronic PID.
- Fibroids.

Further reading

RCOG (2012). Chronic pelvic pain: initial management. Green-top guideline no. 41.
⚕ www.rcog.org.uk/womens-health/clinical-guidance/initial-management-chronic-pelvic-pain-green-top-41

Psychological associations with CPP

- A number of studies have shown that women with CPP have ↑ number of −ve cognitive and emotional traits, although it is not known whether these are the causes or consequences of pain.
- History of abuse (physical, sexual, and psychological) also associated with CPP, but may not be revealed at the first consultation.

Chronic pelvic pain: non-gynaecological causes

Gastrointestinal causes

- *Irritable bowel syndrome:* common, occurring in ~20% of women of reproductive age.
- *Constipation:* common cause of pelvic pain that is easily treated.

▶ Opiate analgesics should not be prescribed without a laxative.

- *Hernia:* abdominal or pelvic hernias may cause pain.

Urological causes

Interstitial cystitis

- Inflammatory disorder causing pain and urinary frequency.
- Diagnosed on cystoscopy.
- Pain is often relieved by voiding.

Urethral syndrome

- Associated with frequency/dysuria in absence of infective cystitis.
- Aetiology is not known, possibly due to a chronic low-grade infection of the paraurethral glands ('female prostatitis').

Calculi

- May occasionally trigger a chronic pain cycle.

Musculoskeletal causes

Fibromyalgia

- Widespread pain especially in the shoulders, neck, and pelvic girdle.
- Characterized by tender points and a reduced pain threshold.
- Often shows cyclical exacerbations.
- Chronic PID.
- Fibroids.

Neurological causes

Nerve entrapments

- Trapped in fascia or narrow foramen or in scar tissue after surgery.
- Classically results in pain and/or dysfunction in nerve distribution.

Neuropathic pain

- Results from actual damage to the nerve (surgery, infection, or inflammation).
- Classically described as shooting, stabbing, or burning.

Chronic pelvic pain: diagnosis and treatment

History

As for acute pelvic pain, but also including:

- A detailed history of the pain, including events surrounding its onset, site, nature, radiation, time course, exacerbating and relieving factors, and any cyclicity.
- A sexual history and future fertility wishes should be explored (it may be possible to discuss abuse at this point).

Examination

- As for acute pelvic pain.
- Speculum may not be appropriate if history of vaginismus or pain to difficult smear or abuse.

Investigations

Be careful not to over-investigate initially.

Treatment

Analgesia

- Pre-emptive analgesia may prevent emergency admissions.
- Opiates may be required for severe, acute exacerbations, but if needed regularly, referral to a dedicated pain clinic should be made.
- Neuropathic treatments such as amitriptyline, gabapentin, and pregabalin can be useful.

Hormonal treatments

- The COCP, progestogens, and GnRH analogues can be effective.
- If pain is improved with a GnRH analogue then this can be combined safely with low-dose HRT for at least 2yrs.

Complementary therapy

- A variety of complementary therapies can produce good results and should be encouraged if the woman suggests them.
- Support groups can also give reassurance.
- Digital distension of painful pelvic structures was more effective for pain when compared with counselling.

Surgery

This has a limited role to play, but hysterectomy can be helpful, as above.

Further reading

RCOG (2012). Chronic pelvic pain: initial management. Green-top guideline no. 41.

🔊 www.rcog.org.uk/womens-health/clinical-guidance/initial-management-chronic-pelvic-pain-green-top-41

Therapeutic trial of GnRH analogues

With clearly cyclical pain, a trial of a GnRH analogue can be a useful diagnostic tool:

- Women requesting hysterectomy with bilateral salpingo-oopherectomy can be reassured that it may be a successful treatment if their pain is relieved with a GnRH analogue.
- If their pain persists on GnRH analogue treatment, they should be counselled that hysterectomy is unlikely to remove their pain and other causes for it should be explored

Subfertility and reproductive medicine

Polycystic ovarian syndrome: overview

Background

- PCOS is the most common endocrinopathy affecting reproductive aged women with an estimated prevalence of 8–13%.
- Responsible for 80% of all cases of anovulatory subfertility.
- USS evidence of polycystic ovaries is seen in 20–30% of women.

Aetiology

The pathogenesis of PCOS is not well understood and thought to be multi-factorial. There is hypersecretion of LH in ~60–75% of PCOS patients (LH stimulates androgen secretion from ovarian thecal cells). Elevated LH:FSH ratio is often seen, but is not needed for diagnosis.

The following factors have been implicated:

- Genetic (familial clustering).
- Insulin resistance with compensatory hyperinsulinaemia.
- Hyperandrogenism (elevated ovarian androgen secretion).
- Obesity:
  - BMI >30kg/m² in 35–60% of women with PCOS
  - central obesity
  - worsens insulin resistance.

Investigations

- Basal (day 2–5): LH, FSH.
- TFTs, prolactin, testosterone, and SHBG to calculated free androgen index (FAI).
- If clinical or biochemical hyperandrogenism detected, check serum:
  - dehydroepiandrosterone sulphate (DHEAS)
  - androstenedione.
- Exclude other causes of 2° amenorrhoea.
- Pelvic USS in those >8yrs past menarche.

Examination

- BMI.
- Physical examination for signs of hyperandrogenism:
  - hirsutism (standardized visual scales are preferred when assessing hirsutism, such as the modified Ferriman–Gallwey score (mFG) with a level ≥4–6 indicating hirsutism)
  - acne
  - alopecia
  - acanthosis nigricans.

Rotterdam criteria for diagnosing PCOS

Requires the presence of two out of the following three variables and exclusion of other disorders:
- Irregular or absent ovulations (cycle <21 days or >35 days).
- Clinical or biochemical signs of hyperandrogenism:
  - acne
  - hirsutism
  - alopecia.
- Polycystic ovaries on pelvic USS: >20 antral follicles or ovarian volume >10mL in one or more ovary.

Long-term health consequences of PCOS

- Obesity, insulin resistance, and metabolic abnormalities including dyslipidaemia are all risk factors for cardiovascular disease. The risk in women with PCOS remains unclear pending high-quality studies; however, prevalence of cardiovascular disease risk factors is ↑ warranting consideration of screening.
- Women with PCOS should be aware that, regardless of age, the prevalence of gestational diabetes, impaired glucose tolerance, and type 2 diabetes are significantly ↑ in PCOS, with risk independent of, yet exacerbated by, obesity.
- Pregnant women with PCOS are at ↑ risk of gestational diabetes (➔ Gestational diabetes, p. 276).
- Women diagnosed with PCOS should be asked (or their partners asked) about snoring and daytime fatigue/somnolence, informed of the possible risk of sleep apnoea, and offered investigation and treatment when necessary.
- Long periods of 2° amenorrhoea, with resultant unopposed oestrogen, are a risk factor for endometrial hyperplasia and, if untreated, endometrial carcinoma.
- There is an ↑ risk of anxiety/depressive disorders, psychosexual dysfunction, and disordered eating in women with PCOS.

Polycystic ovarian syndrome: management

Lifestyle modification

This is the cornerstone to managing PCOS in overweight women. Even a modest weight loss (5%) can improve symptoms. Moreover, weight loss through exercise and diet has been proven effective in restoring ovulatory cycles and achieving pregnancy. Weight loss through diet and exercise should be encouraged, and patients should feel supported.

Improving menstrual regularity

- Weight loss.
- COCP.
- Metformin in combination with the COCP.

Controlling symptoms of hyperandrogenism

- Cosmetic (depilatory cream, electrolysis, shaving, plucking).
- Antiandrogens such as eflornithine facial cream, finasteride, or spironolactone:
  - can be used to help with acne and hirsutism
  - can take 6–9mths to improve hair growth
  - avoid pregnancy (feminizes a male fetus).
- COCP:
  - ↓ serum androgen levels by ↑ SHBG levels
  - co-cyprindiol combines ethinylestradiol and cyproterone acetate, providing a regular monthly withdrawal bleed and beneficial antiandrogenic effects.

Subfertility

- Weight loss alone may achieve spontaneous ovulation.
- Ovulation induction with antioestrogens (letrozole 1st line) or gonadotropins (➔ Ovulation induction, p. 678).
- Laparoscopic ovarian diathermy.
- IVF if ovulation cannot be achieved or does not succeed in pregnancy.

⚠ Women with PCOS who undergo IVF are at ↑ risk of ovarian hyperstimulation syndrome (➔ Ovarian hyperstimulation syndrome, p. 686).

Insulin sensitizers

Metformin has been most widely used (unlicensed in the UK):

- In those with resistant anovulation, metformin combined with letrozole or clomifene citrate improves ovulation and pregnancy rates.
- Does not significantly improve hirsutism, acne, or weight loss, despite lowering androgen levels and improving insulin sensitivity.

Psychological impact of PCOS
- PCOS can be difficult to manage and patients may require additional motivation.
- Symptoms can be distressing and result in low self-esteem.
- It is therefore important to manage patients sensitively, and to adopt a holistic approach, incorporating all members of the MDT.

Hirsutism and virilization: overview

Background

Vellus hair (prepubertal, unpigmented, downy hair) is irreversibly transformed into *terminal hair* (pigmented, coarse) through either ↑ free androgen or ↑ sensitivity of 5α-reductase (conversion of testosterone to the more potent dihydrotestosterone) in the skin. In women, testosterone originates either directly from the ovaries (25%) and adrenal glands (25%) or from peripheral conversion of androstenedione or dehydroepiandrosterone (-sulphate), which are produced in the ovaries and adrenal glands (50%). Testosterone is bound to SHBG (80%) and albumin (19%). In women, only 1% is free (active). LH stimulates ovarian theca cells and ACTH the adrenal glands to synthesize androgen.

Hirsutism

- *Hirsutism*: presence of excessive facial and body hair in women.
- Caused by ↑ of systemic or local androgen, resulting in a male hair growth pattern.
- Incidence of hirsutism is estimated to be ~10% in developed countries.
- Most commonly found in patients with PCOS, together with acne, alopecia, and acanthosis nigricans.
- Even mild forms of hirsutism are often felt unacceptable by the patient and may cause mental trauma.
- Should also not be confused with hypertrichosis, which is a very rare, androgen-independent disorder:
  - hypertrichosis can involve vellus, lanugo, and terminal hair occupying the entire body surface including the face ('werewolf appearance')
  - congenital forms have been described (usually more severe)
  - can be caused by drugs (phenytoin, ciclosporin, glucocorticoids), hypothyroidism, and anorexia nervosa.

Virilization

- Can be distinguished from hirsutism by the presence of:
  - clitoromegaly
  - balding
  - deepening of the voice
  - male body habitus.
- Is relatively rare and usually 2° to androgen-producing tumours or CAH.

Causes of hirsutism

Ovary
- PCOS; 95%.
- Androgen-secreting tumours: <1%.
- Luteoma: <1%.

Adrenal gland
- CAH: <1%.
- Cushing's syndrome: <1%.
- Androgen-secreting tumours: <1%.
- Acromegaly: 1%.

External causes
- Iatrogenic hirsutism: <1%.
- Drugs with androgenic effects (anabolic steroids, danazol, testosterone): <1%.

Reasons for ↑ androgen levels

↓ SHBG levels
- Hyperinsulinaemia.
- Liver disease.
- Androgens.
- Hyperprolactinaemia.
- Hypothyroidism.

↑ production
- Tumours.
- Enzyme defects (including CAH).
- Cushing's syndrome.
- Hyperinsulinaemia.
- ↑ LH levels stimulate theca cells.

External androgen sources
- Androgens:
  - progestogens with androgenic potential
  - ↑ 5α-reductase sensitivity
  - insulin-like growth factor 1 in patients with insulin resistance or hyperinsulinaemia.

Hirsutism and virilization: clinical appearance and investigations

Women mostly present with coarse and pigmented (terminal) hair on the face (upper lip, chin), chest, abdomen, back, and thighs. Ethnic differences in the severity of hair growth are common. Fair-skinned white women show less hair growth, while Mediterranean women have the greatest amount of terminal hair. Genetic differences in the activity of 5α-reductase seem to correlate with the severity of disease. Hirsutism is often accompanied by seborrhoea, acne, and male pattern alopecia.

History

- Age:
  - children with non-classical CAH
  - pregnant women with luteoma.
- *Rate of onset of symptoms:* rapid onset of severe symptoms may indicate an androgen-producing tumour.
- *Menstrual cycle:* oligo- or amenorrhoea.
- Genetic factors:
  - PCOS
  - enzyme deficiencies
  - type 2 diabetes.
- Drugs:
  - COCPs with androgen effects
  - drug abuse (body builders).
- General health and other symptoms:
  - Cushing's syndrome
  - acromegaly
  - liver disease.

Physical examination

- Exclude hypertrichosis.
- Signs of virilization should prompt a search for an androgen-producing tumour.
- BP:
  - ↑ with Cushing's syndrome and acromegaly
  - ↓ in hypothyroidism and CAH.
- Look for acanthosis nigricans:
  - marker of insulin resistance and hyperinsulinaemia
  - skin grey-brown, velvety appearance mainly in the neck, axillae, vulva, and groin.

Ferriman–Gallwey score to grade hirsutism

Nine locations are evaluated and each receives a score between 0 (no growth) and 4 (complete hair cover):
- Upper lip.
- Chin.
- Chest.
- Upper abdomen.
- Lower abdomen.
- Upper back.
- Lower back.
- Upper arms.
- Thighs.

A score >8 is considered androgen excess.

💧 This score is subjective, difficult to compare between different ethnic groups, and has a ↓ validity in pre-treated women. It is therefore, usually reserved for clinical studies.

Investigations for hirsutism

- *Testosterone:* measure of ovarian and adrenal activity.
- *DHEAS:* measure of adrenal activity.
- *OGTT:* in women with indication of hyperinsulinaemia/insulin resistance.
- *17-hydroxyprogesterone (17-OHP):* to rule out CAH, if indicated.

▶ TVS/USS to visualize polycystic ovaries is not necessary to diagnose PCOS in a woman with hirsutism and oligo-/amenorrhoea. However, TVS/USS should always be done to both exclude any ovarian tumours and help in confirming the diagnosis.

▶ Investigations to rule out rare causes of hirsutism such as Cushing's syndrome and acromegaly should be undertaken if clinically indicated.

Hirsutism: first-line treatment

Treatment is aimed at the underlying cause (especially important for the non-ovarian causes such as Cushing's syndrome or CAH).
- Lifestyle changes aiming at weight reduction in women with PCOS.
- COCP:
  - treatment of choice in women not trying to conceive
  - progestational component—LH suppression; 5α-reductase inhibition
  - oestrogenic component—SHBG ↑
  - COCP with ethinylestradiol + drospirenone
  - ethinylestradiol + cyproterone acetate (co-cyprindiol) licensed in the UK for facial hirsutism (not for contraception!).
- Medroxyprogesterone acetate:
  - if COCP is contraindicated
  - LH suppression (less than COCP)
  - SHBG ↓ (counterproductive)
  - testosterone clearance ↑ (induction of liver enzymes)
  - overall, similar results to COCP.

▶ Discontinue treatment after 1–2yrs to observe if ovulatory cycles occur. Suppression of testosterone will last for 6–12mths after discontinuation in anovulatory patients.

Cosmetic approaches
- Hair removal will only be permanent if dermal papilla is destroyed.
- Non-permanent approaches, such as shaving and waxing, do not worsen hirsutism.

Permanent measures
Laser
- 694–1064nm.
- Uses melanin in hair bulb as chromophore.
- Heat causes papillar destruction.
- Works best on fair-skinned women with dark hair.
- Dark-skinned patients at higher risk of dermal damage (scarring and discomfort as more energy is needed).

Electrolysis
- Fine probe inserted into skin.
- Short-wave radio frequency causes heat, thereby destroying dermal papilla.
- Only permanent measure approved by the US Food and Drug Administration (FDA).

Non-permanent measures
- Local chemical depilatories (not for face).
- Bleaching.
- Waxing.
- Tweezing.
- Mechanical epilators.

Hirsutism: second-line treatment

- *Spironolactone* (50–200mg daily, ↓ to 25–50mg qds after a few wks):
  - aldosterone antagonist (diuretic)
  - inhibits ovarian/adrenal androgens
  - competes for androgen receptor in skin
  - inhibits 5α-reductase in skin
  - slow onset (at least 6mths)
  - hyperkalaemia possible (watch renal function)
  - add contraceptive as may cause feminization of male fetus.
- *Cyproterone acetate* (2mg plus 35 micrograms ethinylestradiol in co-cyprindiol):
  - progestational agent with antiandrogenic potency
  - inhibits LH secretion and binds to androgen receptor
  - best after 3mths of treatment
  - side effects—fatigue, oedema, weight gain, libido loss, mastalgia.
- *Finasteride* (5mg daily):
  - inhibits 5α-reductase (type II > type I; type I in skin, therefore limited potency for hirsutism and alopecia)
  - few side effects
  - best after 6mths
  - teratogenic—contraception needed.
- *Flutamide* (250mg daily):
  - non-steroidal antiandrogen
  - best after 6mths, also for treatment of alopecia
  - hepatotoxicity (monitor liver enzymes regularly)
  - add contraceptive as may cause feminization of male fetus.
- *Eflornithine hydrochloride* (cream topically bd):
  - inhibits ornithine decarboxylase, responsible for hair growth
  - ↓ speed of hair growth and hair becomes less coarse
  - works within 8wks, but quick recurrence after cessation
  - may worsen acne (obstructing pilosebaceous glands)
  - recommended for postmenopausal hair growth on upper lip.
- *GnRH agonists* (depot prescriptions):
  - suppress gonadotropins, thereby suppressing ovarian androgens
  - should be combined with add-back HRT
  - expensive and equally effective as other approaches.

Last-resort treatment

- *Ketoconazole* (400mg daily):
  - antifungal agent
  - ↓ androgen levels by inducing hepatic cytochrome p450 metabolic pathways
  - hepatotoxicity (monitor liver enzymes regularly)
  - loss of scalp hair.

⚠ Most of the drugs mentioned are not licensed for this indication. Cyproterone acetate/ethinylestradiol, and eflornithine are the exceptions.

Hirsutism and the menopause

About 17% of patients are menopausal, mainly with facial hirsutism.

Treatment
- Eflornithine cream.
- Spironolactone.
- Cyproterone acetate with HRT (not ethinylestradiol).
- Estradiol + drospirenone HRT.

Endometriosis: overview

Endometriosis is the presence of endometrial-like tissue outside the uterine cavity. It is oestrogen dependent, and therefore mostly affects women during their reproductive years. If the ectopic endometrial-like tissue is within the myometrium itself it is called *adenomyosis*. If the ectopic endometrial-like tissue is present in the ovary itself it is called *endometrioma*. It is hormone mediated and is often associated with menstruation.

Aetiology

The exact aetiology remains unknown, various theories exist, but none accounts for all aspects of endometriosis. There may be one or a combination of theories may contribute.

- Retrograde menstruation with adherence, invasion, and growth of the tissue (*Sampson*): most popular theory; however, >90% show menstrual blood in pelvis at time of menstruation.
- Metaplasia of mesothelial cells (*Meyer*).
- Systemic and lymphatic spread (*Halban*).
- Impaired immunity (*Dmowski*).
- Embryological theory (*Knapp*).

Incidence of endometriosis
- General female population: 10–12% (estimated).
- Infertility investigation: 20–50%.
- Sterilization: 6%.
- Chronic pelvic pain investigation: 20–50%.
- Dysmenorrhea: 40–60%.

Typical presentation of endometriosis (often combination)
- Pelvic pain:
  - cyclic or constant (ectopic endometrial tissue undergoes same cycle, causing repeated inflammation, which may result in the formation of adhesions)
  - severe dysmenorrhoea (period-related pain affecting quality of life and daily activities)
  - dyspareunia (deep pain during or after sexual intercourse)
  - dysuria (pain passing urine) or haematuria (blood in the urine)
  - dyschezia (pain during or after bowel movement) and cyclic rectal bleeding (associated with rectovaginal nodules with invasion of rectal mucosa)
  - change of bowel habits (cyclical diarrhoea or constipation).
- Heavy menstruation (may related to adenomyosis).
- Infertility.

⚠ Pain symptoms are often non-specific, resulting in the delay of the diagnosis by up to 12yrs.

Location of endometriosis

Common sites
- Pelvis (common):
  - ovaries
  - pouch of Douglas
  - broad ligaments
  - uterosacral ligaments
  - uterus
  - rectovaginal space
  - rectosigmoid colon
  - bladder.

Rare sites
- Lungs.
- Liver and diaphragm.
- Abdominal wall—associated with previous surgical incisions.
- Brain.
- Muscle.
- Eye.
- Pelvic nerves.
- Perineum—around episiotomy scar.

▶ Endometriosis has been described in girls prior to menarche, and in men.

Appearance of endometriosis

- *Peritoneal endometriotic lesions:* appear as minuscule (powder burn) to 1–2cm lesions (red, bluish, brown, black, white; vesicular, cystic, petechial).
- Ovarian endometriotic cysts:
  - endometriomas can be >10cm in size
  - usually filled with brownish fluid ('chocolate cysts'; old blood and tissue)
  - often associated with local fibrosis and adhesions.
- *Deep infiltrating endometriosis:* rectovaginal nodules can frequently result in fibrosis of surrounding tissue and often have a solid appearance.

Further reading

European Society of Human Reproduction and Embryology (2022). Endometriosis.
🖰 www.eshre.eu/Guidelines-and-Legal/Guidelines/Endometriosis-guideline.aspx

NICE (2017). Endometriosis: diagnosis and management. NICE guideline [NG73].
🖰 www.nice.org.uk/guidance/ng73

Endometriosis: diagnosis

History
- Menstrual cycle.
- Nature of the pain:
  - site
  - relationship to cycle (mid cycle/dysmenorrhoea)
  - deep dyspareunia.
- Haematuria or rectal bleeding during menstruation.

Examination
- Bimanual pelvic examination for:
  - adnexal masses (endometriomas) or tenderness
  - nodules/tenderness in the posterior vaginal fornix or uterosacral ligaments
  - fixed retroverted uterus
  - rectovaginal nodules.
- Speculum examination of vagina and cervix (rarely, lesions may be visible and bluish black patches at the posterior vaginal fornix).

Investigations
- TV USS:
  - endometriosis located in pelvic organs, bladder, distal ureters, bowels with a sensitivity of 80%.
- Laparoscopy with biopsy for histological verification:
  - especially important for deep infiltrating lesions
  - +ve is confirmative, −ve does not rule it out
  - endometriomas >3cm should to be resected to rule out malignancy (rare).
- Laparoscopy should not be performed within 3mths of hormonal treatment (leads to underdiagnosis).
- Indications for laparoscopy:
  - NSAID-resistant lower abdominal pain/dysmenorrhoea
  - pain resulting in days off work/school or hospitalization
  - pain and infertility investigation.
- It is good practice to document the extent of disease (photos or DVD).
- MRI, intravenous urography (IVU), or barium enema (to assess extent of rectovaginal, bladder, ureteric, or bowel involvement).
- Serum CA125 is sometimes elevated with severe endometriosis, but there is no evidence that it is a useful screening test for this condition.

Grading of endometriosis

The current system (Revised American Society of Reproductive Medicine classification (rASRM), 1996) classifies the extent of endometriosis on a point system, taking into account:

Location
- Peritoneal.
- Ovarian.
- Pouch of Douglas.

Size
- <1cm.
- 1–3cm.
- >3cm.

Depth of infiltration
- Superficial.
- Deep.

Adhesions
- Filmy or dense.
- Extent of enclosure (<1/3; 1/3–2/3, >2/3).
- Colour and form.

The points are added up and the stage of endometriosis is graded accordingly:
- *Stage I:* minimal endometriosis (1–5 points).
- *Stage II:* mild endometriosis (6–15 points).
- *Stage III:* moderate endometriosis (16–40 points).
- *Stage IV:* severe endometriosis (>40 points).

This system of values is highly controversial because of its subjectivity. The severity of disease has not been shown to have any correlation with the severity of pain. It may be of value in infertility prognosis and management

Endometriosis: treatment

The approach should be determined by:
- Reason for treatment (pain, fertility, and heavy periods).
- Side effect profile.
- Cost-effectiveness of each drug.

▶ All drugs are effective in relieving pain and are associated with up to 50% recurrence after ~12–24mths after stopping.

▶ It is acceptable to treat women empirically with progestogens or COCP without a laparoscopic diagnosis. COCP, ideally administered continuously, should be considered as 1st-line agents. NSAIDs are effective and may be used with hormonal drugs.

▶ Severe cases of endometriosis should be referred to a centre with expertise in advanced laparoscopic surgery.

Treatments for pain

Medical treatment
See Table 18.1.

Surgical treatment
- Surgical management is indicated once medical treatment has failed in most of the minimal to moderate endometriosis cases.
- There are no data supporting preoperative hormonal treatment.
- Postoperative 6mth treatment with GnRH analogues is effective in delaying recurrence at 12 and 24mths (not the case with COCP).
- Coagulation, excision, or ablation are recommended surgical techniques and should be done by laparoscopy.
- Laparoscopic excision of deep infiltrating lesions has been reported to provide symptomatic relief lasting >2yrs.
- Risk of complications of laparoscopic surgery is 1–2:1000, but may be ↑ to 7:100 if the disease is widespread or involving pelvic organs. The risk of damaging to internal organs such as bladder, ureters, blood vessels, nerves, and bowel (1–2:100) is small but might require intraoperative temporary colostomy 1–2:100 times.
- As a last resort, hysterectomy may be considered in patients with severe, treatment-refractory dysmenorrhoea: if performed, bilateral oophorectomy should be considered with add-back HRT.

Treatments for subfertility

- Spontaneous pregnancy rate after surgical removal of endometriotic lesions is probably ↑ in minimal/mild endometriosis.
- Spontaneous pregnancy rate after surgical removal of deep infiltrating endometriotic nodules/lesions is probably ↑ in severe disease by 50%.
- Unclear efficacy for moderate/severe disease as no RCTs exist.
- Endometriomas (≥3cm) should be removed: best by cystectomy rather than drainage to ↓ recurrence rates.

▶ Fertility-sparing surgery should be the goal, to ↑ chance of conception. In moderate to severe disease, IVF may be the choice.

Table 18.1 Medical treatment for pain from endometriosis

Drug	Applications/ duration	Effect	Side effects
COCP	Continuous >> cyclic Long term	Ovarian suppression	Headaches Nausea VTE Stroke
Medroxy-progesterone acetate or other progestogens	Orally or IM/SC injection (depot) Long term	Ovarian suppression	Weight gain Bloating Acne Irregular bleeding Depression
GnRH analogues	2nd-line therapy SC/IM injection or nasal spray Short or long term Should never be used without add-back HRT	Ovarian suppression	Loss of bone density (reversible) Hot flushes Vaginal dryness Headaches Depression
Levonorgestrel-releasing IUCD	Intrauterine Long term (change every 5yrs if age <40)	Endometrial suppression; sometimes ovarian suppression	Irregular bleeding Spontaneous expulsion
Danazol	Oral 6mths (longest experience)	Ovarian suppression	Acne Hirsutism Irreversible voice changes
Aromatase inhibitors	Oral Probably 6mths (still experimental and not licensed)	Local oestrogen suppression in endometrial lesions	Ovarian cysts Loss of bone density (reversible)

Gonadotropin-releasing hormone in health and disease

Biochemistry

- GnRH is a decapeptide synthesized in the hypothalamus.
- Released in a pulsatile manner in both males and females.
- Acts on G protein-coupled receptors in the anterior pituitary.
- Has a short half-life ($t_{1/2}$) of 2–4min.

Physiological functions

The frequency and amplitude of the GnRH pulses are more important than absolute hormonal levels. During the fetal and neonatal periods, GnRH is involved in normal development. The amplitude of pulsatile release is then ↓ during childhood until puberty. It is not known what factor(s) trigger the ↑ frequency and amplitude of secretion seen during puberty, but this results in the release of gonadotropins (high-frequency pulses of LH and low-frequency pulses of FSH) from the anterior pituitary gland and subsequently sex steroids from the ovary. A complex system of +ve and −ve feedback loops between GnRH, LH, FSH, progesterone, and oestrogen regulate the normal menstrual cycle (⊙ Physiology of the menstrual cycle, p. 574).

Congenital GnRH deficiency

- Congenital hypothalamic hypogonadism is usually only diagnosed in females when a delay in puberty is noted, as female infants are phenotypically normal.
- When associated with an absence of the sense of smell (anosmia) it is known as Kallman's syndrome.
- It can be difficult to distinguish hypothalamic hypogonadism from delayed puberty; however, in the former, pubic hair is present as adrenarche occurs normally and children are usually of normal height for their age.

Acquired GnRH deficiency

Acquired GnRH deficiency can be due to:
- Damage to the hypothalamus by:
  - trauma
  - tumour.
- Disruption of the hypothalamic–pituitary axis can occur 2° to:
  - intense physical training
  - anorexia nervosa.

GnRH as a treatment

- Pulsatile IV infusions of GnRH can be used to induce puberty and ovulation with a congenital deficiency.
- If deficiency is acquired, it is more usual to use oestrogen and progesterone on a long-term basis, or LH/FSH to induce ovulation.

Gonadotropin-releasing hormone agonists and antagonists

The short half-life of natural GnRH restricts its pharmacological use to IV pulsatile use. However, longer-acting GnRH analogues (agonists) or receptor antagonists can be used to induce a temporary, reversible menopausal state as a treatment for a number of conditions.

GnRH analogues

A number of different GnRH analogues exist, including:
  * goserelin acetate
  * leuprorelin acetate
  * nafarelin.
* Administration:
  * SC injection (daily, monthly, or 3-monthly)
  * intranasally
  * intravaginally.
* They produce a prolonged activation of the GnRH receptor, resulting in an initial ↑ in FSH and LH secretion: this may cause a worsening of symptoms ('initial flare').
* Continued activation of the receptor leads to ↓ LH/FSH secretion:
  * serum oestradiol levels are suppressed by ~21 days
  * remain at similar levels to postmenopausal women with continued dosing.
* Indications and adverse effects are shown in Boxes 18.1 and 18.2.
* Adequate barrier contraception should be used during treatment as there is a theoretical risk of teratogenicity and miscarriage.

Bone mineral density (BMD)
* Up to 6% BMD may be lost after the 1st 6mths of treatment.
* If treatment is to be continued for >3mths, the use of 'add-back' HRT is recommended: combined GnRH agonist and HRT add-back has been shown to be safe for a period of up to 5–10yrs.
* Resumption of menstruation and return of fertility occur soon after stopping treatment.

GnRH antagonists

GnRH antagonists, such as cetrorelix, bind to receptors without activation and therefore do not cause an initial worsening of symptoms. They are currently licensed for assisted conception protocols and are used experimentally in endometriosis treatments. However, their effect on BMD and other side effects are similar to agonists.

Box 18.1 Indications for GnRH analogue treatment
- Pre-surgery:
  - endometrial thinning prior to ablation/resection
  - fibroid shrinkage prior to myomectomy/hysterectomy.
- Endometriosis.
- Adenomyosis.
- Assisted reproduction: pituitary down-regulation prior to superovulation.
- Diagnostic tool in chronic pelvic pain (➔ Chronic pelvic pain: diagnosis and treatment, p. 648).
- Breast cancer.
- Prostate cancer.

Box 18.2 Adverse effects of GnRH agonists/antagonists
- Hot flushes.
- Mood swings.
- Vaginal dryness.
- Abnormal vaginal bleeding.
- ↓ Libido.
- Breast swelling/tenderness.
- ↑ Low-density lipoprotein, ↓ high-density lipoprotein.
- Insomnia.
- Headaches.
- Loss of BMD.
- Alterations in eyesight.
- Initial flare (agonists only).
- Bruising at injection site.

Female subfertility: overview

- Infertility is very common, with 1 in 6 couples seeking specialist help.
- ~84% will achieve a pregnancy in 1yr of regular unprotected intercourse: this ↑ to 92% after 2yrs.
- Referral for specialist advice should be considered after at least 1yr of trying, though in certain situations prompt investigations and referral may be recommended:
  - female age >35yrs
  - known fertility problems
  - anovulatory cycles
  - severe endometriosis
  - previous PID
  - fertility preservation
- Treat couples on an individual basis. There is not necessarily a right answer as to when investigations and treatment should start.
- The management of subfertility aims to correct any specific problem that may or may not be diagnosed.

Causes of subfertility
- Ovulatory disorder: 20%.
- Tubal factor: 15–20%.
- Male factor: 25%.
- Unexplained: 28–35%.

Causes of anovulation

1° ovarian disorders

- Premature ovarian insufficiency.
- *Genetic:* Turner's syndrome (45XO).
- Autoimmune.
- Iatrogenic:
  - surgery
  - chemotherapy.

2° ovarian disorders

- PCOS.
- Excessive weight loss or exercise.
- Hypopituitarism:
  - tumour
  - trauma
  - surgery.
- Kallman's syndrome (anosmia; hypogonadotropic hypogonadism).
- Hyperprolactinaemia.

Causes of tubal blockage

- Previous pelvic surgery.
- Endometriosis.
- Previous PID.
- Iatrogenic: surgery (bilateral salpingectomy for EPs or hydrosalpinges).

Causes of male factor infertility

- Varicocoele.
- Cryptorchidism.
- Prior chemotherapy or radiotherapy.
- Current medications (e.g. sulfasalazine).
- Vasectomy.
- Genetic (e.g. CF carrier, Y-microdeletions).

Female subfertility: diagnosis

History

Couples are often seen together and sometimes it can be difficult to ask about sensitive issues; if necessary, each partner can be seen alone, though this is not ideal.

- Age.
- Duration of subfertility.
- Menstrual cycle regularity and LMP (pregnancy test?).
- Coital frequency.
- Pelvic pain (dysmenorrhoea; dyspareunia).
- Cervical smear history.
- Previous pregnancies.
- History of EP.
- Previous tubal or pelvic surgery.
- Previous or current STIs and PID.
- Any relevant medical or surgical history.
- Drug history (any prescription drugs that may be contraindicated in pregnancy and ask about recreational drug use).
- Smoking.
- Number of units alcohol/week.
- Advise the female patient to take folic acid if not already doing so.

Clinical examination

General examination

- BMI.
- *Signs of endocrine disorder:* hyperandrogenism (acne, hair growth, alopecia), acanthosis nigricans (see ➲ Polycystic ovarian syndrome: overview, p. 652); thyroid disease (hypo- and hyperthyroidism); visual field defects (?prolactinoma).

Pelvic examination

- Exclude obvious pelvic pathology (adnexal masses, uterine fibroids, endometriosis (painful, fixed uterus), vaginismus).

Investigations

1° care

- Chlamydia screening.
- Baseline (day 2–5) hormone profile including FSH, LH (↑ in premature ovarian insufficiency; ↓ in hypothalamic hypogonadism), TSH, prolactin, testosterone.
- Rubella immunity status.
- Mid-luteal progesterone level (to confirm ovulation >30nmol/L).
- Semen analysis (see ➲ Male subfertility, p. 680).
- Cervical smear if not up to date.

2° care

- Ideally a specialist clinic with appropriately trained MDT staff.
- History should be confirmed with the couple and any missing details checked.

Assessment of ovarian reserve
- AMH.
- Antral follicle count.
- Together currently considered the most accurate indirect markers of ovarian reserve.

Assessment of tubal patency

Hysterosalpingography (HSG)
- Easily done.
- Good sensitivity and specificity.
- Can be uncomfortable.
- May have false +ve results (suggesting tubal blockage due to spasm).

Laparoscopy and dye test
- Day-case procedure that can be combined with a hysteroscopy to assess the uterine cavity if necessary.
- 'Gold standard.'
- Pelvic pathology (endometriosis, peritubular adhesions) can be diagnosed and treated.
- Requires GA.
- Carries surgical risks.

Hysterosalpingo contrast sonography (HyCoSy)
- USS with galactose-containing contrast medium.
- Similar sensitivity to HSG.
- No radiation exposure.

Female subfertility: management

Management depends on duration and possible cause of subfertility. Couples should be informed of their options and given relevant evidence-based advice so they can make an informed choice.

Lifestyle modification

- Healthy diet.
- Stop smoking/recreational drugs.
- Reduce alcohol consumption.
- Regular exercise.
- Folic acid.
- Regular unprotected sexual intercourse every 2–3 days.

Ovulation induction

- PCOS is the most common cause of 2° amenorrhoea and is responsible for 75–80% of anovulatory subfertility.
- Weight loss/gain as appropriate.
- Aromatase inhibitor/antioestrogens (e.g. letrozole 5mg/clomifene 50mg days 2–6):
  - ↑ Endogenous FSH levels via −ve feedback to pituitary
  - 8–10% multiple pregnancy rate
  - side effects (hot flushes, headache, nausea, lethargy)
  - offer 6–12 cycles
  - needs USS follicle tracking (abandon cycle if over-response).
- Gonadotropins:
  - used for letrozole or clomifene-resistant PCOS
  - injections
  - expensive
  - multiple pregnancy risk
  - needs USS monitoring (abandon cycle if over-response)
  - dose more easily titrated.
- Laparoscopic ovarian diathermy:
  - aims to restore ovulation in patients with PCOS
  - effect lasts 12–18mths if successful.
- Insulin sensitizers (metformin 500mg tds):
  - used in women with PCOS
  - may achieve spontaneous ovulation
  - can be combined with letrozole or clomifene to ↑ efficacy
  - unlicensed
  - weight loss is more effective.

Surgery

- Preferably laparoscopic.
- Treat endometriosis (laser/diathermy/excision).
- Tubal surgery (microsurgery/adhesiolysis).

Assisted conception

- Intrauterine insemination (IUI).
- IVF.

Psychological issues
- Subfertility and its management can be very distressing.
- Some treatments have side effects and are not guaranteed to be successful.
- The stress of this and disappointment of failed treatment needs to be addressed.
- Couples should be offered counselling before and after treatment, along with information regarding patient support groups.

Further reading

NICE (2013, updated 2017). Fertility problems: assessment and treatment. Clinical guideline [CG156].
⅋ www.nice.org.uk/guidance/cg156

Male subfertility

Accounts for 20–25% of cases of subfertile couples. Investigation should start in primary care after 1yr, or earlier if history of genital surgery, cancer treatment, or previous subfertility. Trend of declining sperm concentration is not affecting global fecundity but there is ↑ 'testicular dysgenesis syndrome' with an ↑ in cryptorchidism, testicular cancer, and hypospadias. Normal male fertility is dependent on normal spermatogenesis, erectile function, and ejaculation.

Normal semen analysis (WHO criteria 2009)

- Volume >1.5mL.
- Concentration >15 × 10⁶/mL.
- Progressive motility >32%.
- Total motility >40%.

Azoospermia: no sperm in ejaculate.
Oligozoospermia: ↓ number of sperm in ejaculate.

Investigations

- *FSH:LH* ↑ in testicular failure.
- *Testosterone:* ↓ in testicular failure.
- *Karyotype:* exclude 47XXY.
- *CF screen:* congenital bilateral absence of the vas deferens (CBAVD).
- *Y-microdeletions* (AZF-a and -b complete arrest in spermatogenesis, AZF-c variable phenotype from oligo-azoospermia).

Management

- Treat any underlying medical conditions.
- Address lifestyle issues (↓ alcohol <14 units/week, stop smoking).
- Review medications:
  - antispermatogenic (anabolic steroids, sulfasalazine)
  - antiandrogenic (cimetidine, spironolactone)
  - erectile/ejaculatory dysfunction (α- or β-blockers, antidepressants, diuretics, metoclopramide).
- Medical treatments:
  - gonadotropins in hypogonadotropic hypogonadism
  - sympathomimetics (e.g. imipramine) in retrograde ejaculation.
- Surgical:
  - relieve obstruction
  - vasectomy reversal.
- ▶ Surgical treatment of varicocele does not improve pregnancy rates.
- Sperm retrieval:
  - from postorgasmic urine in retrograde ejaculation
  - surgical sperm retrieval from testis with up to 50% chance of obtaining sperm (greater if FSH is normal).
- Assisted reproduction:
  - IUI (suitable for erectile or ejaculatory dysfunction)
  - IVF-ICSI.
- Donor sperm.
- Adoption.

Pathogenesis of male subfertility

Semen abnormality (85%)
- Idiopathic oligoasthenoteratozoospermia (OATS).
- Testicular cancer.
- Drugs (including alcohol, nicotine).
- Genetic.
- Varicocoele.

Azoospermia (5%)
- *Pretesticular:* idiopathic hypogonadotropic hypogonadism, e.g. Kallmann's syndrome; pituitary adenoma; anabolic steroid abuse.
- *Non-obstructive:* cryptorchidism, orchitis, 47XXY, chemoradiotherapy.
- *Obstructive:* CBAVD, vasectomy.

Immunological (5%)
- Antisperm antibodies.
- Idiopathic.
- Infection.
- Unilateral testicular obstruction.

Coital dysfunction (5%)
- Mechanical/erectile dysfunction with normal sperm function.
- With normal ejaculatory function (hypospadias, phimosis, disability).
- Retrograde ejaculation (diabetes, bladder neck surgery, phenothiazines).
- Absent ejaculation (multiple sclerosis, spinal cord/pelvic injury).

Assisted conception: *in vitro* fertilization and intracytoplasmic sperm injection

Assisted reproductive technologies refer to all fertility treatments in which sperm and oocytes are handled with the aim of achieving pregnancy. It includes IVF, ICSI, preimplantation genetic diagnosis, preimplantation genetic screening, egg donation, and surrogacy.

In vitro fertilization

Indications may include:
- Tubal disease.
- Male factor subfertility.
- Endometriosis.
- Anovulation.
- ↓ Fecundity observed with ↑ maternal age.
- Unexplained infertility for >2yrs.

Success is dependent on many factors including:
- *Duration of subfertility:* ↓ success with ↑ duration.
- Maternal age:
  - pregnancy rates are highest between 25 and 35yrs with a steep decline thereafter
  - elevated basal FSH and/or low AMH/antral follicle count levels may indicate a poor response to ovarian stimulation.
- Previous pregnancy: ↑ chance of successful IVF outcome.
- Previous failed IVF cycles: ↓ chances of success.
- Presence of hydrosalpinx: unilateral and bilateral up to 20% and 40% ↓ in success rate respectively.
- Smoking and BMI >30kg/m²: ↓ success rates.

Intracytoplasmic sperm injection

- A single sperm is injected into the ooplasm of the oocyte in ICSI.
- Used for men with abnormal semen parameters.
- Can be tried when failed fertilization has occurred in IVF cycles.
- Higher fertilization rates if the selected sperm exhibit progressive motility, but otherwise there are no strict selection criteria.
- ↑ Success of IVF with severe male factor subfertility.
- Sperm may be retrieved from ejaculate or surgically from epididymis or testes.

⚠ There are concerns regarding transmission of genetic mutations when using ICSI. Sperm containing DNA damage induced from ↑ oxidative stress are capable of fertilizing oocytes.

⚠ There is also an ↑ incidence of Y-chromosome microdeletions in subfertile men (AZF-c mutation has variable phenotype) and this may be further propagated by transmission to the offspring born by ICSI.

IVF: how it's done

In preparation, the HFEA consents and 'Welfare of the Child' issues must be considered.

- Down-regulation of the HPO axis using GnRH analogues from day 21 (luteal phase) of the previous cycle: alternatively, in antagonist cycles ('short protocol') GnRH antagonists are co-administered with gonadotropins from day 2 of the cycle during ovarian stimulation.
- Ovarian stimulation achieved with recombinant FSH or human menopausal gonadotropins: response is monitored by ultrasound follicle tracking.
- Follicular maturation by administration of hCG, or GnRH analogue in an antagonist cycle, when mature-sized follicles are seen on USS.
- TV oocyte retrieval by needle-guided aspiration (36h after hCG).
- Sperm sample collected (or thawed if frozen), prepared, and cultured with oocytes overnight (standard IVF) or oocytes injected with a single sperm and cultured (ICSI).
- Fertilization checks of embryos the following day.
- Embryo transfer by a fine catheter through cervix on day 2–3 (cleavage stage) or day 5 (blastocyst stage):
  - a maximum of two embryos are transferred in women <40yrs and there is an NHS elective single embryo transfer criteria given ↑ neonatal morbidity/mortality and ensuing costs of multiple pregnancy
  - blastocyst transfer ↑ the success rates of IVF.
- Surplus embryos may be cryopreserved for future frozen embryo replacement cycles.
- Luteal support given in form of progestogens.
- Pregnancy test 11–13 days later depending on age of embryo transferred.

Assisted conception: other techniques

Intrauterine insemination

- Couples who may benefit include:
  - those with coital difficulties
  - same-sex couples.
- Sperm is prepared and placed into the uterus to aid conception.
- The lower threshold for sperm concentration suitability for IUI has been suggested as a total motile count of >10M/mL.
- NICE recommends up to six cycles of IUI.

 There is no consensus on the role of simultaneous ovarian stimulation, but this should be considered in endometriosis and unexplained infertility when outcome is less favourable.

▶ If >3 mature follicles develop, the treatment cycle should be cancelled as there is a high rate of multiple pregnancies (>25%).

Donor insemination

- Indicated in men with azoospermia and failed surgical sperm recovery.
- Single women with no male partner.
- Same-sex couples.
- Insemination is usually intrauterine: with/without ovarian stimulation and 24–36h after hCG administration.

  Success rates vary from 4% (aged 40–44yrs) to 12% (<34yrs) per cycle.

Egg donation

- May offer a chance of pregnancy for women previously considered to be irreversibly infertile.
- This includes women with:
  - ovarian insufficiency (premature ovarian insufficiency, gonadal dysgenesis, iatrogenic causes such as surgery and chemoradiotherapy)
  - older women (>45yrs)
  - those with repeated IVF failure.

Special concerns regarding donation of gametes

There are strict criteria for gamete donation, which is regulated by the HFEA.

- Ideally, donors should have no severe medical, psychiatric, or genetic disorders.
- Donors must be counselled.
- Donors must undergo a full infection screen.
- Donors may be known or anonymous to the recipient.
- Egg donors should ideally be <35yrs old.
- Each donor can only be used in up to ten families within the UK.

In April 2005, donor anonymity was lifted in the UK, meaning that when children born from the use of donor gametes reach the age of 18yrs, they can contact the HFEA for identifying information regarding the donor.

▶ The supply of donor gametes in the UK is limited. The HFEA may authorize the procurement of gametes from abroad if the supplying clinic fulfils the same quality of standards as the UK.

Surrogacy

IVF surrogacy

- The couple who want the child provide both sets of gametes.
- Following IVF, the embryos are transferred to the surrogate.
- This accounts for <0.1% of the total IVF cycles in the UK.
- Indications include women who have congenital absence of the uterus (Rotikansky's syndrome), following hysterectomy, or with severe medical conditions incompatible with pregnancy.

'Natural surrogacy'

- The surrogate is inseminated by the sperm of the male partner of the couple wanting the child.

⚠ Counselling and legal advice is necessary for all parties involved in the surrogacy.

Preimplantation genetic diagnosis

- Aims to reduce the transmission of genetic disorders to children in couples known to carry a heritable genetic condition.
- Many couples are fertile, but IVF allows embryo biopsy, single cell diagnosis, and the transfer of unaffected embryos.
- Biopsies are usually done at the blastocyst stage and next-generation sequencing used for genetic diagnosis.

Ovarian hyperstimulation syndrome

Ovarian hyperstimulation syndrome (OHSS) is a complication of ovarian stimulation. Incidence varies from 0.5% to 33% and in 1–3% of cases it is severe, requiring hospitalization. Vascular endothelial growth factor (VEGF) and other vasoactive substances are central to the underlying pathophysiology.

- It is characterized by:
  - ovarian enlargement
  - shifting of fluid from the intravascular to the extravascular space.
- Fluid accumulates in the peritoneal and pleural spaces.
- There is intravascular fluid depletion, leading to:
  - haemoconcentration
  - hypercoagulability.
- Risk factors include:
  - polycystic ovaries
  - younger women with low BMI
  - previous OHSS.

Prevention

Management is focused on risk assessment and active prevention. This may involve adopting the antagonist protocol with use of GnRH analogues trigger, low-dose gonadotropins, cycle cancellation, 'coasting' during stimulation, or elective embryo cryopreservation for replacement in a subsequent frozen cycle.

In vitro maturation may also be used in women with polycystic ovaries, with high antral follicle counts, collecting immature eggs, thus avoiding ovarian stimulation and the risk of OHSS.

Treatment

- Is supportive, with the aims of:
  - symptomatic relief
  - prevention of haemoconcentration and thromboembolism
  - maintenance of cardiorespiratory function.
- Daily assessment of:
  - hydration status (FBC, U&E, LFTs, and albumin)
  - chest and respiratory function (pleural effusions)
  - ascites (girth measurement and weight)
  - legs (for evidence of thrombosis).
- Strict fluid balance with careful maintenance of intravascular volume.
- Thromboprophylaxis:
  - compression stockings
  - LMWH.
- Paracentesis for symptomatic relief (± IV replacement albumin).
- Analgesia and antiemetics.

Sexual dysfunction: overview

Sexual health is a state of physical, emotional, mental, and social well-being in relation to sexuality, not merely the absence of disease or dysfunction. Sexual health necessitates the possibility of having pleasurable and safe sexual experiences, free of coercion, discrimination, and violence. Sexual rights must therefore be respected, protected, and fulfilled.

- The prevalence of female sexual dysfunction (FSD) is highly definition dependent (whether dissatisfaction and disinterest constitute FSD is debated).
- Rates are up to 43% in women aged 18–59 compared with 31% in men. Increasing age is inversely proportional to sexual activity. 1/3 of all women >60yrs may be sexually active (55% if married). Up to 50% of men will have some degree of erectile dysfunction, which rises to 67% by 70yrs.
- Menopause is associated with deterioration of sexual function, with one study suggesting an ↑ in FSD from 42% to 88% (45–55yr-olds).
- Dyspareunia is common and may be present in up to 1/3 of women.

Normal sexual function

Masters and Johnson proposed four components of the sexual response: arousal/excitement, plateau, orgasm, and resolution (based on biological, predominantly male, responses). More recently, intimacy-based models include features of satisfaction, pleasure, and relationship context. Overall, the 'normal' for female sexuality is not well characterized and currently FSD is under construction.

Diagnosis

See the woman as she chooses to present herself, with or without a partner, and explore 'Why now?' Many present when not in relationships, concerned about their sexual responses.

Presentation may be overt or covert—it is often useful to give the patient time to explore this and always think of the possibility of somatization of problems.

> **Vital questions in a psychosexual history**
> - Are you sexually active/do you have a partner?
> - Do you have any difficulties?
> - Are they a problem for you?
> - Do you have pain associated with intercourse?

Examination

'The moment of truth' is a frequent occasion for disclosure of sexual problems manifesting as difficulties with examination, exposure, humiliation, or fantasies of disease or disgust.

Tips on handling consultations
- Be led by the patient.
- The patient is the expert—help her understand her behaviour.
- Reflect your thoughts and feelings.
- Try to understand the relationship between the physical findings, such as prolapse, and the psychological reaction to them.
- Be aware of powerful subconscious defences in the patient, especially with lack of libido and desire disorders.

Consider discussing possible fantasies
- Feeling too small.
- Feeling too big.
- Feeling too loose.
- Vagina with teeth.
- Sharp penis.

Further reading
British Association of Sexual & Marital Therapy.
ⅆ www.basrt.org.uk

Institute of Psychosexual Medicine.
ⅆ www.ipm.org.uk

Mary Clegg—devices.
ⅆ www.maryclegg.com

Vulval Pain Society
ⅆ www.vulvalpainsociety.org/

Sexual dysfunction: classification of disorders

Desire disorder

Persistent or recurrent deficiency (or absence) of sexual fantasies/thoughts and/or desire for or receptivity to sexual activity, which causes personal distress (75% of women and 25% of men attending a psychosexual clinic).

The majority of women who have little or no desire are able to derive pleasure from sexual activity. Presentation itself indicates sufficient interest to be hopeful of cure.

Arousal disorder

Persistent or recurrent inability to attain or maintain sufficient sexual excitement, causing personal distress, which may be expressed as a lack of subjective excitement or genital (lubrication/swelling) or other somatic responses. Understanding the sequence of sexual events and the interplay of physical factors (pain, lubrication, environment) helps to deal with the root cause. Lack of sensation is a common presentation of 2° personal or relationship issues.

Orgasmic disorder

Persistent or recurrent difficulty, delay in, or absence of attaining orgasm following sufficient sexual stimulation and arousal, which causes personal distress.

7–10% of women never achieve orgasm with or without a partner. This may not be a concern. Those who can achieve orgasm with masturbation but not with a partner may need to explore their ability to let go or lose control. Up to 25% of women with lifelong anorgasmia have been sexually abused. Women with acquired orgasmic difficulties should explore hormonal status, concomitant medications, and relationship issues. Up to 5% of women with anorgasmia will have an organic cause.

Sexual dysfunction 2° to a general medical condition

Endocrine disorders, psychiatric disorders, and a number of medications will interfere with the sexual response cycle. Treatment of the condition or alteration of therapies may help, but education and explanation may minimize the impact on sexual relationships.

Sexual pain disorders

Dyspareunia

- Dermatological disorders, e.g. psoriasis and lichen sclerosis, infections, such as thrush and recurrent herpes, and atrophic vaginitis are treatable causes of superficial dyspareunia, but may have significant psychological sequelae.
- Poor arousal may be the result or cause of sexual pain: lubricants and topical anaesthetic gels may help break the cycle.
- Deep dyspareunia may be related to a number of medical conditions (endometriosis, PID, adhesions) determined by examination, USS, and, if necessary, laparoscopy.
- Pelvic floor muscle pain could contribute to dyspareunia.

Vaginismus

- Difficulty of the woman to allow vaginal entry of a penis, finger, or object despite the wish to do so.
- This can involve pelvic floor and/or adductor thigh muscle spasm.
- Vaginismus should be regarded as a symptom or sign and not a diagnosis.
- It is generally 2° to another cause—physical, psychological, or both.
- Fear of pain and anticipation of difficulty evolves into avoidance behaviour.
- Check at examination for the presence of anatomical problems, e.g. vaginal septum.

Non-coital sexual pain disorders

- Vulval vestibulitis is the most common pain disorder, but it is frequently difficult to treat.
- Treatment of any skin condition, desensitization, and treatment with topical anaesthetics and lubricants is 1st-line therapy in conjunction with an exploration of the psychosexual issues.
- Amitriptyline and gabapentin can be considered short term to interrupt the pain cycle.

Sexual dysfunction: treatment

Lifestyle

Address issues including those affecting body image and general well-being, ↓ of stress, and dealing with relationship/marital issues.

Education

- Teach people about their bodies and encourage exploration.
- Using 'bibliotherapy' for those needing 'permission' to look at erotic and sexual education material.
- Personal lubricants can be useful for those with arousal difficulties and atrophy (recommend oils or special preparations, but be aware of mineral oil damage to condoms).

Hormonal treatments

- Oestrogen replacement in menopausal women may improve sexuality as well as symptoms of vaginal atrophy: vaginal oestrogens can be used long term.
- Testosterone implants have been used successfully in those who have been oophorectomized and have hypoactive sexual desire disorder (HSDD).
- Testosterone patches are also licensed in the UK.
- Tibolone is licensed for treatment of loss of desire in postmenopausal women.

Complementary therapies

No good evidence for yohimbine, gingko, khat, or ginseng.

Behavioural therapy

Most sex therapists will use a combination of psychotherapeutic techniques and behavioural interventions. Sensate focus uses a programme of exercises building up in stages:
- Non-genital sensate focus.
- Genital sensate focus.
- Vaginal containment.
- Vaginal containment with movement.

Devices for anorgasmia

- Clitoral stimulators.
- Vibrators.

Vaginal trainers or dilators

May be of use for women with vaginismus and are recommended for those having prolapse procedures and postradiotherapy.

Perineal injections

100mg hydrocortisone, 10mL 0.5% bupivacaine, and 1500U hyaluronidase—may be of value for perineal injuries or for pain trigger points.

Surgery

Rarely necessary—may be for those with a rigid hymen, significant skin webs at the fourchette post surgery or childbirth, or septa.

Prognostic factors for the success of FSD interventions
- Motivation for treatment (especially in the male partner).
- Quality of the non-sexual relationship.

Sexual dysfunction: male disorders

If you have elicited a problem in a sexually active couple, the difficulties of both partners should be gently sought.

Male sexual disorders

- Erectile dysfunction most common.
- Desire disorders.
- Ejaculatory disorders.

Erectile dysfunction

Routine tests recommended

- Serum glucose.
- Lipids.
- Testosterone (early morning).
- BP.
- Pulse.
- Weight.
- Genitalia.
- Prostate.

⚠ New-onset erectile dysfunction may be a marker for cardiovascular disease.

Treatment options

- Phosphodiesterase inhibitors:
  - sildenafil and vardenafil ↑ erectile function in 60–70%
  - they act in 20–60min and last for up to 8h.
- Tadalafil may be useful for premature ejaculation.
- Apomorphine:
  - dopamine agonist
  - less efficacious (40–50%).
- Androgens: for men with hypogonadism.
- Intracavernous prostaglandin injections.
- Intraurethral prostaglandin pellets.
- Vacuum devices.
- Penile implants.

⚠ It is important to remember the psychosexual aspects of sexual difficulties for both partners, as well as concentrating on pharmacological treatments.

Chapter 19

Sexual assault

Sexual assault: overview

Sexual offences and rape definitions vary from country to country.

Sexual Offences Act 2003 (UK)

- *Rape:* is defined as non-consensual penetration of mouth, vagina, or anus by a penis. It is important to note that the legal definition of 'vagina' includes the vulva, and ejaculation need not have occurred.
- *Sexual assaults:* are acts of sexual touching without consent. Sexual assault by penetration involves insertion of an object or body parts other than a penis into a vagina or anus (previously indecent assault).
- Children <13yrs cannot legally consent to sexual activity and therefore do not need proof of consent. Mistaken belief of age is not a valid defence.

In assessing a potential victim, it is important to establish:
- Whether a sexual act has occurred.
- Ability of client to give consent to forensic examination: age, understanding, language, maturity, injury, or intoxication.
- Need for interpreters, 'appropriate adult', or advocate if under age of 16yrs, or has learning difficulties.
- Need of assessment for any acute psychiatric or physical symptoms must always take precedence over forensic examination if needed.
- If reported to the police or victim wants to report it to the police.

It is crucial that advice is sought from the police or a sexual assault referral centre (SARC) *before* any examination is undertaken, to preserve possible evidence available.

Presentation

Acute on chronic is also common, particularly with children.

Acute

Victims of acute sexual assault may report to the police directly, or to A&E, GUM, gynaecological, or psychiatric services with covert or overt symptoms. It is crucial to any criminal case that evidence is gathered appropriately and the chain of evidence maintained.

Always consult with the police/SARC if there is any doubt about an individual's presentation.

Delayed

Abuse can present with a number of symptoms (recent or historical). GUM, gynaecology, and psychiatry are frequent specialties for disclosure of sexual assault or abuse. There is a significant ↑ in domestic violence and assault during pregnancy so antenatal services must include screening and referral facilities.

Sexual assault: facts and figures

- The lifetime risk of sexual assault is 1 in 4–6 for women.
- Only 17% of people who have experienced sexual assault report it to the police.
- 10% of victims of sexual assault are men.
- 12% of assaults are by strangers.
- 45% are by acquaintances and 43% by intimate partners.
- 45% involve vaginal rape, 10% anal rape, 15% oral rape, and 25% digital penetration.
- 30% of rape victims will have anogenital injuries.
- 80% will have other bodily injuries.
- The incidence of child sexual abuse is unknown and possibly only 1 in 20–50 assaults of children are known to supervising authorities.
- The prevalence is far higher than that reflected in numbers reported.
- 75% had met the perpetrator before the sexual assault, with nearly 50% reporting that the perpetrator was a current or former boyfriend, family member, or someone they considered a friend.
- >40% of young women had consumed >5 units of alcohol.
- These women were more often sexually assaulted by a stranger or someone they met within 24h prior to the assault.

Sexual abuse in children

Concern for children is heightened by:
- Repeated A&E attendances.
- Poor parent–child interactions or behaviour.
- Child known to social services.
- Any injuries to child <1yr.
- History of domestic abuse.
- Explanation inconsistent with injuries.
- Disclosure of abuse by child.
- Delay in presentation.

⚠ Any concerns should be passed onto the local safeguarding lead—this may be a nurse, midwife, or paediatrician in your local organization.

Sexual assault: history and examination

History

- Establish when it occurred, what happened, where it happened, and who did it. The history should be contemporaneous with the date and time it was taken, and be countersigned.
- *Written consent:* taken before any forensic medical examination:
  - 16–18yr-olds can give or withhold consent even if their parents disagree
  - children <16yrs old, who are considered mature enough to understand, can give or withhold consent even if parents object.
- *Confidentiality issues:* victim may agree to only partial release of information and samples, but can change this decision later:
  - forensic samples can be stored for up to 30yrs or 30yrs after their 18th birthday
  - the SARC would take and store such samples.

Examination

- Examination can be performed by the SARC team at the same time as a gynaecological/general examination if necessary, although it is usually done in the SARC suite.
- If the victim is <13yrs a paediatrician will normally be in attendance as well as a forensic medical examiner.
- The time of the examination and sampling should be noted.
- The presence of pre-existing conditions such as skin problems or markers of self-harm must also be documented.

Collecting evidence

- Early evidence kits should be available in all A&E departments or can be brought by the police/forensic examiner:
  - if at all possible, evidence should be obtained by someone trained in this procedure, to ensure the highest quality evidence is obtained.
- Evidential samples for sexual offences are likely to be:
  - semen
  - saliva
  - vaginal samples
  - urine, blood
  - faeces
  - hair
  - fibres
  - vegetation
  - sanitary pads and/or tampons
  - toilet paper
  - clothes
  - condoms.

Key examination points
- Demeanour.
- Intoxication.
- Height/weight/BP/pulse/temperature.
- General findings.
- Injuries (record accurately with diagrams—photographs may be used (involvement of police photographer is preferred):
  - *non-genital:* none, bruising, petechiae, abrasions, lacerations, incisions, defence injuries
  - *genital and anal:* none, bruising, abrasions, lacerations, incisions, structure of hymen/remnants in those sexually active (or not)
  - *oral:* mucosa, teeth, tongue.
- Clothes may also be important for evidence.

Key samples for reported sexual assault
- *Oral intercourse:* mouth swab/saliva/mouth wash ± appropriate skin swab.
- *Vaginal intercourse:*
  - swabs: vulval and perineal (both ×2), low vaginal (×2), high vaginal with a Cuscoe's speculum (×2), endocervical (×2), from speculum (×1)
  - lubricant used is also sent.
- *Anal intercourse:*
  - swabs: perianal (×2), rectal (×2), and anal (×2) with proctoscope.
- Buccal swabs are taken for victim DNA.
- Double swabs = 1 dry + 1 wet with saline as these have shown the best return of DNA.
- Fingernail (×2) and hand (×2) swabs and skin (×2 from each site) if stranger assailant.

Timescales
- Penile oral penetration within 48h. Penile vaginal penetration within 168h. Penile anal penetration within 72h. Digital penetration of any orifice within 48h. Skin swabs within 48h, or up to 168h if not washed.
- Toxicology samples should be taken, blood within 72h and urine within 120h.

▶ Forensic examination at >7 days for women and >72h for men is unlikely to provide useful DNA evidence; however, it may still be appropriate for documentation of injuries.

Sexual assault: management

Emergency contraception

- Should be given if there has been any vaginal contact in women or menstruating girls, irrespective of stage of menstrual cycle.
- Current recommendations:
  - levonorgestrel 1500 micrograms stat within 72h of sexual act (doubled if postexposure prophylaxis (PEP) is used)
  - or IUCD insertion with antibiotic cover within 5 days
  - ulipristal can now also be considered within 120h.

Principles of management

- Resuscitation/usual 'ABC' measures are of overriding importance.
- Consideration of collection of evidence.
- Prophylactic antibiotics.
- PEP for HIV.
- Emergency contraception.
- Hepatitis B vaccination.
- Analgesia.
- General advice and support.
- Follow-up including counselling.

Child sexual abuse

- Difficult to know proportions of extra-familial and intra-familial sexual abuse because of underreporting (possibly 2/3 to 1/3, respectively, of reported abuse).
- Most children do not present acutely and may present because of social services or medical concerns regarding chronic physical illness, failure to thrive, or neglect.

⚠ Emergency contraception must be remembered in pubescent girls.

- STIs diagnostic for child sexual abuse are:
  - gonorrhoea (if >1yr)
  - syphilis and HIV (if congenital infection excluded)
  - chlamydia (if >3yrs).
- Any victim who has children or any young person <16yrs should be automatically referred to social services.
- All children <13yrs are followed up by the community paediatrician responsible for safeguarding in their area.
- Those >13yrs can be followed up in the SARC if appropriate.

Psychological care after sexual assault

⚠ *Trauma related to sexual violence is considered one of the most significant risk factors for suicide.*

- Those at immediate risk of self-harm or suicide must be referred to on-call psychiatric services.
- Others may be referred to local counselling or support services as well as being given details of emergency out of hours contacts (see Further reading).
- Counselling should aim to contain the trauma of the experience and help the victim bear the 'unbearable'.
- Those with persistent symptoms after 6mths may have post-traumatic stress disorder and need referral to psychiatric services.
- Be aware of local services and charities in your area that may provide support to victims of sexual assault and give the victim their details.

Further reading

Brook—helpline and online enquiry service for the under-25s. Tel. 020 7284 6040.
🖰 www.brook.org.uk
Rape Crisis Federation (local telephone numbers available from website).
🖰 www.rapecrisis.org.uk
Rights of Women. Tel. 020 7251 6577.
🖰 www.rightsofwomen.org.uk
Samaritans. Tel. 08457 90 90 90.
🖰 www.samaritans.org.uk
Suzy Lamplugh Trust—for issues of personal safety. Tel. 020 8392 1839
🖰 www.suzylamplugh.org.uk
The Havens—London SARCs.
🖰 www.thehavens.co.uk
Victim Support: for victims of all crimes including sexual assault. Tel. 0845 30 30 900.
🖰 www.victimsupport.org.uk

Sexual assault: sexually transmitted infections

- Risk is estimated at 4–56% depending on the local prevalence and degree of trauma.
- Consider prophylactic antibiotics particularly if the victim is unlikely to attend for follow-up:
  - 1g azithromycin + 500mg ciprofloxacin or follow local guidelines.
- STD screening 2wks after the assault is recommended.
- Hepatitis B vaccination should be discussed and given where indicated.
▶ PEP of HIV should always be considered and discussed.

HIV and sexual assault

- Risk depends on population prevalence and trauma of assault.
- Prescribing of PEP must be carefully balanced against the side effects and risks of taking them.
- Consider the higher risk factors:
  - assailant HIV +ve or in risk group
  - anal rape
  - trauma and bleeding
  - multiple assailants.
▶ If in doubt, seek advice from a local HIV physician.

PEP

- Currently three antiretroviral drugs taken ASAP (within 1h if possible) and within 72h.
- Appropriate follow-up within the wk must be arranged for:
  - a baseline HIV test
  - U&E, LFTs, FBC (because of the toxicity of the drugs).
- PEP is taken for 1mth and involves several follow-up visits.
- Full compliance is essential to prevent the emergence of resistant HIV strains.
- A follow-up HIV test after 6mths is recommended.
- Counselling is therefore essential prior to prescription of PEP.

💣 There are no studies of the efficacy of PEP after sexual exposure.

Risk of transmission of HIV with single exposure (higher if traumatic)

- Receptive vaginal intercourse: 1:1000.
- Receptive anal intercourse with ejaculation: 1:65.

Chapter 20

Contraception

Combined oral contraceptive pill: overview

The COCP provides reliable, effective contraception, with a failure rate of 0.2–0.3 per 100 woman-yrs, until 50yrs of age. Modern COCPs all contain ethinylestradiol (20–35 micrograms) and are classified by the type of progestogen they contain. The newer quadriphasic COCP Qlaira® is an exception—it contains estradiol valerate.

Type of progestogen in the COCP

2nd generation
- Norethisterone.
- Levonorgestrel (LNG).

3rd generation
- Desogestrel.
- Gestodene (less androgenic).
- Norgestimate (metabolized to LNG).

Yasmin®
- Contains drospirenone (antiandrogenic and weak antidiuretic properties).

Co-cyprindiol
- Contains cyproterone acetate (antiandrogenic).
- Useful in the treatment of hirsutism and acne.

Mode of action
- Ovulation inhibition (–ve feedback on hypothalamus + pituitary).
- Thickened cervical mucus preventing sperm penetration.
- Thin endometrium preventing implantation.

Side effects

Breakthrough bleeding
- May occur especially in the 1st 3 months.
- Missed pills, STIs, and pregnancy should all be considered.

Headache
- Change dose of ethinylestradiol or progestogen.

Weight gain
- There is no evidence of additional weight gain due to COCP.

Contraindications to the COCP

- Pregnancy.
- Personal history of thromboembolic disease.
- Undiagnosed genital tract bleeding.
- Cardiovascular disorders.
- Migraine with aura.
- Oestrogen-dependent tumours.
- Active hepatobiliary disease or liver tumours.
- Hypertension and diabetes.
- ≥35yrs old who smoke (may use 1yr after cessation).
- BMI ≥35kg/m².

Advantages and disadvantages of the COCP

Advantages
- ↓ Menstrual blood loss and pain.
- Menstrual cycle can be regulated and controlled.
- ↓ Risks of benign ovarian tumours.
- ↓ Incidence of PID.
- Improvement in skin condition in acne vulgaris.
- Possible ↓ symptoms:
  - premenstrual syndrome
  - endometriosis.
- ↓ Risks of colorectal cancer.
- ↓ Ovarian cancer risk ≥50% during use and for >15yrs after.

Disadvantages
- ↑ risks (although absolute risk is very low):
  - VTE
  - stroke
  - cardiovascular disease.
- Small ↑ risk of breast cancer: returns to the background risk 10yrs after stopping.
- Very small association with ↑ risk of cervical cancer if taken for >5yrs.

The COCP and VTE

The absolute risk of VTE is:
- *Background risk:* 5:100,000 women/yr.
- *2nd-generation COCP:* 10–15:100,000 women/yr.
- *3rd-generation COCP:* 25:100,000 women/yr.
- *Pregnancy:* 60:100,000 women/yr.

Combined oral contraceptive pill: regimens

Assessment of suitability of COCP for an individual woman
- Assessment of medical eligibility should include:
  - medical conditions
  - lifestyle factors
  - family medical history
  - drug history
  - a recent accurate BP and BMI.

'Pill-teach'
- Contraception is immediate if the woman starts the COCP between days 1 and 5 of her cycle taken daily at the same time.
- If 1st pill is after day 5, other contraception is needed for 7 days.
- One pill daily for 21 days followed by 7 pill-free days:
  - some formulations have seven 'dummy pills', rather than the pill-free interval.
- If vomiting or diarrhoea, use extra contraception from the onset of illness and continue it for the next 7 days.

Special circumstances
- Postpartum (not breast-feeding):
  - start day 21 after delivery.
- Post-termination:
  - within 7 days of termination.
- Switching from other oral hormonal contraception:
  - start immediately if using other contraception reliably.
- Switching from implant or injectable progestogens:
  - start at any time up to removal of implant or when injection due.

Drug interactions
- No additional contraception is needed if taking antibiotics unless associated with diarrhoea/vomiting.
- COCP should not be prescribed to lamotrigine users as it ↓ serum drug concentration and therefore can ↑ seizure frequency.
- Patients taking enzyme-inducing medication should be offered alternative contraceptive method due to ↓ efficacy:
  - if she decides to continue the COCP, the ethinylestradiol should be ↑ to 50 micrograms, or the pill-free interval ↓ to 4 days.

Missed pill rules
- Missed pills may lead to failed contraception.
- The risk of pregnancy is greatest at the beginning and the end of the pack.

If 1 pill is missed
- Take the missed pill as soon as possible.
- Continue the rest of the pack as usual.
- No additional contraception is required

If ≥2 pills are missed
- Take the most recent missed pill as soon as possible.
- Continue the rest of the pack as normal.
- Additional contraceptive cover is required until seven consecutive pills have been taken.
- *If the missed pills are in day 1–7:*
  - emergency contraception should be considered.
- *If the missed pills are in day 8–14:*
  - emergency contraception not needed.
- *If the missed pills are in day 15–21:*
  - omit the pill-free interval.
- Qlaira® has different missed pill rules (see manufacturer's advice).

Other combined hormonal contraceptives
Vaginal ring
- Ethinylestradiol with etonogestrel.
- Remains *in situ* for 21 days, then removed for 7 days to induce a withdrawal bleed.

Transdermal patch
- Ethinylestradiol with norelgestromin.
- Replaced weekly for 21 days, then 7 patch-free days to induce a withdrawal bleed.

▶ Efficacy and side effect profile as for COCP.

Progestogen-only pill

- POPs currently marketed contain either LNG, norethisterone, or desogestrel.
- If used reliably, at the same time every day, POPs are >99% effective.
- Failure rate 0.3–4.0% per 100 woman-yrs:
  - ↓ with age.
- Cerazette®, a POP (75 micrograms desogestrel), reliably blocks ovulation, ↑ efficacy.

Mode of action

- Thickened cervical mucus (4h after dose).
- Thin endometrium preventing implantation.
- Inhibition of ovulation (60% old POP, 97% desogestrel).

Indications

Useful in conditions where COCP is contraindicated:
- During lactation—has no effect on quality or quantity of milk.
- History or current VTE.
- BMI >35kg/m².
- Maternal medical conditions including AF, cardiomyopathy with impaired cardiac function, hypertension, complicated valvular heart disease, SLE, and migraine with aura.

Side effects

- Menstrual disturbance:
  - common reason cited for cessation of POPs
  - prolonged bleeding and breakthrough bleeding or spotting.
- Headaches, mood changes, and weight changes have been reported with the use of POPs but not been supported by definitive evidence.

Drug interactions

- Broad-spectrum antibiotics do not affect the efficacy of POP.
- Rifampicin and other enzyme-inducing drugs ↑ the metabolism of POP and have the potential to ↓ its efficacy.

Contraindications to the POP

- Pregnancy.
- Undiagnosed genital tract bleeding.
- Current breast cancer.
- Severe arterial disease.
- Active hepatic disease.

How to take the POP
- Take the pill daily, at the same hour.
- If started on day 1 of the cycle, no extra contraception is required.
- If started after day 5, extra contraception should be used for 48h.
- After miscarriage or TOP:
  - start on the day of the miscarriage or TOP.
- After delivery:
  - start on day 21 (whether breast-feeding or not).
- From COCP to POP:
  - if the 1st POP is taken the day after the last active COCP, no other contraception is needed.

Missed POP rules
- If >3h late or 27h since last dose:
  - take missed pill as soon as possible
  - take subsequent pill at the usual time
  - use extra contraception for the next 48h.
- If woman vomits within 2h of ingestion:
  - take another pill now
  - use extra contraception for the next 48h.

▶ For Cerazette®, the same rules apply if missed pill is >12h late.

Long-acting reversible contraceptives

Injectable progestogen

Depo-Provera® (MDPA) (given 12-weekly):
- Useful for women who are unable or unwilling to take a pill.
- Contains 150mg of medroxyprogesterone.
- When used as recommended failure rate is <0.2%:
  - with typical use failure rate is 6%

Side effects
- Menstrual disturbance (regular, irregular, or even amenorrhoea).
- Delayed conception (fertility may not return for 6–12mths).
- Weight gain ↑ particularly in <18yr-olds with BMI >30kg/m².
- Small loss of BMD ↓ recovered after stopping.

Progestogen-only subdermal implant

Nexplanon® (has replaced Implanon® in the UK):
- Contains etonogestrel 68mg.
- Insertion and removal involving a small procedure under local anaesthetic (inserted into the inner, upper arm).
- Single non-biodegradable, radio-opaque rod that lasts for 3yrs.
- Highly effective (failure rate reported as <0.1 per 100 woman-yrs).

Side effects
Menstrual disturbance—20% amenorrhoea, 50% erratic bleeding.

Copper intrauterine contraceptive device (Cu-IUCD)

- Provides instant, long-term reversible contraception, up to 10yrs.
- Also serves as emergency contraception within 120h of UPSI.
- Easily inserted and contains 380mm² copper.
- Very effective (failure rate of 0.6–0.8 per 100 woman-yrs).

Mode of action
- Foreign body reaction in the endometrium prevents implantation.
- Copper acts on the cervical mucus inhibiting sperm penetration.

Complications
- Irregular PV bleeding, especially 1st 3–6mths.
- Risk of infection: screen for *Chlamydia* prior to insertion.
- IUCD expulsion: most common in the 1st 3mths after insertion.
- Perforation: poor insertion technique or <4wks postpartum.
- Dysmenorrhoea.

Timing of IUCD insertion
- Insert any time during cycle (as long as pregnancy excluded).
- Post-partum: safe to insert IUCD within 48h of delivery or from 4wks after delivery.
- Following TOP: ideally at the end of the procedure or after the passage of products of conception have been confirmed.
- Switching from other contraception: any time as long as not pregnant.

Contraindications to Cu-IUCD

- Pregnancy.
- Undiagnosed genital tract bleeding.
- Active genital tract infection or PID.
- Uterine anomalies or fibroids distorting cavity.
- Gestational trophoblastic disease with elevated hCG levels.
- Endometrial/cervical cancer.
- Copper allergy.

Levonorgestrel-releasing system (Mirena® IUS)

- T-shaped rod containing 52mg LNG (20 micrograms released daily).
- It is a reversible, highly effective contraceptive with a failure rate of 0.18 per 100 woman-yrs.
- Due to its progestogenic content, menstrual blood loss is ↓ by >90%.
- It is as effective as endometrial ablation in the management of menorrhagia at 1yr.
- Timing of insertion is similar to the Cu-IUD; however, it is not used as an emergency contraceptive.

Mode of action

- Acts on the endometrium, → endometrial atrophy and preventing implantation.
- Thickened cervical mucus inhibits sperm penetration.
- It is particularly useful when oestrogen is contraindicated.
- May be used in patients with a history of breast cancer:
  - no disease for 5yrs and after consultation with breast surgeon.
- Breast-feeding:
  - can be inserted ≥4wks postpartum.
- May be used as part of HRT.

Side effects

- Irregular PV bleeding is common in the 1st 3–4mths: amenorrhoea in up to 30% by 1yr.
- Hormonal symptoms: nausea, headache, breast tenderness, bloating, and acne.

Other IUS brands

▶ Two further LNG IUS contraceptives have been released, a 13.5mg LNG IUS (Jaydess®) and a 19.5mg LNG IUS (Kyleena®).

- Cumulative pregnancy rate of 0.9 per 100 women over 3yrs.
- Effects on the endometrium and cervical mucus are similar for the 13.5mg, 19.5mg, and 52mg LNG-IUS.
- Only licensed as contraceptives (not as part of HRT regimen).

Barrier contraception: types

Types

- *Male condom:* latex, non-latex and deproteinized latex varieties.
- *Female condoms ('femidom'):* nitrile or latex.
- *Spermicides:* Gygel® vaginal cream, is the only licensed spermicide available in the UK.
- *Diaphragm/cervical cap:* latex, silicone.
- *Sponge:* silicone.

Mode of action

Inhibits fertilization by preventing sperm reaching the female upper genital tract.

Background

Condoms

- Both male and female condoms prevent fertilization by providing a barrier to the ejaculate, pre-ejaculate secretions, and cervicovaginal secretions.
- ↓ The risk of STIs.
- Use of condoms lubricated with nonoxinol-9 is not recommended.

Spermicides

- A spermicide is a chemical that inactivates sperm and effective for ~1h.
- Mostly containing nonoxynol-9, it comes as foams, creams, gels, suppositories, and films.

Diaphragms and caps

- Fit into the vagina to cover the cervix, to provide a physical barrier to sperm reaching the cervix.
- Using with a spermicide can ↑ efficacy.

Sponge

- A round device made of soft foam that contains spermicide and acts by covering the cervix.

How to use barrier contraceptives correctly

Condoms

- A new condom should be used for each episode of sexual intercourse.
- The male condom should be rolled down to the base of the penis before there is genital contact.
- After ejaculation, men should withdraw before the penis goes soft.
- There are several lubricated female condoms that are inserted into the vagina before sex.
- Female condoms can have a ring or sponge within the closed end of the sheath.
- The open end of the sheath, which remains outside the vagina, is formed either by a larger ring or flexible 'V' frame.

▶ Care should be taken so as not to tear them due to their delicate nature.

Diaphragms and caps

- Can be inserted with 2cm strips of spermicide any time before intercourse.
- Diaphragms are usually inserted dome down but some types can be inserted dome up.
- When using a cap, the inside of the cap should be filled about a 1/3 with spermicide.

▶ Spermicide should not be put on the rim of a cervical cap.

- Additional spermicide should be applied before sex is repeated or if the diaphragm or cervical cap has been *in situ* for ≥3h before sex takes place.
- The diaphragm or cervical cap must be left *in situ* for at least 6h after the last episode of intercourse (sperm in the lower reproductive tract are unlikely to be alive after 6h).
- Nurses and doctors can provide the initial fitting of a diaphragm and cervical cap.

Barrier contraception: considerations

Efficacy

Condoms

- Male condoms are 98% and female condoms are 95% effective at preventing pregnancy, when used consistently and correctly.
- Condoms are also the most efficient means of protecting against HIV and STIs like *Chlamydia trachomatis*, *Neisseria gonorrhoeae*, *Trichomonas vaginalis*, HSV, genital HPV, syphilis, and HBV.

Diaphragms and cervical caps

- When used consistently, correctly, and with spermicide, estimated to be between 92% and 96% effective at preventing pregnancy.

Sponge

- Less effective in women who have given birth specially 6wks postnatally.

⚠ If a failure is encountered with any method, then need to consider, emergency contraception, testing for STIs, and PEP for HIV.

Sensitivity

- Women with sensitivity to latex proteins may use a silicone diaphragm, cervical cap, non-latex male or female condoms, or deproteinized latex male condoms.

Contraindications

- Latex allergy.
- Recurrent UTIs, uterine prolapse, and an aversion to touching the genitals are all contraindications to diaphragm/cap use.

Relative contraindications

- Women with a history of toxic shock syndrome (TSS) may use male or female condoms.
- For women with a history of TSS, the use of the diaphragm or cervical cap is a UK Medical Eligibility Criteria (UKMEC) Category 3 method (a condition where the theoretical or proven risks usually outweigh the advantages of using the method).
- For women living with HIV or at high risk of HIV infection, the use of either a diaphragm or cervical cap is also UKMEC Category 3.

Male condoms

Advantages

- Easy to obtain and use.
- Client choice.
- Intermittent, infrequent, and predictable intercourse.
- Effective in preventing pregnancy if used correctly.
- Provide significant protection against most STIs, including HIV.
- May protect against cervical cancer.
- Adverse effects are rare.

Disadvantages

- Forward planning and may interrupt sex.
- Requires participation and commitment of both partners.
- Motivation at each act of intercourse.
- Careful disposal.
- Less effective at preventing pregnancy compared to hormonal and intrauterine methods.
- Can break or slip off.
- Loss of sensitivity during intercourse may occur.
- Men who sometimes lose their erection during sex may find it difficult to use a male condom correctly.
- Allergy to latex can occur (rare).

Female condoms

Advantages

- Reduce the risk of most STIs, including HIV.
- Protect against cervical cancer.
- Used with oil-based lubricants because they are made of polyurethane.
- Can be used if either partner is allergic to latex.
- Inserted up to 8h before sex.
- Female condoms are less likely to tear than the latex male condom.
- Some men prefer the freer sensations during the penetration.
- There are no known adverse effects.

Disadvantages

- Require careful insertion.
- Require motivation at each act of intercourse.
- Can be dislodged, or the penis can be inserted between the vaginal wall and the female condom.
- Can be noisy during intercourse.
- May cause discomfort during sex due to the inner ring.
- Are not as effective at preventing pregnancy as hormonal and intrauterine methods.

Fertility awareness contraception

Sometimes also known as 'natural family planning'. These methods involve the avoidance of sexual intercourse during the fertile phase of the menstrual cycle.

Natural methods

- The calendar method (rhythm method).
- Basal body temperature method.
- Billings method (ovulatory mucus).
- Cervical palpation method.
- The lactational amenorrhoea method (only possible after childbirth).

Mode of action

The calendar (rhythm method)

- Based solely on the length of the menstrual cycle and the lifespan of sperm in the female genital tract (5–7 days).
- Intercourse should be avoided around the predicted time of ovulation.

Using biological indicators of ovulation

- More accurate than a pure calculation based on the expected 1st day of menstruation.
- Mobile phone applications support users in identifying their 'safe' days through a combination of these factors.
- Fertility tracking devices are also available which rely on daily urine dipsticks to identify the LH surge and predict ovulation.

Efficacy

- Low compared to other methods.
- Methods can be combined to ↑ effectiveness.
- Failure rate can vary between 0.4% and 24%.

Advantages

- May be an option for couples with religious or cultural beliefs which prevent other methods.
- No side effects.
- No need to seek medical support.
- Makes women aware of their ovulation cycle and natural fertility when they wish to become pregnant.
- Can enhance communication and cooperation within a relationship.

Disadvantages

- Removes spontaneity as intercourse needs to be restricted to occur on 'safe days' only.
- There is variation in length of the follicular phase of the menstrual cycle which ↑ risks of conception.
- Reliability of fertility awareness methods is likely to be ↓ during breastfeeding, when discontinuing hormonal methods or during the perimenopause.

Female sterilization: preoperative considerations

Sterilization has become ↑ popular since the late 1960s and it is now the most commonly used method of contraception in women >40yrs of age.

History

- This includes:
  - reasons for sterilization
  - menstrual history
  - current contraception
  - obstetric history
  - previous abdominal/pelvic surgery
  - chronic medical conditions
  - drug history.

Examination

- BMI.
- Abdominal examination to look for:
  - scars from previous surgery
  - pelvic masses.

⚠ Previous surgery, endometriosis, PID, or fibroids may make the procedure technically challenging.

Counselling

- It is important to establish that the woman is taking the decision of her own free will.
- Alternatives to procedure must be discussed, including long-acting reversible contraceptives (LARCs) and vasectomy.
- Must use effective contraception until her 1st period following sterilization:
  - most common reason for failure is already being pregnant when the procedure is performed or in the same cycle!

Procedure

- Laparoscopy and tubal occlusion with Filshie clips used to be the method of choice.
- More recently, bilateral salpingectomy has been adopted; this has the benefit of:
  - improved contraceptive efficacy
  - ↓ ovarian cancer rate
  - no change in ovarian reserve
  - ↓ risk of EP in the case of failure.
- Counselling must be supported by printed information leaflets.

Consent for female sterilization

- Written informed consent must be taken from the woman prior to procedure:
  - in case of doubt regarding mental capacity, the case should be referred to court for judgement.
- Patient must fully understand that the procedure is intended to be permanent:
  - success rates with reversal procedures are very small and not provided by the NHS.
- Lifetime risk of failure with tubal occlusion is 1:200, rates for bilateral salpingectomy not known at present but likely to be less than for tubal occlusion:
  - pregnancies can occur several years after procedure—longest follow-up data available for Filshie clips suggest failure rate after 10yrs of 2–3 per 1000 procedures.
- In case of failure: ↑ risk of EP—advise women to seek medical attention if pregnant/have abnormal pain and bleeding.
- There is a risk of injury to:
  - blood vessels
  - bowel
  - bladder.
- Women must be warned about the possibility of conversion from laparoscopy to a laparotomy, particularly if they have had previous abdominal surgery.

Women at higher risk of regret

Care must be taken when considering sterilization for women from the following groups, as they are more likely to have regret and present requesting reversal:
- Women <30yrs old.
- Women who do not have children.
- Women who decide during pregnancy.
- Women who have had recent relationship loss.

Female sterilization: procedure

Mandatory preoperative checklist
- Document LMP.
- Check current contraception has been used to date.
- Pregnancy test must be performed:
  - a −ve test does not exclude the possibility of a luteal phase pregnancy.
- If any doubt exists about certainty of wishes or risk of pregnancy, the procedure should be abandoned.

Intraoperative
- Day case laparoscopic procedure is the mainstay and associated with quicker recovery rates and less morbidity than mini-laparotomy.
- Usually GA.
- Laparoscopic mechanical occlusion of the tubes by either Filshie clips or rings or bilateral salpingectomy are the available techniques.
- Diathermy occlusion ↑ the risk of EPs and is less easy to reverse.
- A modified Pomeroy procedure (resection of a portion of the fallopian tube) may be preferable for postpartum sterilization or at the time of CD due to lower failure rates.

🔹 Bilateral salpingectomy can be considered if the operator is skilled in performing this.

Postoperative
- The woman must be informed about the method of occlusion used and any procedural complications.
- She must be advised to use effective contraception until her next menstrual period.

Special circumstances
- Tubal occlusion should ideally be performed after an appropriate interval following pregnancy.
- Sterilization postpartum or postabortion carries:
  - ↑ risk of regret
  - possibly ↑ failure rates.
- In cases of sterilization at the time of CD, counselling and consent should be taken at least 2wks before the procedure.

Emergency contraception

Emergency contraception (EC) is licensed for use to protect women from unwanted pregnancy following UPSI or contraceptive failure.

The two main forms are:
- *Oral*: LNG EC or ulipristal acetate (EllaOne®).
- *Intrauterine*: Cu-IUCD EC.

Levonorgestrel EC

- Consists of a single oral dose of 1.5mg of LNG.
- Licensed up to 72h; if taken within this time, it is estimated to prevent 85% of expected pregnancies.
- Evidence suggests it is ineffective after 96h.
- It may also be used more than once in a cycle if clinically indicated.
- It does not provide contraceptive cover for the remainder of the cycle—another method of contraception must be used.

Side effects

- Nausea is common after ingestion.
- Vomiting only affects 1%.
- If a woman vomits within 2h of ingestion, she should take a further dose as soon as possible.
- Erratic PV bleeding is common in the 1st 7 days following treatment.

Ulipristal acetate EC

- Progesterone receptor modulator oral tablet, evidence suggests more effective than LNG-EC.
- Licensed for use within 120h of UPSI.
- Can only be used once per cycle.
- Not suitable for patients with severe asthma controlled by oral glucocorticoids.
- Due to mode of action may impair the effectiveness of progestogen-containing contraceptives for the remainder of the cycle and so alternative contraceptive methods are advised.

Cu-IUCD EC

- IUCD acts as an emergency contraceptive by inhibiting fertilization by direct toxicity.
- It is the most effective method of EC and should be offered 1st line.
- Affects implantation by inducing an inflammatory reaction in the endometrium.
- The copper content may also inhibit sperm penetration.
- IUCD EC can be inserted within 120h following UPSI.
- Failure rates are <1%.
- The risks and complications are similar to IUCD use in general.
- It can be removed after the next menstruation provided that no UPSI has occurred since menstruation, or retained for ongoing contraception.

Chapter 21

Menopause

Menopause: overview

All women will go through the menopause and the average age is 51yrs. The menopause is the cessation of the menstrual cycle and is caused by ovarian failure → oestrogen deficiency. Worldwide life expectancy is ↑ and women live longer than men. A woman's average life expectancy at birth in the UK is currently 82.9yrs and is estimated to reach 85yrs by 2031. Thus, UK women can expect >30yrs of postmenopausal life. This population expansion will lead to an ↑ importance of the health problems that affect postmenopausal women.

Definitions

Menopause

• Permanent cessation of menstruation that results from loss of ovarian follicular activity. Natural menopause is recognized to have occurred after 12 consecutive mths of amenorrhoea for which no other obvious pathological or physiological cause is present.

Perimenopause

• Includes the period beginning with the first clinical, biological, and endocrinological features of the approaching menopause, such as vasomotor symptoms and menstrual irregularity, and ends 12mths after the last menstrual period.

Pre-menopause

• Term often used to refer either to the 1–2yrs immediately before the menopause or to the whole of the reproductive period before the menopause. Currently, this term is recommended to be used in the latter sense.

Post-menopause

• Should be defined from the final menstrual period regardless of whether the menopause was induced or spontaneous.

Menopausal transition

• Period of time before the final menstrual period, when variability in the menstrual cycle usually is ↑.

Climacteric

• Phase encompassing the transition from the reproductive state to the non-reproductive state. The menopause itself thus is a specific event that occurs during the climacteric, just as the menarche is a specific event that occurs during puberty.

Menopause: short-term consequences

Vasomotor symptoms

Hot flushes and night sweats are the most common symptoms of the menopause, and, although they may begin before periods stop, the prevalence of flushes is highest in the 1st yr after the final menstrual period. Although they usually are present for <5yrs, up to 8% of women suffer hot flushes for up to 20yrs after the menopause.

Sexual dysfunction

Changes in sexual behaviour and activity are common. The term female sexual dysfunction (FSD) is now used. The percentage of women with sexual dysfunction rises from 42% to 88% during the early to late menopausal transition. The underlying reasons for FSD are commonly multifactorial, e.g. vaginal dryness, which results from declining levels of oestrogen, can cause dyspareunia. Low androgen levels have been implicated in low sexual desire though the evidence is conflicting. Non-hormonal factors, such as conflict between partners and life stress or depression, are important contributors to a woman's level of interest in sexual activity. In addition, male sexual problems should not be overlooked.

Sexual problems are classified into various types:
- Loss of sexual desire.
- Loss of sexual arousal.
- Problems with orgasm.
- Sexual pain such as painful sex or dyspareunia.

Psychological symptoms

Psychological symptoms associated with the menopause include:
- Depressed mood.
- Anxiety.
- Irritability and mood swings.
- Lethargy and lack of energy.

Fortunately, only a minority of women experience debilitating changes in mood at the time of menopause and psychological problems are thought to be associated with past problems and current life stresses.

Menopause: long-term consequences

Osteoporosis

Osteoporosis affects 1 in 3 women and 1 in 12 men. It is as a skeletal dis-order characterized by compromised bone strength predisposing to an ↑ risk of fracture (Table 21.1). Bone strength reflects the integration of two main features: bone density and bone quality. Bone density is expressed as grams of mineral per area or volume and, in any given individual, is deter-mined by peak bone mass and amount of bone loss. A BMD scan is used to measure the thickness of the bone in the hip and lumbar spine. Bone quality refers to architecture, turnover, damage accumulation (e.g. microfractures), and mineralization. A fracture occurs when a failure-inducing force, which may or may not involve trauma, is applied to osteoporotic bone. Thus, osteoporosis is a significant risk factor for fracture. Fractures are the clinical consequences of osteoporosis.

The most common sites of osteoporotic fractures are:
- Lower end of radius (wrist or Colles' fracture).
- Proximal femur (hip).
- Vertebrae.

Cardiovascular disease

Myocardial infarction and stroke are the 1° clinical endpoints. Cardiovascular disease is the most common cause of death in women aged >60. Oophorectomized women are at an almost 2-fold higher risk of coronary heart disease than age-matched pre-menopausal women.

Urogenital atrophy

The lower urinary and genital tracts have a common embryological origin and are approximated closely in adult women. Oestrogen receptors and progesterone receptors are present in the vagina, urethra, bladder, and pelvic floor musculature. Oestrogen deficiency after menopause causes atrophic changes within the urogenital tract and is associated with urinary symptoms, such as frequency, urgency, nocturia, incontinence, and recur-rent infection. These symptoms may coexist with those of vaginal atrophy, including dyspareunia, itching, burning, and dryness.

Table 21.1 Risk factors for osteoporosis

Risk factor	Example
Genetic	• Family history of fracture (particularly a 1st-degree relative with hip fracture)
Constitutional	• Low BMI • Early menopause (<45yrs of age)
Environmental	• Cigarette smoking • Alcohol abuse • Low calcium intake • Sedentary lifestyle
Drugs	• Corticosteroids, >5mg prednisolone or equivalent daily • Aromatase inhibitors • GnRH analogues
Disease	• Rheumatoid arthritis • Neuromuscular disease • Chronic liver disease • Chronic renal failure • Malabsorption syndromes • Hyperparathyroidism • Hyperthyroidism • Hypogonadism • Diabetes mellitus

Menopause: history taking and investigations

History

Symptoms, periods, and contraception
- Hot flushes and night sweats.
- Vaginal dryness.
- Other symptoms.
- Date of LMP (could she be pregnant?).
- Frequency, heaviness, and duration of periods.
- Contraception.

Gynaecological history
- Hysterectomy.
- Oophorectomy.

Past medical and surgical history
- Risk factors for osteoporosis (➔ Table 21.1).
- Confirmed DVT or PE.
- Risk factors for cardiovascular disease (e.g. smoking, hypertension, diabetes).
- Breast cancer, benign breast disease, and date of last mammogram (if applicable).
- Does she have migraines?
- Current medications.
- Does she take alternative or complementary therapies?

Family history in close family members
- Breast, ovarian, or bowel cancer.
- Confirmed DVT or PE.
- Cardiovascular disease.
- Osteoporosis.

Investigations
- FSH only helpful if diagnosis is in doubt, such as age <45yrs and levels in menopausal range (>30IU/L).
- LH, oestradiol, and progesterone are of no value in the diagnosis of ovarian failure.
- TFTs (free T_4 and TSH) as abnormalities of thyroid function can be confused with menopausal symptoms.
- Testosterone levels are of uncertain value.
- BMD if significant risk factors for osteoporosis (Table 21.2).

Table 21.2 Bone mineral density

Description	Definition
Normal	A BMD value between −1 and +1 SD of the young adult mean (T score −1 to +1)
Osteopenia	A BMD reduced between −1 and −2.5 SD from the young adult mean (T score −1 to −2.5)
Osteoporosis	A BMD reduced by equal to or more than −2.5 SD from the young adult mean (T score 2.5 or lower)

Premature menopause

Ideally, premature menopause should be defined as menopause that occurs at an age >2 SDs below the mean estimate for the reference population. However, the term 1° ovarian insufficiency is now considered a more appropriate term to use. The age of 40yrs is used frequently as an arbitrary limit below which the menopause is said to be premature. Between 40 and 45yrs, menopause would be termed early. It affects 1% of women <40yrs and 0.1% of those <30yrs. In most cases no cause is found.

Causes of premature ovarian failure

1° causes
- Chromosome abnormalities.
- FSH receptor gene polymorphism and inhibin B mutation.
- Enzyme deficiencies.
- Autoimmune disease.
- Family history of early/premature menopause.

2° causes
- Chemotherapy and radiotherapy.
- Bilateral oophorectomy or surgical menopause.
- Hysterectomy without oophorectomy.
- Infection.

Presentation and assessment

- Most common presentation is 2° amenorrhoea or oligo-menorrhoea (which may not necessarily be accompanied by hot flushes).
- Coexisting disease may be detected, particularly:
  - hypothyroidism
  - Addison's disease
  - diabetes mellitus
  - any chromosome abnormalities (especially in those who have not achieved successful pregnancy).

🌢 The diagnostic usefulness of ovarian biopsy outside the research setting has yet to be proved.

Management issues in premature menopause

Fertility and contraception
- Reduced fertility.
- May require assisted conception.
- Need for contraception if no fertility goals.

Oestrogen replacement
▶ Women need oestrogen replacement until average age of natural menopause, which is usually regarded as 51yrs.
- HRT.
- COCP without gaps (back-to-back).
- No evidence regarding use of bisphosphonates, strontium ranelate, or raloxifene.

💣 No evidence regarding usefulness of alternative and complementary therapies.

Consequences of premature menopause

- Women with untreated premature menopause (no oestrogen replacement) are at ↑ risk of osteoporosis and cardiovascular disease, but at ↓ risk of breast malignancy.
- ↑ Risks of persistent vasomotor symptoms.
- Premature menopause can lead to ↓ peak bone mass (if <25yrs old) or early bone loss thereafter.

⚠ Mean life expectancy in women with menopause before the age of 40yrs is 2.0yrs shorter than that in women with menopause after the age of 55yrs.

Hormone replacement therapy: overview

There are >50 HRT preparations available, which feature different strengths, combinations, and routes of administration. HRT can be given either systemically for vasomotor symptoms and osteoporosis or vaginally (or topically) for local symptoms such as vaginal dryness. In non-hysterectomized women, HRT consists of an oestrogen combined with a progestogen.

Oestrogens

Oestrogens used in HRT include estradiol, oestrone, and estriol, which, although chemically synthesized from soya beans or yams, are molecularly identical to the natural human hormone. Conjugated equine oestrogens containing about 50–65% oestrone sulphate, with the remainder being equine oestrogens (mainly equilin sulphate), are also used.

Progestogens

The progestogens used in HRT are almost all synthetic and derived from plant sources. They are structurally different from progesterone. 17-Hydroxyprogesterone and 19-nortestosterone derivatives are the progestogens used most commonly in HRT.

17-Hydroxyprogesterone
- Dydrogesterone.
- Medroxyprogesterone acetate.

19-Nortestosterone derivatives
- Norethisterone.
- LNG.

Other hormones used at the menopause

Tibolone
A synthetic steroid compound that is inert, but is converted to metabolites with oestrogenic, progestogenic, and androgenic actions. It is classified as HRT in the *British National Formulary*. It is used in postmenopausal women. It may ↑ the risk of stroke in women >60yrs and also ↑ the recurrence risk in women with a previous history of breast cancer.

Testosterone
Patches and implants may be used to improve sexual function.

Treatment of local symptoms

Synthetic or conjugated equine oestrogens should be avoided, as they are well absorbed from the vagina. The options available are low-dose natural oestrogens, e.g. vaginal estriol by cream or pessary or estradiol by tablet or ring. Treatment is needed long term as symptoms return on cessation of treatment. With the recommended dose regimens, no adverse endometrial effects should be incurred, and a progestogen need not be added in non-hysterectomized women. Routine monitoring of endometrial thickness is not recommended.

Micronized progesterone
Thought to have less −ve effects on mood, lipid levels, VTE, and possibly breast cancer.

▶ Bazedoxifene is a selective oestrogen receptor modulator approved as a progesterone alternative for HRT in the intact uterus.

Types of systemic oestrogen-based HRT
- Oestrogen alone in hysterectomized women.
- Oestrogen plus progestogen in non-hysterectomized women:
  - oestrogen and cyclical progestogen in perimenopausal women
  - continuous combined oestrogen–progestogen ('no bleed' HRT) in postmenopausal women.
- Routes of administration of oestrogen:
  - oral
  - transdermal
  - SC
  - vaginal.
- Routes of administration of progestogen:
  - oral
  - transdermal
  - intrauterine (LNG).

Minimum bone-sparing doses of HRT
- Estradiol oral: 0.5mg.
- Estradiol patch: 14 micrograms.
- Estradiol gel: 1–5g.*
- Estradiol implant: 25mg every 6mths.
- Conjugated equine oestrogens: 0.3mg daily.

* Depends on preparation: lower doses may be effective.

Side effects of systemic HRT
- *Oestrogen related:* fluid retention, bloating, vaginal bleeding*, breast tenderness or enlargement, nausea, headaches, leg cramps, and dyspepsia**.
- *Progestogen related:* fluid retention, breast tenderness, headaches or migraine, mood swings, depression, acne, lower abdominal pain, vaginal bleeding*, and backache**.

◆* There is no evidence for weight ↑ compared to the non-HRT age-matched cohort.

* May need investigation
** Changing dose, type, and route of administration may help.

Hormone replacement therapy: benefits

Two large studies—the randomized Women's Health Initiative (WHI) and the observational Million Women Study (MWS)—undertaken in women aged >50yrs resulted in controversy about use of HRT. There are benefits and risks in its use, and some uncertainty concerning some claims made about HRT.

Benefits of HRT

- Vasomotor symptoms.
- Urogenital symptoms and improved sexuality.
- Risk of osteoporosis.
- Risk of colorectal cancer.

Relief of vasomotor symptoms

- Oestrogen is effective in treating hot flushes:
  - improvement usually is noted within 4wks
  - maximum therapeutic response usually achieved by 3mths
  - should be continued for at least 1yr or symptoms often recur
  - the most common indication for a prescription of HRT
  - often is used for <5yrs.
- Oestrogen more effective than SSRIs or clonidine (largely ineffective).

Urogenital symptoms and sexuality

- Urogenital symptoms respond well to oestrogen (which may be given vaginally or systemically).
- Improvement may take several months.
- Long-term treatment often is needed, as symptoms can recur.
- Urinary incontinence is not improved by systemic therapy.
- Sexuality may be improved with oestrogen alone, but may need addition of testosterone, especially in young oophorectomized women.

Osteoporosis

- HRT ↓ the risk of spine and hip and other osteoporotic fractures.
- Most epidemiological studies suggest continuous and lifelong use is required for HRT to be an effective method of preventing fracture.
- Bisphosphonates are effective for management of osteoporosis during menopause, but used with caution in women <65yrs.
- HRT is significantly cheaper than alternative therapies, such as bisphosphonates, strontium ranelate, and parathyroid hormone.

Colorectal cancer

- HRT ↓ the risk of colorectal cancer by about 1/3.
- Little known about risk when treatment is stopped or in high-risk populations.
- Currently, prevention of colonic cancer is not an indication for HRT.

Hormone replacement therapy: risks

Risks of HRT
- ↑ Risk of breast cancer.
- ↑ Risk of endometrial cancer with unopposed oestrogen.
- ↑ Risk of VTE.
- ↑ Risk of gallbladder disease.

Endometrial cancer
- Unopposed oestrogen ↑ the risk of endometrial cancer:
  - the relative risk (RR) is 2.3
  - risk ↑ with prolonged use (RR 9.5 for ≥10yrs)
  - risk remains ↑ for ≥5yrs after stopping (RR 2.3).
- This risk is not eliminated completely with the addition of monthly sequential progestogen (especially if used for >5yrs).
- No risk has been found with continuous combined HRT.

Venous thromboembolism
⚠ HRT more than doubles the risk of VTE, but absolute risk remains small.
- For non-users, over a 5yr period, the incidence of VTE will be:
  - 3:1000 women aged 50–59yrs
  - 8:1000 women aged 60–69yrs.
- The number of additional VTE events in healthy women on HRT ≥5yrs is estimated to be:
  - 4:1000 women aged 50–59yrs
  - 9:1000 women aged 60–69yrs.
- The VTE is more likely in the 1st yr of HRT.
- ↑ Age, obesity, and thrombophilia significantly ↑ risk of VTE.
- For combined oral HRT regimens, conjugated equine oestrogens with medroxyprogesterone acetate noted the highest risk of VTE.
- Transdermal preparations (combined or oestrogen only) is not associated with an ↑ risk of VTE.

Gallbladder disease
☞ HRT appears to ↑ the risk of gallbladder disease, but:
- Risk ↑ with age and obesity.
- Women who use HRT may have silent pre-existing disease.

Duration of HRT
- Discontinuation suggested after 5yrs or age 60yrs.
- Risks ↑ with age and duration of use.

Risk of breast cancer with HRT

- HRT usage for <1yr appears to confer little ↑ risk of breast cancer.
- Risk of breast cancer with HRT is dependent on the regimen:
  - greatest with combined oestrogen–progestogen HRT
  - less with unopposed oestrogen (but ↑ risk of endometrial cancer).
- Women who use HRT for 1–4yrs will have an ↑ risk of:
  - 2 per 100 women using oestrogen and daily progestogen
  - 1 per 200 women using oestrogen-only preparations.
- The risk is dependent on duration of HRT.
- It was thought that the effect was not sustained once HRT was ceased; however, there is now evidence suggesting that some risk persists after 10yrs, dependent on duration of usage.

💣 All risk estimates are based on starting HRT at 50yrs; this effect is not seen in women who start it early for premature menopause (therefore duration of exposure to female sex hormones is probably relevant).

💣 The ↑ in risk of breast cancer found in nulliparous women, those with a high BMI, those who delay their first birth, and those who have a family history may be higher than that conferred by HRT.

Hormone replacement therapy: uncertainties

Uncertainties concerning HRT

- Cardiovascular disease.
- Dementia.
- Ovarian cancer.
- Quality of life.

Cardiovascular disease

- The role of HRT in 1° or 2° prevention is uncertain, and it should not be used primarily for this indication.
- Timing, dose, and possibly type of HRT, however, may be critical in determining cardiovascular effects: women in the WHI who started HRT within 10yrs of the menopause had a lower risk of coronary heart disease than women who started later.

Dementia and cognition

- Oestrogen may delay or ↓ the risk of Alzheimer's disease, but it does not seem to improve established disease.
- It is unclear if there is a critical age to start HRT or an optimal duration of treatment to prevent dementia.

Ovarian cancer

- There is ↑ risk in the very long term (>10yrs) with oestrogen alone.
- This risk is not seen with continuous combined therapy.

💥 Currently insufficient evidence is available to recommend alterations in HRT prescribing practice.

Quality of life

💥 Studies are conflicting as this area is difficult to evaluate because of the different measures used, varying levels of menopausal symptoms, a large placebo effect, and extrinsic factors that may alter responses.

Non-pharmacological treatments for vasomotor symptoms

Moderate evidence
- Cognitive behavioural therapy.
- Hypnosis.

Some evidence
- Diet and supplementary phyto-oestrogens.
- Acupuncture.

Minimal evidence
- Mindfulness/relaxation and weight loss.
- Lifestyle changes (e.g. layered clothing, paced breathing, yoga).
- Black cohosh.
- Vitamin E.

Alternative medical treatments to hormone replacement therapy

Publication of the WHI and the MWS studies led to women stopping HRT and considering alternative medical treatments to alleviate menopausal symptoms.

Treatment of vasomotor symptoms

- *SSRIs:* citalopram, escitalopram, fluoxetine, and paroxetine.
- *Serotonin and norepinephrine reuptake inhibitors (SNRIs):* venlafaxine, desvenlafaxine.
- *Clonidine (α-agonist):* once mainstay treatment, but now shown as having limited effect.
- *Anticonvulsants:* gabapentin, pregabalin.

⚠ Fluoxetine and paroxetine should be avoided with tamoxifen use as they can impair conversion to its active metabolite.

Prevention and treatment of osteoporosis

- Agent used to either inhibit bone resorption or stimulate bone formation.
- Calcium and vitamin D.
- Bisphosphonates (inhibits osteoclasts).
- Selective oestrogen reuptake modulators (SERMs).

Urogenital symptoms

Oestrogen

- Cream, intravaginal sustained-release estradiol ring, or estradiol vaginal tablets are the most effective treatment for vaginal atrophy and dyspareunia.
- Woman can be reassured of minimal systemic absorption and no need for added progestogen.
- Safety noted in one trial in women with breast cancer.

Ospemifene

- SERM.

Alternative treatments to alleviate dyspareunia

- Bioadhesive moisturizers (Replens™, RepHresh™).
- Vaginal lubricants: water based, silicon based, or oil based.

💧 Silicon-based may be more effective than water-based lubricants.

Vaginal laser treatment

- Insufficient evidence, may be a placebo effect, therefore not recommended by professional bodies yet.

Chapter 22

Urogynaecology

Classification of urinary incontinence

Urinary incontinence is the complaint of any involuntary leakage of urine. It can result from a variety of different conditions and it is useful to classify them accordingly.

Stress urinary incontinence

The involuntary leakage of urine on effort or exertion or on sneezing or coughing. Commonly arises from urethral sphincter weakness.

Urge urinary incontinence

The involuntary leakage of urine accompanied by, or immediately preceded by, a strong desire to pass urine (void). Urgency, with or without urge urinary incontinence, usually with frequency and nocturia is also defined as overactive bladder (OAB) syndrome.

Mixed urinary incontinence

The involuntary leakage of urine associated both with urgency and with exertion, effort, sneezing, or coughing. Usually, one of these is predominant, i.e. either the symptoms of urge incontinence, or those of stress incontinence, are most bothersome.

Overflow incontinence

Occurs when the bladder becomes large and flaccid and has little or no detrusor tone or function. This is usually due to injury or insult, e.g. after surgery or postpartum. The condition is diagnosed when the urinary residual is >50% of bladder capacity. The bladder simply leaks when it becomes full.

Continuous urinary incontinence

The complaint of continuous leakage. Classically it is associated with a fistula or congenital abnormality, e.g. ectopic ureter.

Other types of incontinence

- Incontinence arising from UTIs, medications, immobility, or cognitive impairment.
- Situational incontinence, e.g. giggle incontinence.

Urinary symptoms

- *Urinary incontinence*: the complaint of involuntary urinary leakage, which can be divided, broadly, into stress incontinence and urge incontinence.
- *Daytime frequency*: the number of times a woman voids during waking hours—normally between 4 and 7 voids/day. ↑ daytime frequency is when a woman perceives she voids too often.
- *Nocturia*: the complaint of having to wake at night one or more times to void. Up to the age of 70yrs, more than a single void is considered abnormal.
- *Nocturnal enuresis*: urinary incontinence occurring during sleep.
- *Urgency*: sudden compelling desire to pass urine, which is difficult to defer. Urgency is most frequently 2° to detrusor overactivity, although inflammatory bladder conditions such as interstitial cystitis may also present with this.
- *Voiding difficulties* include:
  - hesitancy (difficulty in initiating micturition)
  - straining to void
  - slow or intermittent urinary stream.

▶ These are all suggestive of urethral obstruction, underactive detrusor muscle, or loss of coordination between detrusor construction and urethral relaxation.

- *Post-micturition symptoms* include:
  - feeling of incomplete bladder emptying
  - terminal dribble (a prolonged final part of micturition)
  - post-micturition dribble (the involuntary loss of urine immediately after passing urine).
- *Absent or ↓ bladder sensation*: usually due to denervation caused by spinal cord injuries or pelvic surgery. Leads to infrequent micturition and large-capacity bladder, and is often associated with overflow incontinence.
- *Bladder pain*: felt suprapubically or retropubically. Typically occurs with bladder filling and is relieved by emptying it. Pain is indicative of intravesical pathology, such as interstitial cystitis or malignancy, and warrants further investigation.
- *Urethral pain*: felt in urethra, can be before, during, or after voiding (the woman indicates this as the site of the discomfort).
- *Dysuria*: pain experienced in bladder (suprapubically) or urethra on passing urine. Most frequently associated with UTIs.
- *Haematuria*: presence of blood in urine; can be micro- or macroscopic (frank). Always significant and warrants further investigation.

Assessment of the lower urinary tract: history and examination

History

- The onset of urinary symptoms, their duration, and their severity should be recorded (the predominant bother symptom, e.g. urgency, urge incontinence, or stress incontinence, should be identified).
- Different underlying conditions can cause similar urinary symptoms; history alone is often a poor predictor of pathophysiology.
- Check for coexisting medical conditions and optimize their treatment (the onset of diabetes significantly ↑ urine output and many pharmaceutical agents can alter bladder function).
- Enquire about colorectal symptoms and genitourinary prolapse.

Quality of life assessment

- A good clinical history will enquire how symptoms affect aspects of daily life and social, personal, and sexual relationships.
- Disease-specific quality of life questionnaires allow in-depth assessment of the impact-specific symptoms on a woman's life: validated questionnaires are available from the International Consultation on Incontinence (⌕ www.iciq.net).

Frequency/volume chart

- The frequency/volume chart (Fig. 22.1) is a simple and practical method of obtaining objective quantification of fluid intake and voiding behaviour.
- Fluid intake, frequency, times of voiding, and leakage episodes (day and night) are recorded for at least 24h (typically 3 days).

Physical examination

General examination

- Weight (BMI), BP, urinalysis.
- Check for signs of systemic disease.
- Mobility and mental state.
- Motivation and manual dexterity.
- Neurological examination, if there are any symptoms that point to a possible neurological cause.

Abdominal examination

- Exclude an abdominal or pelvic mass (⚠ including pregnancy).
- Exclude a full bladder (obstruction/retention).

Pelvic examination

- Condition of the vulval skin (any atrophy, erythema, or oedema).
- Presence and degree of any concurrent uterovaginal prolapse.
- Assessment of urethral and bladder neck descent on straining.
- Assessment of pelvic floor muscle strength (graded 0–5 on a modified Oxford scale; ➔ Prolapse: clinical assessment, p. 768).

Frequency/Volume Chart

Name: *Mrs Smith* Patient No. *1234567* Week commencing *20 June 2022*

Time	Date:20.06.22 Day 1			Date:21.06.22 Day 2			Date:22.06.22 Day 3		
am	In	Out	Wet	In	Out	Wet	In	Out	Wet
1		300	X		500	X			
2		300	X						
3					600	X		700	X
4		350	X						
5									
6					600	X		600	X
7		500	X						
8				250	300			500	X
9	250	300		200			250		
10								300	
11							200		
12				200				100	
pm									
1	200	100			100				
2							200	300	
3									
4				200					
5	250	120						200	
6							200		
7				200	100				
8									
9		200			100				
10									
11		100			200		200	200	
12									
Total	650	2270		1050	2500		1050	2800	

Fig. 22.1 A 3-day frequency/volume chart showing severe nocturia.

Information obtainable from a frequency/volume chart
- Functional bladder capacity.
- Volumetric summary of diurnal urinary frequency.
- Volumetric summary of nocturnal urinary frequency.
- Quantification of total fluid intake.
- Distribution of fluid intake throughout the day.
- Total voided volume and diurnal distribution of voiding.
- Evaluation of the severity of urinary incontinence.

Assessment of the lower urinary tract: investigations

Basic investigations

Urinalysis
Reagent strip testing of urine for leucocyte esterase, nitrites, protein, blood, and glucose is a sensitive and cheap screening test.

Urine specimen
Bacteriological analysis of a MSU for microscopy, culture, and sensitivity is reserved for those with a +ve screening test.

Residual check
A post-void residual check should be carried out (either by USS or by catheterization) to exclude incomplete bladder emptying.

Pad test
This is a simple method of detecting and quantifying urinary leakage based on weight gain of absorbent pads during a set period of time.

▶ It is not helpful in determining the cause of urinary leakage and is not recommended as a routine investigation.

Cystourethroscopy
- Allows visualization of all the lower urinary tract: urethra, bladder mucosa, trigone, and ureteric orifices.
- Can be performed using a rigid or flexible cystoscope, with or without anaesthesia.
- Bladder biopsies can be taken to obtain histological diagnosis and exclude malignancy.
- In cases of suspected interstitial cystitis, a 2nd-look cystoscopy should be performed after the initial bladder distension to detect any glomerulations or petechial haemorrhages.

⚠ This requires GA.

Indications for cystourethroscopy
- Recurrent UTIs.
- Haematuria.
- Bladder pain.
- Suspected urinary tract injury or fistula.
- To exclude bladder tumour or stones.
- If interstitial cystitis is suspected.
- To exclude mesh complication, i.e. mesh extrusion.

Assessment of the lower urinary tract: imaging

Imaging of the lower urinary tract is not justified as a routine investigation in all women presenting with urinary symptoms, but should instead be targeted at specific indications.

Ultrasonography

- Is widely used to:
  - exclude incomplete bladder emptying
  - check for congenital abnormalities, calculi, tumours
  - detect cortical scarring of the kidneys.

Plain abdominal radiograph

- Useful for screening for a variety of conditions, including foreign bodies and calculi.

Contrast-enhanced CT

- Imaging modality of choice for detecting and characterizing renal masses and renal tract calculi, as well as ureteric or bladder lesions.
- Commonly performed to investigate haematuria.

IV urography

- Used in women with neuropathic bladder or suspected congenital and acquired abnormalities, e.g. uterovaginal fistulae.
- Contrast-enhanced CT provides more accurate and rapid detection.

Micturating cystourethrography

- Useful to demonstrate bladder and urethral fistulae, vesicoureteric reflux, and anatomical abnormalities of the lower urinary tract, such as urethral diverticula.

MRI

- Remains predominantly a research technique for incontinence and prolapse, because of its cost and availability.
- Mainly used for characterization of renal or pelvic masses and tumour staging.

Conditions requiring imaging of urinary tract

- Recurrent UTIs.
- Haematuria.
- Urethral diverticula, which need to be differentiated from paravaginal cysts.
- Suspected ureteric injuries.
- Suspected urethral or vesical fistulae.
- Suspected malignancy or renal stones.

Assessment of the lower urinary tract: urodynamic investigations

Definition

'Urodynamics' describes a combination of tests that look at the ability of the bladder to store and void urine. The tests include uroflowmetry, post-void residual measurement, and cystometry. In addition, urethral pressure profilometry and video-urodynamic investigations may be undertaken.

Uroflowmetry

Simple, non-invasive investigation that can be used to screen for voiding difficulties. The patient voids in privacy on a commode incorporating a urinary flow meter, which measures voided volume over time, and plots it on a graph (Fig. 22.2).

Cystometry

- Involves measuring the pressure/volume relationship of the bladder during filling and voiding and is a useful test of bladder function.
- The bladder is filled with saline via a catheter, and the 1st sensation of filling, 1st desire to void, and any strong desire to void are recorded (Fig. 22.3).
- Electronic subtraction of the intra-abdominal pressure from the intravesical enables the detrusor pressure to be calculated (Fig. 22.4).
- During filling, the patient is asked to cough at regular intervals to check the quality of the subtraction.
- The presence of detrusor contractions during filling and leakage through the urethra are noted.
- Once the bladder is full tests of provocation are carried out, such as coughing, standing, jumping, and listening to running water.
- The woman is then asked to void at the end of the test, for pressure/flow analysis.

Video-urodynamics

- Combines fluoroscopic imaging of the bladder neck with cystometry, while filling the bladder with an iodine-based contrast medium.
- Enables detection of detrusor-sphincter dyssynergia, vesicoureteric reflux, or presence of abnormalities in the renal tract that are commonly seen in women with neurogenic bladder problems.

Ambulatory urodynamic monitoring

- A small recording device is worn and the information is later downloaded to a computer for analysis and review.
- The bladder is filled naturally and the woman should carry out her normal daily activities, including those that provoke symptoms.
- This approach is particularly useful for investigating detrusor overactivity when standard laboratory urodynamics have failed to replicate the symptoms experienced by the woman in her normal environment.

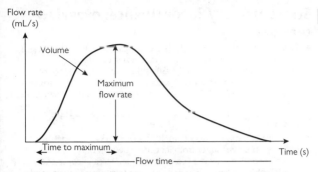

Fig. 22.2 Diagrammatic representation of normal urinary flow rate. *Voided volume*: total volume expelled via the urethra, the area beneath the flow-time curve. *Maximum flow rate*: maximum measured value of the flow rate. *Average flow rate*: volume voided divided by the flow time. *Flow time*: the time over which measurable flow actually occurs.

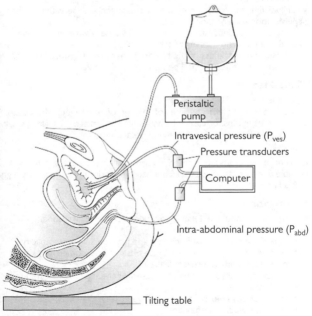

Fig. 22.3 Schematic drawing showing catheter positions during cystometry. Three catheters are required: the 1st in the bladder to fill it; the 2nd in the bladder to measure vesical pressure; and the 3rd in the rectum to measure abdominal pressure. Reproduced with permission from Cardozo L, Staskin D (2001). *Textbook of female urology and urogynaecology*, published by Taylor and Francis, London.

Stress urinary incontinence: overview

Definitions

- *Stress urinary incontinence (SUI):* is the complaint of involuntary leakage of urine on effort or exertion, or on sneezing or coughing.
- *Urodynamic stress incontinence (USI):* is the involuntary leakage of urine during ↑ intra-abdominal pressure in the absence of detrusor contractions. Unlike SUI, it can only be diagnosed by urodynamic testing (Fig. 22.4).

Incidence

- The most common urinary complaint for which women seek advice.
- 1 in 10 women will suffer from it at some point in their lives.
- 50% of incontinent women complain of pure stress incontinence.
- 30–40% of incontinent women have mixed symptoms of urge and stress incontinence.

Pathophysiology and aetiology

- SUI occurs when the intravesical pressure exceeds the closing pressure on the urethra.
- Childbirth is the most common causative factor, → denervation of the pelvic floor, usually during delivery.
- Oestrogen deficiency at the time of menopause → weakening of the pelvic support and thinning of the urothelium.
- Occasionally, weakness of the bladder neck can occur congenitally, or through trauma from radical pelvic surgery or irradiation.

Clinical features

Symptoms

Typically, a woman will complain of leakage of urine when she coughs, sneezes, runs, jumps, or carries heavy loads. The leakage is usually a small, discrete amount, coinciding with the physical activity.

Signs

Descent of the urethra and anterior vaginal wall may be present. It may be possible to demonstrate stress incontinence by asking the woman to cough with a fairly full bladder.

Investigations

- *MSU sample* should be taken to exclude infection or glycosuria.
- *Frequency/volume chart:*
  - typically shows normal frequency and functional bladder capacity
  - slightly ↑ diurnal frequency may be observed, as women may void more frequently to prevent leakage.
- *Urodynamic studies* should be considered when surgery is indicated to:
  - confirm the diagnosis
  - check for any coexisting detrusor overactivity
  - check for voiding dysfunction.

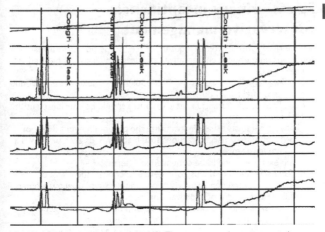

Fig. 22.4 Urodynamic trace showing USI. The upper trace shows intravesical pressure (P_{ves}) and the middle trace shows pressure within the abdomen (P_{abd}), both measured against time. The lower trace, obtained by subtracting intra-abdominal pressure from intravesical pressure ($P_{det} = P_{ves} - P_{abd}$), shows the detrusor pressure. During the test there is no change in detrusor pressure, despite provocation with coughing, and leakage occurs only as a result of the momentary ↑ in intra-abdominal pressure caused by the coughing.

Stress urinary incontinence: conservative management

SUI interferes with a woman's quality of life, but is not a life-threatening condition and therefore conservative measures should always be tried 1st. They include:

- *Lifestyle interventions:* weight ↓ if BMI >30kg/m², smoking cessation, and treatment of chronic cough and constipation.
- *Pelvic floor muscle training:* for at least 3mths should be considered as the 1st-line treatment:
  - physiotherapists usually individualize the programme, but 3 sets of 8–12 slow maximal contractions sustained for 6–8s each per day is a common regimen
  - the exercises need to be continued long term.
- *Biofeedback:* refers to the use of a device to convert the effect of pelvic floor contraction into a visual or auditory signal to allow women objective assessment of improvement.
- *Electrical stimulation:* can assist in production of muscle contractions in women who are unable to produce muscle contraction.
- *Vaginal cones:* have been developed as a way of applying graded resistance against which the pelvic floor muscles contract.

Pharmacological management of SUI

Duloxetine is the only drug licensed for the treatment of moderate to severe SUI:

- It is an SNRI that enhances urethral striated sphincter activity via a centrally mediated pathway.
- However, it is associated with significant side effects. It is not recommended for 1st-line use by NICE.
- Nausea is the most frequently reported side effect (up to 25%).
- Other side effects include dyspepsia, dry mouth, insomnia or drowsiness, and dizziness.

Indications for conservative treatment of SUI

- Mild or easily manageable symptoms.
- Family incomplete.
- Symptoms manifest during pregnancy.
- Surgery contraindicated by coexisting medical conditions.
- Surgery declined by patient.

Stress urinary incontinence: surgical management

Surgery may be considered when conservative measures have failed and the woman's quality of life is compromised. Before attempting surgical repair, it is important to be clear about the underlying cause of the incontinence: USI may be successfully treated surgically, but detrusor overactivity may be made worse, and the effects are largely irreversible.

Periurethral injections

- Injectable periurethral bulking agents have lower immediate success rate (20–40%) and effects wear off over time.
- The procedure has low morbidity and can be performed under local anaesthetic in outpatient settings.
- Injectables or bulking agents may be appropriate for:
  - frail, older, or unfit women
  - young women who have yet to complete their family
  - patients at higher risk of voiding dysfunction.
- The most commonly used periurethral bulking agents are:
  - glutaraldehyde cross-linked bovine collagen
  - water-based gels (Bulkamid®).

Burch colposuspension

- Largely replaced by tension-free vaginal tape (TVT), but having a resurgence in popularity.
- The retropubic space is entered through a low transverse suprapubic incision and two or three sutures placed between the paravaginal fascia and ipsilateral iliopectineal ligament (Cooper's ligament) at the level of the bladder neck.
- Complications may include haemorrhage; injuries to the bladder or ureter; voiding difficulties; de novo detrusor overactivity; enterocele or rectocele formation.
- Overall, meta-analysis of published data suggests that the efficacy of the Burch colposuspension as a 1° procedure is 90% and as a repeat procedure is 83% (Table 22.1).

Laparoscopic colposuspension

- Efficacy and complications similar to those of the open procedure.
- The surgery is technically more demanding and requires considerable laparoscopic expertise.

Autologous fascial sling

- A strip of rectus fascia is harvested and inserted in a similar fashion to performing a TVT.
- Success rates are quoted as up to 93%.
- Surgical morbidity is higher (wound complications, hernia) and rates of voiding dysfunction are ↑.
- In the current climate of controversy surrounding mesh surgery, some patients are requesting this as an alternative to TVT.

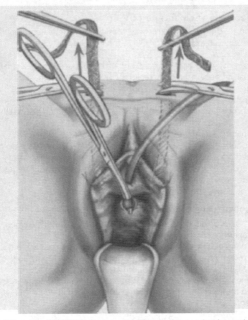

Fig. 22.5 Insertion of TVT. The tape is placed in a U-shape under the urethra and the tension adjusted to prevent leakage as the woman coughs. Illustration reproduced by courtesy of ETHICON Women's Health and Urology.

Tension-free vaginal tape (TVT)

▶ Prior to the mesh controversy, this was the most commonly performed surgical procedure for USI in the UK.

- See Fig. 22.5.
- A polypropylene tape is placed under the mid-urethra via a small vaginal incision, using local, regional, or general anaesthesia.
- Cystourethroscopy is carried out to ensure no damage to the bladder or urethra.
- The procedure is minimally invasive and most women return to normal activity within 2wks.
- *Complications:*
  - moderately high risk of bladder injuries 5–10%, but these do not seem to have long-term sequelae, if treated appropriately
  - bleeding in retropubic space, infection, and voiding difficulties
  - tape erosion into the vagina and urethra has also been reported.
- The objective cure rate is 82–98% (mean 94%).

Transobturator tape (TOT)

- The polypropylene tape is passed via a transobturator foramen, through the transobturator and adductor muscles.
- The main difference from TVT is that the retropubic space is not entered and the risk of bladder perforation is low. It may be preferred if there has been extensive abdominal/pelvic surgery.
- Potential disadvantages of transobturator slings are a higher risk of nerve trauma, with chronic groin pain described in up to 20% of patients.

The UK 'mesh controversy'

- At the time of publication, all vaginally inserted mesh procedures are suspended by NHS England due to concerns about complications.
- NICE guidance published in 2019 recommends offering patients a choice of incontinence procedure after detailed discussion about risks and benefits.

Further reading

NICE (2019). Urinary incontinence and pelvic organ prolapse in women: management. NICE guideline [NG123].
℞ www.nice.org.uk/guidance/ng123

Overactive bladder syndrome: overview

Definition

- OAB is a chronic condition, defined as urgency, with or without urge incontinence, usually with frequency or nocturia.
- It is used to imply probable underlying detrusor overactivity, but this is a diagnosis only made on urodynamic testing (Fig. 22.6).

Aetiology

- Idiopathic in most cases.
- Neurogenic detrusor overactivity is found in the presence of conditions such as multiple sclerosis, spina bifida, and upper motor neuron lesions.
- 2° to pelvic or incontinence surgery.
- OAB due to outflow obstruction is uncommon in women.

Clinical features of OAB

- Symptoms of OAB include urinary frequency, urgency, urge incontinence, and nocturia.
- Provocative factors often trigger it, such as cold weather, opening the front door, or hearing running water.
- Bladder contractions (detrusor overactivity) may also be provoked by ↑ intra-abdominal pressure (coughing or sneezing), which must be distinguished from SUI.
- Quality of life can be significantly impaired by the unpredictability and large volume of leakage.

Investigations

Urine culture

To exclude infection, as symptoms overlap those of UTI.

Frequency/volume chart

- Typical features are ↑ diurnal frequency associated with urgency and episodes of urge incontinence.
- Voids are frequently small in volume.
- Nocturia is a common feature of OAB.

Urodynamics

- Involuntary detrusor contractions during the filling phase of the micturition cycle, which may be spontaneous or provoked.
- Video-urodynamic testing is better in women with neurological diseases, to exclude vesicoureteric reflux or renal damage 2° to a persistent significant rise in intravesical pressure.

Diagnosis

- Urodynamic assessment is helpful for the diagnosis of OAB in women with multiple and complex symptoms.
- Other factors, such as metabolic abnormalities (diabetes or hypercalcaemia), physical causes (prolapse or faecal impaction), or urinary pathology (UTI or interstitial cystitis), need to be excluded before the diagnosis of OAB is made.

Key points
- OAB is a common condition affecting ~1 in 6 women.
- Incidence of OAB ↑ with age.
- OAB is the 2nd most common cause of urinary incontinence.
- OAB is the most common cause of incontinence in older women.
- Urodynamic assessment is required to make a diagnosis of detrusor overactivity.
- Quality of life is often severely affected by OAB symptoms.

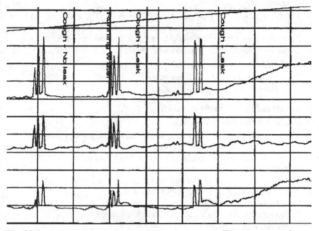

Fig. 22.6 Urodynamic trace showing detrusor overactivity. The upper trace of intravesical pressure (P_{ves}) vs time shows a sharp ↑ of pressure within the bladder. The middle trace of pressure within the abdomen (P_{abd}) shows no similar ↑. The lower trace, obtained by subtracting intra-abdominal pressure from intravesical pressure ($P_{det} = P_{ves} - P_{abd}$), shows significant detrusor overactivity.

Overactive bladder syndrome: management I

Conservative management

Behavioural therapy
- Advice to consume 1–1.5L of liquids per day.
- Avoid caffeine-based drinks (tea, coffee, cola) and alcohol.
- Various drugs, such as diuretics and antipsychotics, alter bladder function and should be reviewed.

Bladder retraining
- The principles of bladder retraining are based on the ability to suppress urinary urge and extend the intervals between voids.
- Reported cure rates using bladder retraining alone are 44–90%.
- It may be offered in conjunction with pelvic floor muscle training.

Hypnotherapy and acupuncture
- These can be successful in some cases.
- The relapse rate is very high.

Pharmacological interventions

Anticholinergic (antimuscarinic) drugs
- The mainstay of pharmacotherapy; they block the parasympathetic nerves, thereby relaxing the detrusor muscle.
- Advise about the side effects before starting treatment (some may be better tolerated than others) (Table 22.1).
- Dosage needs to be titrated against efficacy and adverse effects.
- Adverse effects of anticholinergics may include:
  - dry mouth (up to 30%)
  - constipation, nausea, dyspepsia, and flatulence
  - blurred vision, dizziness, and insomnia
  - palpitation and arrhythmias.
- Some data are emerging, suggesting a link between long-term anticholinergic medication use (anticholinergic burden) and an ↑ incidence of dementia. Women on long-term treatment should have their medication reviewed annually, or every 6mths if >75yrs.

β_3-adrenoceptor agonists
- These activate β_3-adrenoceptors, causing the bladder to relax, thus aiding filling and storage of urine.
- Mirabegron (25–50mg od) is recommended for use where anticholinergics are not tolerated, ineffective, or contraindicated.

Oestrogens
- Intravaginal oestrogens may be tried in women with vaginal atrophy.
- Treatment with vaginal oestrogen often helps with symptoms of urgency, urge incontinence, frequency, and nocturia.
- Systemic HRT is not recommended for treatment of urinary symptoms.

Contraindications to anticholinergics

- Acute (narrow-angle) glaucoma.
- Myasthenia gravis.
- Urinary retention or outflow obstruction.
- Severe ulcerative colitis.
- Gastrointestinal obstruction.
- Use with caution in dementia or cognitive impairment.

Table 22.1 Anticholinergic drugs and their doses

Drug	Dose (adult)	Selectivity	Notes
Oxybutynin	2.5–5mg, 2–4 times/ day	Selective, M1, M3	• Use ↓ dose in elderly and avoid if frail (risk of falls and confusion) • Transdermal patch available (may have ↓ side effects)
Tolterodine	2mg, bd	Non-selective	
Fesoterodine	4–8mg, od	Selective, M3	
Solifenacin	5–10mg, od	Selective, M3	
Darifenacin	7.5–15mg, od	Selective, M3	
Trospium	20mg, bd	Non-selective	• Less likely to cross blood–brain barrier

Overactive bladder syndrome: management II

Use of botulinum toxin A

- Botulinum toxin A blocks neuromuscular transmission, causing temporary paralysis.
- Increasingly used as an intervention for refractory OAB, with an efficacy of up to 90%.
- It is injected cystoscopically into the detrusor, usually under local anaesthetic.
- It can cause urinary retention in 5–10% of cases, in which case intermittent self-catheterization may be required.
- Repeat injections are required every 6–12mths.
- The long-term effects of repeat injections are unknown and are the subject of ongoing research.

Neuromodulation and sacral nerve stimulation

- Provides continuous stimulation of the S3 nerve root via an implanted electrical pulse generator and is thought to improve the ability to suppress detrusor contractions.
- It is being ↑ used in the treatment of refractory detrusor overactivity.
- Overall, neuromodulation has up to 50% clinical success rate.

Surgical management of OAB

- Surgery is reserved for those with debilitating symptoms and who have failed to benefit from medical, behavioural, and/or neuromodulation therapy.
- Procedures such as detrusor myomectomy and augmentation cystoplasty have limited efficacy and complication rates are high, hence they are rarely indicated.
- Permanent urinary diversion is occasionally indicated in women with intractable incontinence.

Anatomy of the pelvic floor

The pelvic floor consists of muscular and fascial structures that provide support to the pelvic viscera and the external openings of the vagina, urethra, and rectum (Fig. 22.7). The uterus and vagina are suspended from the pelvic side walls by endopelvic fascial attachments that support the vagina at three levels.

Levels of vaginal support

Level 1
The cervix and upper 1/3 of the vagina are supported by the cardinal (transverse cervical) and uterosacral ligaments. These are attached to the cervix and suspend the uterus from the pelvic sidewall and sacrum.

Level 2
The mid portion of the vagina is attached by endofascial condensation (endopelvic fascia) laterally to the pelvic side walls.

Level 3
The lower 1/3 of the vagina is supported by the levator ani muscles and the perineal body. The levator ani, together with its associated fascia, is termed the pelvic diaphragm.

▶ The axis of the vagina is also important. It normally lies horizontally on the levator muscles. This protects it during coughing and other activities that ↑ intra-abdominal pressure (Fig. 22.7).

▶ Damage occurring at the different levels of vaginal support causes different types of prolapse. It is therefore important to have an understanding of this anatomy.

Aetiology of prolapse

- *Pregnancy and vaginal delivery*: prolapse is uncommon in nulliparous women. Vaginal delivery may cause mechanical injuries and denervation of the pelvic floor. The risk is ↑ with large babies, prolonged 2nd stage, and instrumental delivery (forceps).
- *Congenital factors*: abnormal collagen metabolism, e.g. Ehlers–Danlos syndrome can predispose to prolapse.
- *Menopause*: the incidence of prolapse ↑ with age. This may be due to the deterioration of collagenous connective tissue that occurs following oestrogen withdrawal.
- *Chronic predisposing factors*: prolapse is aggravated by any chronic ↑ in intra-abdominal pressure, resulting from factors such as obesity, chronic cough, constipation, heavy lifting, or pelvic mass.
- *Iatrogenic factors*: pelvic surgery may also influence the occurrence of prolapse:
  - hysterectomy is associated with subsequent vaginal vault prolapse (particularly when the original indication was prolapse)
  - continence procedures, although elevating the bladder neck, may lead to defects in other pelvic compartments (Burch colposuspension may predispose to rectocele and enterocele formation).

(a)

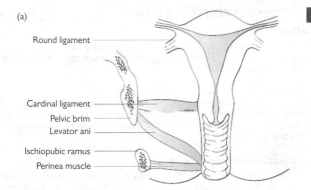

Round ligament

Cardinal ligament
Pelvic brim
Levator ani

Ischiopubic ramus
Perinea muscle

(b)

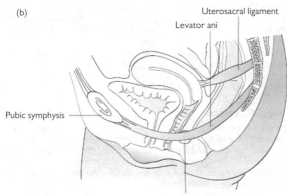

Uterosacral ligament

Levator ani

Pubic symphysis

Perineal body

Fig. 22.7 (a) Coronal view of the pelvis, showing cardinal ligaments and levator ani. (b) Lateral view of the pelvis, showing the uterosacral ligaments and levator ani. Reproduced with permission from Impey L. (1999). *Obstetrics and Gynaecology*. Oxford: Wiley-Blackwell Publishing.

Prolapse: classification

Definition

Prolapse is defined as protrusion of the uterus and/or vagina beyond normal anatomical confines. The bladder, urethra, rectum, and bowel are also often involved.

Incidence

The incidence of prolapse is difficult to define, as many women do not seek help and clinical examination does not necessarily correlate with symptoms. It is probably extremely common and is present in varying degrees in older parous women.

Classification of prolapse

Types of uterovaginal prolapse are classified anatomically, according to the site of the defect and the pelvic viscera that are involved (Fig. 22.8).
- Cystocele is prolapse of the anterior vaginal wall, involving the bladder. Often there is an associated prolapse of the urethra, in which case the term cysto-urethrocele is used.
- Uterine (apical) prolapse is the term used to describe prolapse of the uterus, cervix, and upper vagina. If the uterus has been removed, the vault or top of the vagina, where the uterus used to be, can itself prolapse.
- Enterocele is prolapse of the upper posterior wall of the vagina. The resulting pouch usually contains loops of small bowel.
- Rectocele is prolapse of the lower posterior wall of the vagina, involving the anterior wall of the rectum.

Grading of prolapse

There are many grading systems. None is perfect, and some are complex and impractical. In 1996, the International Continence Society (ICS) Committee for Standardization published its Pelvic Organ Prolapse Quantification (POP-Q) scoring system which compares a number of points in the vagina to the level of the hymen. Another frequently used system is the Baden–Walker classification.

Grading of prolapse (Baden–Walker classification)

- *1st degree:* the lowest part of the prolapse descends halfway down the vaginal axis to the introitus.
- *2nd degree:* the lowest part of the prolapse extends to the level of the introitus and through the introitus on straining.
- *3rd degree:* the lowest part of the prolapse extends through the introitus and lies outside the vagina.

▶ Procidentia describes a 3rd-degree uterine prolapse.

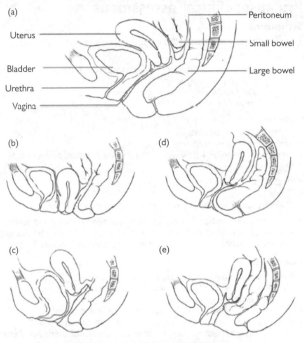

Fig. 22.8 Types of prolapse. (a) Normal pelvis, (b) uterine prolapse, (c) cystocele, (d) rectocele, (e) enterocele. Reproduced with permission from Impey L. (1999) *Obstetrics and Gynaecology*. Oxford: Wiley-Blackwell Publishing.

Prolapse: clinical assessment

Symptoms

Symptoms may be absent, but the most commonly reported are:

General
- Dragging sensation, discomfort, and heaviness within the pelvis.
- Feeling of 'a lump coming down'.
- Dyspareunia or difficulty in inserting tampons.
- Discomfort and backache.

Cysto-urethrocele
- Urinary urgency and frequency.
- Incomplete bladder emptying.
- Urinary retention or ↓ flow where the urethra is kinked by descent of the anterior vaginal wall.

Rectocele
- Constipation.
- Difficulty with defecation (may digitally reduce it to defecate).

▶ Symptoms tend to become worse with prolonged standing and towards the end of the day. In case of grade 3 or 4 prolapse, there may be mucosal ulceration and lichenification, resulting in vaginal bleeding and discharge.

Examination

- Exclude pelvic masses with a bimanual examination.
- Vaginal examination is best carried out with the woman in the left lateral position, using a Sims speculum.
- The walls should be checked in turn for descent and atrophy.
- If absolutely necessary, an Vulsellum forceps may be applied to the cervix so that traction will demonstrate the severity of uterine prolapse (this can cause marked discomfort, perform very gently).
- Sometimes, prolapse may only be demonstrated with the woman standing or straining.
- An assessment of pelvic floor muscle strength should be carried out (Box 22.1).

Quality of life assessment

- Symptoms can affect quality of life, causing social, psychological, occupational, or sexual limitations to a woman's lifestyle.
- Self-completion questionnaires allow a comprehensive assessment of prolapse symptoms and their impact, such as the Vaginal Symptoms module of the International Consultation on Incontinence Questionnaire (ICIQ-VS) (🖰 www.iciq.net).

Investigations

- USS to exclude pelvic or abdominal masses (if suspected clinically).
- Urodynamics are required if urinary incontinence is present.
- ECG, CXR, FBC, and U&E (if appropriate pre-surgery).

Box 22.1 Modified Oxford system for grading pelvic floor muscle strength

A system of grading using vaginal palpation of the pelvic floor muscles:
- 0: no contraction.
- 1: flicker.
- 2: weak.
- 3: moderate.
- 4: good (with lift).
- 5: strong.

Prevention of pelvic organ prolapse
- Ensure excessively long labour is prevented.
- Careful consideration of pelvic anatomy when performing instrumental deliveries.
- Encouraging persistence with postnatal pelvic floor exercises.
- Weight ↓.
- Treatment of chronic constipation.
- Treatment of chronic cough (including smoking cessation).

Prolapse: conservative management

Physiotherapy

Physiotherapy has a role in the management grade 1 and 2 prolapse:

- *Pelvic floor muscle exercises:* are most effective when taught under the direct supervision of a physiotherapist; these will improve the tone in young parous women, but are unlikely to benefit women with more significant uterovaginal prolapse.
- *Biofeedback and vaginal cones* (→ Stress urinary incontinence: conservative management, p. 752).

Intravaginal devices (pessaries)

Vaginal pessaries (Fig. 22.9) offer a further conservative line of therapy for women who decline surgery, who are unfit for surgery, or for whom surgery is contraindicated. They should be changed 6-monthly and topical oestrogen may be given to ↓ the risk of vaginal erosion.

- *Ring pessary:* is most commonly used and is available in a number of different sizes (52–129mm); the ring is placed between the posterior aspect of the symphysis pubis and the posterior fornix of the vagina. Patients may be taught to self-insert and remove the device to facilitate sexual activity.
- *Shelf pessary:* can be used when a correctly sized ring pessary will not sit in the vagina and/or where the perineum is deficient (it may be difficult to insert and remove and its use precludes penetrative intercourse).
- *Hodge pessary:* can be used to correct uterine retroversion. It is of classical interest, but in practice is virtually never used now.
- *Cube and doughnut pessaries:* are, very rarely, used for significant prolapse, when others are not retained.

Factors influencing management of prolapse

- Severity of symptoms.
- Grade of prolapse (asymptomatic grade 1 prolapse does not require treatment).
- Age, parity, and wish for further pregnancies.
- Patient's sexual activity.
- Presence of aggravating features such as smoking and obesity.
- Urinary symptoms.
- Other gynaecological problems such as menorrhagia.
- Comorbidity and previous surgeries.

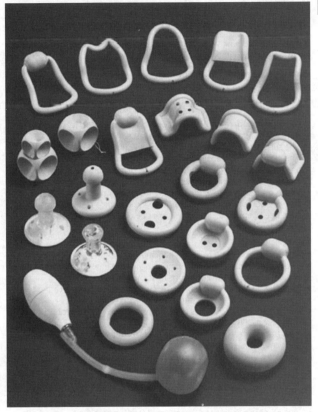

Fig. 22.9 Types of pessary for uterine prolapse include rings, cubes, shelf, and doughnuts. Reproduced by courtesy of Milex Products Inc., Chicago © 2002.

Prolapse: surgical management, anterior and posterior compartments

Surgery offers definitive treatment of prolapse. Choice of procedure depends on patient and type of prolapse that exists.

Anterior compartment defect

Anterior colporrhaphy (anterior repair)
- Appropriate for the repair of a cysto-urethrocele.
- A longitudinal incision is made on the anterior vaginal wall and the vaginal skin separated by dissection from the pubocervical fascia.
- Buttressing sutures are placed on the fascia.
- The surplus vaginal skin is excised and the skin is closed.
- The repair is traditionally performed under regional or general anaesthesia; however, it can also be performed under local anaesthesia, allowing early mobilization and discharge home.
- While morbidity is low, the long-term success rate of conventional anterior colporrhaphy is disappointing; recurrence rates of up to 30% have been reported. This may in part be due to failure to identify a coexisting apical defect.

Paravaginal repair
- Abdominal approach to correct an anterior defect.
- The retropubic space is opened through a Pfannenstiel incision and the bladder is swept medially, exposing the pelvic sidewall.
- The lateral sulcus of the vagina is elevated and reattached to the pelvic sidewall using interrupted sutures.
- A cure rate of 70–90% has been reported (may also be done laparoscopically).
- It isn't a commonly performed procedure, it is very invasive if performed via laparotomy, and the author's personal experience suggests higher recurrence rates than published data suggest.

Posterior compartment defect

Posterior colpoperineorrhaphy (posterior repair)
- Appropriate for correction of a rectocele and deficient perineum.
- It involves the repair of a rectovaginal fascial defect and removal of excess vaginal skin.

▶ Care must be taken when removing redundant vaginal skin, as vaginal narrowing can result in dyspareunia.

▶ Perineoplasty is performed by placing deeper sutures into the perineal muscles, building up the perineal body to provide additional support.

Prolapse: surgical management, uterovaginal and vaginal vault

Uterovaginal (apical) prolapse

Vaginal hysterectomy
- May be combined with the procedures previously described (➔ Prolapse: surgical management, anterior and posterior compartments, p. 772), in cases of significant uterine descent or menstrual problems (Table 22.2).

Manchester repair (or Fothergill repair)
- Now rarely performed.
- Cervical amputation is followed by approximation and shortening of the cardinal ligaments anterior to the cervical stump.
- This is combined with an anterior and posterior colporrhaphy.

Hysteropexy/sacrohysteropexy
- Can be performed if patient wishes to preserve uterus as an open or laparoscopic procedure (Fig. 22.10).
- Uterus and cervix are attached to sacrum using bifurcated non-absorbable mesh.
- Theoretical advantage of hysteropexy is stronger apical support when compared with vaginal hysterectomy.

Vaginal vault prolapse

Sacrospinous ligament fixation
- Involves suturing the vaginal vault to the sacrospinous ligaments, using a vaginal approach.
- Low immediate postoperative morbidity; success rate 70–85%.

⚠ As vaginal axis is changed by this procedure, there is risk of postoperative dyspareunia.

Sacrocolpopexy
- The vault is attached to the sacrum using a non-absorbable mesh, and if can be performed either as an open procedure or laparoscopically.
- It has a higher success rate, of ~90%, and a better anatomical result than sacrospinous fixation.

⚠ Mesh erosion into the vagina, or rarely into the bladder or bowel, is a possible late complication.

Table 22.2 Operations available for uterovaginal prolapse

Defect	Vaginal route	Abdominal route (open or laparoscopic)
Anterior	• Anterior colporrhaphy • Transvaginal mesh repair (currently suspended)	• Paravaginal repair • Sacrocolpopexy with placement of mesh over anterior vaginal wall
Apical	• Vaginal hysterectomy • Sacrospinous fixation	• Hysteropexy (laparoscopic or open) • Sacrocolpopexy
Posterior	• Posterior repair • Transvaginal mesh repair (currently suspended) • Perineal body reconstruction	• Sacrocolpopexy to correct recto/enterocele

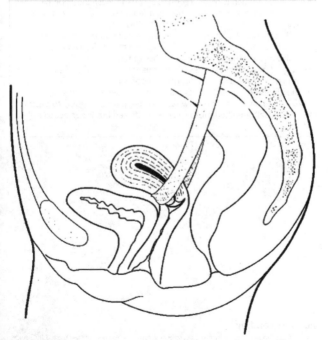

Fig. 22.10 Bifurcated mesh in position for sacrohysteropexy. Reproduced from Springer-Verlag London Ltd., Female Pelvic Reconstructive Surgery, 2002, p 187, Figure 13.10 Stanton and Zimmern. With kind permission of Springer Science and Business Media.

Recurrent urogenital prolapse

- ~1/3 of all prolapse surgery is for recurrent defects.
- Vaginal epithelium may be scarred and atrophic:
  - making surgical correction technically more difficult
  - ↑ the risk of damage to the bladder and bowel.

▶ Use of synthetic meshes was common for repair of recurrent prolapse, as they may offer more support where endopelvic fascia has proved to be deficient.

☛ Due to concerns regarding complications all vaginally inserted meshes are currently suspended by NHS England.

Use of 'mesh' in urogynaecological surgery

- This has been the source of much attention from patients and the media.
- Concerns have been raised due to potential adverse effects, including pain, mesh erosion, and sexual dysfunction.
- NICE recommends that surgeons performing mesh insertion have had specialist training and carry out a sufficient case load to maintain their skills:
  - all surgeons should maintain audit data and contribute to national audit databases (such as the British Society for Urogynaecology)
  - all surgeons should work within the context of the MDT.
- Patients must be provided with information about risks of surgery and should be made aware of alternative procedures.
- NHS England 'paused' all vaginal mesh surgeries (as of July 2018) pending further review (still paused at time of going to press).
- Abdominally inserted mesh can still be offered but is subject to high vigilance.

Further reading

NICE (2019). Urinary incontinence and pelvic organ prolapse in women: management. NICE guideline [NG123].
🔗 www.nice.org.uk/guidance/ng123

Chapter 23

Benign and malignant gynaecological conditions

Benign neoplasms of the lower genital tract

Benign neoplasms are very common in the genital tract; most are innocent and easy to recognize.

Vulva

(See Fig. 14.3, p. 541.)

- *Bartholin's cyst:* arises from blocked Bartholin's duct. Bartholin's gland normally <1cm and located deep to posterior ends of each vestibular bulb. Glands open bilaterally into posterolateral vaginal orifice (between the hymen and labium minus) via a 2cm long duct. It may present as a simple lump or an acute abscess after infection:
  - *conservative treatment*—cyst incised under local anaesthesia and a Word catheter placed for 7 days to facilitate drainage of the cyst
  - *surgical treatment*—incision and marsupialization.

⚠ Send pus to microbiology if infected (some are due to gonococcal infection and may need treatment and referral to GUM for contact tracing).

- *Sebaceous cysts, boils, and carbuncles:* very common and if symptomatic should be treated by incision and drainage. Tend to recur.
- *Cysts of the canal of Nuck* (embryological remnants): appear in the anterior part of the vulva.
- *Mucinous cysts:* may arise from the minor vestibular glands.
- *Mesonephric cysts:* generally seen on the labia majora.
- *Endometriotic lesions:* especially on an episiotomy wound.
- *Lipomas and fibromas:* also common.
- *Condylomata acuminata* (HPV 6/11):
  - sessile polypoidal mass on the vulva
  - 1/3 people will clear warts spontaneously
  - topical treatments include podophyllotoxin (Warticon® and Condyline®) or imiquimod 5%
  - excision using laser or electro-diathermy under local anaesthesia reserved for larger lesions
  - prevention involves vaccination prior to exposure—HPV subtypes 6/11 included in HPV vaccine since 2012.

Urethra

- *Urethral caruncle:* most common in postmenopausal women and children. Appears as a bright red, tender swelling at the posterior margin of the urethral meatus. May present with dysuria, bleeding, and dyspareunia. The treatment is excision using diathermy.
- *Prolapse of the urethra:* presents as red lesion involving entire circumference of the urethral meatal margin. May be acute or chronic. Again, diathermy of the prolapsed mucosa is curative.

Vagina

- *Endometriotic deposits:* may present as small brown-black nodules.
- *Simple mesonephric (Gartner's) cysts and paramesonephric cysts:* usually appear in the fornices of the vagina. If symptomatic they should be marsupialized rather than excised.
- *Inclusion cysts:* can arise where vaginal epithelium is embedded under surface during perineal surgery. Treatment warranted only when patients are symptomatic.

Cervix

- *Cervical polyps (adenoma):* common; due to overgrowth of the endocervical mucosa. Sometimes arise from the endometrium (pedunculated) and protrude through cervix. Very rarely malignant (1:6000), but they should be removed and hysteroscopy to rule out further polyps should be considered if symptoms warrant it. ➲ Colour plate 1.
- *Nabothian cysts:* very common; mucous-retention cysts caused by blockage of endocervical mucous glands due to squamous metaplasia of the transformation zone, a normal physiological process. Treatment is not required. Can appear white or blueish due to mucous and can calcify. ➲ Colour plate 2.

Further reading

British Association for Sexual Health and HIV. Guidelines.
ℛ www.bashh.org/guidelines

NHS (2019). HPV vaccine overview.
ℛ www.nhs.uk/conditions/vaccinations/hpv-human-papillomavirus-vaccine/

NICE (2009). Guidance on the Word catheter.
ℛ www.nice.org.uk/guidance/ipg323/evidence/overview-pdf-314093341

Benign neoplasms of the uterus

Uterine fibroids

These are the most common benign tumours arising from the myometrium of the uterus. Also called *leiomyomata*, they are composed mainly of smooth muscle cells, but may contain fibrous tissue. Present in 20–40% of women in the reproductive age group, they have an ↑ incidence in Afro-Caribbean women and those with a family history of fibroids. Many women are asymptomatic, but may present with dysmenorrhoea, menorrhagia, pressure symptoms (especially urinary frequency), and pelvic pain. Infertility may be associated and, in <10% cases, caused solely by fibroids. In pregnancy can cause pain from degeneration, abnormal lie, and obstruction if cervical, and difficulty at CD. Not associated with ↑ risk of miscarriage.

> ### Types of uterine fibroids
> - *Submucous:* >50% projection into the endometrial cavity.
> - *Intramural:* located within the myometrium.
> - *Subserous:* >50% of the fibroid mass extends outside the uterine contours.
> - *Cervical:* relatively uncommon and can cause surgical difficulty due to the proximity to the bladder and the ureters.
> - *Pedunculated:* mobile and prone to torsion.
> - *Parasitic:* have become detached from the uterus and attached to other structures.
> - *IV leiomyomatosis:* very rare, spread through the pelvic veins and vena cava to involve the heart.

Diagnosis

Clinical examination (hard, irregular uterine mass) may be sufficient. TV or abdominal USS can differentiate the types and dimensions of the fibroids. Rarely, MRI may be needed when the scan is inconclusive.

⚠ Leiomyosarcomas are very rare—consider if fibroid painful/rapidly growing/bleeding—imaging cannot reliably diagnose or exclude.

Endometrial polyps (adenoma)

These are focal overgrowth of the endometrium and are malignant in <1%. They are more common in women >40yrs, but may occur at any age. Treatment is usually resection during hysteroscopy and the polyp should be sent for histological assessment to exclude malignancy.

Treatment options for uterine fibroids

- *No treatment:* if minimal symptoms.
- *Mirena® IUS:* 1st line if heavy bleeding and fibroids <3cm.
- *GnRH analogues:* shrink fibroids, but should only be used for this purpose prior to surgery.
- *Myomectomy:* open, laparoscopic, or hysteroscopic depending upon location (especially when wish to preserve fertility and when the fibroids are distinctly isolated on scan—fibroids often recur).

⚠ Caution with morcellation as will disseminate disease if unsuspected leiomyosarcoma.

- *Hysterectomy:* women who have either completed their family or are >45yrs—guaranteed cure of fibroids.
- *Uterine artery embolization:* uterine artery is catheterized generally using the unilateral approach; embolic agent with a diameter of 300–750µm used, e.g. polyvinyl alcohol powder or gelatin sponge (minimally invasive procedure with avoidance of a GA).
- *MR-guided focused ultrasound therapy:* non-invasive procedure using high doses of focused ultrasound waves to destroy fibroids.

Benign neoplasms of the fallopian tube

Hydrosalpinx, pyosalpinx, and tubo-ovarian masses following PID or endometriotic adhesions may present as a benign mass in the pelvis. The diagnosis is essentially by ultrasound and laparoscopy. Most tumours of the fallopian tubes are malignant. Although they were thought to be rare, data from series of breast cancer gene (*BRCA*) +ve women undergoing prophylactic bilateral salpingo-oophorectomy (BSO) suggest that many of what were thought to be ovarian cancers arise from serous tubal intraepithelial carcinoma (STIC lesions) in the fimbriae of fallopian tubes.

Further reading

NICE (2018, updated 2021). Heavy menstrual bleeding: assessment and management. NICE guideline [NG88].
🔗 www.nice.org.uk/guidance/ng88/

RCOG (2013). Uterine artery embolisation in the management of fibroids.
🔗 www.rcog.org.uk/guidance/browse-all-guidance/other-guidelines-and-reports/uterine-artery-embolisation-in-the-management-of-fibroids/

RCOG (2014). The distal fallopian tube as the origin of non-uterine pelvic high-grade serous carcinomas.
🔗 www.rcog.org.uk/globalassets/documents/guidelines/scientific-impact-papers/sip44hgscs.pdf

RCOG (2019). Morcellation for myomectomy or hysterectomy.
🔗 www.rcog.org.uk/globalassets/documents/guidelines/consent-advice/consent-advice-no-13-morcellation-myomectormy-hysterectomy.pdf

Benign ovarian tumours: diagnosis

Ovarian cysts are frequently physiological, due to follicular cyst (≤3cm) and corpus luteal cyst (≤5cm) formation during the menstrual cycle. In a woman who is having periods, a cyst of <5cm should not cause concern (or referral), unless there are other suspicious features or she is symptomatic (e.g. pain). Large cysts (≥5cm), are at risk of torsion. Small cysts (>1cm) are frequently seen in postmenopausal women (up to 14%) on TVS.

Presentation

- Asymptomatic.
- Chronic pain:
  - dull ache
  - pressure on organs (urinary frequency or bowel disturbance)
  - dyspareunia (endometrioma)
  - cyclical pain (endometrioma).
- Acute pain (cyst accident):
  - bleeding (into the cyst or intra-abdominal)
  - torsion
  - rupture.
- Abnormal uterine bleeding.
- Hormonal effects.

History and investigation

History

Menstrual history (LMP, cycle length, menorrhagia); pain (site, nature, radiation—typically down leg/s, duration, precipitating factors); bowel/bladder function; abdominal distension; medical and family history. Acute presentation of cyst accident often associated with nausea, vomiting, and loss of appetite (rule out appendicitis).

Examination

- *Systemic:* pulse, BP, anaemia, temperature.
- *Abdominal:* mass arising from pelvis, tenderness, signs of peritonism, upper abdominal masses or ascites suggest cyst less likely to be benign.
- *Pelvic:* PV discharge/bleeding, cervical excitation, adnexal mass or tenderness (mobile or fixed, smooth or nodular, size).

Haematological tests

- FBC.
- Tumour markers:
  - CA125 (consider CA19-9 and CEA if suspicious USS)
  - add AFP, hCG, LDH in a woman <40yrs as higher risk of germ cell tumours (➔ Ovarian cancer: presentation and investigation, p. 826)
  - consider inhibin, if abnormal bleeding and solid ovarian mass.

Non-gynaecological causes of pelvic masses

Other benign masses due to non-gynaecological conditions in the pelvis should always be borne in mind as a differential diagnosis:
- Bladder tumours.
- Pelvic kidney.
- Intestinal tumours.
- Diverticular disease.
- IBD.
- Pregnancy

Benign ovarian tumours: imaging

Ultrasound features and the tumour marker CA125 are used to determine the risk of malignancy index (RMI; Box 23.1). This is useful for identifying patients with a high risk of cancer who should be referred to a cancer centre for treatment (sensitivity 87.4%, +ve predictive value (PPV) 86.8% in recent series) (Table 23.1).

Abdominal/pelvic USS

- Presence and appearance of pelvic mass ± ascites.
- 'Whirlpool' sign in case of ovarian torsion.

MRI

- If cyst >7cm due to difficulty visualizing entire cyst at time of ultrasound, if not considering surgical management.

Box 23.1 Modified RMI

$RMI = U \times M \times CA125$
- U = ultrasound score (0, 1, or 3).
- M = menopausal status (1 = premenopausal, 3 = postmenopausal).
- CA125 = serum cancer antigen 125 level (U/L).

Ultrasound scoring system
- Features looked for on USS:
  - multilocular cyst
  - evidence of solid areas
  - evidence of metastases
  - ascites
  - bilateral lesions.
- Final U score:
  - 0 if no features
  - 1 if 1 feature
  - 3 if 2 or more features.

Reproduced from Tingulstad S, Hagen B, Skjeldestad FE, et al. (1996). 'Evaluation of a risk of malignancy index based on serum CA125, ultrasound findings and menopausal status in the pre-operative diagnosis of pelvic masses' *BJOG* 103(8): 826–31 with permission from Wiley.

Table 23.1 RMI score and ovarian cancer risk

Risk	RMI score	Risk of cancer
Low	<25	<3%
Moderate	25–250	20%
High	>250	75%

International Ovarian Tumor Analysis (IOTA) rules
- An alternative scoring system is the IOTA rules (Table 23.2).
- This recommends referral to gynae-oncology if there are any M rules present:
  - sensitivity 95%
  - specificity 91%
  - +ve likelihood ratio of 10.37
  - −ve likelihood ratio of 0.06.

Table 23.2 IOTA USS features

Benign (B) rules	Malignant (M) rules
Unilocular cyst	Irregular solid tumour
Solid components where the largest solid component <7mm	Ascites
	At least 4 papillary structures
Presence of acoustic shadowing	Irregular multilocular solid tumour—largest diameter ≥100mm
Smooth multilocular tumour—largest diameter <100mm	
No blood flow	

Source: data from Timmerman et al. (2000) Terms, definitions and measurements to describe the sonographic features of adnexal tumors: a consensus opinion from the International Ovarian Tumor Analysis (IOTA) Group. *Ultrasound Obstet Gynecol* 16:500–505.

Further reading
RCOG (2011). Management of suspected ovarian masses in premenopausal women. Green-top guideline no. 62.
ℂ www.rcog.org.uk/globalassets/documents/guidelines/gtg_62.pdf

Benign ovarian tumours: histology

Histology

It is difficult to know the true incidences of benign ovarian tumours, as many are functional cysts and not removed; hence, ratios of functional/benign/malignant tumours are highly dependent on the age and selection of the population studied.

Non-neoplastic

- Functional:
  - follicular cysts (normally <3cm)
  - corpus luteal cysts (normally <5cm (may show signs of haemorrhage into cyst or even cause haemoperitoneum)).
- Pathological:
  - *ovarian endometriotic cyst* (filled with old altered blood, 'chocolate cyst'; ➔ Endometriosis: overview, p. 664)
  - *polycystic ovarian syndrome* (generally bulky ovaries with >12 small follicles (2–9mm), fibrotic capsule, and smooth surface, 'string of pearls' sign on TVnUSS)
  - *theca leutin cysts* (multiple ovarian cysts, occur in conditions with ↑ hCG, e.g. hydatidiform molar pregnancy—resolve if ↑ hCG levels fall)
  - *ovarian oedema* (2° to ovarian torsion, the ovary is enlarged and boggy—exclude germ cell tumour in young woman).

Benign neoplastic

- *Epithelial tumours:*
  - *serous cystadenoma* (usually unilocular and 20–30% are bilateral, may have septations)
  - *mucinous cystadenoma* (often multiloculated, but usually unilateral (5% bilateral)—can get extremely large, >150 kg)
  - *Brenner tumours* (1–2% of ovarian tumours, unilateral, and have solid grey, white, or yellow appearance to cut surface, fibrous elements, and transitional epithelium).
- *Benign germ cell tumours:* mature teratoma or dermoid cyst:
  - 10% are bilateral
  - 90% occur in women of reproductive age
  - usually full of sebaceous material and hair, but may contain teeth, skin, cartilage, fat, or bone
  - can cause chemical peritonitis if contents spill.
- *Sex-cord stromal tumours* (➔ Rare ovarian tumours: other, p. 834):
  - *fibroma* (most common stromal tumour, up to 40% present with Meig's syndrome, ascites, and pleural effusion)
  - *Sertoli–Leydig cell tumour* (1% of ovarian tumours; produce androgens and present with virilization)
  - *thecoma* (produce oestrogens—present with abnormal vaginal bleeding)
  - *lipoma.*

Benign ovarian tumours: management

Most cysts will present with lower abdominal pain, but no peritonism or systemic upset. Most will resolve spontaneously with analgesia.

⚠ If presentation is an acute abdomen and/or any systemic upset, due to ovarian torsion, rupture, or haemorrhage of a cyst, urgent diagnostic laparoscopy or laparotomy may be required.

⚠ Peritoneal washings should be taken and blood sent for tumour markers at the time of surgery, if not benign, this will aid follow-up.

Adolescent women

* Manage as for premenopausal women.
* Germ cell tumours are more common in this age group (up to 20% in some series), especially in with ovarian torsion.
* Aim for conservative surgery (cystectomy, if possible) to diagnose, but preserve fertility.

Premenopausal women

* Malignant tumours rare in this age group (0.4–9:100,000).
* Aim to exclude malignancy and preserve fertility.
* If simple cyst, CA125 not necessary.
* If asymptomatic simple cyst <5cm, no follow-up is indicated as they normally resolve over 2–3 cycles.
* Asymptomatic 5–7cm simple cysts require a rescan in 12mths.
* If cyst is complex, but low RMI, monitor with USS and CA125 (e.g. 3× over 12mths).

Management of symptomatic low-risk cysts in premenopausal women

⚠ If suspected torted ovarian cyst can be 'de-torted' surgically—treat as emergency to preserve ovarian function.

* TV cyst aspiration under USS guidance has no advantage over expectant management.
* If cyst still persists, ↑, or is >5cm, then consider surgical management, e.g. laparoscopic cystectomy/oophorectomy depending on age.

✹ Maximum size for laparoscopy is controversial; with cysts >7cm, inadvertent rupture is more common in laparoscopic surgery:

  * *if cyst <5cm and simple:* cyst fenestration and wall biopsy for histology is acceptable.
  * *if cyst >5cm or is a dermoid:* aim to prevent spillage of contents, e.g. cystectomy and removal of cyst in an 'endobag'
  * *if suspicious findings at laparoscopy:* abandon procedure (take peritoneal biopsy for diagnosis). Refer to cancer centre for full staging laparotomy.

⚠ Caution with morcellator—use in bag and avoid spilling contents.

* If a dermoid cyst, this can cause a chemical peritonitis.
* If cyst ruptured and contents spill out, this can disseminate an otherwise early ovarian cancer (although rare in this age group).

Postmenopausal women

Should be managed according to RMI score (➲ Table 23.1, p. 784).

Low RMI (<25)

- Simple, <5cm cyst and normal CA125.
- Follow-up over 1yr with 3× USS and CA125, e.g. every 4mths.
- If no change, then discontinue monitoring.
- If change and RMI still low, or woman requests removal, laparoscopic salpingo-oophorectomy (usually bilateral) is appropriate.

Moderate RMI (25–250)

- Salpingo-oophorectomy (usually bilateral) in cancer centre recommended.
- May be acceptable to perform laparoscopically in some cases.
- If malignancy found then full staging laparotomy will be needed.

High RMI (>250)

- Refer to a cancer centre for a full staging laparotomy.

Further reading

RCOG (2011). Management of suspected ovarian masses in premenopausal women. Green-top guideline no. 62.
ℐ www.rcog.org.uk/globalassets/documents/guidelines/gtg_62.pdf

RCOG (2016). Ovarian cysts in post-menopausal women. Green-top guideline no. 34.
ℐ www.rcog.org.uk/guidance/browse-all-guidance/green-top-guidelines/ovarian-cysts-in-pos tmenopausal-women-green-top-guideline-no-34/

Vulval dermatoses: lichen sclerosus

Skin conditions of the vulva can cause distressing symptoms, and be difficult to diagnose and manage. Irritation leads to scratching and excoriation, which may make it clinically difficult to differentiate, especially following 2° infection or use of topical creams.

Vulval dermatoses refers to a range of benign skin conditions, which generally cause white thickening of the vulval skin: *lichen sclerosus*, *lichen planus*, *vulval dermatitis*, and *vulval psoriasis*.

Lichen sclerosus

- Chronic inflammatory condition (lymphocyte mediated).
- May be hereditary (association with HLA-DQ7).
- Usually confined to anogenital area.
- More common in women.
- Incidence estimated as 1:300–1:1000 women.
- Normally in perimenopausal women, but can occur in young girls (2/3 improve at puberty—may be misdiagnosed as signs of abuse).
- Associated with other autoimmune diseases:
  - e.g. thyroid disease, diabetes, vitiligo, pernicious anaemia
  - 20–34% have association with autoimmune disease
  - up to 74% have autoantibodies.

Clinical presentation of lichen sclerosus

- Burning pain or itch, occasionally asymptomatic.
- Figure-of-8 appearance around vulva and anus.
- White, shiny, wrinkly, atrophic appearance 'like tissue paper':
  - may have white patches, purpura, or telangiectasia
  - hyperkeratosis and lichenification if chronic scratching
  - over time, can develop loss and fusion of labia minora, narrowing of introitus, resulting in problems with intercourse and micturition.
- ➔ Colour plates 3 and 4.

⚠ Long-term risk of vulval squamous cell carcinoma (VSCC) (2–5%), so need long-term observation, follow-up, and biopsy of suspicious lesions. This can be in 1° care if symptoms well controlled.

⚠ Differentiated vulval intraepithelial neoplasia (dVIN) can develop (not associated with HPV infection). Very high risk of progression to cancer—recommend excision.

⚠ Women with combination of lichen sclerosus and usual-type vulval intraepithelial neoplasia (uVIN; associated with HPV) have ~19% risk of progression to cancer over 10yrs—specialist long-term follow-up recommended.

Management of lichen sclerosus

⚠ Biopsy suspicious lesions (risk of vulval cancer) or if not responding to treatment made on clinical diagnosis.

▶ Take biopsy from edge of lesion and photograph with diagram to accurately indicate site of biopsy.

- Check ferritin levels and treat if low.
- Screen for autoimmune conditions, if suggestive symptoms (FBC, TFTs, glucose, serum iron, autoimmune antibodies, intrinsic factor, and vitamin B_{12}).
- Ultra-potent corticosteroids: clobetasol propionate 0.05% initially once a night for 4wks, alternate nights for 4wks, once or twice weekly for 4wks, then use weekly maintenance or 'as required' for flares; the shiny appearance will remain.
- Follow-up at 3mths to check response.
- Annual review with GP and advise urgent contact if ulcers, bleeding, or suspicious lesions.
- Referral to specialist unit for tacrolimus if symptoms not responding.

⚠ Data suggest good control of lichen sclerosus with ultra-potent topical steroids may ↓ the risk of progression to squamous cell carcinoma.

▶ Encourage appropriate use—as long as no more than 30g tube of clobetasol propionate 0.05% over 3mths.

Further reading

Association for Lichen Sclerosus.
🖰 www.lichensclerosus.org

British Association for Sexual Health and HIV (2014). 2014 UK national guideline on the management of vulval conditions.
🖰 www.bashhguidelines.org/media/1056/vulval-conditions_2014-ijstda.pdf

British Association of Dermatologists.
🖰 www.bad.org.uk

Macmillan Cancer Support. Vulval lichen sclerosus.
🖰 www.macmillan.org.uk/Cancerinformation/Cancertypes/Vulva/Pre-cancerousconditions/Vulvallichensclerosuslichenplanus.aspx

Other vulval dermatoses

Vulval dermatitis

- Dermatitis or eczema.
- If scratched so much that skin thickens → lichen simplex chronicus.
- Association with other atopic illnesses (asthma, hay fever, eczema).
- Common irritants:
  - soaps, shower gels, condoms, deodorants, creams
  - if diagnosed as candidiasis, topical creams can be irritant.

Clinical presentation of vulval dermatitis
- Itch, burning, and pain 2° to scratching.
- Erythema ± scaling of skin.
- No loss or fusion of labia.

Management
- Avoid irritant and apply general vulval skin care (Box 23.2).
- LVSs for 2° infection (e.g. *Candida*).
- Severe disease—treat with steroid cream:
  - clobetasol propionate or betamethasone valerate, if less severe
  - use bd initially; ↓ to od, then twice weekly, as condition improves.
- Consider sedating antihistamine (e.g. chlorphenamine 4 mg) at night to prevent scratching.
- Referral to dermatology for patch testing.

Lichen planus

- Rare condition. ◗ Colour plate 5.

Clinical presentation of lichen planus
- Purplish papules and plaques; can have white streaks on top—'Wickham's striae'.
- May involve mouth too.
- May cause painful, red, ulcerated areas around introitus.
- Occasionally can cause severe desquamative vaginitis.
- Cause itch, pain, PCB, or discharge.

Management
- As for lichen sclerosus, including follow-up, as also have an ↑ risk of developing vulval cancer (up to 3%).
- Biopsy; ultra-potent steroids (clobetasol proprionate, e.g. Dermovate®); good vulval skin care; local anaesthetic ointment.

Vulval psoriasis

Clinical presentation of vulval psoriasis
- Classically well-defined erythematous patches, may have scaling on pubic area, but not necessarily on vulval skin.

Management
- Good vulval skin care:
  - bland emollients
  - mild topical steroids.
- Other psoriatic medications often too harsh for vulval skin.

Box 23.2 Vulval skin care advice

- Keep area clean but avoid soap:
  - *use soap substitutes*—soap-free shower gels, bath oil, just water
  - salt baths *may* help.
- Do not soak in hot bath.
- Allow air circulation to avoid sweating:
  - loose underwear and bed clothes
  - avoid jeans, etc.
- Wear cotton next to skin:
  - avoid synthetics (especially nylon) and wool (intrinsically itchy!).
- Avoid vaginal lubricants:
  - may be irritating
  - can use saliva or oil (vegetable, olive, almond) but avoid perfumed oil.

⚠ Warn that oils weaken condoms therefore an alternate method of contraception might be advisable
- Refer for patch testing if vulval dermatitis.

Further reading

Association for Lichen Sclerosus.
🔗 www.lichensclerosus.org

British Association for Sexual Health and HIV (2014). 2014 UK national guideline on the management of vulval conditions.
🔗 www.bashhguidelines.org/media/1056/vulval-conditions_2014-ijstda.pdf

British Association of Dermatologists.
🔗 www.bad.org.uk

Macmillan Cancer Support. Vulval lichen sclerosus.
🔗 www.macmillan.org.uk/Cancerinformation/Cancertypes/Vulva/Pre-cancerousconditions/Vulvallichensclerosuslichenplanus.aspx

Idiopathic vulval itch and pain

Pruritis vulvae

- Common (1 in 10 women).
- Persistent itch, often worse at night and may disturb sleep.

Management

- Identify cause and treat appropriately: may need swabs, skin scrapings, skin biopsy, U&E, LFTs.
- General vulval skin care and bland emollients.
- Short course of weak steroid cream (hydrocortisone 1–2wks).
- Sedating antihistamine at night (e.g. chlorphenamine 4mg) (break itch/scratch/itch cycle).

Vulvodynia/vestibulodynia

These are dysaesthesia, which involve pain in the vulva or around the introitus in the absence of a specific cause.

- Burning, stinging, or raw discomfort.
- Typically worse when sitting down.
- May occur as sequelae to inflammatory vulval condition, e.g. lichen sclerosus.
- Neuropathic pain.

Management

- Investigate and exclude other causes.
- General vulval skin care.
- Topical local anaesthetic ointment.
- Amitriptyline; start on low dose (10mg) 3h before bed (to avoid morning 'hangover') and ↑ as tolerated/required by ~10mg/wk up to 80mg, reduce gradually after 3mths.
- Antiepileptics (used rarely and with specialist referral, e.g. chronic pain service): gabapentin and pregabalin.

Ulcers

- Aphthous ulcers.
- Infectious:
  - *HSV*—multiple, extremely painful ulcers
  - *syphilis* 1° *chancre*—painless unless infected
  - *tropical* (chancroid, granuloma inguinale, lymphogranuloma venereum).
- Inflammatory/autoimmune:
  - Crohn's disease
  - Behçet's disease (causes orogenital ulcers and ophthalmic inflammation, uncommon in women, HLA-B51 association).

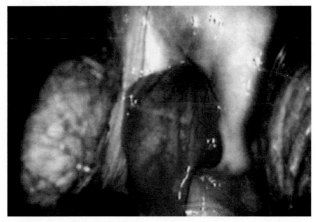

Colour plate 1 Cervical polyp.

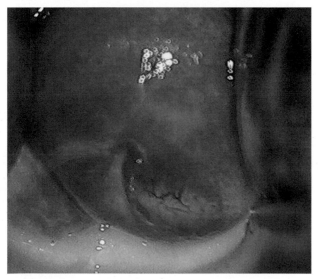

Colour plate 2 Nabothian follicle (note swelling to right of os with normal branching vessels over top).

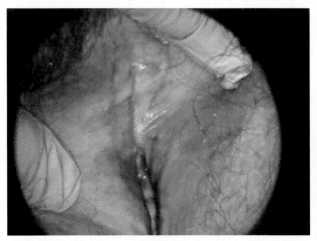

Colour plate 3 Lichen sclerosus (note the labial fusion and leukoplakia).

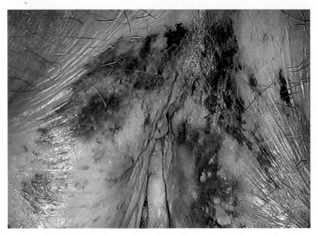

Colour plate 4 Lichen sclerosus (extensive ecchymoses, whitening, and cigarette-paper skin. Raised area concerning for dVIN).

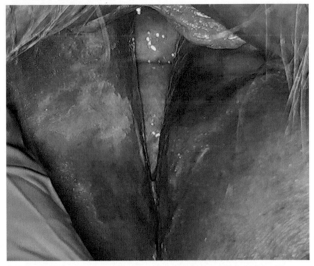

Colour plate 5 Lichen planus—note red erosive areas at introitus with white striations and halos.

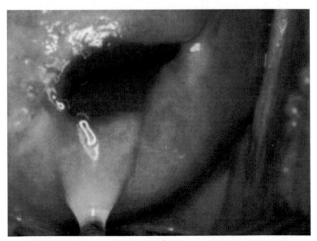

Colour plate 6 Normal cervix (squamocolumnar junction where lighter pink of ectocervix meets darker pink of endocervix).

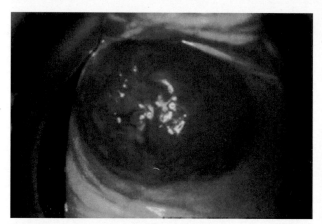

Colour plate 7 Ectropion in a nulliparous woman.

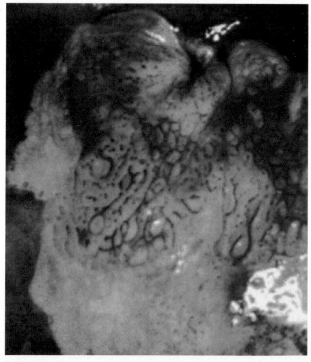

Colour plate 8 Abnormal transformation zone (stained with acetic acid).

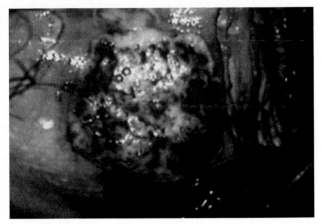

Colour plate 9 Squamous cell carcinoma of the cervix.

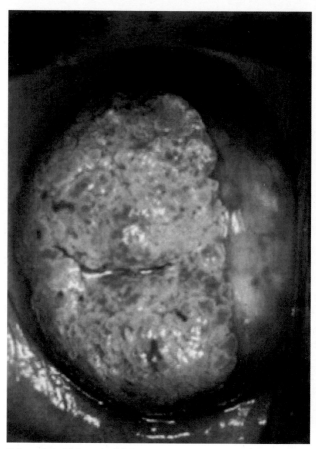

Colour plate 10 Large cervical wart.

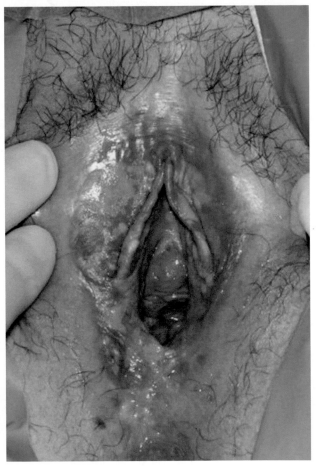

Colour plate 11 Extensive uVIN.

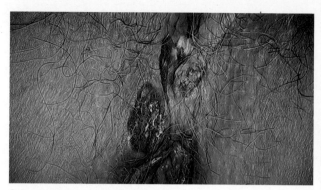

Colour plate 12 Vulval squamous cell carcinoma.

Causes of pruritis vulvae

- Infection:
  - candidiasis
  - threadworms
  - *Phthirus pubis* (genital lice)
  - *Sarcoptes scabiei* (scabies, from Latin 'to itch').
- Vulval dermatoses:
  - lichen sclerosus
  - vulval dermatitis
  - lichen planus
  - vulval psoriasis.
- Systemic conditions:
  - liver failure
  - uraemia.
- Urinary incontinence.
- Medication.
- Pregnancy/menopause.
- Idiopathic.

⚠ VIN or vulval carcinoma.

Further reading

British Association for Sexual Health and HIV (2014). 2014 UK national guideline on the management of vulval conditions.
🔗 https://www.bashh.org/documents/UK%20national%20guideline%20for%20the%20management%20of%20vulval%20conditions%202014.pdf

British Association of Dermatologists
🔗 www.bad.org.uk

Patient (2020). Itchy vulva.
🔗 www.patient.co.uk/health/pruritus-vulvae-vulval-itch

Vulval Pain Society.
🔗 www.vulvalpainsociety.org/

Cancer screening in gynaecology: overview

The intention of screening is early identification of a disease, prompt referral for diagnostic tests, and appropriate intervention and management. Screening does not necessarily diagnose a condition or disease, but may reduce associated incidence, mortality, and morbidity.

WHO principles of screening (1968)

- The condition should be an important public health problem.
- An effective intervention should be available.
- Clear, recognizable early stage and known natural history of condition.
- There should be a suitable screening test available.
- The test should be acceptable to the population.
- Benefits of the test should outweigh the risks.
- There should be an agreed policy on who to treat.
- The total cost of finding a case should be economically balanced.

Sensitivity, specificity, and positive and negative predictive values

- *Sensitivity:* the ability of the screening test to detect the disease—acceptable sensitivity detects most disease.
- *Specificity:* the ability of the screening test not to identify those who do not have the condition—acceptable specificity excludes most without the disease.
- *Positive predictive value (PPV):* the proportion with a +ve test result who have the disease.
- *Negative predictive value (NPV):* the proportion with a −ve test result who do not have the disease.

Ovarian cancer screening

Ovarian carcinoma presents with advanced disease in nearly 75% of cases. A few aetiological factors have been identified.

The main predisposing factors to epithelial cancer of the ovary are:
- Nulliparity.
- Non-use of oral contraceptives (RR 0.40 if used for >36mths).
- Family history (*BRCA* gene mutations and Lynch syndrome).

☛ There is lack of robust evidence for other factors such as age at menarche, menopause, and 1st childbirth.

The most common type, *high-grade serous ovarian carcinoma* (HGSOC), commonly arises from STIC lesions in the fimbriae of fallopian tubes and HGSOCs should be regarded as *tubo-ovarian/primary peritoneal cancers*.

Genetic factors

- If a 1st-degree relative develops ovarian cancer aged <50yrs, the risk ↑ 6–10-fold.
- If ≥2 close relatives were affected, the lifetime risk ↑ to 40%:
  - risk is associated with a mutation of the *BRCA* genes and genes encoding the mismatch repair (MMR) proteins (Lynch syndrome)
  - *BRCA1* is a mutation in chromosome 17 (17q21) and *BRCA2* is a mutation in chromosome 13 (13q12.3)
  - ~15% of women with HGSOC have a germline *BRCA* gene mutation with ~7% having a mutation in the tumour
  - genetic testing (tumour testing with germline testing, if indicated) should be offered as this has treatment implications, as well as implications for other family members.

⚠ Women found to have *BRCA* or MMR gene mutations should be offered referral to a clinical geneticist.

- Cumulative risk of ovarian cancer by the age of 70 is:
  - ~40–60% in *BRCA1*
  - ~10–20% in *BRCA2*
  - 9–12% in Lynch syndrome.
- Women with a family history of ovarian cancers in one 1st-degree relative without a *BRCA* mutation absolute risk remains small (lifetime risk of 5–10% vs ~2% in the general population).

Risk-reducing bilateral salpingo-oophorectomy (RRBSO) should be considered in women who have a strong family history and have completed their family.
- There is a residual risk of peritoneal cancer.
- RRBSO ↑ overall survival of ovarian cancer and ovarian cancer-specific survival in *BRCA* mutation carriers.
- May have small beneficial effect on breast cancer risk.

⚠ Bilateral salpingectomy with delayed oophorectomy may overcome the quality-of-life issues of early menopause in premenopausal women.

▶ Consider salpingectomy whenever performing a hysterectomy.

Ovarian cancer screening

⚠ No routine population screening is currently recommended.

- 202,000 women were recruited into the large UK Collaborative Trial of Ovarian Cancer Screening (UKCTOCS) RCT. Multimodal screening using CA125, a risk of ovarian cancer algorithm, and TV USS has not shown a survival benefit on 1° analysis; long-term results are awaited.
- Results of the Prostate, Lung, Colorectal, Ovarian (PLCO) cancer screening trial did not demonstrate reduced mortality from ovarian cancer; surgery for false +ve screening tests caused harm.
- Screening for those at ↑ familial risk is not recommended by RCOG on the basis of the UK Familial Ovarian Cancer Screening Study (UKFOCSS) RCT.

CA125

- CA125 is a glycoprotein shed by 85% of epithelial tumours.
- Normal levels are 0–35IU/mL.
- False +ves are commonly seen in other malignancies (liver, pancreas), as well as benign disease such as endometriosis, fibroids, PID, lung disease (including pneumonia, TB), other causes of ascites (e.g. heart and liver disease), and early pregnancy.
- *Specificity* is especially low in premenopausal women (50%) presenting with ovarian tumours.
- *Sensitivity* is improved using serial measurements and trends.
- Up to 50% of stage 1 tumours will present with a CA125 level of <35IU/mL.
- Both ultrasound examination and CA125 estimation can give rise to a false +ve result in nearly 2–3% of postmenopausal women. The use of the two tests together ↓ the chance of false +ves.
- NICE recommends measurement of CA125 in 1° care in women with symptoms suggestive of ovarian cancer.

▶ If CA125 ↑ in face of symptoms of bloating and no cause found, consider CT scan of chest/abdo/pelvis ± diagnostic laparoscopy.

Further reading

NICE (2011). Ovarian cancer. Clinical guideline [CG27].
℗ www.nice.org.uk/guidance/cg122/evidence/full-guideline-pdf-181688799

Ovarian Cancer Action. What are genetic mutations?
℗ www.ovarian.org.uk/ovarian-cancer/brca/what-are-genetic-mutations/

RCOG (2014). The distal fallopian tube as the origin of non-uterine pelvic high-grade serous carcinomas. Scientific impact paper no. 44.
℗ www.rcog.org.uk/globalassets/documents/guidelines/scientific-impact-pa-pers/sip44hgscs.pdf

RCOG (2015). Management of women with a genetic predisposition to gynaecological cancers. Scientific impact paper no. 48.
℗ www.rcog.org.uk/globalassets/documents/guidelines/scientific-impact-papers/sip48.pdf

Endometrial cancer screening

General population screening

Evidence does not support screening with USS and endometrial sampling in the general population. Endometrial cancer presents early with aberrant bleeding and, as such, often has a good prognosis.

⚠ Women with PMB should be referred for urgent investigation.

Alternative screening with less invasive tests currently under investigation for effectiveness/cost-effectiveness.

Screening high-risk groups

Tamoxifen

- Tamoxifen has a pro-oestrogenic effect on the endometrium and ↑ the risk of endometrial hyperplasia and malignancy.
- Evidence does not support screening in asymptomatic women on tamoxifen.

⚠ *Investigate symptomatic women with hysteroscopy and TV USS.*

Lynch syndrome

- Endometrial cancer can be the index cancer for MMR protein mutations.
- 3% of endometrial cancer patients have Lynch syndrome which supports the role for universal tumour testing for MMR mutation in endometrial cancer patients.

▶ MMR deficiency testing of tumour with immunohistochemistry (IHC) in those diagnosed with endometrial cancer.

- If loss of MLH1, or loss of MLH1 and PMS2 protein expression, do MLH1 promoter hypermethylation testing of tumour DNA.
- If MLH1 promoter hypermethylation not detected, offer germline genetic testing to confirm Lynch syndrome.
- If IHC is abnormal with loss of MSH2, MSH6, or isolated PMS2 protein expression, offer germline genetic testing to confirm Lynch syndrome.

▶ Annual colonoscopy improves overall survival in Lynch syndrome patients.

▶ Offer risk-reducing hysterectomy BSO to those with Lynch syndrome once finished family (laparoscopic if suitable).

▶ If +ve for Lynch syndrome refer to clinical genetics.

💊 Consider annual endometrial sampling + TV USS from 35yrs if risk reduction surgery declined/deferred although evidence of effectiveness lacking and counsel regarding limitations of screening.

Further reading

British Gynaecological Cancer Society (2021). Uterine cancer guidelines: recommendations for practice.
℘ www.bgcs.org.uk/wp-content/uploads/2019/05/BGCS-Endometrial-Guidelines-2017.pdf

NICE (2020). Testing strategies for Lynch syndrome in people with endometrial cancer. Diagnostics guidance [DG42].
℘ www.nice.org.uk/guidance/dg42

Ryan NAJ et al. (2019). The proportion of endometrial cancers associated with Lynch syndrome: a systematic review of the literature and meta-analysis. *Genet Med.* 21:2167–2180.
℘ www.nature.com/articles/s41436-019-0536-8

Cervical cancer: pathology

- HPV is a DNA virus which is spread by skin-to-skin contact.
- There are >100 subtypes, most of which do not cause significant disease in humans.
- There are 15 *high-risk* oncogenic subtypes of HPV (hrHPV), the most common being 16, 18, 31, 33, 45, 52, and 58.
- Almost everyone will be exposed to hrHPV and ~80% will develop evidence of infection.
- Most people clear HPV infection within 6–18mths.

Persistent cervical infection with hrHPV can lead to development of cervical intraepithelial neoplasia (CIN) or cervical glandular intraepithelial neoplasia (CGIN), the precursor lesions for carcinoma of the cervix

Risk factors for CIN

- Persistent hrHPV infection.
- Multiple partners ↑ risk of exposure to hrHPV infection.
- Smoking as a promoter.
- Immunocompromise, e.g. HIV, immunosuppressive agents.
- Use of the COCP is associated, probably due to non-barrier method and exposure to HPV—if women are satisfied with COCP as their contraceptive method, do not change.

Further reading

Public Health England (2015, updated 2021). Cervical screening: implementation guide for primary HPV screening.

℗ www.gov.uk/guidance/cervical-screening-programme-overview

Cervical cancer: prevention

Role of HPV vaccination

- Persistent hrHPV is necessary for the development of CIN and 99.7% of cervical cancer.
- hrHPV predisposes to cervical, vulval, vaginal, anal, penile, and many head and neck cancers.
- Prophylactic HPV vaccines have been developed targeting HPV 16 and 18 which are responsible for ~70% of cervical cancer:
  - they utilize type-specific virus capsid proteins that self-assemble into virus-like particles (VLPs)
  - vaccines include VLP for either HPV 16 and 18 (bivalent), HPV 6, 11, 16, and 18 (quadrivalent), or HPV 6, 11, 16, 18, 31, 33, 45, 52, and 58 (nonavalent).
- HPV 6 and HPV 11 are not oncogenic, but cause most anogenital warts.

In the UK, the HPV vaccine is part of the NHS childhood vaccination programme and has been routinely offered to girls aged 12 and 13 since 2008 and boys since 2019, in two doses. Vaccination is available up to the age of 25 in women, but requires three injections if commenced after the age of 15. Vaccination is extremely effective in those not previously exposed to hrHPV, hence why vaccination is recommended before the aged of onset of sexual activity (9–13yrs in different populations).

HPV vaccines—what we know

- They reliably induce excellent type-specific antibody titres.
- RCT evidence and cohort data for reliable prevention of CIN and anogenital warts; 89% ↓ (95% CI 81–94%) in prevalence of CIN3 or worse from Scottish data.
- Due to type specificity, they will not prevent all cancers—there are 15 hrHPVs (current vaccines target the common seven strains of hrHPV with evidence of cross-reactivity to other subtypes).
- The long-term antibody response is not yet known, although current data suggest it is likely to be good.
- They need to be widely used in young girls before sexual debut to be most effective—recommended at 12yrs in the UK.
- They offer no protection once infected with HPV.

Further reading

Cochrane (2018). Prophylactic vaccination against human papillomaviruses to prevent cervical cancer and its precursors.
🔗 www.cochranelibrary.com/cdsr/doi/10.1002/14651858.CD009069.pub3/full

NHS (2019). HPV vaccine overview.
🔗 www.nhs.uk/conditions/vaccinations/hpv-human-papillomavirus-vaccine/

Cervical screening

The NHS Cervical Screening Programme (NHSCSP) has been systematic since the 1980s and has since shown a 50% ↓ in mortality from cervical cancer.

▶ Regular cervical screening ↓ the risk of death from cervical cancer by 75%. Screening is based on the natural history of cervical cancer where persistent hrHPV infection precedes development of CIN (dysplasia) and overt malignancy. However, CIN can also regress, although the rate of regression ↓ with severity of CIN.

From 2019, NHSCSP brought in to 1° hrHPV testing:

- Samples are tested for hrHPV and if positive, cytology screening is performed.
- Those found to have cytological abnormalities, or persistent hrHPV without cytological atypia over 2yrs, are referred for colposcopic examination (Fig. 23.1).
- hrHPV testing has improved sensitivity compared to liquid-based cytology.

Systematic review of HPV testing vs liquid-based cytology demonstrated ↑ sensitivity for CIN 2+ (1.18 (95% CI 1.10–1.26)) although at a cost of ↓ specificity (0.96 (95% CI 0.95–0.97)), so results in more women being referred for colposcopy.

Current UK criteria for cervical screening

- Women aged 25–64.
- 3-yearly for women aged 25–50, if normal, 5-yearly till 64.

▶ 3-yearly screening identifies >95% of abnormalities tested by annual screening and is cost-effective.

▶ Scotland and Wales have also delayed screening to 25yrs and Scotland switched to 1° HPV testing in March 2020.

⚠ HIV +ve women need annual screening.

Further reading

Cochrane (2017). Human papillomavirus (HPV) test compared to the Papanicolaou (Pap) test to screen for cervical cancer.
℘ www.cochrane.org/CD008587/GYNAECA_human-papillomavirus-hpv-test-compared-papanicolaou-pap-test-screen-cervical-cancer

NHSCSP (2019). Cervical screening: primary HPV screening implementation.
℘ www.gov.uk/government/publications/cervical-screening-primary-hpv-screening-implementation

Public Health Scotland (2022). Cervical screening.
℘ www.healthscotland.scot/health-topics/screening/cervical-screening/cervical-screening-overview

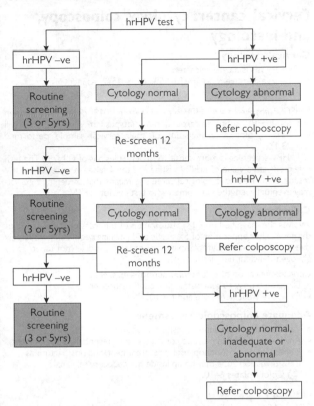

Fig. 23.1 Management of abnormal cervical screening.

Cervical cancer: cytology, colposcopy, and histology

Cervical cytology

- Dyskaryosis is a cytological term.
- False +ve and −ve rates are 10–15% and 5–15%, respectively.
- Abnormal cervical screening is further assessed by colposcopy.

NHSCSP changed to 1° HPV screening from 2019; people who screen −ve for hrHPV subtypes (around ten subtypes are screened for) will not have cytological examination of their cervical sample performed (Fig. 23.1).

1° HPV screening is more sensitive to detect lesions of CIN2+. The high −ve predicative value of hrHPV testing and the ↓ false −ve rates of hrHPV testing compared to cytological screening means that screening intervals may eventually lengthen in women who test −ve for hrHPV.

Colposcopy

Involves the magnified (6–40×) visualization of the transformation zone of the cervix after application of 5% acetic acid (staining neoplastic cells largely due to higher nuclear:cytoplasmic ratio) or Lugol's iodine (not taken up by glycogen-deficient neoplastic cells).

Upon identification of colposcopic abnormalities, either:
- Directed biopsy to gain histological confirmation, *or*
- Definitive treatment ('see and treat').

Adequate colposcopic assessment

- Visualization of the entire transformation zone.
- Any lesion identified must be completely seen (especially upper extent).
- *Problem areas:* postmenopausal, post treatment, and postpartum as transformation zone may be up inside the endocervical canal.
  ➔ Colour plates 6–10.

Histology

CIN is a histological diagnosis and is characterized by loss of differentiation and maturation from the basal layer of the squamous epithelium upwards.
- Bottom 1/3 = CIN 1.
- Bottom 2/3 = CIN 2.
- Full thickness = CIN 3.
- Mitotic figures are present throughout the epithelium in all grades.

Cytological markers seen with abnormal smears

- ↑ nuclear/cytoplasmic ratio.
- Shape of the nucleus (poikilocytosis—abnormal shape).
- Density of the nucleus (koilocytosis—abnormal density).
- Inflammation, infection, and mitoses.

Referral criteria for colposcopy

(See Fig. 23.1.)
- Any cervical screening sample with hrHPV +ve and abnormal cytology.
- Three consecutive cervical screening samples with hrHRV +ve regardless of cytology.
- Three consecutive inadequate cervical screening samples.
- PCB.
- Abnormal-looking cervix.

Colposcopic appearances of CIN

- ➲ Colour plates 6–10.
- Aceto-white epithelium (AWE).
- Iodine-negative.
- Vascular abnormalities, especially mosaic and punctuation.
- Bizarre or grossly abnormal vessels are suggestive of micro-invasive carcinoma.

CIN, VAIN, VIN, and AIN

- The presence of any form of intraepithelial abnormality of the lower genital tract is a marker for a 'field change'.
- The vagina (VAIN), vulva (VIN), and perianal (AIN/PAIN) area are all at risk in the presence of CIN and vice versa.
- When the cervical appearances are normal with abnormal cytology, the abnormal cells may be derived from elsewhere—other potential sites should be examined at colposcopy.

Further reading

Public Health England (2021). Cervical screening: programme and colposcopy management. ℗www.gov.uk/government/publications/cervical-screening-programme-and-colposcopy-management

Marina OC et al. (2012). Effects of acetic acid on light scattering from cells. J Biomed Opt. 17:085002. ℗ www.ncbi.nlm.nih.gov/pmc/articles/PMC3414239/

Management of cervical intraepithelial neoplasia

CIN can be managed conservatively, by excision, by destruction, or rarely by hysterectomy. Management depends upon the grade of CIN and patient preference, but excision is the preferred treatment modality for high-grade CIN (CIN 2–3). This is usually by LLETZ.

Low-grade CIN (CIN 1)

- Spontaneously regress in at least 50–60% of cases within 2yrs.
- Malignant potential is very low but still up to 10× greater than women with normal cytology.
- Management options are:
  - conservative monitoring with repeat hrHPV test after 12mths
  - LLETZ if persistent low-grade CIN.

High-grade CIN (CIN 2+)

- Progress to cancer in up to 3–5% (CIN 2) and 20–30% (CIN 3) within 10yrs.
- Spontaneous regression occurs less often.
- LLETZ recommended.
- Consider conservative management for women <30yrs with CIN 2 who are prepared to attend colposcopy clinic every 6mths for 24mths:
  - regression rates up to 60%
  - if progress, or woman wants treatment at any point in 24mths or sustained high-grade CIN at 24mths, recommend LLETZ.
- Requires colposcopy MDT review.

Follow-up and management after LLETZ for CIN

- If margins involved with CIN 2+ no further excision required if:
  - no evidence of glandular abnormality and
  - no evidence of invasive disease and
  - <50yrs of age.
- Otherwise offer repeat LLETZ or hysterectomy.
- *Follow-up for CIN:* hrHPV test-of-cure 6mths post LLETZ:
  - if –ve, repeat cervical screening in 3yrs
  - if +ve for hrHPV, refer to colposcopy.

Benefits of LLETZ

- Easy and safe.
- Usually possible with local anaesthetic.
- Tissue available for histology and assessment of excision margins.

Complications of LLETZ

Short term

- Haemorrhage.
- Infection (and 2° haemorrhage typically day 7–10 post LLETZ)
- Vaso-vagal reaction.
- Anxiety (disproportionately high in colposcopy clinic attenders).

Long term

- Cervical stenosis (dysmenorrhoea and/or difficulty in follow-up).
- Cervical weakness leading to:
  - 2nd-trimester miscarriage
  - pre-term delivery

💣 Evidence suggests absolute risk of adverse effect on neonatal outcome is very low compared to potential benefit.

Further reading

Cochrane (2017). Obstetric outcomes after conservative treatment for cervical intraepithelial lesions and early invasive disease.
🔗 www.cochranelibrary.com/cdsr/doi/10.1002/14651858.CD012847/

Public Health England (2016). Cervical screening: colposcopy and programme management.
🔗 https://assets.publishing.service.gov.uk/government/uploads/system/uploads/attachment_d
ata/file/856972/Screening_and_colposcopy_pathways.pdf

Public Health England (2021). Cervical screening: programme and colposcopy management.
🔗www.gov.uk/government/publications/cervical-screening-programme-and-colposcopy-man
agement

Management of cervical glandular intraepithelial neoplasia

Dysplasia originating primarily in the glandular epithelium is known as CGIN. It is divided into low and high grade: the latter is a full-thickness abnormality. It can coexist with CIN or stand alone and is associated with hrHPV, especially HPV 18. It poses difficulties in management because:

- The endocervical epithelium extends beyond view of the colposcope into the endocervical canal (up to 10% of CGIN lesions will have higher 'skip' lesions).
- The natural history is less well understood than squamous CIN.
- No specific colposcopic appearances, unlike CIN.
- Follow-up is difficult; may be recommended hysterectomy.
- Incidence of adenocarcinoma has ↑ compared to squamous cell carcinoma, as the screening programme is more effective at detecting squamous lesions.

Management of CGIN

- All glandular cytological abnormalities should be referred for colposcopy.
- Colposcopy ± endometrial sampling may need to be performed.
- Endocervical curettage has a very low yield and is no longer recommended.

▶ A cylindrical-shaped LLETZ or cone with deep 'top hat' is recommended, even if colposcopy is not obviously abnormal for those with cervical screening suggestive of high-grade glandular changes.

▶ Margins should be clear of CGIN and a 2nd LLETZ/hysterectomy should be recommended if margins are not clear.

⚠ Hysterectomy may be required after completion of family or if colposcopic assessment is inadequate with repeated cytological abnormality.

Follow-up after LLETZ for CGIN

- Follow-up hrHPV test-of-cure 6mths post LLETZ:
  - if −ve, a 2nd test-of-cure sample is taken 12mths later (i.e. 18mths after LLETZ)
  - if this is also −ve for hrHPV, the woman can be discharged to recall in 3yrs
  - refer to colposcopy if any test is +ve for hrHPV.

Further reading

Public Health England (2016). Cervical screening: colposcopy and programme management. ℘ https://assets.publishing.service.gov.uk/government/uploads/system/uploads/attachment_data/file/856972/Screening_and_colposcopy_pathways.pdf

Public Health England (2021). Cervical screening: programme and colposcopy management. ℘www.gov.uk/government/publications/cervical-screening-programme-and-colposcopy-management

Gynaecological cancer:
a multidisciplinary approach

Optimal treatment of the gynaecological cancer patient is provided by co-ordination of care within a MDT made up of doctors, nurses, and allied professionals with an interest in treating gynaecological cancer patients (Box 23.3).

Role of the MDT

- Diagnosis, staging, 1° surgical, and adjuvant treatment, and coordination of follow-up care.
- Psychological preparation for anticancer treatment and follow-up:
  - psychosexual support is a vital aspect, since many of the treatments can have major impacts on sexual functioning, either physically and/ or psychologically.
- Information on diagnosis, treatment plans, likely side effects, and follow-up plans.
- Access to financial, social, and psychological support:
  - often required as patients may be young and have either young or older dependants, for whom they may be either the financial provider or 1° carer.
- Advice on future fertility and treatments available.
- Aiding rehabilitation and preventing complications, e.g. provision of vaginal dilators following pelvic radiotherapy.
- Support with issues of survivorship.
- Appropriate and timely transition from active care to palliative care.
- Recruitment to clinical trials.
- Training of junior doctors and nurses.
- Audit of practice.

Cancer nurse specialist

Often the central point of contact for the patient and ideally is trained to fulfil a supportive, advisory, advocacy role, in addition to being experienced in caring for women with complex medical issues and treatments.

Provision of appropriate care within an MDT has been shown to not only improve outcomes in terms of life expectancy and cure rates, but also benefit patients' functional, cosmetic, and psychological well-being.

Further reading

National Cancer Guidance Steering Group, Department of Health (1999). *Improving Outcomes in Gynaecological Cancers—Guidance for Commissioners: The Manual*. London: NHS Executive.

NHS England (2013). Service specification for gynaecological cancers.
℘ www.england.nhs.uk/commissioning/wp-content/uploads/sites/12/2014/04/e10-cancer-gynae-0414.pdf

Box 23.3 Gynaecological cancer MDT

- This should, at a minimum, consist of:
  - two gynaecological oncologists (surgeons)
  - clinical oncologist
  - medical oncologist
  - radiologist
  - histopathologist
  - colposcopist
  - gynaecological cancer nurse specialist
  - MDT coordinator.
- Ideally, because of the complex nature of gynaecological cancer patients, their treatments, and the complications they may encounter, teams should also include or have ready access to:
  - palliative care team
  - dietician; fertility specialist
  - lymphoedema specialist
  - lower gastrointestinal surgeon
  - urological surgeon
  - stoma therapy nurse
  - psychologist
  - psychosexual counsellor.

Sources of information for patients

Excellent patient advice and information leaflets are available from:
- Macmillan Cancer Support: ℅ www.macmillan.org.uk
- Cancer Research UK: ℅ www.cancerresearchuk.org
- Ovacome, an ovarian cancer support network: ℅ www.ovacome. org.uk
- Ovarian Cancer Action: ℅ www.ovarian.org.uk
- Jo's Cervical Cancer Trust: ℅ www.jostrust.org.uk/

Cervical cancer: aetiology and presentation

4th most common cancer in women worldwide with ~570,000 new cancers in 2018 and 311,00 deaths. 2nd most common cancer in women in low- and middle-income countries. Mortality declined in the UK due to the NHSCSP, introduced in the 1980s (from ~4000 to 850 deaths/yr by 2015–2017) (➲ Cancer screening in gynaecology: overview, p. 796).

14th most common cancer in UK ~3200/yr—24% ↓ in incidence since 1990 (although 4% ↑ over past decade due to ↓ screening uptake). There are dual peaks in incidence (25–29yr age group and over 70s). NHSCSP has changed the spectrum of disease: ↑ proportion of microscopic disease and adenocarcinomas, especially in younger women.

Aetiology

99.7% of cervical cancer is associated with persistent infection with hrHPV subtypes (~70% from HPV 16 and 18). The natural history is well known; untreated high-grade CIN leads to cervical cancer in 20–30% of women over 10yrs.

Risk factors for cervical cancer

- Exposure to hrHPV:
  - early 1st sexual experience
  - multiple partners
  - non-barrier contraceptive.
- COCP and high parity—possibly a direct hormonal effect, but difficult to show independent role from indirect effect of sexual behaviour—if women are satisfied with COCP as their contraceptive method, do not change.
- *Smoking*: strong dose/response effect—↓ viral clearance.
- *Immunosuppression*: HIV and transplant patients especially.

Presentation

- Cervical screening demonstrating ?invasion.
- Incidental at treatment for pre-invasive disease (CIN).
- PCB.
- PMB (~1% of women with PMB).
- Rarer presentations (often suggestive of advanced disease):
  - heavy bleeding PV
  - ureteric obstruction
  - weight loss
  - bowel disturbance
  - fistula (vesico-vaginal most common)
  - lymphoedema (of one or both legs).

⚠ Cervical screening can be false −ve if cervical cancer is present.

▶▶ If suspect cancer clinically, refer for colposcopy and biopsy.

Histology of cervical cancers

- Squamous cell carcinoma (67%):
  - more common in early stage screen-detected cancers.
- Adenocarcinoma (20%)
- Adenosquamous (2.3%)
- Undifferentiated (0.2%):
  - more common in those with advanced disease at presentation.
- Neuroendocrine tumour (<1%):
  - originates from argyrophil cells in the cervix
  - may present with carcinoid syndrome (very rare)
  - median survival <2yrs.
- Clear cell carcinoma (<1%):
  - <25yrs 2° to DES exposure *in utero* (not now given)
  - >45yrs not associated with DES
  - treat as per adenocarcinoma, but prognosis worse.
- Glassy cell carcinoma (<<1%):
  - median age 35yrs
  - presents with bleeding—often normal smear history
  - similar prognosis to adenocarcinoma.
- Sarcoma botryoides of the cervix (<<1%):
  - type of embryonal rhabdomyosarcoma
  - median age ~14yrs (range 5mths–45yrs)
  - local excision (conservative surgery if possible)
  - ± chemotherapy.
- Lymphoma of cervix (0.06%):
  - no need for surgical excision
  - responds well to combination chemotherapy.

Further reading

Bray F et al. (2018). Global cancer statistics 2018: GLOBOCAN estimates of incidence and mortality worldwide for 36 cancers in 185 countries. *CA Cancer J Clin.* 68:394–424.
🔗 https://acsjournals.onlinelibrary.wiley.com/doi/epdf/10.3322/caac.21492

British Gynaecological Cancer Society. Guidelines and recent publications.
🔗 www.bgcs.org.uk/professionals/guidelines-for-recent-publications/

Cancer Research UK. Cervical cancer statistics.
🔗 www.cancerresearchuk.org/health-professional/cancer-statistics/statistics-by-cancer-type/cervical-cancer

NHSCSP (2019). Audit report.
🔗 www.gov.uk/government/publications/cervical-screening-invasive-cervical-cancer-audit-2013-to-2016/audit-report

Cervical cancer: diagnosis

History

- Asymptomatic, detected via screening programme (~1 in 6 in UK often at early stage).
- PCB.
- Abnormal menstruation (heavy and/or irregular periods).
- PMB.
- PV discharge.
- Risk factors (smoking, previous CIN, known HPV or HIV infection, vaccination status, and age at vaccination).
- Parity.
- Fertility wishes.

Examination

- *Vaginal and bimanual examination:* roughened hard cervix, ± loss of fornices and fixed cervix, if there is local extension of disease.
- *Colposcopy:* irregular cervical surface, abnormal vessels, dense aceto-white changes.

△ Pelvic USS does not exclude cervical cancer (or endometrial cancer in premenopausal women) and can give false reassurance to doctor and patient.

▶ Clinical examination required to visualize cervix.

Histology

If visible cancer, take multiple punch biopsies or small diagnostic loop biopsy at colposcopy.

▶ May only be diagnosed on histology after LLETZ if not suspected clinically.

△ Can bleed ++ at LLETZ and if clinically obvious cancer, likely to need more extensive treatment so recommend diagnostic biopsies.

Further investigations, if cancer confirmed on biopsy >stage Ia1

- U&E, LFTs, FBC.
- CT chest and abdomen (staging and preoperative assessment).
- MRI pelvis (can be very accurate at staging and examining for suspicious LNs) (Table 23.3).
- EUA:
  - bimanual vaginal examination, cystoscopy, hysteroscopy, and PV/PR examination ± sigmoidoscopy
  - less often performed now as MRI is good and many tumours are microscopic, but it still has an important role when considering surgery: MRI may have false +ve and −ve for vaginal extension
  - can insert fiducial markers (small gold beads) at clinical extent of tumour in advanced disease to aid radiotherapy planning.

Table 23.3 2019 Revised FIGO staging of cervical cancer

Stage		Extent of disease
0		Cervical Intraepithelial neoplasia (CIN)
I		Limited to cervix
IA		Microscopic disease
	IA1	Microscopic disease: invasion ≤3mm
	IA2	Microscopic disease: invasion >3mm and ≤5mm
IB		Invasive carcinoma with measured deepest invasion >5mm (greater than stage IA). Lesion limited to cervix uteri
	IB1	≥5mm depth of stromal invasion and <2cm in dimension
	IB2	≥2cm and <4cm in greatest dimension
	IB3	≥4cm in greatest dimension
II		Extended beyond the uterus, but not onto lower 1/3 of vagina or into pelvic side war
IIA		Involvement of the upper 2/3 of vagina, but no parametrial involvement
	IIA1	Involvement of upper 2/3 of vagina <4cm in diameter
	IIA2	Involvement of upper 2/3 of vagina ≥4cm in diameter
IIB		Parametrial involvement but not into pelvic sidewall
III		Involvement of lower 1/3 of vagina or extends to pelvic side-wall or causes hydronephrotic kidney or lymph nodes
IIIA		Lower 1/3 vagina involved
IIIB		Extension of pelvic sidewall (includes all cases with hydronephrosis)
IIIC		Involvement of pelvic and/or paraaortic lymph nodes, irrespective of tumour size and extent
	IIIC1	Pelvic lymph node metastasis only
	IIIC2	Paraaortic lymph node metastasis
IV		Extension beyond true pelvis or involvement of bladder/bowel mucosa
	IVA	Extension to adjacent organs
	IVB	Distant metastases

Reprinted from Bhatla N. et al. (2019), Revised FIG staging for carcinoma of the cervix uteri. *Int J Gynecol Obstet*, 145: 129–135. doi:10.1002/ijgo.12749, with permission from Wiley.

Cervical cancer: treatment

- Management depends on stage and age.
- Age is not an independent adverse prognostic factor, but is associated with ↑ stage at presentation.
- Early-stage cervical cancers (up to IB2) usually managed surgically, options ranging from a LLETZ to a radical hysterectomy dependent upon FIGO stage (Table 23.3).
- RCTs show that for IB1–2 disease Wertheim's hysterectomy and radiotherapy have equivalent survival.
- If +ve LN on histology, patient will need radiotherapy as well, which ↑ morbidity and mortality, if both treatments required.
- SHAPE RCT—simple hysterectomy vs radical hysterectomy for stage IA2–IB1 cervical cancer—results awaited.

Surgery for recurrent cervical cancer confined to pelvis often involves removal of other structures of the pelvis (anterior, posterior, or total exenteration).

Role of minimal access surgery

⚕ Minimal access surgical techniques (laparoscopic and robotic) have been used in cervical cancer treatment.

⚠ An RCT showed ↓ progression-free survival and ↓ overall survival after minimal access radical hysterectomy compared to open radical hysterectomy—English and US observational data support this.
▶ Caution is advised if considering use of minimal access techniques.

Fertility-sparing surgery

In young women, fertility-sparing surgery (e.g. radical trachelectomy) is an option for early-stage disease (stage IA2 and early stage IB1) if LNs are proven to be –ve following lymphadenectomy.

This is a vaginal or abdominal/minimal access surgery procedure involving the removal of cervix and paracervical tissue, to the level of the internal os, with the introduction of a cerclage suture at the level of the internal os in preparation for subsequent pregnancy.

- Recurrence rates may be higher than open radical hysterectomy.
- Successful pregnancies can be achieved, although ↑ risk of late miscarriage, PPROM, and preterm delivery.
- Fertility rate 55%, live birth rate 70%, and prematurity rate 38% are reported in a systematic review with 2777 participants.
- CD is the required mode of delivery due to the intra-abdominal suture.

Survival

- Survival dependent upon stage and age at diagnosis.
- Overall survival ~66%.
  - stage I: 95% 5yr survival
  - stage II: ~50% 5yr survival
  - stage III: ~40% 5yr survival
  - stage IV: ~5% 5yr survival.

Treatment options for cervical cancer by 2018 FIGO stage

- Stage IA1:
  - local excision or hysterectomy (risk of +ve LN <1%).
- Stage IA2 and IB2:
  - lymphadenectomy + Wertheim's hysterectomy if −ve LN (~5% +ve LN)
  - consider radical trachelectomy.
- Stage IB3 and early IIA:
  - chemoradiotherapy
  - consider lymphadenectomy and Wertheim's hysterectomy in very selected LN −ve cases (PET-CT prior to surgery).
- >Stage IB3:
  - radical chemoradiotherapy.
- Stage IVB:
  - ?chemotherapy and pelvic radiotherapy, if response
  - ?best supportive care ± palliative radiotherapy for symptoms.

Complications of treatment

- Radical (Wertheim's) hysterectomy and lymphadenectomy:
  - bleeding
  - infection
  - DVT/PE
  - vaginal shortening
  - ureteric fistula
  - bladder dysfunction
  - pelvic pain
  - lymphoedema
  - lymphocysts.
- Radiotherapy:
  - acute bowel and bladder dysfunction (tenesmus, mucositis, bleeding)
  - 5% late bowel and bladder dysfunction (ulceration, strictures, bleeding, fistula formation)
  - vaginal stenosis, shortening and dryness.
  - lymphoedema.

Sentinel lymph node biopsy

Sentinel lymph node biopsy (SLNB) in cervical cancer

- Pelvic lymphadenectomy ± pelvic radiotherapy is associated with long-term lymphoedema:
  - significant lymphoedema ~21% following surgery
  - 78% if both surgery and radiotherapy.
- Sentinel lymph node (SLN) algorithms for staging of cervical cancer have high NPV.
- Safety of SLNB for cervical cancer not proven in long-term RCT.
- If considering SLNB, limit to those with tumour size <2cm and recruit to registered clinical trial:
  - >2cm higher false −ve rate.
- Cervical injection of combination of technetium (Tc)-99m colloid with blue dye or near-infrared fluorescence with indocyanine green (ICG) dye have emerged as better than blue dye alone in the detection of SLN in cervical cancer:
  - limited data on ICG alone at present.
- If fail to find SLN—proceed to hemi-pelvic lymphadenectomy on that side.
- Need ultra-staging and IHC protocol for SLN—frozen section not accurate.
- Can consider for those with FIGO stage IA1 and lymphovascular space invasion—use of SLN algorithms can be considered for surgical staging.

Further reading

British Gynaecological Cancer Society. BGCS guidelines.
🔗 www.bgcs.org.uk/professionals/guidelines-for-recent-publications/

British Gynaecological Cancer Society (2019). BGCS position statement on laparoscopic radical hysterectomy for cervical cancer.
🔗 www.bgcs.org.uk/wp-content/uploads/2019/07/NCRAS-mas-v-open-radical-hysterectomy-BGCS-professionals-statement-May-2019-1.pdf

British Gynaecological Cancer Society (2019). Sentinel consensus document for vulval, endometrial and cervical cancer.
🔗 www.bgcs.org.uk/wp-content/uploads/2020/01/BGCS-Sentinel-Consensus-Document-7.5.-2019.pdf

Ovarian cancer: aetiology

Ovarian cancer is the leading cause of death from gynaecological malignancy in the UK, with around 7500 new cases/yr (2014–2016) and 4116 deaths in 2017. 8th most common cancer in women globally, ~300,000 new cases in 2018.

The ovary is a collection of several different cell types, each of which can have neoplastic development. However, 90% are epithelial ovarian cancers thought to arise from the surface layer of the ovary/fimbrial end of the fallopian tube. Peak incidence of ovarian cancer is in women aged 75–84yrs.

Aetiology

Different aetiologies are proposed for the known subtypes. There is now compelling evidence that many of the host common type—HGSOCs—originate from the epithelium of the distal fimbrial portion of the fallopian tube.

Risk factors

- ↑ risk if multiple ovulations and ↓ risk if ovulation suppressed:
  - nulliparity ↑ risk
  - early menarche and/or late menopause ↑ risk
  - COCP ↓ risk (RR 0.5)
  - pregnancy ↓ risk.
  - tubal ligation ↓ risk
  - talcum powder (applied at genital area) ↑ risk.

BRCA mutations
(→ Ovarian cancer screening, p. 798.)
- ~10% of HGSOC associated with *BRCA* mutation.
- Patients with HGSOC should be offered tumour testing for *BRCA* mutations and referred for germline testing, as indicated.
- *BRCA1* and *BRCA2* gene products involved in repair of DNA.
- Mutations lead to ↑ risk of ovarian and breast cancer.
- Cumulative risk of ovarian cancer by the age of 70 is ~40–60% with *BRCA1* mutations; ~10–20% with *BRCA2* mutations (Table 23.4).

Lynch syndrome
Identified in families with strong history of colorectal, uterine, and ovarian cancer.
- Rarer than *BRCA1* and *BRCA2* mutations.
- Lifetime risk of ovarian cancer 9–12% in Lynch syndrome.
- If prophylactic surgery for Lynch syndrome, recommend hysterectomy in addition to BSO once finished having children.

Screening of genetically high-risk individuals
- Need a blood sample from a consenting affected relative (often a problem as may have died).
- Mutations may occur anywhere within the *BRCA1* and *BRCA2* genes, so the entire sequence should be screened.
- Even if a deletion is not found, the patient is still at moderately high risk.

Table 23.4 Ovarian cancer risk for *BRCA1* and *BRCA2*

Cumulative risk by age	BRCA1	BRCA2
30	0%	0%
40	3%	2%
50	21%	2%
60	40%	6%
70	46%	12%

Source: data from King MC, Marks JH, Mandell JB, et al. (2003). Breast and ovarian cancer risks due to inherited mutations in BRCA1 and BRCA2. *Science* 302(5645): 643–646.

Clinical genetics counselling

Refer for if:
- Two 1° cancers (breast and/or ovary) in one 1st- or 2nd-degree relative, at any age.
- Three 1st- and 2nd-degree relatives with any of the following cancers at any age:
  - breast
  - ovary
  - colorectal
  - stomach
  - endometrial.
- Two 1st- or 2nd-degree relatives, one with ovarian cancer at any age, *and one* with breast cancer <50yrs.
- Two 1st- or 2nd-degree relatives with ovarian cancer at any age.

Further reading

Ovarian Cancer Action. What are genetic mutations?
℘ https://ovarian.org.uk/ovarian-cancer/brca/what-are-genetic-mutations/

RCOG (2014). The distal fallopian tube as the origin of non-uterine pelvic high-grade serous carcinomas. Scientific impact paper no. 44.
℘ www.rcog.org.uk/globalassets/documents/guidelines/scientific-impact-pa-pers/sip44hgscs.pdf

Management of *BRCA* mutation

General lifestyle

- Advice to ↓ risk of cancer:
  - smoking cessation
  - maintain a normal BMI.

COCP

- Or alternate contraceptive method that prevents ovulation, e.g. long-acting progesterone implant.

Surveillance

- Repeated CA125 and TV USS (➔ Ovarian cancer screening, p. 798).
- UKFOCSS showed 4-monthly screening with the risk of ovarian cancer algorithm may be an option for these high-risk women until they decide to undergo surgery.

Prophylactic surgery

- RRBSO.
- Evidence that many tumours actually arise from the *fallopian tubes*, so as much tube as possible must be removed.
- Counsel regarding risk of finding occult tumour at surgery.
- Screen with CA125 and USS within 2mths prior to surgery:
  - if evidence of cancer, a full staging laparotomy is required, not laparoscopic BSO.
- Can develop 1° peritoneal cancer, so cancer risk not ↓ to zero.
- ↓ Breast cancer risk following oophorectomy if premenopausal (even with combined HRT).
- Theoretically ↓ risk of breast cancer further if oestrogen-only HRT but need hysterectomy.

Hysterectomy

- Only recommended if required for other reasons (fibroids, menorrhagia, etc.).

Further reading

RCOG (2015). Management of Women with a Genetic Predisposition to Gynaecological Cancers. Scientific impact paper no. 48.
🖰www.rcog.org.uk/globalassets/documents/guidelines/scientific-impact-papers/sip48.pdf
The Eve Appeal. UKFOCSS
🖰 https://eveappeal.org.uk/our-research/our-research-programmes/ukfocss/

Ovarian cancer: presentation and investigation

Presentation

Women present with a range of vague, common symptoms, which may be misinterpreted as other conditions, e.g. irritable bowel syndrome, diverticular disease, or 'middle-aged spread'.

- ~50% of women will present to a specialty other than gynaecology.
- 75% of women will present once disease has spread to the abdomen (FIGO stage III, see Table 23.5).
- *Common symptoms:* abdominal distension (often described as bloating, but persistent); ↑ girth; urinary symptoms; change in bowel habit; abnormal vaginal bleeding; detection of pelvic mass; early satiety.

Investigation

History

Symptoms; risk factors; comorbidities; family history (if strong, consider referral for genetic screening).

Clinical examination

Pelvic/abdominal mass (fixed/mobile); ascites; omental mass (common site for metastasis, may involve whole omentum—'omental cake'); pleural effusion; supraclavicular LNs.

Haematological tests

- FBC, U&E, LFTs—especially albumin due to ascites.

Tumour markers

- *CA125:* ↑ in 80% of epithelial cancers:
  - RMI useful for identifying patients at high risk of cancer and who should be referred to a cancer centre for treatment (sensitivity 87%, PPV 87% in recent series) (➲ Benign ovarian tumours: imaging, p. 784).
  - NICE guidelines suggest performing CA125 in women with symptoms suggestive of ovarian cancer.
- *Carcinoembryonic antigen (CEA):* raised in colorectal cancers and mucinous ovarian cancer.
- *CA19.9:* may be raised in mucinous or endometrioid tumours, which are more likely to have normal CA125 (also raised in pancreatic and breast cancer).
- *Inhibin:* if granulosa cell tumour suspected.
- Tumour markers for rarer ovarian tumours if <40yrs 'juvenile markers': AFP, hCG, LDH.

Imaging

- Abdominal/pelvic USS: presence of pelvic mass and ascites (NICE guidelines if CA125 raised).
- CT chest/abdomen/pelvis (CAP) if RMI >250: omental cake, peritoneal implants, liver or splenic metastases, and pelvic/para-aortic LN.

Management of ascites and pleural effusion

Diagnosis

- Ascitic or pleural fluid should be sampled and sent for:
  - cytology
  - microbiology
  - biochemistry (U&E).

▶ Send as much fluid as possible as it may be relatively acellular.

- If planning neoadjuvant chemotherapy (NAC), histological diagnosis is needed:
  - image-guided percutaneous biopsy (may need to drain ascites before biopsy)
  - diagnostic laparoscopy.

▶ If patient very poor WHO performance status and biopsy not feasible, CT CAP, cytology, and CA125/CEA ratio may be adequate.

Symptom control

- Drainage of massive tense ascites or a pleural effusion preoperatively.
- For ascitic drainage use a pig-tail drain, aseptic technique with local anaesthesia into skin and through abdominal wall.

⚠ USS guidance recommended—risk of bowel damage.

▶ Albumin may ↓ precipitously following ascitic drainage due to 3rd spacing. Suggest dietitian referral and use of high-protein supplements to avoid problems with hypoalbuminaemia and severe generalized oedema. Albumin infusion not recommended.

Ovarian cancer: treatment

Surgery

- Current standard care for a high RMI is a staging laparotomy performed through a midline incision.
- Should be at a cancer centre by a gynaecological oncologist—↑ prognosis.
- Laparotomy should aim to remove as much tumour as possible, ideally leaving no macroscopic tumour.
- Achievement of macroscopic debulking (no residual disease visible to naked eye) is a +ve prognostic factor.
- Full staging in stage Ia cancers affects whether adjuvant chemotherapy is required.

▶ Women with advanced ovarian cancer (bulky stage IIIc or IV) may benefit from NAC before interval debulking surgery (IDS) after 3 cycles, followed by an additional 3 cycles postoperatively. Survival rates are similar, with reduced morbidity in the NAC group.

IDS (after 3 cycles of chemotherapy), may benefit those where debulking not attempted at 1° surgery.

✸ Ultra-radical surgery (diaphragmatic resection, peritoneal stripping, liver resection, splenectomy, ± bowel resection etc.) has a role in those fit enough to consider it.

Surgical staging laparotomy for tubo-ovarian cancer
- Hysterectomy.
- BSO.
- Omentectomy.
- LN sampling (pelvic and para-aortic) if no obvious extra-ovarian disease, otherwise debulk bulky nodes only.
- Peritoneal biopsies.
- Pelvic washings/ascitic sampling.
- Debulking tumour deposits with attempt at macroscopic debulk.

Pseudomyxoma peritonei

Mucinous cystadenocarcinomas may present with a thick, jelly-like ascites with tumour deposits throughout the abdominal cavity. Frequently these may arise from a 1° tumour of the appendix and an appendicectomy is recommended as part of limited debulking surgery for diagnosis.

⚠ Specialist centres exist in the UK. Optimal treatment requires extensive abdominal surgery (Sugarbaker technique) and heated intraperitoneal chemotherapy. Diagnosis should be made before surgery and patients referred for 1° surgery at a specialist centre. If found intraoperatively, the main masses should be removed (including ovaries and appendix) and the abdomen thoroughly washed out to remove as much jelly-like material as possible. More extensive 1° surgery can limit ability of specialist centre to perform radical debulking and should be avoided.

Table 23.5 FIGO staging of ovarian/fallopian tube cancer (2018)

Stage			Extent of disease	5yr survival
I			Limited to ovaries (negative washings)	75–90%
	IA		One ovary or fallopian tube	
	IB		Both ovaries or fallopian tubes	
	IC		One or both ovaries	
		IC1	Surgical spill	
		IC2	Ruptured capsule, tumours on ovarian or fallopian tube surface	
		IC3	+ve peritoneal washings/ascites	
II			Pelvic extension	45–60%
	IIA		Extension/implants on uterus	
	IIB		Extension/implants on other pelvic structures	
III			Extends beyond pelvic brim limited to abdomen (including retroperitoneal regional LN metastases)	30–40%
	IIIA		+ve retroperitoneal LN only	
		IIIA1	IIIA1i <10mm	
			IIIA1ii >10mm	
		IIIA2	Microscopic metastases	
	IIIB		Macroscopic metastases <2cm	
	IIIC		Macroscopic metastases >2cm	
IV			Distant metastases outside abdominal cavity	<20%
	IVA		Pleural effusion with +ve cytology	
	IVB		Metastasis to liver, spleen, inguinal LNs, and extra-abdominal organs	

Source: data from J. S., Kehoe, S. T., Kumar, L. and Friedlander, M. (2018), Cancer of the ovary, fallopian tube, and peritoneum. *Int J Gynecol Obstet*. 143:59–78. doi:10.1002/ijgo.12614

Ovarian cancer: chemotherapy and follow-up

Adjuvant chemotherapy

Adjuvant chemotherapy is recommended for all patients other than those with low-risk early-stage disease (stage IA–B low-grade disease).

- For advanced disease (≥stage II) platinum agents are superior and carboplatin ≈ cisplatin in terms of prognosis, but has ↓ side effects.
- 6 cycles of carboplatin ± paclitaxel every 3wks.
- Patients with bulky stage IIIc/IV may benefit from NAC prior to IDS (3 cycles chemo, IDS, 3 cycles chemo).
- Paclitaxel is standard of care for women with adequate performance status as it gives small additional survival benefit, however it:
  - uniformly causes alopecia
  - ↑ side effects caused by platinum agents.

💉 Intraperitoneal chemotherapy may improve survival (improved regional pharmacokinetics), although has ↑ side effects (many related to the intraperitoneal catheter or ↑ absolute dose of chemotherapy with intraperitoneal)—should only be used as part of a clinical trial.

> ### Investigations before starting chemotherapy
>
> - Baseline CT scan (to assess response).
> - Assess renal function (to determine platinum agent dosing):
>   - creatinine clearance, *or*
>   - isotope EGFR.
> - Histological diagnosis.

Follow-up

- Patients are monitored using clinical examination ± tumour markers (if previously raised):
  - every 3mths for 1st yr
  - every 4mths for 2nd yr
  - if no recurrence, every 6mths for up to 5yrs.

💉 No evidence of benefit from monitoring CA125 in asymptomatic women during follow-up but the evidence pre-dates 2° debulking surgery and poly-ADP ribose polymerase inhibitor (PARPi) studies (➲ Classes of chemotherapy agents, p. 870).

▶ PARPi maintenance treatment is used for recurrence after response to chemotherapy of platinum-sensitive, BRCA-mutated ovarian cancer.

⚠ Biological agents for 1°, relapsed disease and maintenance include agents targeted against vascular endothelial growth factor (VEGF; e.g. bevacizumab) ↑ risk bowel fistula.

Further reading

NICE (2020). Olaparib for maintenance treatment of relapsed platinum-sensitive ovarian, fallopian tube or peritoneal cancer. Technology appraisal guidance [TA620]
🔗 https://www.nice.org.uk/guidance/ta620

NICE (2022). Niraparib for maintenance treatment of relapsed, platinum-sensitive ovarian, fallopian tube and peritoneal cancer. Technology appraisal guidance [TA784].
🔗https://www.nice.org.uk/guidance/ta784

Rare ovarian tumours: germ cell

See Table 23.6.

Germ cell tumours account for <5% of ovarian tumours. Can arise anywhere down tract of embryological genital ridge, along which primordial germ cells migrate from yolk sac, although most occur in the ovaries. Degree of differentiation of primordial germ cell affects type of cancer produced: undifferentiated germ cells cause dysgerminomas; cells that have undergone initial differentiation can undergo embryonal or extra-embryonal differentiation, to produce choriocarcinoma/endodermal sinus tumours (yolk sac) or teratomas, respectively. Germ cell tumours most commonly occur in young women and account for 70% of ovarian tumours in the under 20s, when ~30% of these are malignant.

Dermoid cyst

Common benign ovarian tumour, often bilateral (10%), and commonly contain sebaceous material; sometimes hair and teeth.

Dysgerminoma

- Commonest malignant germ cell tumour.
- Female equivalent of a seminoma.
- 80% present at stage I and so treat with conservative surgery.
- Can be bilateral (10–20%) and require close follow-up of the conserved ovary.
- Common in XY karyotypically abnormal gonads, e.g. XO/XY Turner's syndrome mosaic, and prophylactic removal should be recommended.

⚠ Dysgerminomas may require chemotherapy, if more advanced. Combination chemotherapy regimens include bleomycin, etoposide, and cisplatin (BEP); vinblastine, bleomycin, and cisplatin (VBP); and cisplatin, vincristine, methotrexate, bleomycin, dactinomycin, cyclophosphamide, and etoposide (POMB/ACE).

⚠ Aim is to conserve fertility if appropriate in young women, but ↑ risk of 2° malignancies following chemotherapy.

Immature teratomas

- Present most commonly in girls aged 10–20yrs.
- Conservative surgery/chemotherapy unless stage Ia (BEP regimen).

Endodermal sinus tumours (previously yolk sac tumours)

- Median age 18yrs at presentation.
- Raised AFP levels.
- Conservative surgery and chemotherapy (BEP or POMB/ACE).
- 2yr median survival 60–70%.

Choriocarcinoma of ovary and embryonal carcinoma

- Presentation in women <20yrs.
- Raised hCG levels (choriocarcinoma) or hCG and AFP (embryonal carcinoma).
- Treat as other germ cell tumours.

Table 23.6 Ovarian cancer: histological subtypes

Epithelial (85–90%)	Sex-cord stromal (5%)	Germ cell (5%)
Serous cystadenocarcinoma (75%)	Granulosa-stromal cell tumours	Dysgerminoma
Mucinous cystadenocarcinoma	Granulosa cell	Embryonal carcinoma
Endometrioid adenocarcinoma	Thecoma	Immature teratoma
Clear cell	Fibroma	Mature teratoma
Undifferentiated	Androblastomas	Struma ovarii
	Sertoli cell	Carcinoid
	Sertoli–Leydig cell	Endodermal sinus tumour (yolk sac)
	Leydig cell	Choriocarcinoma

5% of ovarian tumours are 2° tumours: endometrium; cervix; fallopian tube; Krukenberg tumours (breast, stomach, colon); lymphoma; melanoma; carcinoid.

Rare ovarian tumours: other

Sex-cord stromal tumours (~5%)

➲ Table 23.6.

Granulosa cell tumour
- Solid ovarian tumours, which commonly produce oestrogens.
- Peak incidences in young girls and postmenopausal women.
- Present with PMB, menstrual problems, or precocious pseudo-puberty, depending on age.
- May be associated with concurrent endometrial cancer (2° to unopposed oestrogens).
- Often have ↑ inhibin (produced by granulosa cells to cause −ve feedback on FSH levels from pituitary gland) and oestradiol levels—used as tumour markers for monitoring recurrence.
- Treat with surgery (conservative surgery in young woman, i.e. remove affected ovary, biopsy omentum and LN ± biopsy other ovary) as most (~80%) present at stage I and so fertility can be preserved.
- Often recur, which may be many years later and may require repeated surgical debulking.

Sertoli–Leydig cell tumour
- Produce androgens.
- Present with hirsutism, amenorrhoea, and virilization (male pattern baldness, clitoromegaly, deepening voice, hairiness, oily skin, etc.).
- Normally benign tumours—treat surgically.

Fibroma
- Benign solid tumour.
- May present with ascites and pleural effusion (R > L)—Meig's syndrome.

Borderline ovarian and low-grade serous ovarian tumours

Borderline ovarian tumours (BOTs) arise from the ovarian surface epithelium. They are not benign tumours, and are staged as for ovarian cancer. They were previously known as 'tumours of low malignant potential' and account for ~15% of ovarian epithelial cancers, although they are more common in younger women (average 10yrs earlier than epithelial ovarian cancer).

Borderline tumours

- Often confined to ovary (unilateral in mucinous BOT).
- Occur in premenopausal women: even in girls and teenagers.
- Challenging to diagnose histologically:
  - serous > mucinous histology.
- CA125 or CA19-9 may be elevated and if so, can be useful tumour markers for recurrence.
- Can have metastatic implants:
  - these may be non-invasive or invasive.
- BOTs without invasive implants do not benefit from chemotherapy.
- Surgical debulking is the recommended treatment:
  - in young women conservative surgery is valid, with the aim of preserving fertility (i.e. oophorectomy with staging biopsies)
  - high recurrence if unilateral salpingo-oophorectomy (26.0%)—follow-up with TV USS with fertility-conserving surgery
  - frozen section can be useful to plan intraoperatively
  - no indication for LN sampling unless bulky nodes
  - recommend appendicectomy, if mucinous tumour.
- In stage I disease conservative treatment is safe:
  - relapse rate of 8% over 2–18yrs.
- May relapse at a very late stage:
  - after the traditional 5yr follow-up
  - can be >25yrs after initial presentation.

⚠ Very high recurrence if ovarian cystectomy alone (41%).

▶ May be diagnosed after surgery with non-gynae oncologist. Refer for discussion of pros/cons regrading formal staging surgery.

Survival

- 5yr and 10yr survival rates:
  - stage I: 99% and 97%
  - stage II: 98% and 90%
  - stage III: 96% and 88%.

Further reading

British Gynaecological Cancer Society (2017). BGCS epithelial ovarian/fallopian tube/primary peritoneal cancer guidelines.
🔗 www.bgcs.org.uk/wp-content/uploads/2019/05/BGCS-Guidelines-Ovarian-Guidelines-2017.pdf

Low-grade ovarian carcinoma

⚠ BOT with invasive implants classified as low-grade ovarian cancer.

Low-grade serous ovarian carcinoma (LGSOC)

Rarer than HGSOCs and often in younger women. LGSOCs are believed to arise in a stepwise fashion from a benign serous cystadenoma through a serous borderline tumour to an invasive low-grade serous carcinoma. Serous BOT can recur as LGSOC in rare cases.

▶ High-grade serous carcinomas are not related to serous borderline tumours.

▶ BOTs/LGSOCs are not associated with BRCA mutations.

• Slow-growing and may present after vague symptoms over many years.
• CA125 often raised and tumour deposits may be highly calcified—consider diagnosis from CT appearance.
• Management predominantly surgical—debulking laparotomy.
• ↓↓ response rates to chemotherapy cf. HGSOC.
• ~25% response rate to platinum-taxane regimen.
• Consider hormone treatment as adjuvant or maintenance after chemotherapy (e.g. letrozole).

Mucinous ovarian carcinoma

1° ovarian mucinous tumours are rare:
• 3–5% of all ovarian carcinomas.
• Typically confined to the ovary at presentation.
• May be large with continuum of architectural features—benign, borderline, and malignant areas.
• Usually exhibit a CK7+/CK20−/CDX2− immunoprofile.
• Invasive pattern more aggressive than those with expansile growth pattern.
• Debulking laparotomy standard of care—consider fertility sparing in younger women.
• Exclude other more common 1° site for mucinous adenocarcinoma (appendix; colorectal; stomach—oesophagogastroduodenoscopy and colonoscopy).
• Respond less well to chemotherapy than non-mucinous types although platinum-taxane normally 1st-line treatment with lack of evidence for other combinations as rare.

Endometrial hyperplasia

Endometrial hyperplasia is a premalignant condition that can predispose to, or be associated with, endometrial carcinoma. It is characterized by the overgrowth of endometrial cells and is caused by excess unopposed oestrogen, either endogenous or exogenous, similar to endometrial cancer, with which it shares a common aetiology (➔ Endometrial cancer: aetiology and histology, p. 840).

Presentation

Endometrial hyperplasia most commonly presents with heavy ± irregular menstruation or PMB.

Histology

- Endometrial biopsy necessary for diagnosis.
- Endometrial hyperplasia divided into:
  - hyperplasia without atypia
  - atypical hyperplasia.
  - atypia is abnormal appearance of individual glandular cells.
- If atypical glandular cells are back-to-back (i.e. no stromal component between layers), it is endometrial carcinoma.

Management of endometrial hyperplasia *without* atypia

- Risk of progression to cancer <5% over 20yrs.
- Management depends on age of patient, histology, symptoms, and desire for retaining fertility.
- Treat causes of unopposed oestrogens: obesity; PCOS; HRT (especially oestrogen-only HRT); oestrogen-secreting tumour (e.g. granulosa cell tumour of ovary).
- Consider observation alone, if reversible cause.
  - majority of cases of endometrial hyperplasia without atypia
  - regress spontaneously.
- Treat with progestogens has higher regression rate:
  - LNG-IUS (e.g. Mirena®)
  - 1st line for minimum 6mths (most effective)
  - continuous oral progestogens (medroxyprogesterone acetate (MPA) 10–20mg/day or norethisterone 10–15mg/day), if decline LNG-IUS.
- Endometrial sampling 6-monthly until 2× normal biopsies—consider long-term follow-up with annual biopsy (especially if ↑ BMI).
- Consider hysterectomy if:
  - progression to atypical hyperplasia
  - no regression despite 12mths of progestogen treatment
  - relapse after progestogen treatment
  - persistent bleeding symptoms
  - woman declines treatment or surveillance.

⚠ Avoid endometrial ablation—does not adequately treat and makes adequate endometrial surveillance problematic.

Atypical endometrial hyperplasia

⚠ 43% of women with atypical hyperplasia undergoing hysterectomy will have a concurrent adenocarcinoma and, if not concurrent, there is a high risk the woman will develop adenocarcinoma (28% over 19yrs in one case series).

▶ Counsel about high risk of underlying/developing endometrial carcinoma.

▶ Unless fertility is desired or unacceptably high operative risk, recommend hysterectomy ± salpingectomy/BSO (recommend BSO if postmenopausal). Laparoscopic route, if possible. Lymphadenectomy not indicted.

⚠ Treat underlying cause (e.g. refer to bariatric team, if obesity)

If fertility conservation desired

▶ Counsel regarding risk of underlying endometrial cancer.

▶ Treat underlying cause (e.g. refer to bariatric team, if obesity).
• Imaging and formal hysteroscopy and further biopsies, if pipelle only for initial diagnosis, and MDT review:
  • CA125
  • TV USS and/or MRI pelvis.
• LNG-IUS 1st-line treatment—continuous oral progestogens less effective.
• MPA 10–20 mg/day or norethisterone 10–15 mg/day, if decline LNG-IUS.
• 3-monthly surveillance until 2× normal biopsies then 6–12-monthly until fertility not required and recommend hysterectomy.
• Recommend disease regression on at least one endometrial sample before trying for pregnancy (also better implantation rates if assisted reproduction).
• Refer to fertility specialist.

If conservative treatment due to comorbidities

As per conservative treatment described above.

▶ Urgent indication for bariatric referral alongside progestogen treatment, if clinically appropriate.

Can consider higher-dose MPA, especially if continued bleeding (➔ Endometrial cancer: non-surgical treatment, p. 846).

Further reading

Cochrane (2017). Metformin for treatment of endometrial hyperplasia
Ⓡwww.cochranelibrary.com/cdsr/doi/10.1002/14651858.CD012214.pub2/full

Cochrane (2018). Oral and intrauterine progestogens for atypical endometrial hyperplasia
Ⓡwww.cochranelibrary.com/cdsr/doi/10.1002/14651858.CD009458.pub3/full

RCOG (2016). Management of endometrial hyperplasia. Green-top guideline no. 67.
Ⓡ www.rcog.org.uk/guidance/browse-all-guidance/green-top-guidelines/management-of-endo
metrial-hyperplasia-green-top-guideline-no-67/

Endometrial cancer: aetiology and histology

Endometrial cancer is the 4th most common cancer in women in the UK with ~9500 cases in 2016. Incidence ↑ by 57% since the 1990s in the UK. Endometrial cancer predominantly affects postmenopausal women (91% of cases in >50yr olds) and is the 6th most common cancer worldwide: prevalence reflect differences in risk factors and incidence is ↑ with ↑ obesity.

Aetiology

Presence of unopposed oestrogen (i.e. no protective effect of progestogen), whether endogenous or exogenous:
- Endogenous:
  - peripheral conversion in adipose tissue of androstenedione to oestrone (obesity)
  - oestrogen-producing tumour (granulosa cell tumour)
  - PCOS or anovulatory cycles at menarche or during climacteric period (lack of progesterone as no luteal phase).
- Exogenous:
  - oestrogen-only HRT
  - tamoxifen (acts as oestrogen agonist in endometrial tissue).

Histology

- Endometrial cancer arises from the uterine lining.
- The major prognostic indicators in endometrial cancer are their grade of differentiation and FIGO stage of disease.
- These factors guide use of adjuvant treatment.

⚠ Atypical endometrial hyperplasia is a premalignant condition and may have coincidental cancer in almost 50% at time of hysterectomy.

Molecular profiling

▶ Tumour testing for MMR IHC is recommended as routine for newly diagnosed endometrial cancer.
- Allows identification of those with Lynch syndrome and guides management.
- Molecular profiling includes:
  - tumour testing for MMR deficiency with 4-panel IHC (➔ Endometrial cancer screening, p. 800)
  - testing for p53 mutation
  - testing for *POLE* mutation (where available).

Further reading

NICE (2020). Testing strategies for Lynch syndrome in people with endometrial cancer. Diagnostics guidance [DG42].
ℛ https://www.nice.org.uk/guidance/dg42

Risk factors for endometrial cancer

- Obesity and conditions predisposing or associated with obesity (including type 2 diabetes mellitus, hypothyroidism, hypertension).
- Reduced endogenous progesterone production:
  - nulliparity (pregnancy associated with ↑ progesterone levels)
  - PCOS (anovulatory cycles—no corpus luteum, no progesterone)
  - early menarche/late menopause (anovulatory cycles).
- *Genetic predisposition:* Lynch syndrome with high risk of colorectal, endometrial, and ovarian tumours (40–60% lifetime risk of endometrial cancer; inherited as autosomal dominant condition; inherited mutation in one copy of a MMR gene)
- ➔ Endometrial cancer screening, p. 800.
- Breast cancer (shared lifestyle risk factors and tamoxifen usage).

Protective factors

- Parity (high progesterone dose in pregnancy).
- COCP (50% ↑ with up to 4yrs of use up to 72% with ≥12yrs) (progesterone effect).

Histological types of endometrial cancer

Adenocarcinoma

- Endometrial adenocarcinoma: 87%.
- Adenosquamous carcinoma*: 6%.
- Clear cell or serous carcinoma*: 6%.
- Carcinosarcoma*: 1%.

*High risk of advanced disease at presentation and recurrence—all G3 (see Box 23.4).

Box 23.4 Histological grading of endometrial cancer

- Well differentiated (G1).
- Moderately differentiated (G2).
- Poorly differentiated or high-risk cell type (G3).

Endometrial cancer: presentation and investigation

Presentation

Most commonly presents with PMB. Younger women present with menstrual disturbance (heavy ± irregular periods).

▶ 1% are picked up on routine cervical smear tests.

▶ 1 in 10 women with PMB will have endometrial cancer or atypical hyperplasia (Table 23.7).

▶ Endometrial sampling required for women >45yrs with abnormal menstrual symptoms or in those <45yrs with abnormal menstrual bleeding and failure of medical treatment.

▶ PV discharge and pyometra may occur instead of bleeding—have a ↑ index of suspicion in postmenopausal women with ↑ PV discharge (50% of postmenopausal women with pyometra have carcinoma).

Investigation

History
- Presenting symptoms.
- Menstrual history.
- Parity.
- Comorbidities.
- Drug history (COCP, HRT, tamoxifen, antihypertensives, oral hypoglycaemics).
- Family history.

Examination
- Rule out other causes of bleeding (vulval, vaginal, and cervical pathology) with clinical examination.

⚠ Check anterior and posterior vaginal walls carefully when withdrawing the speculum to ensure there are no vaginal lesions.
- *Bimanual examination:* uterine size, mobility, adnexal masses.

Haematological investigations
- FBC, U&E, LFTs.

Imaging—TV USS
- <4mm ET/echo ↓ very low risk of endometrial pathology in postmenopausal women (96% NPV)—no requirement for endometrial sampling unless recurrent bleeding.

Endometrial biopsy
- Perform endometrial sampling if ET ≥4mm or persistent bleeding in woman with ET <4mm (or consider formal hysteroscopy):
  - blind outpatient sampling (e.g. pipelle, Vabra®)
  - hysteroscopy: under local anaesthesia or GA with targeted sampling and pipelle/general curettage.

Further imaging investigations if cancer diagnosed

- CXR (staging) G1 endometrial cancer on biopsy.
- CT CAP: G2–G3 disease for preoperative staging as ↑ risk of disease outside of uterus.
- MRI pelvis:
  - can be useful to determine local extent of tumour and presence of grossly involved pelvic LNs
  - may be useful to stratify to pathway of care
  - necessary, if considering fertility-preserving treatment

Table 23.7 Histopathology findings in women with PMB

Histological diagnosis	%
Atrophy	49.9
Proliferative/secretory	5.5
Benign polyps	9.2
Hyperplasia without atypia	27.8
Atypical hyperplasia	5.5
Adenocarcinoma	8.1
Not diagnostic	14.2
Other disorders	3.3

Source: data from Gredmark T, Kvint S, Havel G, et al. (1995). Histopathological findings in women with postmenopausal bleeding. *Br J Obstet Gynaecol.* 102(2):133–136.

Further reading

British Gynaecological Cancer Society (2017). BGCS endometrial guidelines 2017.
℅ www.bgcs.org.uk/wp-content/uploads/2019/05/BGCS-Endometrial-Guidelines-2017.pdf

Endometrial cancer: surgical treatment

Surgery

Hysterectomy and BSO and pelvic washings

See Table 23.8 for FIGO staging.

- For G1–G2 endometrial cancer thought to be confined to uterus.
- G3 serous histological subtype also need omental biopsy for staging as ↑ risk of transcoelomic spread.
- Total laparoscopic hysterectomy (TLH) or laparoscopic-assisted vaginal hysterectomy (LAVH) preferred route as no difference in survival outcomes and ↓ morbidity.
- Abdominal via transvers or midline incision if uterus too large to be removed PV/more extensive disease or patient unable to tolerate pneumoperitoneum.
- Robotic surgery may have a role in morbidly obese patients as ↓ pneumoperitoneal pressures required and fewer short-term complications but evidence on longer-term outcomes limited and costs higher.
- Debulking surgery may have a role in advanced disease, similar to ovarian cancer, in selected cases before/after chemotherapy.

Pelvic lymphadenectomy

- No survival advantage of routine lymphadenectomy of non-bulky LN in presumed early disease.

🌢 G3 disease included in studies, but numbers smaller and practice variable.

SLNB

🌢 Studies of cervical injection of ICG or a combination of blue dye and Tc99m-labelled colloid demonstrate high NPVs.

- Significantly ↓ morbidity cf. systematic lymphadenectomy.
- Ultra-staging of LN picks up more +ve nodes than conventional histology.
- Impact of SLNB on survival outcomes is being tested in RCTs and will provide prognostic information to guide adjuvant treatment.
- Consider SLNB in G3 endometrial cancer.

Table 23.8 FIGO staging of endometrial cancer

Stage			Extent of disease	5yr survival
I			Tumour limited to uterine body	85%
	Ia		<1/2 myometrial depth invaded	
	Ib		>1/2 myometrial depth invaded	
II			Tumour invades cervical stroma but no extension beyond uterus*	75%
III			Local and/or regional extension to uterine serosa, peritoneal cavity, and/or LNs	45%
	IIIa		Extension to uterine serosa and/or adnexae	
	IIIb		Extension to vagina and/or parametrium	
	IIIc		Pelvic or para-aortic LNs involved	
		IIIc1	Pelvic node involvement	
		IIIc2	Para-aortic node involvement	
IV			Extension beyond true pelvis and/or involvement of bladder/bowel mucosa	25%
	IVa		Extension to bladder and/or bowel mucosa	
	IVb		Distant metastases or +ve inguinal LNs	

* Endocervical involvement without stromal invasion now included in stage I.

Source: data from Amant, F., Mirza, M. R., Koskas, M. and Creutzberg, C. L. (2018), Cancer of the corpus uteri. *Int J Gynecol Obstet.* 143:37–50. doi:10.1002/ijgo.12612

Further reading

ASTEC Study Group (2009). Efficacy of systematic pelvic lymphadenectomy in endometrial cancer (MRC ASTEC trial): a randomised study. *Lancet.* 373:125–136.
ℰ www.thelancet.com/journals/lancet/article/PIIS0140-6736(08)61766-3/fulltext#articleInformation

British Gynaecological Cancer Society (2017). BGCS endometrial guidelines 2017.
ℰ www.bgcs.org.uk/wp-content/uploads/2019/05/BGCS-Endometrial-Guidelines-2017.pdf

British Gynaecological Cancer Society (2019). Sentinel consensus document for vulval, endometrial and cervical cancer.
ℰ www.bgcs.org.uk/wp-content/uploads/2020/01/BGCS-Sentinel-Consensus-Document-7.5.-2019.pdf

Cochrane (2021). Sentinel node biopsy for diagnosis of lymph node involvement in endometrial cancer.
ℰ www.cochranelibrary.com/cdsr/doi/10.1002/14651858.CD013021.pub2/full

Endometrial cancer: non-surgical treatment

Adjuvant radiotherapy

- Adjuvant radiotherapy limited to vault brachytherapy, if intermediate risk (see below).
- External beam radiotherapy (EBRT) ± vault brachytherapy boost for high-risk (G3, stage Ib) or locally advanced disease.

PORTEC-3 RCT

- RCT of adjuvant chemotherapy + EBRT in high-risk endometrial cancer.
- 5% 5yr survival advantage of chemoradiotherapy over radiotherapy alone (hazard ratio 0.70; 95% CI 0.51–0.97).
- Consider it in stage III and those with serous histological subtype.
- Role for NAC in those not suitable for 1° debulking surgery, although efficacy data limited.
- Carboplatin/paclitaxel normal 1st-line treatment for endometrial cancer in adjuvant or NAC setting.

Hormonal treatment

- No role for adjuvant progestogen therapy after 1° treatment.
- High-dose progesterone may be used for advanced and recurrent disease or those unfit for active treatment:
  - megestrol (160mg daily), or
  - MPA (200mg/400mg daily).

⚠ Risk of VTE or heart failure—reduced dose (MPA 10–20 mg/day) or aromatase inhibitors are an alternative.

- LNG-IUS and bariatric surgery in morbidly obese can make some fit enough to have subsequent surgical treatment:
  - ~50% response rate in small studies.

Palliative radiotherapy

- If not fit for surgical treatment.
- EBRT given at lower dose and in few fractions to control local symptoms (e.g. bleeding).

Molecular profiling

- Tumour testing for MMR IHC (➔ Endometrial cancer screening, p. 800), and testing for p53 mutation (and *POLE* mutation where available) can stratify by risk of recurrence and guide adjuvant treatment.

⚠ Risk groups are now complex—refer to latest guidelines (see ESGO/ESTRO/ESP endometrial cancer guidelines: ℘ https://ijgc.bmj.com/content/31/1/12.long).

Fertility-sparing treatment

➔ Endometrial hyperplasia, p. 837.

Conservative management may be safe in selected women with G1 endometrial cancer and superficial myometrial invasion (completion hysterectomy strongly recommended in medium term).

▶ Counsel regarding risk of progression of endometrial cancer during conservative management which may ↓ likelihood of curative treatment—fatal consequences have been reported.

▶ Treat underlying cause (e.g. refer to bariatric team, if obesity)

- Imaging CT CAP and MRI pelvis to exclude deep myometrial invasion and lymphadenopathy.
- MPA 400–600 mg/day or megestrol (160–320 mg/day)
- LNG-IUS may be as effective, with better compliance.
- Regression rate 76%; relapse rate 26%; live birth rate 26%.
- 3-monthly surveillance until 2× normal biopsies then 6-monthly until fertility not required and recommend hysterectomy ASAP.
- Recommend disease regression on at least one endometrial sample before trying for pregnancy (also better implantation rates, if assisted reproduction).
- Refer to fertility specialist.
- Omitting BSO at hysterectomy not associated with ↑ cancer mortality.

⚠ Refer to clinical genetics and beware of Lynch syndrome and subsequent ovarian/bowel cancer risk.

PORTEC-2 and ASTEC radiotherapy trials

- These trials compared adjuvant radiotherapy vs no adjuvant radiotherapy in women with intermediate-risk early endometrial adenocarcinoma:
  - G1 with deep myometrial invasion (>50%)
  - G2 with any myometrial invasion (stage Ia or Ib)
  - G3 with superficial invasion (stage Ia).
- Radiotherapy ↓ pelvic recurrences, but gave no survival advantage with stage Ib endometrial cancer and intermediate risk histology.
- Isolated pelvic recurrences were amenable to salvage radiotherapy in previously non-irradiated patients.
- Vault brachytherapy reduced risk of pelvic recurrence.

Further reading

ASTEC/EN.5 Study Group (2009). Adjuvant external beam radiotherapy in the treatment of endometrial cancer (MRC ASTEC and NCIC CTG EN.5 randomised trials): pooled trial results, systematic review, and meta-analysis. *Lancet*. 373:137–146.
🔊www.ncbi.nlm.nih.gov/pmc/articles/PMC2646125/

PORTEC Study Group (2018). Ten-year results of the PORTEC-2 trial for high-intermediate risk endometrial carcinoma: improving patient selection for adjuvant therapy. *Br J Cancer*. 119:1067–1074.
🔊 www.nature.com/articles/s41416-018-0310-8

Rare uterine malignancies

Uterine sarcomas

Uterine sarcomas are very rare, accounting for 3–5% of uterine cancers and have an incidence of 2:100,000 women. Abnormal bleeding is the most common presenting feature; other symptoms include pain and a pelvic mass. Polypoid masses may protrude through the cervical os.

⚠ Uterine corpus sarcomas account for 3–5% of all uterine cancers, but cause 26% of the mortality.

Types of uterine sarcomas
- Leiomyosarcoma (46%).
- Endometrial stromal sarcoma (12%).
- Carcinosarcoma (27%).
- Not specified/others (15%).

- The peak incidence for leiomyosarcoma and endometrial stromal sarcoma is 50–64yrs of age.
- Peak incidence for carcinosarcoma is older, at 65–79yrs.
- ▶ Age, stage, and tumour type are important prognostic factors.
- The 5yr survival figures are:
  - leiomyosarcoma, stage I: 65%; stage IV: 0%.
  - carcinosarcoma, stage I: 62%; stage IV: 17%.
  - endometrial stromal sarcoma, stage I: 85%; stage IV: 37%.

Uterine morcellation and occult uterine sarcomas
The FDA issued an updated safety statement regarding the use of power morcellation in laparoscopic hysterectomy and myomectomy due to the risk of disease spread and subsequent worsening of long-term survival in women with unsuspected uterine sarcomas.

The FDA, therefore, discourages the use of laparoscopic power morcellation during hysterectomy or myomectomy for uterine fibroids.

(See ℜ www.fda.gov/medical-devices/surgery-devices/laparoscopic-power-morcellators)

Vulval intraepithelial neoplasia: overview

Vulval intraepithelial neoplasia (VIN) can occur in any age group, but is more common in postmenopausal women. ↑ incidence of VIN over 30yrs, especially in younger women, reflecting changes in sexual practice, as well as ↑ recognition. The natural history of VIN is not as well understood as CIN, but up to 9% of women with HPV-related usual-type VIN (uVIN) may progress to VSCC over several years. The risk of progression of differentiated VIN (dVIN) to VSCC is much higher (associated with lichen sclerosus; ➔ Vulval dermatoses: lichen sclerosus, p. 790). VIN can be difficult to treat and frustrating to patient and doctor and may represent a field change—recurrence rates are high.

Aetiology

- Dysplastic lesion of the squamous epithelium.
- uVIN linked with high-risk HPV infection, smoking and immunosuppression.
- Associated with persistent infection with HPV in >90% of cases, especially HPV 16.
- HPV infection may cause multifocal disease, and patients with uVIN should be carefully screened for CIN.
- dVIN is associated with an underlying skin condition such as lichen sclerosis or lichen planus.

Histology

The 2004 classification system (ISSVD) now uses VIN to refer to previous VIN II–III, whereas VIN I is now thought to be non-specific inflammatory changes and is not premalignant.

Presentation and investigation

- Symptoms are 1° itch, but include pain and ulceration.
- >20% may be asymptomatic.
- Lesions may be raised, hyperkeratotic, and warty or flat and erythematous frequently found at multiple sites (~50%).
- Diagnosis is made by punch or excision biopsy.
- Since HPV causes multifocal disease, patients are advised to undergo regular cervical screening. ➔ Colour plate 11.

Further reading

British Gynaecological Cancer Society. Vulval cancer guidelines.
℘ www.bgcs.org.uk/professionals/guidelines-for-recent-publications/

Cochrane (2016). Medical and surgical interventions for the treatment of usual-type vulval intraepithelial neoplasia.
℘www.cochranelibrary.com/cdsr/doi/10.1002/14651858.CD011837.pub2/abstract

Vulval intraepithelial neoplasia: management

uVIN

Although small, painful lesions can be excised, there is normally a field change, and so it is difficult to completely excise the VIN, and recurrence rate is high, even after skinning vulvectomy. Treatment should ↓ symptoms and side effects and exclude development of VSCC. If multifocal/recurrent HPV related disease, consider HIV testing as per BASHH guidelines (℞ www.bashhguidelines.org/media/1067/1838.pdf).

Surveillance
- Risk of progression of uVIN to cancer ~2–3% per annum.
- Recurrence rates range between ~30% and 66%.
- If cancer excluded, individualize treatment (can be observation).
- Follow-up is required, suspicious lesions should be biopsied.

Surgery
- Wide local excision (WLE) of painful/irritating lesions.
- Recurrence rate of unifocal lesions 34% vs 66% for multifocal.
- Development of pain is associated with ↑ risk of vulval cancer.

▶▶ Encourage patients to contact urgently if develop symptoms on surveillance and biopsy painful lesions.

Medical treatment
- Imiquimod has been shown to help clearance of genital warts:
  - apply 5% imiquimod cream 3 times weekly for 12–16wks
  - colposcopic assessment at ~6wk intervals during treatment.
  - ~50% response rate
  - treatment can be limited by side effects—soreness and burning.
  - evidence suggests ↓ in need for excision.
- Cidofovir is a topical antiviral agent:
  - response rates similar for 16wk course of imiquimod
  - ↑ maintenance of response to medical treatment cf. surgery (cidofovir = 94% cidofovir (95% CI 78.2–98.5) vs imiquimod = 71.6% (95% CI 52.0–84.3))
  - cidofovir currently unlicensed in UK, only used in clinical trials.

Vaccination
HPV vaccination for prevention of CIN very likely ↓ incidence of uVIN, but as yet no proven role in treatment of existing VIN.

Chemotherapy
☙ Topical fluorouracil (5-FU), usually ineffective and badly tolerated and is no longer recommended.

dVIN

High risk of progression or underlying VSCC—WLE and active treatment of lichen sclerosus with ultra-high potency topical steroids.

Vulval cancer: aetiology and investigation

Rare (1300 per annum in UK). Risk ↑ with age (median age 74yrs), although younger women are at risk, especially those with multifocal VIN. Incidence ↑ 18% since the early 1990s, mainly in association with HPV in younger women. ~90% are squamous cell carcinomas (VSCC) and ~7–10% are vulval melanomas, with basal cell, Bartholin's gland carcinoma, and, rarely, sarcomas accounting for the rest.

Aetiology

VSCC commonly arise on a background of lichen sclerosus or VIN (usual type or differentiated).

Presentation

Vulval cancers commonly present with a lump, pain, irritation, or bleeding. There may be an obvious ulcer present. Older women in particular may delay presentation due to embarrassment. Referral to 2° care may also be delayed if there is not an adequately high index of suspicion.

▶▶ If lesions highly suspicious, refer to gynaecological oncologist without waiting for biopsy results. ◗ Colour plate 12.

Investigation

History

Vulval symptoms, treatments (prescribed or self), past medical history, and performance status/frailty score.

Clinical examination

Palpable groin LN, size and location of lesion, general medical condition. May be too painful for examination unless under GA, so if obvious tumour, refer to gynae oncology for EUA and biopsy.

Haematological investigations

FBC, U&E, LFTs.

Imaging investigations

CT CAP ± MRI (+ CT head if melanoma).

Histology

Punch or wedge biopsy, including the edge of the lesion (in ulcerated lesions, it may be difficult to get a diagnosis from the sloughed central tissue). Avoid excision biopsy.

▶ Labelled, anatomical diagram and clinical photos (ideally pre/post biopsy) to aid accurate location of biopsy site/s.

▶ Ensure each biopsy in separate pot with location clearly described.

⚠ It can be extremely hard to locate biopsy site when seen later, especially as high chance of multifocal disease, and inability to localize may necessitate more extensive treatment.

Staging

See Table 23.9.

Table 23.9 FIGO staging of vulval cancer

Stage		Extent of disease	5yr survival
I		Tumour limited to vulva and perineum (−ve regional (groin/inguinofemoral) LNs)	
	Ia	≤1mm depth of invasion and ≤2cm diameter	86%
	Ib	>1mm depth of invasion and/or >2cm diameter	77%
II		Tumour of any size with spread to lower 1/3 of vagina, lower 1/3 urethra, or anus (−ve regional LNs)	65%
III		Tumour of any size with extension to adjacent perineal structures (lower 1/3 urethra; lower 1/3 vagina; anus), or with any number with +ve regional LNs	
	IIIa	Tumour of any size with extension to adjacent perineal structures (lower 1/3 urethra; lower 1/3 vagina, anus), or regional LN metastasis ≤5mm	60%
	IIIb	Regional LN metastases >5mm	50%
	IIIc	Regional LN metastases with extracapsular spread	31%
IV		Tumour of any size fixed to bone, or fixed or ulcerated regional LN metastases, or distant metastases	
	IVa	Tumour of any size fixed to bone, or fixed or ulcerated regional LN metastases	26%
	IVb	Any distant metastases including pelvic LNs	18%

(See FIGO staging 2021: ◈ https://obgyn.onlinelibrary.wiley.com/doi/epdf/10.1002/ijgo.13880)

Vulval cancer: treatment

Surgery

Surgery is the mainstay, both for curative intent and for palliation.
- Patients with disease >1mm depth of invasion should have groin node sampling/lymphadenectomy performed.
- Lateral disease can have an ipsilateral LN surgery: if +ve LN, bilateral groin LN dissection is required.
- Central disease requires bilateral groin LN surgery.

The importance of lymphadenectomy was recognized in the 1940s by Way and Taussig, who developed the 'butterfly' incision en bloc dissection—removal of entire vulva and inguinal LNs with all connecting tissue. Wounds frequently broke down and took many months to heal by 2° intent. Triple incision vulvectomy, with separate groin incisions, was subsequently developed to ↓ morbidity. Current treatment aims for WLE of the vulval lesion (R0 margins free of microscopic disease) and SLNB ± LN dissection through separate incisions along the inguinal ligament to ↓ morbidity.

▶ Plastic surgical reconstruction may be required.

⚠ Groin recurrence is very difficult to treat and carries a very ↑ rate of mortality.

Complications
- Wound breakdown and infection.
- Lymphocysts.
- Lymphoedema.
- DVT/PE.

SLNB

Now standard of care for small, unifocal disease (>1mm depth of invasion and <4cm diameter), without evidence of LN metastases, that does not encroach urethra, vagina, or anus, and no previous groin node surgery. If lesion within 1cm of midline structure then bilateral SLNB required. ↓↓ morbidity cf. full groin node dissection. SLNB finds LN(s) that 1° drains the tumour. If this is identified, and is −ve, full groin dissection not required. Identify SLN with combination of blue dye and Tc-99m radiolabelled tracer. SLN examined with ultra-staging and IHC. If SLN +ve or no node found then full ipsilateral lymphadenectomy required.

Radiotherapy ± chemotherapy
- Can be used before surgery to shrink 1° to reduced morbidity of surgery (e.g. if urethra or anus involved).
- Is used after surgery if +ve groin LNs, to prevent regional recurrence.
- EBRT given to treat +ve pelvic LN.
- Can combine with chemotherapy.

▶ Should not be used as an alternative to groin dissection (RCT halted early as 5/26 had groin recurrences, compared with none in surgical arm).

Rare vulval malignancies

Vulval/vaginal melanoma

- 7–10% of vulval cancers.
- Staged, like other melanomas, rather than vulval cancer: Breslow depth and American Joint Committee on Cancer (AJCC) staging (2002).
- Most common site is the lower anterior vaginal wall (so easy to miss on speculum examination).
- Melanotic or amelanotic.
- Very poor prognosis.
- Low rate of b-raf and c-kit mutations.
- Role for immunotherapy (nivolumab) in improving recurrence-free survival for patients with node +ve, surgically resected cutaneous melanoma.

(For guideline, see Melanoma Focus (2018). Ano-uro-genital mucosal malignant melanoma guideline: ℜ https://melanomafocus.org/wp-content/uploads/2022/04/aug-executive-summary.pdf)

Vulval Paget's disease

Non-mammary adenocarcinoma *in situ*: in breast, Paget's disease is normally associated with underlying malignancy, whereas only 20% with vulval Paget's disease have invasion into underlying stroma, and another ~8% have another underlying carcinoma (e.g. bladder, uterine, colorectal).

💣 Recent data suggest rate of other malignancy may not be this common and routine screening for other malignancies not required unless symptoms warrant further investigation, although should be considered.

- Postmenopausal women.
- Presents with itching and vulval soreness.
- Eczematous or raised and erythematous, velvety appearance—may weep serous fluid, usually on the labia majora. 'Cake-icing' scaling.
- Extent of disease spreads well beyond clinical lesion—difficult to excise completely.
- Treat with surgical excision ± lymphadenectomy if invasive.
- No data of safety of SLNB.
- Recurrence common (60–70%) and if occurs is normally another adenocarcinoma *in situ*.
- Small studies suggest imiquimod may have good response rates (67% complete response; 21% partial response)—if complete response recurrence rate very low (6%).
- Invasive Paget's disease rare—represents 1–2% of vulval cancers.

Bartholin's gland cancer

- Rare tumours <5% vulval cancers.
- Treatment based on very small case series or extrapolated from VSCC.
- Honan's criteria. Tumour must be:
  - in the correct position
  - deep in the labium majora
  - normal overlying skin
  - still some normal gland present.
- Bartholin's glands and ducts are comprised of several different cell types: stratified squamous epithelium at the vulval surface to transitional epithelium at the terminal ducts.
- Variety of histological types of Bartholin gland cancer: adenocarcinoma, squamous carcinoma, and transitional cell carcinoma.
- Surgical excision involves extensive dissection of ischiorectal fossa and potentially anal sphincter.
- No data on safety of SLNB—full groin node lymphadenectomy required.
- Need preoperative staging CT CAP.
- Likely to need adjuvant chemoradiotherapy as often diagnosed at more advanced stage.

Basal cell carcinoma

- Rare vulval cancer (<5%).
- Mean age of presentation 76yrs.
- Locally invasive and rarely spread to local LNs unless very large and invasive at diagnosis.
- Local excision with microscopic clear margins (R0).
- Groin node dissection only if clinical evidence of local disease.
- Gorlin's syndrome associated with multiple basal cell carcinomas.

Vaginal cancer

1° vaginal carcinomas are rare and account for only 1% of gynaecological malignancies. Most vaginal tumours are metastases from either above (cervical or uterine) or below (vulval). Of the remaining true vaginal tumours, ~90% are squamous cell carcinomas and normally present in older women. Many will have a previous history of intraepithelial neoplasia or invasive carcinoma of the vulva, vagina, or cervix. Other predisposing factors include pelvic radiotherapy and long-term inflammation due to a vaginal pessary or procidentia. Squamous cell carcinoma, similar to cervical carcinoma, is commonly HPV related, especially HPV 16. Most of the remaining 8–10% are adenocarcinomas. Lymphoma, melanoma, and sarcoma extremely rare. The most common site for squamous cell carcinoma is in the upper posterior vagina—easy to miss if obscured by a speculum.

Spread

- Direct extension.
- Upper vagina—pelvic LNs.
- Lower vagina—inguinal LNs.

Investigations

- Biopsy.
- CT CAP and MRI pelvis for local infiltration extent.

Treatment

Surgery

Role of surgery limited due to close proximity of other organs. Largely limited to small tumours confined to vaginal wall or, more rarely, or as exenterative procedure (involving removal of pelvic organs and diversion of bladder ± bowel) in locally advanced disease/pelvic recurrence or palliative diversion of bladder ± bowel.

Upper vaginal cancer—radical hysterectomy (if uterus, *in situ*) with vaginectomy with 1cm disease-free margins and pelvic lymphadenectomy.

Lower vaginal disease—WLE and bilateral groin node dissection.

Radiotherapy

Combination of EBRT to the pelvis plus vaginal brachytherapy. May be given with concurrent cisplatin, extrapolating from treatment of cervical cancer.

Staging

See Table 23.10.

Table 23.10 FIGO staging of vaginal cancer

Stage		Extent of disease	5yr survival
I		Tumour contained within the vagina and no larger than 2cm	85%
II		Tumour grown through the vaginal wall, but not extending to pelvic sidewall or LN	78%
III		Tumour spread to pelvic sidewall, and/or growing into lower 1/3 vagina, and/or causing hydronephrosis, and/or spread to local LN in groins or pelvis	54% for stage III–IVa
IV		Tumour spread beyond true pelvis and/or into bladder/bowel mucosa	
	IVa	Tumour spread to bladder/bowel or directly invading beyond true pelvis	
	IVb	Distant metastases, e.g. to lungs or bones	

Further reading

FIGO Cancer Report (2018). Cancer of the vagina.
https://obgyn.onlinelibrary.wiley.com/doi/epdf/10.1002/ijgo.12610

Rare vaginal cancers

Vaginal clear cell adenocarcinoma

- Occur in younger women and are strongly associated with DES exposure *in utero*.
- DES was administered to several million pregnant women at risk of miscarriage or premature delivery between 1940 and 1971. The critical time for exposure was in the 1st 16wks of pregnancy.
- Most occurred in 14–22yr-olds, but later peak in 40s.
- Screen with annual colposcopy of cervix and vagina.

Treatment of vaginal clear cell adenocarcinoma

- Aim to preserve reproductive function in (often) young women.
- Stage I tumours treated with WLE.
- In more advanced stage disease, radiotherapy is indicated (see Table 23.10).
- Overall 5yr survival ~80–87% when associated with DES exposure.
- Non-DES adenocarcinoma 5yr survival ~34%.

Vaginal malignant melanoma

- Extremely rare—3 in 10 million women.
- Typically in elderly women.
- Treatment largely surgical, colpectomy ± pelvic exenteration.
- 5yr survival ~15%; median overall survival 22mths.

(For guideline, see Melanoma Focus (2018): ℛ https://melanomafocus.org/wp-content/uploads/2022/04/aug-executive-summary.pdf)

Embryonal rhabdomyosarcoma (sarcoma botryoides)

- Rare tumour with a multicystic grape-like form.
- Derived from rhabdomyoblasts.
- Presents in infancy (girls <3yrs).
- Cervical rhabdomyosarcoma can occur in teenagers, and uterine rhabdomyosarcoma has been described in postmenopausal women.
- Presents with a grape-like mass arising from the vagina; can present with vaginal bleeding or a single polyp.
- Treatment—preserve fertility and vaginal function:
  - smaller tumours excised followed by combination chemotherapy (vincristine, dactinomycin, and cyclophosphamide)
  - NAC given for larger tumours, to reduce their size prior to surgery.
- Survival rates of 90% can be achieved.
- Refer to centres with expertise—may need reconstructive surgery.

Gestational trophoblastic disease: hydatidiform mole

Gestational trophoblastic disease (GTD) covers a spectrum of diseases caused by overgrowth of the placenta. This includes hydatidiform mole, persistent trophoblastic disease/gestational trophoblastic neoplasia (GTN), choriocarcinoma, invasive mole, and placental site trophoblastic tumour.

- *Incidence:* molar pregnancy 1 in 590 pregnancies in UK.

⚠ Most GTN follow a molar pregnancy—can occur after miscarriage, EP, or normal pregnancy. Perform urinary pregnancy test if persistent/irregular bleeding after any pregnancy.

Hydatidiform mole

Can be subdivided into complete and partial mole based on genetic and histological features.

Complete mole
- Consists of diffuse hydropic villi with trophoblastic hyperplasia.
- This is diploid, derived from sperm duplicating its own chromosome following fertilization of an 'empty' ovum, it is mostly 46XX with no evidence of fetal tissue.

Partial mole
- Consists of hydropic and normal villi.
- This is triploid (69XXX, XXY, XYY) with one maternal and two paternal haploid sets. Most cases occur following two sperms fertilizing an ovum, and a fetus may be present.

Diagnosis

Symptoms and signs (with approximate frequency)
- Irregular 1st-trimester vaginal bleeding (>90%).
- Uterus large for dates (25%).
- Pain from large theca lutein cysts (20%) resulting from ovarian hyperstimulation by high hCG levels.
- Vaginal passage of vesicles containing products of conception (10%).
- Exaggerated pregnancy symptoms:
  - hyperemesis (10%)
  - hyperthyroidism (5%)
  - early pre-eclampsia (5%).

▶ Serum hCG is excessively high with complete moles, but levels may be within the normal range for partial moles.

Risk factors for hydatidiform mole
- *Age:* extremes of reproductive life (>40yrs and <15yrs of age) in complete moles, not partial moles.
- *Ethnicity:* 2× higher in east Asia, particularly Korea and Japan.
- *Previous molar pregnancy:* 10× higher risk of developing future molar pregnancy.

USS findings
See Fig. 23.2.

Complete mole
- 'Snowstorm' appearance of mixed echogenicity, representing hydropic villi and intrauterine haemorrhage.
- Large theca lutein cysts.

Partial mole
- Fetus may be viable, with signs of early growth restriction or structural abnormalities.

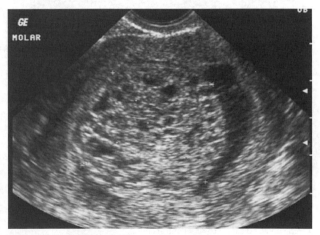

Fig. 23.2 Ultrasound of hydatidiform mole.

Hydatidiform mole: management

Management

- *Complete mole:* surgical curettage performed by an experienced surgeon as risks of uterine perforation and haemorrhage are high. A single dose of oxytocin may be required to ↓ risk of haemorrhage, but is associated with a theoretical ↑ risk of tissue dissemination → metastatic disease to the lungs or brain and should be avoided until uterus is evacuated, if possible, and only used, to control significant bleeding.
- *Partial mole:* surgical evacuation is preferable, unless the size of fetal parts necessitates medical evacuation.
- Histological examination of products of conception is essential to confirm diagnosis.

▶ Anti-D after suction curettage in Rh −ve women.
- Send urinary pregnancy test 3wks after medical management of miscarriage, if no histology sent. If raised consider molar pregnancy.

Treatment of persistent GTD

Risk of requiring chemotherapy is 15% after a complete mole and 0.5% after a partial mole.

Indications for chemotherapy
- Serum hCG levels >20,000IU/L at 4wks after uterine evacuation.
- Static or ↑ hCG after uterine evacuation in absence of new symptoms, e.g. uterine bleeding and/or abdominal pain.
- Evidence of metastases.
- Histological diagnosis of choriocarcinoma.

Prognosis

- With effective registration and treatment programme, cure rate is high (98–100%) with low chemotherapy rates (5–8%).
- Recurrence rate is low (1/55).
- Women should be advised not to conceive until hCG level has been normal for 6mths and follow-up completed; if required chemotherapy 12mths after completion of treatment.
- hCG levels should be checked 6 and 10wks after any subsequent pregnancies with urine and serum hCG.

Contraception and hormone replacement therapy

- No contraindication to oral contraception.
- No evidence of risk with HRT (▶ those who require chemotherapy likely to have earlier menopause).

Specialist follow-up for molar pregnancy

In the UK, all women with any molar pregnancy should be registered at one of the three specialist centres (Sheffield, Dundee, London) who then manage follow-up. Molar pregnancy often associated with variant of hCG so need specialist testing.

Protocols vary slightly between centres

Confirmed partial molar pregnancy (Charing Cross)
- Urine ± serum samples every 2wks until hCG levels normal.
- If another normal sample 4wks later, follow-up complete.

Complete molar pregnancy
- Urine ± serum hCG checked fortnightly until levels are normal.
- If hCG normalizes within 8wks, hCG levels follow-up for 6mths.
- Patients who do not have normal hCG values within 8wks have follow-up until levels normal for 6mths.

▶ Inform specialist centre of any subsequent pregnancy—check hCG 6 and 10wks after any subsequent pregnancies.

Further reading

Braga et al. (2015). Hormonal contraceptive use before hCG remission does not increase the risk of gestational trophoblastic neoplasia following complete hydatidiform mole: a historical database review. BJOG, 123:1330–1335.
⏚https://obgyn.onlinelibrary.wiley.com/doi/full/10.1111/1471-0528.13617

Cochrane (2016). Chemotherapy for resistant or recurrent gestational trophoblastic neoplasia.
⏚ www.cochranelibrary.com/cdsr/doi/10.1002/14651858.CD008891.pub3/abstract

Cochrane (2016). First-line chemotherapy in low-risk gestational trophoblastic neoplasia.
⏚ www.cochranelibrary.com/cdsr/doi/10.1002/14651858.CD007102.pub4/full

Hydatidiform Mole and Choriocarcinoma UK Information and Support Service.
⏚ https://hmole-chorio.org.uk/patients_info/patients_info_timetable/

RCOG (2010). The management of gestational trophoblastic neoplasia. Green-top guideline no. 38.
⏚ www.rcog.org.uk/files/rcog-corp/GT38ManagementGestational0210.pdf.

Sheffield Trophoblastic Tumour Screening and Treatment Centre.
⏚ www.chorio.group.shef.ac.uk/clin.html

Gestational trophoblastic disease: choriocarcinoma

This is a highly malignant tumour consisting of syncytio- and cytotrophoblast with myometrial invasion. Local spread and vascular metastases to the lung are common. 50% of cases are preceded by hydatidiform mole, 40% by normal pregnancy, 5% by miscarriage or EP, and 5% are non-gestational in origin.

Incidence

1:30,000 pregnancies in Western countries and 1:11,000 in East Asia.

Diagnosis

Signs and symptoms
- Vaginal bleeding.
- Abdominal or vaginal swelling.
- Amenorrhoea.
- Dyspnoea and haemoptysis (2° to lung metastases).
- Intra-abdominal haemorrhage (2° uterine perforation by tumour).
- Less common sites for metastases include brain, kidney, liver, or spleen; these present with symptoms related to their site.

Investigations

Persistent trophoblastic disease
- Serum hCG, FBC, U&E, LFTs, clotting, HIV and hepatitis B serology, group and save.
- Doppler USS pelvis.

Additional tests if presumed choriocarcinoma or placental site trophoblastic tumour
- CT CAP.
- MRI head.
- Diagnostic CSF for hCG if lung or brain metastases.
- GFR measurement to guide chemotherapy dosing.

Treatment

The chemotherapy regimen used is determined by a FIGO prognostic scoring system which is based on:
- Age of patient and type of antecedent pregnancy.
- Extent of tumour burden (hCG level, number, site, and size of tumour, site of metastases).
- Interval from antecedent pregnancy.
- Response to previous chemotherapy.

Prognosis

- Overall survival rate is >90%.
- Poorer prognosis is associated with patient aged >40yrs, antecedent pregnancy being term pregnancy, time interval from antecedent pregnancy to chemotherapy >4mths, large tumour burden, and poor response to previous chemotherapy.

Chemotherapy for GTD

- Chemotherapy continued until hCG normal for 6wks.
- More likely to have earlier menopause.
- Low-risk patients (≤6):
  - methotrexate and folinic acid (well tolerated with main side effects of mucositis and pleuritic chest pain)—1st dose at specialist centre
  - may need intrathecal methotrexate if lung metastases for CNS prophylaxis
  - 67% response rate to 1st-line treatment
  - overall cure rate almost 100%.
- High-risk patients (≥7):
  - intensive weekly schedule of EMA (etoposide, methotrexate, and dactinomycin) alternating with CO (cyclophosphamide and vincristine)
  - salvage surgery may be required (craniotomy, pleurotomy, hysterectomy)
  - 17% develop resistance and need 2nd-line chemotherapy—overall cure rate 95%
  - ↑ risk of 2° cancers
  - small ↑ risk of miscarriage and stillbirth, but no ↑ in fetal abnormalities in subsequent pregnancy.
- Placental site trophoblastic tumour:
  - recommend hysterectomy, can be curative if disease confined to uterus
  - EP/EMA chemotherapy if disseminated disease (etoposide, cisplatin/etoposide, methotrexate, dactinomycin)
  - 100% cure rate if present within 4yrs of antecedent pregnancy.

Principles of chemotherapy

Chemotherapy, together with radiotherapy and surgery, is used in the treatment of gynaecological cancers for cure, control, or palliation of symptoms.

The cell cycle

- Chemotherapeutic agents interfere with cell division by acting on a specific phase of the cell cycle (e.g. taxanes active against cells in G2/M) or non-specifically (e.g. alkylating agents exert their effects throughout the cell cycle).
- One of the characteristics of cancer cells is uncontrolled proliferation. As chemotherapy has a propensity for actively proliferating cells, they are more vulnerable than normal cells.
- However, they do act on normal cells, hence common side effects ($\rightarrow$ Side effects of chemotherapy: haematological and gastrointestinal, p. 871).

Practical aspects

Intent of treatment (i.e. curative or palliative) for each patient should be discussed at MDT and clearly explained to the patient to allow them to weigh up the potential risks/anticipated benefits so that optimal survival and quality of life may be achieved. Factors to consider are:

Disease related
- Type and stage of cancer.
- Response to previous treatment.

Patient related
- Performance status (WHO PS; the general condition of the patient) (Table 23.11) ± frailty index (e.g. Rockwood index: $\mathbb{S}$ http://www.frailtytoolkit.org/wp-content/uploads/2016/12/Rockwood.jpg)
- Concurrent medical problems.
- Nutritional status.
- Patient's wishes.

Chemotherapy is generally delivered on an outpatient basis
- For most ovarian chemotherapy, each course of treatment is composed of 6 cycles, depending on response assessed after the 3rd one.
- Each cycle lasts 21–28 days.
- The gap between consecutive cycles enables damaged 'normal' cells to repair and regenerate.
- Some chemotherapy regimens given weekly (e.g. paclitaxel as single agent or in clinical trials).

Response to treatment is assessed by
- Changes in evaluable disease on CT/MRI scans (RECIST (response evaluation criteria in solid tumours) criteria).
- Trends in tumour markers (e.g. CA125 levels for ovarian cancer).
- Patient-reported outcomes—symptoms and quality of life.
- Clinical examination.

Table 23.11 WHO performance status

Grade	Performance criteria
0	Asymptomatic; fully active—capable of heavy work
1	Symptomatic; restricted in strenuous physical activity, but ambulatory and able to perform light work, e.g. light housework, office work
2	Symptomatic; ambulatory >50% of waking hours and capable of all self-care, but unable to carry out work activities
3	Symptomatic; limited self-care, confined to bed or chair >50% of waking hours
4	Totally confined to bed or chair, cannot carry out any self-care
5	Death

RECIST criteria

- *Complete:* disappearance of all lesions with no evidence of new lesions on two occasions of at least 4wks apart.
- *Partial:* ≥30% ↓ in sum of longest diameters of lesions.
- Stable disease.
- *Progression:* ≥20% ↑ in the sum of longest diameters of lesions or presence of new lesions.

Classes of chemotherapy agents

Antimetabolites

- Interfere with DNA and RNA synthesis, e.g. 5-FU, gemcitabine, methotrexate.

Alkylating agents

- Form covalent bonds with DNA bases, e.g. cyclophosphamide, ifosfamide.

Intercalating agents

- Bind to DNA, thus inhibiting its replication, e.g. cisplatin, carboplatin (most widely used in gynaecological cancer).

Anti-tumour antibiotics

- Complex mechanism of action → inhibition of DNA synthesis, e.g. bleomycin, doxorubicin, etoposide.

Drugs against spindle microtubules

- Prevent mitosis, e.g. paclitaxel, vincristine.

Biological agents

Extensive research being done to find targeted agents that act on specific pathways that preferentially affect cancer cells, rather than all dividing cells, to improve activity of cancer cells and reduce side effects of chemotherapy. The most common types currently in gynaecological cancer treatment include:

PARPis

Inhibit poly-ADP ribose polymerase, the enzyme that repairs single-strand breaks in DNA (e.g. olaparib, niraparib). If cells divide with single-strand breaks then multiple double-strand breaks form. BRCA proteins involved in homologous recombinational repair of double-stand breaks in DNA. In tumours with BRCA mutations/deficiency, cells cannot repair breaks and so cells die by apoptosis. Given orally and used in maintenance treatment.

Angiogenesis inhibitors

Block new blood vessel formation to micrometastases and limit growth of new tumour deposits. Cancer cells release VEGF in response to hypoxia. Angiogenic inhibitors either block VEGF or its receptor with an antibody (e.g. bevacizumab) or stop cell signalling of VEGF receptor by blocking its tyrosine kinase activity (e.g. cediranib, sorafenib). May be used during chemotherapy and then for a prolonged maintenance period. VEGF also required to repair wounds, so avoided within several wks of surgery and risk of bowel perforation. Can also commonly cause hypertension.

Side effects of chemotherapy: haematological and gastrointestinal

Chemotherapy is associated with a range of side effects due to its action on normal cells, as well as cancer cells. Patterns of toxicity varies between drugs, as well as between individuals. Most side effects are self-limiting. It is important to recognize and seek ways to prevent and manage them, whenever possible, to maintain good quality of life.

Haematological

Bone marrow suppression leads to a gradual fall in blood count, which eventually recovers. The *nadir* (period of lowest count) typically occurs around 7–14 days after chemotherapy.
- *Neutropenic sepsis:* potentially fatal, urgent action required:
  - neutropenia = neutrophil count ≤1.0 × 10^9/L
  - must have a high level of suspicion in any patient having chemotherapy presenting with a temperature of ≥38°C and feeling unwell
  - *take FBC, cultures*—blood, urine, etc., start IV broad-spectrum antibiotics, as per hospital protocol, and inform acute oncology team
  - prophylaxis with granulocyte colony-stimulating factor (GCSF) and oral antibiotics, as per local protocol, may be appropriate if there have been previous episodes of neutropenic sepsis.
- *Anaemia* (Hb ≤11g/dL):
  - may be seen, especially after several cycles of chemotherapy
  - treatment depends on severity and includes blood transfusion, iron tablets/infusion, erythropoietin.
- *Thrombocytopaenia* (platelet count ≤100 × 10^9/L):
  - common with carboplatin, especially in combination with paclitaxel
  - avoid invasive procedures until counts recovered.

Gastrointestinal

Gastrointestinal side effects are due to loss of epithelial cells.
- *Nausea and vomiting:* can be prevented in most cases with effective antiemetics (e.g. steroids, domperidone, metoclopramide, and/or 5-HT$_3$ antagonists).
- Mucositis:
  - resolves spontaneously with epithelial healing
  - helpful measures are good mouth care, use of local anaesthetic agents, treatment of oral candidiasis
  - commonly occurs with methotrexate and 5-FU.
- *Constipation:* pay attention to diet and fluid intake; short-term use of laxatives.
- Diarrhoea:
  - exclude infection/constipation
  - control with codeine phosphate, loperamide, and rehydration.

Side effects of chemotherapy: other

Alopecia

- Taxanes (e.g. paclitaxel), doxorubicin, and etoposide commonly cause temporary hair loss.
- Carboplatin and cisplatin are not usually associated with this side effect.
- Has a psychological impact on some women. Individual preference for wigs, scarves, or hats.
- Can try to ameliorate with 'cooling cap'.

Neurological

These are dose-related side effects that often slowly subside on dose ↓ or on stopping the offending drug but can be severe and persistent.

- *Peripheral neuropathy:*
  - usually sensory changes such as numbness and tingling
  - commonly seen with paclitaxel and cisplatin.
- *Tinnitus:* associated with cisplatin and taxanes.

Constitutional

These symptoms tend to have cumulative effects as treatment progresses but resolve on its cessation.

- Lethargy.
- Anorexia.

Reproductive function

Fetal abnormality

- Most chemotherapeutic agents are teratogenic and should be avoided during the 1st trimester.
- Some agents may be used after 12wks if necessary—data are generally reassuring but limited.
- Contraception is necessary until a period of time has elapsed following completion of treatment.

Ovarian failure

- More likely to be caused by alkylating agents than other chemotherapy.
- Permanent ovarian failure in premenopausal patients results in early menopause and infertility.
- Young women with premature menopause are predisposed to osteoporosis, cardiovascular disease, and postmenopausal symptoms; HRT can be used without evidence of ↑ risk of cancer recurrence in most cancers.
- Cryopreservation of embryos and ovarian tissue is possible for women who wish to preserve their fertility options prior to chemotherapy—consider urgent referral to fertility services.

Chemotherapy for gynaecological cancer

General points

- Chemotherapy has a narrow therapeutic index; close monitoring while on treatment is essential.
- Before the start of each cycle of treatment, blood tests (FBC, U&E, LFT) are taken, and the patient's performance status and side effects are assessed (see ℘ https://www.nice.org.uk/guidance/ta121/chap ter/Appendix-C-WHO-performance-status-classification)
- Chemotherapy when used alone normally has a palliative rather than curative role, except for persistent GTD/choriocarcinoma, which is highly chemosensitive.
- Response rate is better when chemotherapy is used in combination with surgery or radiotherapy—this may be given as:
  - *neoadjuvant*—before definitive treatment (i.e. surgery or radiotherapy) intended to ↓ tumour bulk
  - *adjuvant*—after definitive treatment to ↓ the risk of recurrence.

Common chemotherapy regimens for gynaecological cancers

Ovarian cancer

- Sensitive to platinum-based regimens, response rate ~70%.
- Carboplatin ± paclitaxel (may be used as neoadjuvant, adjuvant, or palliative treatment).
- >50% of patients will relapse and require further treatment:
  - if >6mths have elapsed since initial chemotherapy then tumour defined as platinum sensitive
  - <6mths since platinum based chemotherapy given defined as platinum resistant.
- Intraperitoneal chemotherapy (section can be useful to directly into the peritoneal cavity) has shown clinical benefit, but with ↑ toxicity (recommended to be used as part of clinical trial only).
- Treatments for recurrence and platinum-resistant disease include pegylated doxorubicin, single-agent paclitaxel, gemcitabine, cisplatin.
- Biological agents: include bevacizumab (angiogenic inhibitor) and PARPis—often used as maintenance treatment ± in combination with conventional chemotherapy.

Endometrial cancer

- Chemotherapy has a limited role, reserved for recurrent or metastatic disease.
- Carboplatin ± paclitaxel 1st line.

Cervical cancer

- Cisplatin combined with radiotherapy has been shown to ↓ risk of relapse for those undergoing radiotherapy after surgery.
- Platinum-based chemotherapy may be used for metastatic disease but the response rate is low.

Vulval/vaginal cancer

- Cisplatin can be used in combination with radiotherapy for patients unfit for surgery.
- Cisplatin may be used as sole therapy for symptom control in metastatic disease.

Trophoblastic tumour

- Chemotherapy alone may be curative.
- Treatment given at specialist centres.

Radiotherapy: principles

Radiotherapy, unlike chemotherapy, is loco-regional and not systemic treatment. It may be used with curative and palliative intent in some gynaecological cancers.

Radiobiology

- Radiotherapy kills cells by the use of ionizing radiation:
  - X-rays
  - gamma-rays
  - β-particles.
- Radiation can lead to double strand breaks DNA directly or indirectly via production of free radicals.
- Sensitivity of any cell to radiation depends on:
  - cell type (e.g. cells of the small bowel have low tolerance to radiation)
  - cell cycle (cells in G0, resting, phase are relatively resistant, whereas cells in G1 and G2 phases are sensitive)
  - micro-environment (cells in areas of low oxygen are radioresistant).
- Many cells are able to repair a certain amount of DNA damage but cancer cells do this less effectively; thus a significantly higher proportion will be destroyed.
- The total dose of radiotherapy that can be given to one area is limited by the tolerance of the surrounding normal tissue of that area.

Delivery of radiotherapy

Radiation may be given by EBRT and/or brachytherapy:
- EBRT:
  - radiation is distant from the patient
  - delivered from a linear accelerator
  - use of conformal radiotherapy (i.e. shaping the radiation beam to shape of tumour) encompasses less normal tissue within the field and therefore reduces side effects.
- Brachytherapy:
  - placement of radioactive source directly within or around the tumour site (e.g. intravaginal/intrauterine brachytherapy for cervical cancer)
  - *advantage*—higher radiation dose to the tumour, lower exposure to normal tissue.
- Side effects may be reduced by giving radiotherapy in divided doses so that normal tissues can recover.

Radiotherapy for symptom palliation

Radiotherapy is used to control some symptoms caused by metastatic disease. Examples are:
- Pain.
- Symptoms from bone/brain metastases.
- Bleeding from fungating tumour.

Radiotherapy: gynaecological cancers

Management of gynaecological cancers is often multimodal in nature, combining surgery, chemotherapy, and radiotherapy. The choice of treatment depends on the type of cancer, the extent of disease, and the patient's fitness and wishes.

Cervical cancer

- Early disease (stage Ib):
  - radiotherapy is as effective as radical hysterectomy
  - for those who have had surgery, radiotherapy may be given afterwards (adjuvant treatment) to reduce the risk of pelvic recurrence if +ve LNs/close margins.
- Locally advanced disease (stage II–IVa):
  - chemoradiotherapy or radiotherapy (including EBRT and intracavity brachytherapy).
- Recurrent disease:
  - localized recurrence may be treated by surgical resection or radiotherapy, depending on previous treatment and extent.
- Distant metastatic disease (stage IVb): best supportive care ± palliative radiotherapy ± palliative chemotherapy.

Endometrial cancer

- Early disease (stage I):
  - if patient unfit for surgery, radiotherapy used as 1° treatment.
  - if fit for surgery, adjuvant brachytherapy (± EBRT), if high-risk features present (e.g. poorly differentiated tumour, deep myometrial involvement).
- Locally advanced disease (stage II–IIIc):
  - postoperative (adjuvant) EBRT and brachytherapy.
- Recurrent disease:
  - as for cervical cancer.

Vulval cancer

- Early disease:
  - 1° radiotherapy if unfit for surgery.
- Locally advanced disease:
  - EBRT (chemo) radiotherapy to groins/pelvis after surgery if LNs found to be involved
  - neoadjuvant chemoradiotherapy to shrink extensive disease before surgery if involves urethra/anus to limit morbidity of surgery.
- Recurrent disease:
  - may be possible depending on previous treatment.

Ovarian cancer

- No evidence to support the use of radiotherapy in the 1° or adjuvant setting.
- Radiotherapy may have a role in the palliation of localized symptoms.

Radiotherapy: side effects

The side effects of radiotherapy depend on the site being irradiated. In gynaecological cancers this is the pelvis, and therefore tissues in this area are prone to damage. Problems may become apparent during and immediately after treatment (early effects) or occur months or years later (late effects).

Early side effects

- Due to damage of rapidly dividing cells such as the mucosa:
  - usually self limiting.
- Skin:
  - *erythema*—moist desquamation
  - management—aqueous cream, hydrocortisone cream.
- Mouth/bowel:
  - *mucositis*—treat with mouthwash, analgesia, nystatin if oral candidiasis present
  - *nausea* (± vomiting)—antiemetics for prophylaxis or treatment
  - *diarrhoea*—exclude infection, treat with loperamide or codeine phosphate.
- Bladder:
  - *cystitis*—frequency and dysuria
  - management—exclude infection, ensure adequate fluid intake, oxybutynin may help.
- Tiredness/fatigue:
  - treat anaemia, if present, and gentle exercise.
- Bone marrow suppression.

Late effects

Cumulative over time due to induction of cytokines and growth factors in normal tissues causing fibrosis, lack of tissue compliance and new vessel formation (telangiectasia).

Skin

- Fibrosis, (e.g. → vaginal stenosis and shortening), telangiectasia, lymphoedema (fibrosis of lymphatic channels), vaginal dryness, dyspareunia.

Bladder

- Radiation cystitis: pain, bleeding (due to telangiectasia), urinary infections, difficulty voiding, urinary urgency, and incontinence.

Bowel

- Radiation proctitis: pain, diarrhoea, rectal bleeding (due to telangiectasia), urgency, faecal incontinence.
- Small bowel—stenosis, adhesions, and fibrosis → small bowel obstruction.

Pain

- Abdominal and pelvic pain due to effects on small bowel and pelvic nerves; microinstability fractures in pelvis; leg pain due to lymphoedema.

Hormone replacement therapy after gynaecological cancer treatment

- Menopausal symptoms may have a significant detrimental impact on quality of life and premature ovarian failure (POF) can ↓ overall survival without adequate HRT.
- 2-fold ↑ in age-specific mortality from POF.
- Quality of life important factor in those with advanced disease.
- Treatment for many gynaecological cancers may make women menopausal—surgery (oophorectomy) ± chemotherapy ± pelvic radiotherapy ± steroids (e.g. for nausea in chemotherapy).
- Gynaecologists and GPs may be reluctant to prescribe HRT when in many cases it is not contraindicated.
- Menstruation can restart if POF due to chemotherapy—depending on age and other treatment may need to counsel regarding contraception.
- Consider ovarian transposition—to move away from intended radiation field.
- If fertility desired, options include oocyte/embryo freezing, ovarian harvesting, oocyte/embryo donation, surrogacy, adoption, fostering.
- Menopausal—FSH >25 on two occasions 4wks apart and low oestradiol.
- Menopause leads to more rapid loss of (trabecular) spinal than cortical bone (femoral neck).
- Surgically induced menopause associated with more rapid bone loss than natural menopause: BSO <40yrs → 3× ↑ risk of ischaemic heart disease than >50yrs but minimal ↑ risk with other causes of POF.
- If POF may need higher oestrogen than postmenopausal; use 'body identical' hormones:
  - *if no uterus:* 75–100 micrograms estradiol patch; 3–4 doses gel; 2–4 mg oral
  - *if uterus:* LNG-IUS or Utrogestan® 200 mg od day 15–26 of each 28-day oestrogen HRT cycle, or 100 mg od day 1–25 of each 28-day oestrogen HRT cycle; Femoston® HRT
  - HRT better than COCP at protecting bone density.

Factors in HRT and cancer

- Patient views.
- Severity of symptoms and effect on quality of life.
- Risks of POF.
- Malignancy—type and hormone receptor status (e.g. breast cancer).

▶ Can use HRT in *BRCA* gene mutation carriers after RRSO if no personal history of cancer.

- Lifestyle factor modification: smoking, adequate exercise, avoid excess alcohol, ensure vitamin D and calcium.

HRT and ovarian cancer

Tubo-ovarian epithelial cancer
- HRT associated with improved overall survival in epithelial ovarian cancer.

Germ cell/sex cord/ borderline
- Minimal evidence—consider clinical situation and weigh pros/cons.

HRT and endometrial cancer

- Low risk of recurrence in early stage G1 endometrial cancer.
- Data do not demonstrate significant harm of HRT.
- Can be used immediately after curative surgery.
- Theoretical advantage of combined HRT if concern of residual disease but weak data and no data in more advanced disease.

HRT and cervical cancer

Squamous cell carcinoma
- Not oestrogen sensitive.
- No change in disease-free survival for HRT vs no HRT with FIGO stage I/II.

Adenocarcinoma
- Minimal evidence—consider clinical situation and weigh pros/cons.

HRT and vulval/vaginal cancer

No data but unlikely to be significant effect in squamous cell carcinoma.

Alternatives to HRT
- Clonidine.
- Venlafaxine.
- Gabapentin.
- Oxybutynin.
- Vaginal oestrogen—minimal systemic uptake if on maintenance treatment.

Further reading

Alternatives to HRT for management of menopausal symptoms:
- www.rcog.org.uk/globalassets/documents/guidelines/scientific-impact-papers/sip_6.pdf
- www.bgcs.org.uk/members-area/webinars-and-journal-clubs/
- https://thebms.org.uk/publications/consensus-statements/premature-ovarian-insufficiency/
- https://obgyn.onlinelibrary.wiley.com/doi/full/10.1111/tog.12607

Principles of palliative care

The WHO defines palliative care as the 'active, holistic care of patients with advanced, progressive illness'.

▶ Good communication with the person (and family/caregivers) are essential to facilitate frank discussion of prognosis and formulate a plan of care that is most suited to her.

▶ Communication with person and family/caregivers regarding treatment escalation plan and regular review for ceilings of appropriate treatment for anyone with a life-limiting illness, not just those for end-of-life care.

▶ Palliative care is everyone's responsibility—palliative care team available for specialist support and advice. In advanced cancer, early palliative care can improve life expectancy, as well as quality of life, and can be delivered alongside active treatment. Explain to patients who may confuse palliative care with end-of-life care (as do some clinicians). Explain limitations of care, including attempted resuscitation, especially in the over 80s.

Goals of palliative care
- To achieve optimal symptom relief.
- To promote the best quality of life.

In order to palliate effectively, it is necessary to individualize each person's care and take her wishes into account.

Aspects to explore include
- Physical symptoms.
- Psychological symptoms.
- Social issues.
- Spiritual issues.

Multidisciplinary approach
- Symptoms may be controlled by pharmacological or non-pharmacological means (e.g. fan and low-dose morphine for breathlessness).
- The expertise of different specialties may be needed depending on the nature of the patient's problems, not just palliative care team, e.g. clinical oncologists, general surgeons, interventional radiology, urology, occupational therapy, dietitians/gastroenterology.
- Palliative care can be delivered at home, hospice, or in hospital.

End-of-life care

- Aim for a peaceful and dignified death.
- Communication with person and family, exploring aims, hopes, fears, expectations.
- Maintain comfort and offer psychosocial/spiritual support.
- Avoid unnecessary/uncomfortable procedures.
- Discuss/re-evaluate treatment escalation plan.
- Review medication. Most can be stopped, but continue analgesics, antiemetics, anxiolytics, anticonvulsants,

Pain and its management

Most patients with advanced cancer experience moderate to severe pain that can be attributed directly to the cancer.

Principles

- Treat different types of pain differently.
- Multimodal approach.
- Give regular medication—aim for baseline control with additional treatment as required for breakthrough pain.
- Least invasive delivery method—consider sublingual, oral, topical (patches/creams) before SC/IV.
- Individualize to patient—be guided by patient-reported symptoms.
- Consider other supportive care—e.g. massage, heat, meditation, spiritual care.
- Anticipatory prescribing for side effects of analgesia—antiemetics, laxatives.
- Adaptive treatment and adjust to varying symptoms.

Types of pain

- Neuropathic (e.g. lumbosacral plexus involvement, often described as burning, sharp): anticonvulsants, antidepressants, gabapentinoids, transcutaneous stimulation.
- Acute inflammation: corticosteroids, NSAIDs.
- Anxiety and depression: anxiolytics and antidepressants.
- Tissue damage pain (nociceptive): ladder of paracetamol, NSAIDs, weak opiates, strong opiates.
- Bone metastases/brain metastases: consider local radiotherapy.
- Localized pain: consider blocks and indwelling epidural analgesia.

Assessment

- Ask questions about pain ('SOCRATES') to assess its nature and distinguish whether acute or chronic.
- Measurement of pain may be done using scales; e.g. by asking the patient to score her pain out of 10.
- Consider psychological factors that might contribute to or exacerbate pain, such as anxiety and depression.

'SOCRATES'

- **S**ite.
- **O**nset.
- **C**haracter.
- **R**adiation.
- **A**ssociations.
- **T**iming.
- **E**xacerbating/relieving factors.
- **S**everity.

WHO analgesic ladder
- *Step 1:* non-opioid (e.g. paracetamol, NSAIDs).
- *Step 2:* weak opioid (e.g. codeine) + non-opioid.
- *Step 3:* strong opioid (e.g. morphine) + non-opioid.

Side effects of opioids
- Commonly:
  - nausea
  - constipation
  - sedation (advise amitriptyline should be taken 3h before bed to avoid morning 'hangover').
- Inform patient of potential problems.
- Give antiemetics and laxatives.

⚠ *Do not allow concerns about potential dependence prevent you from prescribing adequate amounts of opiates in palliative treatment.*

Other symptoms in advanced gynaecological cancer

Gastrointestinal symptoms

Nausea and vomiting

- Causes:
  - ascites
  - constipation
  - metabolic (e.g. ↓ Na, ↑ Ca^{2+})
  - bowel obstruction
  - brain metastases
  - medication.
- Treat cause, if possible:
  - radiotherapy and corticosteroids for brain metastases
  - paracentesis for ascites—consider indwelling, tunnelled drain in those with recurrent ascites without active treatment options
  - hydration and bisphosphonates for hypercalcaemia.
- Antiemetics: metoclopramide, hyoscine butylbromide, haloperidol, 5-HT_3 antagonists, steroids, proton pump inhibitors.

Constipation

- Causes:
  - ↓ fluid intake
  - immobility
  - lethargy
  - bowel obstruction
  - metabolic (e.g. Ca^{2+})
  - medication (especially opioids).
- Treat cause, if possible.
- Laxatives (senna, sodium docusate, macrogols, lactulose, glycerol suppositories, enemas).

(Subacute) bowel obstruction

- Caused by tumour seedling within the peritoneum or adhesions following treatment.
- Exclude constipation with abdominal X-ray.
- Initially manage medically; however, if patient is reasonably fit and there is a transition point, surgery may be an option, although prognosis poor in recurrent disease ± surgery—median survival only ~60 days in systematic review.
- Total parenteral nutrition in rare situations.

Diarrhoea

- Exclude incontinence with overflow.
- Loperamide/codeine.
- Good skin care and hygiene crucial, if faecal incontinence.
- Depending on prognosis/situation diversion with stoma may be considered.

Fistulae

- Difficult to manage, limited role for surgery unless well enough to consider surgical diversion (stoma/urostomy).

Fatigue

- Dexamethasone may give a sense of well-being.

Vaginal discharge and bleeding

- May be due to necrotic and infected consider antibiotics, e.g. metronidazole.
- Tranexamic acid (up to 1g qds).
- Topical clotting agents and vaginal packs (e.g. Surgicel®).
- Palliative radiotherapy.
- Consider interventional radiology and embolization for bleeding—often multiple feeding vessels to tumour so may be challenging.
- Massive haemorrhage may be terminal event and can be extremely traumatic—prepare person, family, and carers; 'just in case' medications including analgesia and anxiolytics, dark towels (to camouflage blood loss).

Anorexia and cachexia

- Caused by the secretion of pro-inflammatory cytokines.
- Normal part of dying process—explanation and support to family/ caregivers.
- Dexamethasone or megestrol/MPA may improve appetite short term.

Dyspnoea

- Causes—pleural effusion, cachexia, lymphangitis, anaemia, lung metastases, PE.
- Suspect PE, if acute onset of shortness of breath.
- Low-dose opioids, fans, anxiolytics.

Anxiety and depression

- Psycho-spiritual care.
- Anxiolytics and antidepressants.

Chapter 24

Miscellaneous gynaecology

Injuries in obstetric and gynaecological practice: overview

Because of their close anatomical relationship, operating on the genital tract may also incur injury to the urinary tract. Complicated gynaecological procedures ↑ the risk of urinary tract injury. If an injury occurs, prompt recognition and appropriate management are important to prevent long-term sequelae (urinary incontinence, fistulae, and, rarely, renal failure) and to ↓ litigation.

Medico-legal implications

Up to 6% of all medical malpractice claims in gynaecological practice are related to urinary tract injuries. The quantum of claims is probably related to the degree of suffering or perceived suffering by the patient. Thus, urinary tract injuries that lead to litigation are likely to be associated with significant physical and psychological morbidity or loss of income.

Claims have ↑ over time and every attempt should be made to ↓ the risk. Despite every effort, occasional injury is inevitable, particularly with highly challenging surgery.

> **In the event of an adverse event**
> - Remember the GMC guidance on being open and honest with patients, the *duty of candour.*
> - If a patient under your care has suffered harm or distress:
>   - you must act immediately to put matters right, if that is possible
>   - you should offer an apology and explain fully and promptly to the patient what has happened, and the likely short-term and long-term effects.
> - Patients who complain about the care or treatment they have received have a right to expect a prompt, open, constructive, and honest response including an explanation and, if appropriate, an apology.
> - You must not allow a patient's complaint to affect adversely the care or treatment you provide or arrange.
>
> ▶ Remember, doctors who are open, honest, and non-defensive are less likely to be sued for negligence and less likely to have formal complaints made about them, regardless of what has gone wrong.

Further reading

Care Quality Commission (2022). Health and Social Care Act 2008. Regulations 2014: Regulation 20: Duty of candour.
🖰 www.cqc.org.uk/guidance-providers/regulations-enforcement/regulation-20-duty-candour

Ureteric injury

Incidence

0.5–2.5% of iatrogenic ureteric injuries occur during routine pelvic surgery, mainly gynaecological. Ureteric injury occurs in 0.03% of CDs compared with 0.001% of vaginal births.

Mechanism of injury

- *Avulsion:* liable to occur when tissues are fragile.
- *Transection commonly at:*
  - the pelvic brim (vascular ovarian pedicle is close to the ureter)
  - the base of the broad ligament where the uterine arteries cross (commonly during hysterectomy as the ureters enter the bladder above the lateral vaginal fornix just 2cm lateral to the cervix)
  - the ureterovesical junction.
- *Ligation:* especially during vaginal hysterectomy and repair of procidentia when the ureters also prolapse.
- *Crush:* by clamps causing necrosis or stricture.
- *Devascularization:* causing ischaemia and necrosis.

Presentation

Only 15–20% of iatrogenic injury presents at the time of surgery.

Diagnosis

- IVU or CT urogram.
- Cystoscopy and bilateral retrograde pyelography to identify site of injury, extravasation, or ureteric dilatation.
- CT for suspected urinoma.
- USS may also diagnose hydronephrosis or urinoma.

Treatment

⚠ Intraoperative repair has a better long-term prognosis than postoperative interval repair. Assistance from the urological team should be requested as soon as injury is suspected.

Injuries at or below the pelvic brim

- *Psoas hitch:* shortens the ureterovesical gap and ↓ tension.
- *Boari flap:* creation of a tension-free anastomosis.

Higher-level injuries

- May require nephrostomy or downward displacement of the kidney with end-to-end ureteric anastomosis with the ipsilateral ureter.
- Ureteroileal anastomosis may be necessary in extensive upper ureteral injury (very rare).
- May need cutaneous ureterostomy or transureteroureterostomy.

Presentation

Postoperatively, ureteric injury presents with:

- Fever (sepsis),
- Flank pain from hydronephrosis.
- Vaginal fistulae.
- Non-specific symptoms of malaise, ileus, or the presence of a pelvic mass ('urinoma').
- Bilateral ureteric injury is very rare, so renal function is usually normal.

Risk factors for ureteric injury

- Previous surgery.
- Bulky tumours distorting anatomy and/or displacing ureters.
- Endometriosis with peritoneal scarring or frozen pelvis.
- PID and tubo-ovarian abscesses.
- Carcinoma of the cervix with parametrial involvement.
- Situations that require haste (e.g. emergency CD).
- Angular or broad ligament tears during CD.

Prevention is better than cure!

▶ Identification of the ureters prior to ligation of the uterine and ovarian arteries during hysterectomy should be routine practice. If difficult surgery is anticipated or encountered, identification aids include:

- Preoperative ureteric stents (can be 'lighted').
- IV administration of 10mL indigo carmine or methylene blue with 20mg of furosemide. Leakage of dye or contrast is demonstrated with ureteric injury.
- Retrograde pyelography under fluoroscopic guidance (identifies ureteric strictures).

Bladder and urethral injury

Incidence

~50% of all bladder injuries are the result of surgical procedures (may occur during hysterectomy and usually involves the anterior bladder wall). Obstetric bladder injury occurs in 1.4% of CDs compared with 0.01% of vaginal deliveries.

Mechanisms of injury

- Mobilization of the bladder to expose the cervix or the lower uterine segment during a hysterectomy. Previous scarring (CD, myomectomy, PID, or endometriosis) contributes to ↑ risk.
- Perforation of the bladder may occur during laparoscopy, hysteroscopy, and sling procedures (TVT).
- Ischaemic injury result from an inadvertent suture in the bladder.
- Prolonged and obstructed labour may compress the bladder → avascular necrosis and vesicovaginal fistula.
- High forceps deliveries (↑ if the bladder is not emptied beforehand).

Presentation

Bladder injuries commonly present with haematuria and abdominal pain, but can present with abdominal distension, suprapubic tenderness, leakage of urine PV, and an inability to void.

Diagnosis

- Bladder injury may be obvious at the time of surgery as the catheter balloon may become visible.
- Instillation of methylene blue dye into the bladder through a Foley's catheter may demonstrate leakage into the peritoneal cavity under direct visualization at surgery.
- Cystoscopy is commonly used when bladder injury is suspected postoperatively.
- A cystogram will also demonstrate urinary leakage.
- Instillation of methylene blue dye into the bladder through a Foley's catheter with swabs inserted into the vagina may help identify a vesicovaginal fistula ('three-swab test').

Treatment

- Iatrogenic injuries may be repaired surgically or managed with catheter drainage depending on size and location of injury.
- Bladder perforation is repaired in two layers using absorbable sutures.
- Foley catheter is recommended for 7–14 days with antibiotic cover.
- Thorough assessment of whether the ureteric orifices have been involved needs to be made at time of repair particularly if injury is large, posterior, or basal.

▶ It is good practice and medico-legally prudent to involve specialist urological advice and help when there has been an inadvertent urinary tract injury.

Urethral injury at a glance

Female urethral injuries are rare, and they occur commonly with urethral instrumentation, vaginal surgery, and obstetric complications. Most commonly the result of difficult catheterization where it is forced and there is rupture or subsequent scarring of the urethra.

Presentation
- Diagnosis can be difficult, but they can present with urethral bleeding or an inability to void (retention or poor stream/dribbling)
- Fistulae will present with labial swelling or with leaking of urine through the vagina.

Diagnosis
- IVU.
- Voiding cystourethrography.
- MRI.
- Cystoscopy.

Treatment
- For most cases urethral catheterization is sufficient if this is possible.
- Suprapubic catheterization may be necessary prior to repair.
- Larger tears are surgically repaired using layered closure.
- Proximal damage to the urethra requires reconstruction surgery including bladder flap–urethral tube reconstruction and vaginal flap urethroplasty.
- Long-term suprapubic catheterization may be necessary in the small group of women for whom urethral repair is unsuccessful.

⚠ Urethral surgery is very difficult and requires expert urological input.

Risk factors during Caesarean delivery
- Emergency CD, particularly category 1.
- Low station of the presenting part (especially at full dilatation as the bladder is stretched up the lower segment and is 'higher than expected').
- Prolonged labour prior to CD.
- Preterm delivery (<32wks gestation).
- Previous CD (risk ↑ with ↑ number of CD).
- Previous extensive abdominal and pelvic surgery, especially previous myomectomy.
- The presence of lower uterine and cervical fibroids.
- Suboptimal operator skill.

Communication and record keeping

Good communication is as highly valued by patients as any knowledge or technical ability. Repeatedly, the biggest cause of complaints is poor communication (patients will rarely complain about a doctor they like!). Just about every patient complaint, regardless of the underlying issue, is compounded by perceived gaps in communication. The biggest cause of lost medico-legal cases is poor documentation.

Good communication

- Treat your patients as you would like to be treated yourself.
- Always introduce yourself and explain the purpose of any consultation.
- Generally, ask 'open' questions ('Could you describe the pain you have?') and signpost changes of enquiry ('Can I now ask you about any medication you are taking?').
- Give the patient time to talk (it is her story, not yours, and remember, the patient knows her symptoms better than you do!).
- Listen to the answers (if you don't listen, why ask the question?)— patient complaints frequently cite that 'The doctor just wasn't listening' or 'Nobody was listening to me'.
- Summarize your history and invite questions from the patient.
- Always close the consultation with a clear plan of action.
- Acknowledge fear, upset, or if someone looks worried—do not avoid it; the patient nearly always feels better for discussing it.
- Do not be dismissive or appear rushed.
- Doctors who come across as arrogant or patronizing induce anger and resentment in their patients—be wary of this, you will also be complained about or sued if you make a mistake!
- Don't take anger or criticism personally (part of a doctor's job is listening, even when we don't want to hear it).
- Be honest at all times, including when things go wrong or if you are unsure about a particular problem or management plan—patients understand that things sometimes go wrong and that doctors don't know everything.
- Apologize when appropriate. Often this is all a patient wants—things do go wrong, and apologizing is not an admission of guilt or culpability.

Good documentation

- Always record correct date and time of every patient encounter.
- Ensure name, date of birth, and identifying number are on every sheet of paper (both sides if possible as the notes may be photocopied).
- Always write legibly in black ink.
- If entries need to be changed/altered then cross out old entry, but leave it visible and legible and sign and date new changes.
- Never alter or remove pages from notes when things may have gone wrong—they have usually been photocopied already!
- Always identify yourself by signature, printed name, and position.
- Identify all people present for any discussions (especially interpreters).
- Keep notes contemporaneously wherever possible (you never remember things quite as they were if there is a time delay).
- If you need to back-date an entry (e.g. if you are called to deal with an emergency), then indicate that this is back-dated and what time the actual event refers to.
- Document discussions fully, particularly possible complications; 'complications of laparoscopy explained' will not stand up to scrutiny or challenge after a bowel injury! (**→** Consent to treatment, p. 900.)
- For operative procedures or diagnostic imaging, take hard-copy prints or preferably archive images wherever possible—a diagram may also be useful.
- If you need to deviate from a guideline then fully document your reasons for doing so in the given clinical situation including when discussed with a colleague.
- Avoid abbreviations and acronyms wherever possible, or explain them (IUD = intrauterine device or intrauterine death!?).
- Never make jokes or flippant comments: they are distasteful, notes are a legal document, and patients can access their files—how would you feel if your notes said 'needs a check-up from the neck up'?

Medico-legal aspects of obstetrics and gynaecology: overview

It is good medical practice for all doctors to have a basic understanding of the law and its relationship with medicine. For the obstetrician and gynaecologist it is essential, because of the many complex medico-legal issues dealt with on a daily basis. The two largest areas for medico-legal claims are A&E and obstetrics.

UK law and the court system

The legal system in England and Wales is quite different from that in Scotland, although many of the principles are the same. What is described here is the English system. Medico-legal cases may be heard in different types of court. The court system is hierarchical. The Supreme Court is the most senior court in the land followed by the Court of Appeal and the High Court. Laws are made in a variety of different ways.

Common law

This is law that is developed over time through decisions made by judges. These decisions establish legal principles or 'precedent' which can be applied to future cases. Precedent set by a higher court such as the Supreme Court overrules that of a lower court. Medical law regarding clinical negligence is largely derived from common law.

Statute law

These are laws made by parliament. Statute law overrides common law developed by the courts. Many medico-legal issues in obstetrics and gynaecology are governed by statutes, such as the Abortion Act 1967.

Medical negligence

In order to establish that negligence has occurred, it must be shown that on the balance of probabilities:
- The doctor or hospital had a duty of care.
- There was a breach of that duty.
- The breach of duty caused harm to the patient.

What is medical negligence?

- Claims for medical negligence are both more common and more costly in obstetrics and gynaecology than in any other specialty.
- The National Health Service Litigation Authority (NHSLA) has dealt with nearly £2 billion of claims by patients since 1995.
- Claims are usually made against doctors (in practice, a claim is made against a hospital trust) in civil law rather than criminal charges.
- Medical negligence is the legal term used when harm arises because of a breach of duty by an individual clinician or a hospital:
  - an inappropriate treatment or failure to make a correct diagnosis may be found negligent if the patient suffers harm as a result
  - it may be judged negligent to fail to warn a patient about a risk inherent in an operation, e.g. ureteric injury during hysterectomy.
- The standard used to decide if a doctor breached his or her duty of care is whether a responsible body of medical opinion, acting in a logical manner, would have acted differently in the same circumstances.
- It also has to be proved that, on the balance of probabilities, it was the breach of duty that caused the harm. Thus, where an abnormal CTG was not acted upon and a baby develops CP, negligence will only be established if the CP is shown to be caused by hypoxia during labour and not another cause.

Consent to treatment

Treating an adult without her consent (Box 24.1) may lead to claims of negligence or, more rarely, a claim of battery.

Capacity

- The Mental Capacity Act 2005 has defined capacity in law.
- The pain and distress caused by labour is not enough to determine that a woman lacks capacity to consent (Box 24.2.)

If a patient lacks capacity but treatment is being considered, initially there should be appropriate dialogue with family/carers in the context of a multidisciplinary team. If there are differences of opinion regarding the patient's best interest, the doctor can seek legal advice and/or apply to the court. The Mental Capacity Act 2005 allows for the appointment of an Independent Mental Capacity Advocate (IMCA).

Voluntary consent

Consent must be given freely, without undue influence or pressure from others.

Information

To avoid a claim of battery, a patient must be aware of the nature and purpose of any procedure to which she consents. For example, when a medical student is to perform a vaginal examination, it must be clear to the patient that the purpose is to enhance the student's training and not for the benefit of the woman. More commonly, lack of information during the consent procedure may give rise to a claim of negligence.

Consent for operations

The law does not specify who can take the consent for an operation, but the person obtaining consent should, at the very least, be familiar with the procedure and be able to explain it in detail. Thus, in complex cancer or laparoscopic surgery it may be wise for the operating surgeon to obtain the patient's written consent.

The Department of Health has published guidance on what information should be given to patients before an operation. This includes:
- Details of the proposed procedure.
- The nature of the condition being treated.
- The benefits of treatment.
- Alternative treatments.
- Serious and frequently occurring risks.
- Additional procedures that may be necessary, e.g. blood transfusion.

Box 24.1 Consent

In order for consent to be valid the patient must:
• Have the capacity to give consent.
• Give consent voluntarily.
• Be given appropriate information regarding the procedure.
• Given time to reflect on their decision 'cooling off period'.

Box 24.2 Assessment of capacity

The person will lack capacity if there is a disturbance in the functioning of the mind or brain so she cannot:
• Understand the information relevant to the decision.
• Retain the information.
• Use or weigh up the information.
• Communicate the decision.

Montgomery and informed consent

Bolam test
• Was previously applied to litigations in cases of medical negligence.
• An action is reasonable if a body of doctors of similar experience would have made the same decision.

Montgomery's principle
• Has recently replaced the Bolam test:
  • based on a pivotal case involving a pregnant patient with diabetes who expressed concern about her ability to deliver vaginally, and was not counselled regarding the risks of shoulder dystocia
  • she had a shoulder dystocia and her son developed CP
  • she claimed that she would have asked for a CD had she known of the ↑ risk of shoulder dystocia with diabetes.
• Now doctors must provide information about all 'material risks', and any alternative course of action.
• A material risk is:
  • what a reasonable person in the patient's position would be likely to attach significance to the risk
  • or what the doctor should reasonably judge the individual patient would likely attach significant risk to.
• In essence, the focus has shifted from what a body of doctors would deem reasonable to what a patient would deem reasonable.

Consent: other issues

Refusal of treatment

The law allows a competent adult to refuse medical treatment without reason or justification.

Blood products

Religious groups such as Jehovah's Witnesses may refuse all blood products and it is essential that such wishes are very carefully documented. In cases where advanced refusal of blood products is known and the potential for bleeding anticipated (e.g. laparoscopy for EP) the most senior person available should perform the procedure.

Caesarean delivery

Several cases have been brought to court challenging a woman's right to refuse a CD thought by doctors to be in the best interests of her or her fetus. ▶ The law is clear that the fetus *in utero* has no legal rights up until the moment of birth. Therefore, a woman may refuse to consent to CD even if the consequences for herself or the fetus are death or severe injury.

Subfertility

The Human Fertilization and Embryology Authority (HFEA) Act 1990 regulates the area of reproductive medicine covering:
- Infertility treatments using donated genetic material.
- Infertility treatments involving stored genetic material.
- The creation of embryos outside the body.
- Embryo research.

The Act established the HFEA. This body licenses, monitors, and reports on establishments that provide fertility treatments. Individuals undergoing fertility treatments covered by the Act must give written consent to treatment as well as to storage of gametes and embryos. When couples have fertility treatment together, both must consent to the treatment and either may withdraw their consent at any time.

Consent in under 16s (*Fraser competence*)

▶ It is not uncommon for a child <16yrs to request contraception or a TOP without parental knowledge.

In the case of *Gillick v West Norfolk and Wisbech AHA* (1985), the courts ruled that doctors may treat children without parental consent if certain conditions are fulfilled (often colloquially referred to as *Fraser competence*):

- The child understands the advice or treatment being given.
- Attempt has been made to persuade the child to inform the parents.
- In case of seeking contraception, the child is likely to have unprotected intercourse whether or not contraception is prescribed.
- The physical or mental health of the child is likely to suffer if the treatment is not provided.

Consent for common gynaecological procedures: overview

The principles of consent are universal for all procedures and outlined in the GMC guidance on decision-making and consent.

Consent

Patients and doctors must make decisions together:
- You must work in partnership with your patients.
- You should discuss their condition and treatment options in a way they can understand.
- You should respect their right to make decisions about their care.
- Gaining their consent is an important part of the process of discussion and decision-making, not something that happens in isolation.
- The information you share should be in proportion to the nature of their condition, the complexity of the proposed investigation or treatment, and the seriousness of any potential side effects, complications, or other risks.
- *Risks of procedures will usually include:*
  - side effects
  - complications
  - failure of an intervention to achieve the desired aim.
- In the event an adult patient cannot consent, e.g. they are unconscious, remember the laws on capacity and that nobody can consent on behalf of another adult without power of attorney.
- All necessary information on consent in difficult circumstances, e.g. in children <16yrs, or those without capacity, can be found in the GMC's guidance (see 'Further reading').

Some practical tips on consent

- If you are the surgeon, consent the patient personally, do not delegate the responsibility unless unavoidable.
- If consent has already occurred, but there is a significant time gap (>1mth), then check it is still clinically appropriate and consider reconsent for the procedure.
- If you do not document what you have discussed, it didn't occur!
- 'Risks of procedure fully discussed' is not adequate—you need to be procedure specific including realistic possible outcomes.
- Even if a patient's decisions about her procedure seem inappropriate, they are her right to make

⚠ If you feel uncomfortable about a patient's decision or are feeling manipulated into performing something you do not feel is appropriate, then do not do the procedure!—get a 2nd opinion.

- Always record their LMP and current method of contraception in the reproductive age group.
- If there is even a remote chance the patient may be pregnant (especially in the luteal phase), then it is better to postpone the procedure—the most common reason for a pregnancy post sterilization is that the patient was pregnant at the time of the procedure!

⚠ If you are in any doubt about the appropriateness of surgery, the patient's decision, or unexpected anaesthetic issues on the day (e.g. temperature or unexpected low Hb) at the time of consent, then it is generally better to postpone the operation—if something adverse occurs, the first question will always be 'Did she need an operation at all or on that day?'

Further reading

GMC (2019). Good medical practice.
ℬ www.gmc-uk.org/ethical-guidance/ethical-guidance-for-doctors/good-medical-practice

GMC (2020). Decision making and consent.
ℬ www.gmc-uk.org/ethical-guidance/ethical-guidance-for-doctors/decision-making-and-consent

RCOG (2015). Obtaining valid consent. Clinical Governance Advice No. 6.
ℬ www.rcog.org.uk/guidance/browse-all-guidance/clinical-governance-advice/obtaining-valid-consent-clinical-governance-advice-no-6/

Consent for surgery that breaches the peritoneum

Laparoscopic, open abdominal procedures and vaginal procedures that breach the peritoneum (e.g. vaginal hysterectomy) are some of the commonest in the specialty. The following need to be discussed and documented with the patient's full understanding:

- *Proposed method of incision:* e.g. Pfannenstiel/midline/either if decision is genuinely uncertain and dependent on EUA for instance.
- *1° purpose of procedure:* e.g. diagnostic/therapeutic/both.
- *Which, if any, organs will be removed:* including making the patient aware this may change depending upon intraoperative findings, e.g. total abdominal hysterectomy with ovarian conservation unless ovary(ies) abnormal at procedure.
- *Likely possibilities when the intra-abdominal pathology is genuinely unknown:* e.g. laparoscopy for pelvic pain of uncertain aetiology—diagnostic laparoscopy ± adhesiolysis ± diathermy endometriosis.
- *Risks of all intra-abdominal procedures:* haemorrhage/infection (abdominal, skin, urinary)/injury to bowel, bladder, ureters, major blood vessels.
- *Risks of visceral injury ↑ in the presence of:* endometriosis, known adhesions, cancer or distorting pathology, multiple previous surgeries.
- *Larger procedures:* e.g. gynae-oncology debulking procedures, extra visceral risks, e.g. liver, spleen, may need discussion.
- *In the case of laparoscopy, the small risk of conversion to laparotomy in the event of:* inadvertent visceral injury/intractable bleeding/operative inability to complete the procedure due to difficulty.
- *The small possibility of the need for blood transfusion:* in the event of unexpected bleeding.
- *If the patient refuses blood products:* then a preoperative meeting is mandatory with the surgeon, anaesthetist, and haematologist to establish what is and is not acceptable to the patient, sign advance directives, and re-evaluate risks.
- *The type of anaesthetic to be used:* individual anaesthetic risks should be explained by the anaesthetist.
- *Concurrent medical comorbidities:* need preoperative assessment and appropriate specialty input to establish operative risk.

Consent issues specific to laparoscopic sterilization

The following are mandatory for anyone requesting sterilization:
- Absolute certainty that their family is complete.
- The irreversible nature of sterilization.
- A recognized failure rate of 1:200.
- That male sterilization is a less risky procedure, done under local anaesthesia, and has a failure rate of 1:2000 after two negative semen analyses.
- There has been a full consideration of all LARCs, e.g. IUCD, Mirena®, implants.

▶ Current recommendations are that sterilization should almost never be considered in patients <30yrs as later regret is common. A 2nd opinion, at minimum, is good practice in these circumstances.

Further reading

RCOG (2015). Obtaining valid consent. Clinical Governance Advice No. 6.
🔗 www.rcog.org.uk/guidance/browse-all-guidance/clinical-governance-advice/obtaining-valid-consent-clinical-governance-advice-no-6/

Consent for surgery that enters the uterine cavity

Procedures involving entry to the uterine cavity include hysteroscopy, surgical management of miscarriage, and TOP procedures.
- *1° purpose of procedure:* e.g. diagnostic/therapeutic/both.
- *What if anything will be removed:* including making the patient aware this may change depending upon intraoperative findings, e.g. hysteroscopy ± endometrial biopsy ± resection of polyp ± fibroid resection.
- *Specifically consent for operative resection:* if this is a realistic possibility.
- *Risks of all intrauterine procedures:* haemorrhage/infection (endometritis)/small risk of uterine perforation with a small risk of injury to bowel, bladder, ureters, major blood vessels.
- *Specifically for SMM/TOP:* procedures the small risk of incomplete evacuation.
- Risks of intra-abdominal injury ↑ when operative resection and/or other energy sources are used.
- Small risk of the need for laparoscopy ± laparotomy and repair in the event of uterine perforation.

Endometrial ablation procedures

In addition to the above issues the following are mandatory for anyone requesting endometrial ablation:
- Absolute certainty that their family is complete.
- The continued need for contraception post procedure.
- The possibility (procedure type dependent) of amenorrhoea.
- The possibility of the need for a 2nd procedure in the next 5yrs.

Further reading

RCOG (2015). Obtaining valid consent. Clinical Governance Advice No. 6.
🔗 www.rcog.org.uk/guidance/browse-all-guidance/clinical-governance-advice/obtaining-valid-consent-clinical-governance-advice-no-6/

Considerations for preoperative assessment in gynaecology

Preoperative assessment has all of the same general considerations as for all other surgical procedures—the majority of procedures are now done in day surgery. In terms of specific considerations, they are procedure specific, but consider the following:

Specific gynaecological issues

- All women in the reproductive age are pregnant till proven otherwise— ensure that contraception and last normal menstrual period are clearly sought and documented in clinic and again immediately preoperatively (➔ Consent to treatment, p. 900).
- The above is especially true in those having surgery for fertility reasons—a preoperative pregnancy test is mandatory, but also *beware* unprotected sex in the cycle of the procedure—her pregnancy test may not be +ve yet!
- If there is any doubt regarding possible pregnancy or the viability of a pregnancy prior to SMM then do not continue until your doubts have been answered.
- *NEVER* assume a woman's future reproductive wishes—*always* ask them and document them.
- Do not operate on a pregnant woman unless that is the indication for surgery (e.g. SMM) or the benefits outweigh the risks.
- Do *not* forget anti-D administration for all Rh −ve women who have a uterine evacuation procedure or surgery for EP.
- Where the uterine cavity is instrumented, consider chlamydial prophylaxis to prevent ascending infection unless the patient has been screened recently and is −ve—the default position is to give it!
- Many of the women will *de facto* have risk factors for VTE, e.g. pregnancy, pelvic surgery, COCP use:
  - *all* need a WHO VTE assessment.
- Woman having intraperitoneal surgery need consideration for bowel preparation if multiple previous abdominal surgery, endometriosis, known adhesions, or cancer.
- The need for specific preoperative investigations (e.g. ECG, CXR) is otherwise similar to general surgery, though nearly all will require an FBC and group and save at minimum.
- The majority of women will require USS (or more rarely other imaging, e.g. CT/MRI) as part of their clinical pathway to provide information regarding their procedure—ask yourself: 'Has this woman had an USS?', and if not, 'Does she need one?'

Clinical risk management: identifying and analysing risks

Clinical risk management is a mechanism for improving the quality of patient care. There are several steps in the process.

Identifying risk

What went wrong or what could go wrong

The local and national sources used to identify risk issues are outlined in Box 24.3.

Completing an incident reporting form

Most trusts have a dedicated reporting form to complete. These should be available in all clinical areas. All members of staff of all grades should be encouraged to complete forms when they are aware of risk incidents. A form should be completed for all actual adverse incidents affecting patients, as well as near misses.

Many units have a list of specific risk triggers that should prompt completion of a risk form. These might include an unplanned return to theatre, cord pH <7.10, or an operative blood loss of >800mL.

Serious incidents must be reported immediately to the local lead for clinical risk. All hospitals will have definitions for what constitutes such a serious untoward incident. When a serious incident has occurred, all staff concerned should prepare contemporaneous statements of their involvement while the incident is still fresh in their mind.

When writing incident reports and statements, only an account of the facts should be documented, *not* an opinion of what went wrong.

Risk analysis

Root cause analysis is a structured investigation that aims to identify the true cause of a problem and the actions necessary to eliminate it.

Adverse incidents rarely occur as a result of individual error alone. Factors contributing to the incident should be identified and an analysis report submitted. A good root cause analysis removes biases, employs the correct context, and interviews the key people involved, and is as factual as possible.

Risk management score

Often a score is used to determine if an event is unacceptable. This is calculated using the likelihood of the event occurring and the severity of the event.

Incident form information
- Full patient details.
- Date, time, and location of incident.
- All staff involved (statements may be requested at a later date).
- Brief factual report of the incident.

Box 24.3 Possible sources of risk identification
Local sources for identifying risk
- Incident report forms.
- Patient complaints.
- Audit results.

National sources for identifying risk
- National Patient Safety Agency alerts.
- Reports of national confidential enquiries.
- Care Quality Commission.

Possible contributory factors to a risk incident
- The patient.
- Individual staff.
- Communication.
- Team working (or not).
- Education and training of staff.
- Equipment and resources.
- Working conditions.

Risk analysis report
Will contain:
- Obvious outcomes that occurred.
- The chronology of events.
- The care management problems identified.
- A list of contributing factors.
- Recommended actions required.
- A timetable for implementation of recommendations.

Clinical risk management: risk reduction

Risk reduction

May be achieved by:
- Training, e.g. simulation.
- Introduction of guidelines.
- ↑ resources.

Risk elimination

May mean ceasing to provide a particular service.

Acceptance of risk

- There is an acceptance that some risk cannot be ↓ or eliminated.
- Hospitals attempt to keep litigation costs to a minimum by joining the Clinical Negligence Scheme for Trusts (CNST—see Box 24.4).

Dissemination of lessons learned

Local level
- Sharing information with other units in the hospital.

National level
- Through bodies such as the National Patient Safety Agency and Royal Colleges.

▶ Sharing information should always include good practice points.

What risk management is not!

- 'Big brother'.
- A vehicle for individual blame or recrimination.
- An audit or research tool.
- A management policing policy (it is for everyone to learn from).
- Only designed to highlight bad care (good care should also be commended and fed back to staff, even if the outcome is poor or risk has occurred).
- A legal or negligence body.

Box 24.4 The Clinical Negligence Scheme for Trusts

- The CNST handles clinical negligence claims against member NHS bodies.
- Membership is voluntary, but currently all NHS and primary care trusts in England belong.
- The costs of the scheme are met by membership contributions:
  - the total projected claim costs are assessed in advance each year and contributions are determined for each trust (influenced by a range of factors including type of trust and specialties it provides)
  - discounts are available to trusts that achieve the relevant NHSLA risk management standards and to those with a good claims history.
- When a claim is made against a member of the CNST, the body remains the legal defendant, but the NHSLA is responsible for handling the claim and associated costs.

Gynaecological imaging I

Gynaecological practice has changed enormously over the last 20–30yrs principally due to improvements in pelvic imaging, particularly TV USS.

Early pregnancy

USS is the imaging modality of choice for early pregnancy, allowing assessment of pregnancy location, viability, and gestational age. The main diagnostic criteria used are as follows:
- In a normal intrauterine pregnancy, a gestational sac should be visible from 5wks gestation and fetal heart pulsations visible from 6wks using TVS.
- In the 1st trimester, accurate dating is performed by measuring the CRL (optimum time is 11–13+6wks gestation).
- NICE guidelines (2019) for the diagnosis of miscarriage: CRL ≥7mm with no FH or mean gestational sac diameter ≥25mm with no fetal pole.
- It should be possible to identify up to 90% of EPs on TVS.
- Other pathology may also be discovered, usually as an incidental finding, e.g. ovarian cysts.

Menstrual disorders

TVS can be used to reliably diagnose anatomical abnormalities such as:
- Endometrial polyps.
- Fibroids.
- Adenomyosis.

Other causes of bleeding disturbance, such as hormonal dysfunction, hormonal treatment, and infections, cannot be reliably established using imaging methods.
- TVS and saline infusion sonography allow assessment of endometrial pathology, such as polyps and submucous fibroids.
- USS and MRI have a similar ability to diagnose uterine fibroids, but MRI is superior to USS in determining the exact location, especially with a large uterus (>4 fibroids).

Postmenopausal bleeding

⚠ ~10% of women with PMB will have gynaecological cancer, most of which is endometrial cancer.

▶ A TVS examination with measurement of ET can discriminate between women at high and low risk.

Using a cut-off of an ET of 4mm:

- 96% of endometrial carcinomas can be identified using TVS.
- Endometrial cancer and hyperplasia can be suspected on TVS, but need a biopsy to confirm them histologically.
- If the ET is <4mm it is extremely unlikely that the woman has endometrial cancer: <1% (very high −ve predictive value) so further investigation is usually not required.
- Up to 55% of women with no disease will also have a +ve result (much lower +ve predictive value).
- If the ET is >4mm and there is a global thickening, a biopsy should be taken.
- Polyps may also be picked up as focal entities and require hysteroscopic removal.
- Incidental ET measurements >4mm do not generally need further investigation in the absence of PMB.
- These ET measurements, in women before they are officially menopausal, cannot be used as their ET will vary depending upon cyclical activity.
- Although the −ve predictive value is high for ET <4mm, in the presence of recurrent PMB the patient should have hysteroscopy.

Other methods for assessing the endometrium

- *Saline infusion sonography:*
  - infusion of saline into uterine cavity during scanning
  - allows assessment of focal endometrial lesions
  - agreement between saline infusion sonography and hysteroscopy is excellent.
- *MRI:*
  - may be indicated in the presence of fibroids if hysteroscopy is unhelpful.

Gynaecological imaging II

Pelvic pain

Acute pelvic pain

- USS is the diagnostic imaging method of choice.
- The following can reliably be diagnosed on TV USS:
  - ovarian cysts
  - some sequelae of PID (including pyosalpinx and tubo-ovarian abscess)
  - hydrosalpinges
  - fibroid degeneration.

▶ Colour Doppler may aid in adnexal torsion, but the findings are not specific enough and the diagnosis is usually made on clinical findings.

▶ Haemorrhagic ovarian cysts and ruptured ovarian cyst accidents have typical appearances on TVS.

Chronic pelvic pain

- Endometriosis may be diagnosed by the finding of endometriomas and occasionally by the visualization of endometriotic nodules elsewhere in the pelvis such as the rectovaginal septum, although these may be better visualized with MRI or rectal USS.
- Adenomyosis is associated with a thickening of the myometrium, uterine asymmetry, and with areas of mixed echogenicity and a 'rays through the forest' appearance.
- Imaging has a role in assessing pelvic adhesions.
- 'Soft markers' including immobile ovaries, site-specific tenderness, and loculated pelvic fluid may indicate pathology confirmed by laparoscopy.

Subfertility

- USS is used in both the diagnosis and the management of infertility. It can be used to diagnose conditions such as polycystic ovarian disease and hydrosalpinx and to track follicular growth and rupture during normal and stimulated cycles during infertility treatment.
- Oocyte retrieval for assisted conception techniques is performed under USS guidance.
- Complications such OHSS can also be assessed by USS.
- HSG using radio-opaque dye and image intensification used to be the imaging method of choice to assess the uterine cavity and fallopian tubes:
  - has now been superseded by HyCoSy where a solution is infused into the uterine cavity while performing a TVS
  - combines a baseline TVS, assessment of the fallopian tubes, and possibly even ovulation if the investigation is correctly timed.
- TVS is used to confirm viable or non-viable intrauterine pregnancy and indeed EP as a result of IVF or other assisted reproduction techniques.

Gynaecological imaging III

Ovarian masses and gynaecological malignancy

- Experienced sonographers use pattern recognition to make a diagnosis.
- USS has been shown to be as good as or even superior to CT for the discrimination between different types of pelvic mass.
- When a pelvic mass is large and extending out of the pelvis, a combined TVS and transabdominal scan (TAS) approach will ensure the whole mass is imaged.
- The following masses generally have characteristic sonographic appearances:
  - functional and luteal cysts
  - serous and mucinous cystadenomata
  - endometriomata
  - haemorrhagic cysts
  - teratomas (dermoids)
  - hydrosalpinges and para-ovarian cysts
  - tubo-ovarian abscess
  - 'typical' fibroids (when fibroids have undergone degeneration they can appear mixed solid/cystic and even have bizarre appearances—differentiation between fibroid and leiomyosarcoma cannot be made on TVS in these circumstances)
  - adhesional pockets of fluid.
- The following features are more suggestive of a malignant ovarian mass:
  - complex morphology—mixed solid/cystic appearance
  - large papillary cyst wall projections (>6mm)
  - thickened and irregular septations
  - ascites
  - evidence of peritoneal disease
  - highly vascularized solid elements or projections/septations.
- TVS or TAS can also be used to safely guide diagnostic ascitic taps or symptomatic drainage.
- MRI is superior to CT for discriminating between benign and malignant masses and may be better than USS due to a lower false +ve rate.
- MRI can identify fat-containing fluid typical of dermoid cysts and blood typical of endometriomata due to their physical properties.
- Plain abdominal X-ray may occasionally give further information about pelvic mass:
  - fibroids may have become calcified
  - dermoid cysts may contain radio-opaque material (teeth or bone).
- MRI and CT are used in the imaging and staging and subsequent follow-up of gynaecological malignancies.
- A CXR is part of the routine assessment in cases of suspected malignancy (may show pleural effusions or metastases).

⚠ No single imaging modality can reliably distinguish between all benign and malignant masses even in the best hands.

Gynaecological imaging IV

Urogynaecology

- USS may be used to assess:
  - residual bladder volumes
  - the bladder neck in cases of incontinence.
- Urodynamic flow/pressure studies can be combined with the use of X-ray screening to gain additional information about the anatomy of the bladder and urethra (video-cystourethrography).
- IVU may be used to investigate continuous incontinence following childbirth, radiotherapy, or gynaecological surgery, which may be due to fistula formation between the ureters or bladder and the genital tract.
- Three-dimensional TVS is being used in some centres to aid in the diagnosis of pelvic floor dysfunction.

Other uses

- USS can be used to visualize intrauterine devices within the uterus:
  - lost IUCDs may be located on plain abdominal X-ray
  - Mirena® devices are radio-opaque.
- Congenital abnormalities of the uterus can be diagnosed on USS (especially if three-dimensional), HSG, and MRI.
- Contrast studies of the renal tract (e.g. IVU) should be considered when congenital malformations of the reproductive tract are diagnosed, as up to 40% are associated with abnormalities of the urinary tract.

Index

For the benefit of digital users, indexed terms that span two pages (e.g., 52–53) may, on occasion, appear on only one of those pages.

Note: Tables, figures, and boxes are indicated by an italic *t*, *f*, and *b* following the page number.

Common drugs: safety and usage in pregnancy and breast-feeding (Cont.)

Drug	Risk*	Conclude	Alternatives	Breast-feeding
Psychiatric medications				
Tricyclics	Largely safe	Use if high risk of relapse	Sertraline	Safe
SSRIs	Paroxetine teratogenic (3% risk) Others probably safe	Use if high risk of relapse (avoid paroxetine, fluoxetine best)	Sertraline	Safe
Lithium	Teratogenic (cardiac) (10% risk)	Use only if high risk of relapse	Difficult	Watch for toxicity
Neuroleptics	Possible very mild teratogenicity Largely unknown (avoid clozapine)	Usually continue because of risk of relapse	Difficult	Probably safe
Fundamentals: psychiatric disease is a major problem during/after pregnancy so treatment may need to continue				
Antiepileptics				
Sodium valproate	Impaired childhood cognition Teratogenic (4–9% risk)	Minimize combinations	Carbamazepine	Safe
Carbamazepine	Teratogenic (1–3% risk)	Consider change if <12 weeks Usually continue	N/A	Safe
Lamotrigine	Teratogenic (1–5% risk)	Usually continue	N/A	Safe
Fundamentals: best sorted preconceptually. Seizure control imperative, but minimize combinations and doses. High-dose folic acid				
Other drugs				
Steroids (lung maturation; β- and dexamethasone)	Nil known with single course	Use if high risk for preterm delivery Betamethasone best	N/A	N/A
β-agonists	Nil known at anti-asthmatic doses	Use if indicated, e.g. asthma	N/A	Safe
Ursodeoxycholic acid		Use if indicated, e.g. cholestasis	N/A	Not indicated

*Note background risk of congenital malformations 1–2%